KU-165-478

*Made available by an educational grant of*

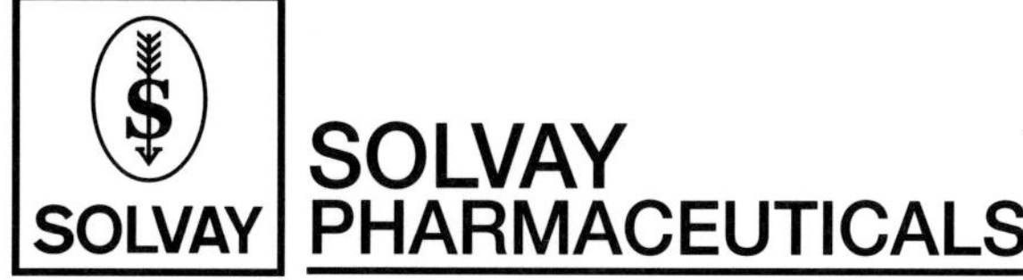

*A mia madre*

*Editor*
Corazziari Enrico
Dipartimento Scienze Cliniche
Clinica Medica II
Università "La Sapienza" Roma - Italy

*Editorial Assistant*
Crescini Emanuela

Cataloging-in-Publication Data

APPROACH TO THE PATIENT WITH CHRONIC GASTROINTESTINAL DISORDERS
Enrico Corazziari, Editor
- Bibliographical references
- Index
- ISBN 88-87830-00-2
1. Gastrointestinal System - Chronic diseases
2. Gastrointestinal diseases - Diagnosis - Therapy
3. Gastrointestinal diseases - Chronic
4. Gastrointestinal diseases - Biopsychosocial approach


*Via G. Sismondi, 44 20133 Milano Tel +39 02 76110205 Fax +39 02 7381635*



ISBN 88-87830-00-2

First edition, November 1999, Printed in Italy

*Notice*
Every effort has been made from the authors to ensure the accuracy of the information herein. However, appropriate information sources should be consulted, especially for new or unfamiliar drugs or procedures. It is the responsibility of every practitioner to evaluate the appropriateness of a particular opinion in the context of actual clinical situations and with due consideration to new developments. Authors, editor, and the publisher cannot be held responsible for any typographical or other errors found in this book.

*On the front cover*
"*The Man in Oxford*", 1292. Oxford, UK: Bodleian Library. Miniature of an anatomy table, *modified.*

Printed by EverPrint Via G. Rossa, 3 Carugate (MI)
Giancarlo Bausano, Arké, Graph Italia have contributed to the book
Marian Shields has revised the English language.

*Price* ITL 96,000 € 49.58

APPROACH TO THE PATIENT WITH

# CHRONIC GASTROINTESTINAL DISORDERS

Edited by *E Corazziari*

***MESSAGGI***

**AGGADI Y**
Gastroenterology Unit
CHU Rangueil
Toulouse, France

**BADIALI D**
Dipartimento di Scienze Cliniche
Clinica Medica II
Università di Roma "La Sapienza"
Roma, Italia

**BARBARA G**
Dipartimento Medicina Interna
e Gastroenterologia
Università di Bologna
Policlinico S. Orsola - Malpighi
Bologna, Italia

**BIANCHI PORRO G**
Unità di Gastroenterologia
Università di Milano
Ospedale "L. Sacco"
Milano, Italia

**BIANCONE L**
Dipartimento di Medicina Interna
Università di Roma "Tor Vergata"
Roma, Italia

**BRACCI F**
Dipartimento di Scienze Cliniche
Clinica Medica II
Università di Roma "La Sapienza"
Roma, Italia

**CAMILLERI M**
Mayo Clinic
Gastroenterology Research Unit
Rochester, Minnesota USA

**CAMPIERI M**
Dipartimento di Medicina Interna
e Gastroenterologia
Università di Bologna
Bologna, Italia

**CAPRILLI R**
Dipartimento di Scienze Cliniche
Cattedra di Gastroenterologia I
Università di Roma "La Sapienza"
Roma, Italia

**CAPURSO L**
Dipartimento Malattie Digestive
e Nutrizionali
Azienda Complesso Ospedaliero
"San Filippo Neri"
Roma, Italia

**CORAZZIARI E**
Dipartimento di Scienze Cliniche
Clinica Medica II
Università di Roma "La Sapienza"
Roma, Italia

**CORINALDESI R**
Dipartimento Medicina Interna
e Gastroenterologia
Università di Bologna
Policlinico S. Orsola - Malpighi
Bologna, Italia

**CREED FH**
Department of Psychiatry
University of Manchester
Manchester, United Kingdom

**D'ALBA L**
Servizio di Gastroenterologia
ed Endoscopia Digestiva
Complesso Ospedaliero
"S. Giovanni - Addolorata"
Roma, Italia

**DELVAUX M**
Gastroenterology Unit
CHU Rangueil
Toulouse, France

**DOLDO P**
Dipartimento di Medicina Sperimentale
Università degli Studi di Catanzaro
"Magna Graecia"
Catanzaro, Italia

**DROSSMAN DA**
UNC Center for Functional
Gastrointestinal and Motility Disorders
Division of Digestive Diseases
University of North Carolina at Chapel Hill
Chapel Hill, North Carolina USA

**EANDI M**
Dipartimento di Anatomia Farmacologia
e Medicina Legale
Università di Torino
Torino, Italia

**ENCK P**
Department of General Surgery
University Hospitals
Tübingen, Germany

**FAVA GA**
Dipartimento di Psicologia
Università di Bologna
Bologna, Italia

**FREXINOS J**
Gastroenterology Unit
CHU Rangueil
Toulouse, France

**GALMICHE J-P**
Department of Hepatology and
Gastroenterology
CHU Hotel Dieu
Nantes, France

**GALMICHE HR**
Department of Hepatology and
Gastroenterology
CHU Hotel Dieu
Nantes, France

**GIONCHETTI P**
Dipartimento di Medicina Interna
e Gastroenterologia
Università di Bologna
Bologna, Italia

**HABIB FI**
Cattedra di Gastroenterologia I
Università di Roma "La Sapienza"
Roma, Italia

**HEADING RC**
University of Edinburgh
Edinburgh, United Kingdom

**HELWIG U**
Dipartimento di Medicina Interna
e Gastroenterologia
Università di Bologna
Bologna, Italia

**IRVINE EJ**
Division of Gastroenterology
McMaster University
Hamilton, Ontario Canada

**JOHANSSON R**
Dipartimento di Medicina Interna
e Gastroenterologia
Università di Bologna
Bologna, Italia

**KESSLER M**
University of Ulm
Ulm, Germany

**KLEIN KB**
International Drug Development
Consulting
Bainbridge Island, Washington USA

**KOCH KL**
Division of Gastroenterology and
Hepatology
The Pennsylvania State University
Hershey, Pennsylvania USA

**KRUSE J**
Department of Psychosomatics
Heinrich-Heine-University Hospitals
Düsseldorf, Germany

**LATELLA G**
Dipartimento Medicina Interna
Unità di Gastroenterologia
Università dell'Aquila
L'Aquila, Italia

**LAZZARONI M**
Unità di Gastroenterologia
Università di Milano
Ospedale "L. Sacco"
Milano, Italia

**LONGSTRETH GF**
Kaiser Permanente Medical Care Program
San Diego, California USA

**MALAGELADA J-R**
Hospital General Vall D'Hebron
Digestive Diseases Department
Barcelona, Spain

**MUSIAL F**
Department of Psychology
Heinrich-Heine-University
Düsseldorf, Germany

**OLDEN KW**
Division of Gastroenterology
Mayo Clinic Scottsdale
Scottsdale, Arizona USA

**PALLONE F**
Dipartimento di Medicina Interna
Università di Roma "Tor Vergata"
Roma, Italia

**PANICHI G**
Dipartimento Malattie Infettive e Tropicali
Università di Roma "La Sapienza"
Roma, Italia

**PAPI C**
Dipartimento Malattie Digestive
e Nutrizionali
Azienda Complesso Ospedaliero
"San Filippo Neri"
Roma, Italia

**PATRICK DL**
Department of Health Services
University of Washington
Seattle, Washington USA

**PELOSINI I**
Dipartimento di Medicina Interna
Laboratorio di Farmacologia Clinica
Università di Parma
Ospedale Maggiore
Parma, Italia

**PRANTERA C**
Divisione di Gastroenterologia
Azienda Ospedaliera S. Camillo-Forlanini
Roma, Italia

**RAO SSC**
Department of Internal Medicine
University of Iowa Hospitals
Iowa City, Iowa USA

**RIZZELLO F**
Dipartimento di Medicina Interna
e Gastroenterologia
Università di Bologna
Bologna, Italia

**RUDISCH T**
Szent-Györgyi Albert University
Szeged, Hungary

**RUGGERI M**
Cattedra di Gastroenterologia I
Università di Roma "La Sapienza"
Roma, Italia

**SCARPIGNATO C**
Dipartimento di Medicina Interna
Laboratorio di Farmacologia Clinica
Università di Parma
Ospedale Maggiore
Parma, Italia

**SCRIBANO ML**
Divisione di Gastroenterologia
Azienda Ospedaliera S. Camillo-Forlanini
Roma, Italia

**STACHER G**
Department of Surgery
Psychophysiology Unit
University of Vienna
Wien, Austria

**STANGHELLINI V**
Dipartimento Medicina Interna
e Gastroenterologia
Università di Bologna
Policlinico S. Orsola - Malpighi
Bologna, Italia

**TACK JF**
Department of Internal Medicine
Division of Gastroenterology
University Hospitals Leuven
Leuven, Belgium

**THOMPSON DG**
Department of Medicine
University of Manchester
Hope Hospital
Salford, United Kingdom

**THOMPSON WG**
Emeritus Professor of Medicine
University of Ottawa
Ottawa, Ontario Canada

**TONER BB**
Department of Psychiatry
Centre for Addiction and Mental Health
University of Toronto
Toronto, Ontario Canada

**TONINI M**
Dipartimento di Medicina Interna
e Terapia Medica
Sezione di Farmacologia Clinica
e Sperimentale
Pavia, Italia

**TORRICO S**
Cattedra di Gastroenterologia I
Università di Roma "La Sapienza"
Roma, Italia

**TRAUE HC**
Department of Medical Psychology
University of Ulm
Ulm, Germany

**VENTURI A**
Dipartimento di Medicina Interna
e Gastroenterologia
Università di Bologna
Bologna, Italia

**VISCIDO A**
Dipartimento di Scienze Cliniche
Cattedra di Gastroenterologia I
Università di Roma "La Sapienza"
Roma, Italia

**WHITEHEAD WE**
Division of Digestive Diseases
University of North Carolina at Chapel Hill
and UNC Center for Functional
Gastrointestinal and Motility Disorders
Chapel Hill, North Carolina USA

**WHORWELL PJ**
Department of Medicine
University Hospital of South Manchester
Manchester, United Kingdom

**ZAMPALETTA C**
Cattedra di Gastroenterologia I
Università di Roma "La Sapienza"
Roma, Italia

**ZARA GP**
Dipartimento di Anatomia Farmacologia
e Medicina Legale
Università di Torino
Torino, Italia

**ZUCCONI EC**
Dipartimento di Medicina Interna
e Gastroenterologia
Università di Bologna
Bologna, Italia

# Contents

PART TWO

## BIOPSYCHOSOCIAL MODEL AND PATIENT EVALUATION



PART THREE

## MECHANISMS OF GASTROINTESTINAL PAIN AND DISCOMFORT

## INDEX

# Preface

"What matters in chronic disorders is the patients' suffering,
not the disease entity"

"La nature m'enseigne aussi par ces sentiments de douleur,
de faim, de soif, etc. que ne suis pas seulement logé dans mon corps,
ainsi qu'un pilote en son navire,
mais outre cela que je lui suis conjoint très-étroitement
et tellement confondu et mêlé
que je compose comme un seul tout avec lui"
*Réné Descartes. Méditations Métaphysiques.* 1641

With economic, scientific, and technological developments, the populations of industrialized countries have experienced a dramatic decrease both in the death rate and in acute infectious diseases as well as an increase in chronic morbid conditions that parallel the prolonged life expectancy and that negatively affect the health status and quality of life. Hence, the main challenge for the health care system of these industrialized countries is to be able to deal with the impact of the chronic diseases as far as concerns high prevalence, elevated degree of individual suffering, high demands on the medical profession, inadequacy of therapeutic means, and elevated costs.

Chronic Gastrointestinal (GI) disorders represent a large proportion of all chronic diseases, with which they share several common features. Not unlike other chronic diseases, the prevalence of Chronic GI Disorders (CGID) is increasing with the increase in life expectancy and improved therapeutic means to cure life-threatening complications. In addition, they present aspects peculiar to the GI tract that, besides being the nutritional organ, is the largest surface of the body exposed to the environment, the largest immune organ and second only to the brain in terms of innervation. It is not surprising that chronic GI disorders can originate from several different conditions: genetical, immunological, nutritional, neuromuscular. The environment, physical and social, as well as psychological conditions play a determinant role in the onset of chronic GI disorders.

Not only are chronic GI disorders numerous and highly prevalent, but the toll paid in terms of individual suffering is considerable although not self-evident. In CGID, the degree of suffering and the disease manifestations themselves are not proportional to the pathophysiologic modifications/impairments, clinical expression and treatment outcome, but are, rather, the end result of the interference of the GI disorder on eating and defaecatory behaviour and their interactions with the psychosocial factors. As far as concerns the latter, an abnormal patient's illness behaviour, sustained by the chronic state of suffering itself, and/or the concomitance of stressful events should be taken into consideration. In this respect, a great deal of attention has been given to the close relationship between physical and/or sexual victimization and health care seeking attitude, chronicization of the disorders, low health status, and poor response to treatment. On account of all these considerations, the impact of CGID on the health status cannot be well assessed by listing symptoms, signs or pathological findings, but rather from assessing the Quality of Life, that takes into consideration several domains of well-being.

The management of patients with chronic diseases differs markedly from that of patients with acute diseases not only in the diagnostic approach and the treatment, but also in terms of outcome. In acute conditions, the widely applied biomedical model centered on identification and removal of causative factors in a condition expected, both by the patient and the physician, to be reversible is usually satisfactory whilst, in chronic conditions, the causative factors cannot always be identified and/or the therapeutic armamentarium is unable to resolve the condition. Consequently, a linear relationship between the identification of causative factors and their resolution is often hairline or totally lacking.

The widely applied, mainly disease-centered, biomedical model is, to a large extent, unsatisfactory in chronic conditions requiring a different medical approach which should be centered on the patient, taking into consideration, together with the disease entity, his/her long-term suffering or disability as well as his/her expectations as far as concerns the persistent state of illness and to the everyday social, physical and emotional aspects.

Until now, initial medical training takes place in teaching hospitals where chronic conditions are not dealt with, except for acute remissions and complications and where the disease-centered biomedical model of the acute condition is learnt as the basic, and often the only prototypic, medical approach to be, from then on, applied, by the practising physician, even in non-acute, non-hospitalized patients. Since 80% of the conditions outside the hospital are chronic, it is self-evident that a disease-centered biomedically based training cannot adequately match the need of the population health status.

Traditional biomedically-centered education and technological diagnostic and therapeutical advancements, mainly directed towards well-defined pathological and functional modifications, have greatly influenced the approach to patients with CGID which differs according to the entity of the disease. The approach to diseases with known structural or biochemical abnormalities is standardized and directed mainly to specific aspects of the pathological condition, such as diagnosis, complications, treatment of the aetiologic and/or pathophysiologic factors, focusing less on the patients' suffering, which is the result of the interactions of the physical alterations with the psychological and behavioural as well as the social/environmental conditions.

Once an organic disease has been excluded, the approach to disturbances with no known structural or biochemical abnormalities, is not standardized and the treatment is often selected in keeping with the physician's specialty rather than with the patients' needs. In these functional conditions, there is also a tendency on the part of some physicians to attempt symptomatic treatment and to minimize issues of suffering "due to stress and/or psychological causes", or, on the contrary,

to focus on the psychological aspects, ignoring the physical dysfunctions. In addition, there is a trend to overlook the fact that organic and functional disorders are frequently associated and each of them may give rise to the other and that CGID may cause such disability as to markedly interfere with everyday life, regardless of the disease entity.
In the attempt to develop awareness on patients presenting with chronic suffering with pain and/or dysfunctions originating from the gastrointestinal tract, ANEMGI (Associazione per la NeUro-Gastroenterologia e la Motilità Gastrointestinale) promoted an interdisciplinary symposium in Baveno, Italy, 10-13 June 1998.
This volume is the outcome of data presented and discussed at the Baveno Symposium.
The contents highlight the basic approach to chronic GI disorders, often referring to the patient-centered biopsychosocial model and the close relationships between functional, organic and psychological disorders.
Several chapters deal with specific disease entity, and in many an effort is clearly made to offer an approach to the chronic conditions which would take into consideration the different life and health domains of the patient.
This volume has been compiled with the collaboration of renowned experts in the field and I am confident that this text will contribute to reinforcing and advancing our knowledge on Chronic Gastrointestinal disorders.

*Enrico Corazziari*

*ANEMGI mission is*

To promote research,
education and care
of visceral dysfunctions related
to nervous system alterations,
psycho-social status,
and environmental conditions

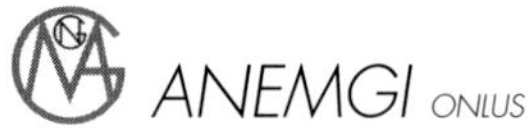

*Associazione per la NeUroGastroenterologia e la Motilità Gastrointestinale*

V.le M. Pilsudski, 118 - 00197 Roma - Italy - Tel. e Fax +39 06 8078303
e-mail: anemgi@mclink.it - http://www.adance.com/anemgi

# PART ONE

# COMMON FEATURES OF CHRONIC GASTROINTESTINAL DISORDERS

# Chronic gastrointestinal disorders
## Individual suffering, social, health and economic burden

*GF Longstreth*

Chronic Gastrointestinal (GI) disorders vary greatly in their pathophysiology, clinical manifestations, epidemiology, and treatment. However, whether the disorders are organic or functional, they are similar in that they create a demand on medical professionals and society (particularly economic effects), cause individual suffering, and are influenced by exogenous factors not subject to control by the health care system.
This review focuses on the epidemiology, high cost (especially of functional disorders), and exogenous determinates of selected chronic gastrointestinal disorders. When pathophysiologic and clinical information are supplemented with knowledge of these aspects, the impact of chronic gastrointestinal disorders on health and the challenge of managing them is more apparent. The disorders given particular emphasis are Irritable Bowel Syndrome (IBS), functional dyspepsia, Gastroesophageal Reflux Disease (GERD), and Inflammatory Bowel Disease (IBD).

### Epidemiology of chronic gastrointestinal disorders

*U.S. national surveys*
The National Health Interview Survey conducted on the U.S. population derives self-reported data on selected chronic conditions from household interviews. In 1989, approximately 30 million people (12% of the population) reported having had a chronic digestive disease during the previous year[1]. By comparison, the figures for some nongastrointestinal diseases were: arthritis, 31 million; heart disease, 18.5 million; asthma, 11.6 million; migraine headache, 10 million; and diabetes mellitus, 6.5 million. Although the accuracy of these data can not be verified, their magnitude indicates that chronic gastrointestinal disorders are among the most common self-reported medical conditions. In the U.S., outpatient care visits are estimated from surveys on a national

sample of office-based physicians in the National Ambulatory Medical Care Survey[1]. In 1985, acute and chronic digestive diseases were the seventh most common diagnostic group. The 1987 National Hospital Discharge Survey in the U.S., based on discharge diagnoses in short-stay, non-Federal hospitals according to the International Classification of Diseases, revealed 1.8 hospitalizations per 1,000 population annually for digestive diseases[1]. This figure comprises many acute and chronic diseases and underestimates the prevalence of many chronic disorders, especially functional disorders, which usually do not cause hospitalization. However, other national surveys have attracted attention to the frequency of care-seeking for the prototypic functional bowel disorder, IBS[2,3].

The surge in research on the functional gastrointestinal disorders during the last two decades has contributed much additional epidemiological data[4]. For example, the U.S. Householders study[5] assessed the prevalence of functional gastrointestinal syndromes by a self-report questionnaire based on multinational (Rome) symptom criteria[6]. Sixty-nine percent of people sampled reported having at least one of 20 functional disorders attributed to various parts of the digestive tract, and there was considerable overlap of symptoms among the anatomic regions involved.

*Surveys on specific disorders*

IBS has been identified in various populations using Manning[7] or Rome[8] symptom criteria. The prevalence among people not seeking medical care in Britain and the U.S. ranges from 14 to 24% of women and 5 to 19% of men, depending in part on the stringency of diagnostic criteria[9]. In addition, the chronic, remittent nature of IBS contributes to its importance as a cause of poor health[10].

GERD has been identified from self-reports of heartburn in about one-third of subjects from surveys in the U.S. and Europe[4,11]. One-fifth of people have weekly heartburn. In the survey conducted in Olmsted County in the U.S., the majority of subjects with heartburn reported the symptom had been present for at least five years[12].

Dyspepsia is a symptom that can be caused by a variety of diseases or can occur in the absence of a structural or biochemical explanation; i.e., functional or nonulcer dyspepsia. In the past, the range of definitions used by some researchers and clinicians has included biliary and gastroesophageal reflux symptoms; however, it is now defined by the Rome criteria as chronic or recurrent pain or discomfort centered in the upper abdomen[13]. In most series that exclude subjects with reflux

symptoms, only a minority of patients have peptic ulcers and few have cancer; the majority have functional dyspepsia[14]. As is the case with IBS, the frequency of dyspepsia determined by population surveys is influenced by the definition used. For example, in Great Britain when reflux symptoms were included, 6-month and 12-month prevalences of 38%[15] and 40% were reported[16]. The annual prevalence of dyspepsia, excluding reflux symptoms, in the U.S. and other Western countries is approximately 25%. Dyspepsia tends to come and go over time and overlap and interchange with IBS[10,17].
Although the prevalence of IBD varies considerably among populations, there are few epidemiologic differences between ulcerative colitis and Crohn's disease in specific populations[18], except for cigarette smoking, which is positively associated with Crohn's disease and negatively associated with ulcerative colitis[19]. This observation suggests that these types of IBD are either different expressions of the same disease or separate diseases with nearly identical risk factors.

## Costs of digestive disease

Consideration of the costs of a particular disorder is important because, in general, the costs reflect the importance of the entity from an overall view. Health costs are of two types: direct and indirect (Table 1).

TYPES OF HEALTH COSTS: DIRECT AND INDIRECT

| Direct costs | Indirect costs |
|---|---|
| Hospital stays | Work absenteeism |
| Medical procedures | Income loss |
| Physician charges | Transportation for medical care |
| Drugs | Arrangements at home |
| | Rehabilitation and retraining |
| | Premature retirement |
| | Premature death |

Table 1

Although analysts can often estimate direct costs with acceptable accuracy, they have more difficulty estimating indirect costs accurately[20]. Furthermore, many factors complicate the generalizability of cost estimates, including wide variations in charges for medical services and drugs, differences in access to care and in the gate-keeper role of general practitioners, and in sick-leave benefits. Moreover, changes in direct costs over time; e.g., with the introduction of new therapies, such as Helicobacter pylori (H. Pylori) eradication and laparoscopic-assisted surgery, can diminish the applicability of cost estimates derived before such advances. Indirect costs can also change over time, even in the population in which they are estimated; e.g., with changes in short-term sick-leave benefits, as has recently occurred in Sweden.

The 1985 economic costs of digestive disease in the U.S. were estimated at $56 billion, of which direct health care costs were more than $40 billion[21]. In addition, functional gastrointestinal disorders are associated with multiple nongastrointestinal complaints that influence costs, such as fatigue, fibromyalgia, and headache. For example, in the U.S. Householder study, subjects with a functional gastrointestinal disorder reported four times as many physician visits for nongastrointestinal as gastrointestinal problems[5]. Studies have been carried out on the costs of some specific disorders (Table 2).

MEDICAL COST ESTIMATES FOR SELECTED DISORDERS

| Disorder, year [ref] | Country / Population | Cost Type | Annual Estimate |
|---|---|---|---|
| IBS, 1992[26] | U.S. 255 million | Direct | $ 8 billion |
| Functional dyspepsia, 1980 - 1982[29] | Sweden 8 million | Direct *and* indirect | $ 348 million |
| IBD, 1994[33] | Sweden 8.8 million | Direct *and* indirect | $ 86 million |
| IBD, 1990[34] | U.S. 249 million | Direct *and* indirect | $ 1.8 to 2.6 billion |

Table 2

In surveys on IBS, physician consulting was reported by 25% of affected U.S. subjects[22] and approximately half of British IBS subjects[23]. Severity of symptoms, especially abdominal pain, was associated with physician consulting. In addition, psychosocial disturbance influences health care seeking[24]. In the U.S. Householder study, people with IBS reported 18 times as many physician visits for gastrointestinal complaints in the year before the survey as subjects without IBS. Furthermore, those with IBS reported nearly three times as many missed days of work due to illness[5]. The predisposition of IBS patients to consult for nongastrointestinal complaints[5] and undergo surgery, particularly hysterectomy[25], also contributes to the costs. The most comprehensive estimate of the direct medical costs attributable to IBS was derived from a community survey by Talley et al.[26] The investigators excluded people with major psychiatric or medical disease, a history of major abdominal surgery, or nursing home residency, and assessed outpatient and inpatient health services charges, except for outpatient drugs. Overall annual medical charges and certain specific types of charges increased progressively in controls, subjects with some gastrointestinal symptoms, and the group with IBS. In this estimation, median annual charges incurred by subjects with IBS were $742, compared with $429 for controls. By extrapolating their results to the U.S. white population, they estimated excess charges of $8 billion yearly. Even more expense would have been estimated if the analysis had included costs of IBS in nonwhites, outpatient drug costs, subjects with major comorbidity or past surgery, and indirect costs[27].

The cost of nonprescription antacid use by people with GERD is high. Among heavy antacid-users, more than 84% reported using the preparation to treat heartburn[28]. The reported proportion of people with GERD who have consulted a physician during the previous year has varied from 5% in the U.S.[12] to 28% in England[11]. The frequency of symptoms[12] and presence of dysphagia and nocturnal heartburn[11] have been associated with seeing a physician.

Nyren et al. studied the costs for the care of functional dyspepsia in Sweden[29]. Their comprehensive analysis included inpatient and outpatient care, prescription drugs, short-term sick-leave, and early retirement. They estimated direct and indirect costs of $33 million and

$315 million, respectively (based on the currency exchange rate in early 1998). Ninety-eight per cent of consultations resulted in a drug prescription. Sick-leave was the most important factor, as dyspepsia patients accounted for 26 more days of lost production than the average employee, which alone resulted in $312 million in indirect costs. In a British study, dyspepsia drugs accounted for over 15% of prescription costs in general practice[20].

Of course, factors influencing the actual costs of dyspepsia include the number of patients who receive diagnostic tests, such as radiography, endoscopy, or noninvasive H. pylori testing, and the number who receive H. pylori eradication therapy or other drugs[20]. In one study, the long-term (6-month) costs were lower after gastroenterology consultation and endoscopy than after barium radiography in patients who had responded incompletely to empiric therapy[30]. However, initial endoscopy in young patients without alarm symptoms rather than empiric therapy has gained support, partly due to a high rate of subsequent endoscopy because of persisting symptoms in patients initially given empiric therapy[14,30]. The advent of noninvasive H. pylori tests has introduced the option of routinely testing patients with dyspepsia and, in those who test positive, of either prescribing eradication therapy or performing endoscopy to evaluate for peptic ulcer disease. These and other management strategies have been assessed by decision analysis, and the results have differed according to the assumptions made concerning the cost of endoscopy, the prevalence rate of peptic ulcer in H. pylori-positive patients, the response rate of functional dyspepsia to eradicaton therapy, and other factors. In view of these variables and the lack of randomized controlled trials of management, an international group of experts recently chose not to advocate a universal policy[14]. Therefore, there may be great inter-regional variation in costs attributed to dyspepsia.

The costs attributed to IBD in Sweden were estimated by Blomqvist and Ekbom[31]. Direct costs accounted for one-third of the total costs, amounting to $27.5 million. Patients with Crohn's disease were hospitalized twice as often as those with chronic ulcerative colitis. The remaining $58.4 million in indirect costs was comprised approximately equally by sick-leave and early retirement. Sick-leave for Crohn's disease was more than four times as common as for ulcerative colitis. Notably, indirect sick-leave comprised a much lower proportion of the total costs than was found in the Swedish study of functional dyspepsia[29]. Hay and Hay estimated the annual direct medical costs for IBD in the U.S. to be $1.0 to 1.2 billion[32]. The indirect cost of lost work productivity was estimated at $0.4 to 0.8 billion, yielding a total annual cost for IBD of $1.8 to 2.6 billion. In their estimate, the top 7% of patients accounted for 50% of expenditures. The total IBD cost estimate was about one-fourth the partial estimate of IBS direct costs in the U.S. provided by Talley et al.[26].

## Exogenous determinants of digestive disease

Sonnenberg and Everhart have emphasized that the impact of digestive disease on society, including the associated costs, is influenced by exogenous factors that are not under the control of medical intervention (Table 3)[33].

DETERMINANTS OF DIGESTIVE DISEASE OUTSIDE THE CONTROL OF THE MEDICAL PROFESSION

- ✓ Temporal trends
- ✓ Seasonal variation
- ✓ Socio-economic variation
- ✓ Variations by age, sex, race
- ✓ Geographical variations
- ✓ Occupational variations
- ✓ Social support

Table 3

Adapted from Sonnenberg A, Everhart JE[33].

They emphasize that the time trend of mortality from all causes in the U.S. had achieved most of its fall since the beginning of this century before the percentage of gross national product spent on health care started to rise rapidly (Figure 1).

Figure 1

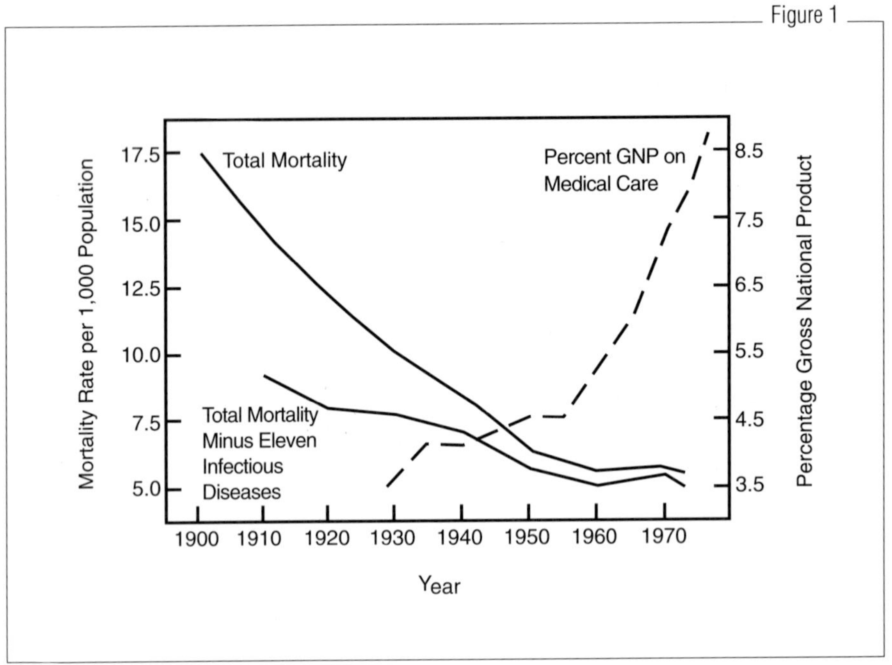


Time trends of mortality from all causes and percentage of the gross national product spent on medical care in the United States.
Reproduced from McKinlay JB, McKinlay SM[45].

Therefore, the authors stated, "...social and environmental conditions have a stronger impact on the economic burden of digestive diseases than the most sophisticated treatments." The importance of temporal trends to gastrointestinal disease is illustrated by their assessment of the factors possibly responsible for the declines in mortality from gastric cancer and gastric ulcer since the 1930's and the decline in duodenal ulcer mortality since 1960. They suggest that lower rates of infection with H. pylori due to improved hygiene, reduced salt intake due to the introduction of the refrigerator for food preservation, reduced occupational work load, and reduced smoking could have contributed to these trends. Notably, the decrease in peptic ulcer disease began long before the major surgical and pharmacological advances in treatment. The incidence of Crohn's disease increased throughout the 1950s and 1960s in the northerly nations of Western Europe and North America but has since leveled off[34]. A similar but less variable time trend also applies to the incidence of ulcerative colitis[34]. A Swedish study revealed a shift toward a higher proportion of cases of colonic Crohn's disease and a reciprocal decrease in ileocecal disease from 1955 to 1989[35]. There is a seasonal effect on mortality from peptic ulcer and other diseases, as it peaks in the winter[33]. In Western countries, the prevalence and mortality of various digestive diseases, including duodenal ulcer, decrease with increasing socio-economic status and educational achievement[33]. The U.S. Householder survey of functional gastrointestinal disorders found greater symptom reporting was associated with low income[5]. Inflammatory bowel disease tends to occur more in higher socio-economic groups[18].

Variations in age, sex, and race are major factors. Most Western surveys of IBS have found a reduced frequency among older subjects. Younger people are most likely to report functional esophageal symptoms, aerophagia, IBS, and proctalgia fugax, but are less likely to have functional fecal incontinence[5]. A survey of health examinees revealed an increase in incontinence with age in women but not in men[36]. In that study, there were declines in self-reporting of a stress effect on both bowel pattern and abdominal pain with increasing age in both sexes, and more women than men at all ages reported these stress effects. Age has an effect on the hospitalization rate and incidence of IBD; both Crohn's disease and ulcerative colitis manifest two peaks in age distribution[18,33]. In contrast to the female predominance of IBS generally found in Western surveys, females represent only 20 to 30% of IBS patients in India and Sri Lanka[37]. Erosive esophagitis and its complications are more common in men than in women and more common in whites than in blacks[33]. Incidence rates for Crohn's disease are approximately 20% higher in women than men, and incidence rates for ulcerative colitis are approximately 20% higher in men[18]. In the U.S., the prevalence of IBS seems similar in whites and blacks[38], but it may be lower in Hispanics[39] and Asians[38]. Ethnic variation in Israel is reflected by higher rates of ulcerative colitis and Crohn's disease in Ashkenazi Jews than in Sephardic Jews[18].

Geographical variaton also influences the reporting of chronic gastrointestinal disorders. In South African blacks, IBS is unusual in rural areas but appears to be common in cities[37], and it is common in Nigerian medical students[40]. It seems less prevalent in Thailand than China, but is prevalent in India and Japan[37]. There is a striking geographic variability in IBD with decreasing incidence from northern to southern latitudes. For example, there are reported incidence rates (per 100,000 population) for ulcerative colitis and Crohn's disease of 14.8 and 5.3 in Norway, 5.0 and 2.7 in Italy, and 2.0 and 0.9 in Spain[18]. Incidence rates of IBD are similar in U.S. blacks and U.S. whites, but very low in African blacks[18]. The geographical variation in celiac sprue has been related to the agricultural revolution in Europe, as the British Isles were the last areas to introduce gluten-containing crops and have the highest prevalence of the disease[33].

An occupational effect is reflected by the association in multiple countries of IBD with a white collar occupation or profession as opposed to a blue collar occupation or manual labor employment[18,33].

The concept of "social support" as a health-promoting factor has undergone rather extensive investigation, although the data apply to illness, in general, rather than gastrointestinal disease, in particular[18,41]. For example, age-adjusted mortality rates from all causes of death are consistently higher among unmarried than married people. Other social ties, including family and friends, church membership, and other group affiliations comprise a "social network" that has been associated with a reduction in mortality of as much as 50% in prospective studies when other demographic, social and medical factors were controlled for. Being widowed seems to be more detrimental to the health of men than women. A mechanism proposed for these observations is that social relationships moderate the deleterious effects of stress or other health hazards. House et al. suggest that reduction in family size and social contacts during the last few decades portends serious consequences for health[41].

In view of the many exogenous factors influencing digestive diseases, Sonnenberg and Everhart suggested that we have reached the point of diminishing returns regarding health expenditure for their management[33]. They acknowledged that advances in science and technology may pay off in the long run, but proposed that improving education, income and social networks are the most promising methods of improving health in the short run.

## Current and future methods of care

Certainly, the goal of altering these exogenous factors is worthy, but achieving it, in many patients, in the near future, could be a daunting task. However, it is clear that patients benefit and money is saved when physicians do their best to make accurate, yet economical diagnoses. For example, IBS should be a symptom-based diagnosis supplemented by a limited laboratory and structural evaluation[42]. Costs can also be saved by avoiding the unnecessary surgery to which patients with IBS are predisposed. A physician-patient interaction that includes a confident diagnosis, reassurance and attention to psychosocial factors results in reduced use of health services by patients with IBS[43]. Promising therapies that are immediately available and inexpensive include low-technology approaches to helping patients cope with chronic digestive disorders, such as the use of healthy life-style instruction[44]. Additional progress in the mangement of various disorders can be expected from randomized, controlled clinical trials.

*REFERENCES*


1. Everhart JE. *Overview.* In: Everhart JE, editor. Digestive diseases in the United States: Epidemiology and Impact. U.S. Department of Health and Human Services, Public Health Service, National Institutes of Health, National Institute of Diabetes, Digestive and Kidney Disease. NIH Publication 94-1447. Washington DC: U.S. Government Printing Office; 1994;3-50.
2. Sandler RS. *Epidemiology of irritable bowel syndrome in the United States.* Gastroenterology 1990; 99:409-15.
3. Everhart JE, Renault PF. *Irritable bowel syndrome in office-based practice in the United States.* Gastroenterology 1991;100:998-1005.

4. Locke GR III. *The epidemiology of functional gastrointestinal disorders in North America.* Gastroenterol Clin N Am 1996;25:1-19.
5. Drossman DA, Li Z, Andreuzzi E, et al. *U.S. householder survey of functional gastrointestinal disorders. Prevalence, sociodemography, and health impact.* Dig Dis Sci 1993;38:1569-80.
6. Drossman DA, Funch-Jensen P, Janssens J, et al. *Identification of subgroups of functional bowel disorders.* Gastroenterol Int 1990;3:159-72.
7. Manning AP, Thompson WG, Heaton KW, et al. *Towards positive diagnosis of the irritable bowel syndrome.* Br Med J 1978; 2:653-4.
8. Thompson WG, Creed F, Drossman DA, et al. *Functional bowel disorders and chronic functional abdominal pain.* Gastroenterol Int 1992;5:75-91.
9. Drossman DA, Whitehead WE, Camilleri M. *Irritable bowel syndrome: a technical review for practice guideline development.* Gastroenterology 1997; 112:2120-37.
10. Talley NJ. *Why do functional gastrointestinal disorders come and go?* (editorial) Dig Dis Sci 1994;39:673-7.
11. Kennedy T, Jones R. *Gastro-esophageal reflux symptoms in the community.* Gut 1998; 42(Suppl 1):A64.
12. Locke GR III, Talley NJ, Fett SL, et al. *Prevalence and clinical spectrum of gastroesophageal reflux: a population-based study in Olmsted County, Minnesota.* Gastroenterology 1997;112:1448-56.
13. Talley NJ, Colin-Jones D, Koch KJ, et al. *Functional dyspepsia: a classification with guidelines for diagnosis and management.* Gastroenterol Int 1991;4:145-60.
14. Talley NJ, Silverstein MD, Agreus L, et al. *AGA technical review: evaluation of dyspepsia.* Gastroenterology 1998;114:582-95.
15. Jones R, Lydeard S. *Dyspepsia in the community: a follow-up study.* Br J Clin Pract 1992; 46:95-7.
16. Penston JG, Pounder RE. *A survey of dyspepsia in Great Britain.* Aliment Pharmacol Ther 1996;10:83-9.
17. Agréus L, Svärdsudd K, Nyrén O, et al. *Irritable bowel syndrome and dyspepsia in the general population: overlap and lack of stability over time.* Gastroenterology 1995; 109:671-80.
18. Lashner BA. *Epidemiology of inflammatory bowel disease.* Gastroenterol Clin N Am 1995;24:467-74.
19. Thomas GAO, Rhodes J, Green JT. *Inflammatory bowel disease and smoking - a review.* Am J Gastroenterol 1998;93:144-9.
20. Jones RH. *Clinical economics review: gastrointestinal disease in primary care.* Aliment Pharmacol Ther 1996;10:233-9.
21. Everhart JE. *Summary.* In: Everhart JE, editor. Digestive diseases in the United States: Epidemiology and Impact. U.S. Department of Health and Human Services,

Public Health Service, National Institutes of Health, National Institute of Diabetes, Digestive and Kidney Disease. NIH Publication 94-1447. Washington DC: U.S. Government Printing Office; 1994, op. IX-XII.

22. Talley NJ, Zinmeister AR, Melton LJ. III *Irritable bowel syndrome in a community: symptom subgroups, risk factors, and health care utilization.* Am J Epidemiol 1995; 142:76-83.
23. Heaton KW, O'Donnell LJD, Braddon FEM, et al. *Symptoms of irritable bowel syndrome in a British urban community: Consulters and nonconsulters.* Gastroenterology 1992;102:1962-7.
24. Drossman DA, McKee DC, Sandler RS, et al. *Psychosocial factors in the irritable bowel syndrome: a multivariate study of patients and nonpatients with irritable bowel syndrome.* Gastroenterology 1988; 95:701-8.
25. Longstreth GF. *Irritable bowel syndrome and chronic pelvic pain.* Obstet Gynecol Surv 1994;49:505-7.
26. Talley NJ, Gabriel SE, Harmsen WS, et al. *Medical costs in community subjects with irritable bowel syndrome.* Gastroenterology 1995;109:1736-41.
27. Longstreth GF. *Irritable bowel syndrome: a multibillion-dollar problem* (editorial). Gastroenterology 1995;109:2029-42.
28. Graham DY, Smith JL, Patterson DJ. *Why do apparently healthy people use antacid tablets?* Am J Gastroenterol 1983;78:25-7.
29. Nyren O, Adami H-O, Gustavsson S, et al. *Social and economic effects of non-ulcer dyspepsia.* Scand J Gastroenterol 1985;20(Suppl 211):21-5.
30. Longstreth GF. *Long-term costs after gastroenterology consultation with endoscopy versus radiography in dyspepsia.* Gastrointest Endosc 1992; 38:23-26.
31. Blomqvist P, Ekbom A. *Inflammatory bowel diseases: health care costs in Sweden in 1994.* Scand J Gastroenterol 1997;32:1134-9.
32. Hay JW, Hay AR. *Inflammatory bowel disease: cost of illness.* J Clin Gastroenterol 1992; 14:309-17.
33. Sonnenberg A, Everhart JE. *Socio-economic determinants of digestive disease.* Gastroenterol Int 1993;6:100-114.
34. Logan RFA. *Inflammatory bowel disease incidence: up, down or unchanged?* Gut 1998; 42:309-11.
35. Lapidus A, Bernell O, Hellers G, et al. *Incidence of Crohn's disease in Stockholm County 1955-1989.* Gut 1997;41:480-6.
36. Longstreth GF. *Bowel patterns and anxiety. Demographic factors.* J Clin Gastroenterol 1993;17:128-32.
37. Thompson WG, Gick M. *Irritable bowel syndrome.* Semin Gastrointest Dis 1996; 7:217-29.
38. Longstreth GF, Wolde-Tsadik G. *Irritable bowel-type symptoms in HMO examinees.*

*Prevalence, demographics, and clinical characteristics.* Dig Dis Sci 1993;38:1581-9.

39. Zuckerman MJ, Guerra LG, Drossman DA, et al. *Comparison of bowel patterns in Hispanics and Non-Hispanic whites.* Dig Dis Sci 1995;40:1763-9.
40. Olubuyide IO, Olawuyi F, Fasanmade AA. *A study of irritable bowel syndrome diagnosed by Manning criteria in an African population.* Dig Dis Sci 1995;40:983-5.
41. House JS, Landis KR, Umberson D. *Social relationships and health.* Science 1988; 241:540-5.
42. Longstreth GF. *Irritable bowel syndrome. Diagnosis in the managed care era.* Dig Dis Sci 1997;42:1105-11.
43. Owens DM, Nelson DK, Talley NJ. *The irritable bowel syndrome: long-term prognosis and the physician-patient interaction.* Ann Int Med 1995;122:107-12.
44. Colwell LJ, Prather CM, Phillips SF, et al. *Effects of an irritable bowel syndrome (IBS) education class on health promoting behaviors and symptoms.* Am J Gastroenterol 1998; 93:901-5.
45. McKinlay JB, McKinlay SM. *The questionable contribution of medical measures to the decline of mortality in the twentieth century.* Milbank Memorial Fund Quarterly 1977;55:405-28.

*ADDRESS FOR CORRESPONDENCE*

**LONGSTRETH GF, MD**

4647 Zion Avenue
San Diego, California 92120 USA
Fax: +1 619 528 5999
E-mail: george.f.longstreth@kp.org

# Quality of life in chronic gastrointestinal disorders

*DL Patrick*

Clinicians, patients and their families, and policymakers recognize increasingly that there should be a greater convergence of biomedical and psychosocial perspectives in the evaluation and treatment of Chronic Gastrointestinal Disorders (CGID). Health-related quality of life (HrQoL) assessments can be used to inform patient management, to evaluate treatment effectiveness, and to influence policy decisions. Potentially, HrQoL information could be helpful whether or not the disorders have recognized organic involvement based on physiologic evaluation such as findings from a colonoscopy or tissue analyses for Inflammatory Bowel Diseases (IBD). HrQoL assessments might also provide useful information when few, if any, biological markers exist, as in functional gastrointestinal disorders. The assessment of quality of life in clinical trials and epidemiological investigations of gastrointestinal disorders are increasing, although clinical practice and policy applications are slower to emerge.

This paper examines the rationale for assessing HrQoL in gastrointestinal disorders, distinguishes relevant HrQoL concepts, explores the types of measures used in HrQoL assessments, and identifies challenges in the development and use of these measures in clinical trials and clinical practice.

### *Why measure HrQoL?*

HrQoL is important for assessing the impact of chronic diseases[1]. Physiologic measures are of limited interest to patients; they often correlate poorly with functional capacity and well-being, the areas in which patients and families are most concerned. Given the lack of clear-cut structural, biochemical, or physiologic bases for many of these disorders, quality-of-life concerns are extremely important to the understanding of how biology intermingles with the cultural, social, interpersonal, and psychological aspects. The disease-related laboratory studies and endoscopic/radiological findings must be complemented by understanding of individual and social perceptions of these disorders and how the disorders, treatment for them, and societal reactions to disease and treatment affect people's lives.

Quality of life can play a central role in how the symptom constellations are perceived by those affected, how these symptoms prompt help-seeking and influence illness behavior, and how effective different treatments are in ameliorating symptoms. Patients' perceptions of well-being, subjective evaluation of symptoms, and ability to function in daily activity are issues of primary importance to the individual patient and their significant others, and to the clinical treatment of CGID. Two patients with the same clinical criteria or gastrointestinal symptom constellation may have dramatically different responses in work, in psychological reaction, and in social life. This variation in response to symptoms may also occur in response to treatment.

Hence, systematic evaluation of HrQoL can be clinically meaningful for both individual patient care and for research. HrQoL measures may be used in clinical trials, epidemiologic investigations, and health policy studies for increasing knowledge about outcomes. Potentially these measures may also be used in clinical practice to monitor individual patient outcomes, negotiate treatment decisions, or improve provider-patient communications.

### *What is health-related quality of life?*

Three concepts are often used interchangeably to refer to the same domain of "health": *health status, functional status, and quality of life*[2]. We use the term *health-related quality of life (HrQoL)* to include both negatively valued aspects of life, including death, and the more positively valued aspects such as role function, happiness, and opportunity[1]. Sometimes death or life expectancy is integrated with other aspects of health to create a composite definition. In one such definition, HrQoL is the duration of survival as modified by the impairments, functional states, perceptions, and opportunities influenced by disease, treatment, or policy. All these concepts are potentially relevant to persons with CGID. Even though these disorders or their treatment do not usually cause death, the length of time patients experience symptoms and their impact during their lifetime can be important considerations for patients and clinicians.

Few measures of quality of life are theory-driven, given the lack of encompassing or even middle-range theories of quality of life. One conceptual approach is the needs-based model that identifies quality of life as the degree to which most or all human needs are met[3]. This approach is similar to that developed by the World Health Organization in the cross-cultural development of a generic quality-of-life measure[4]. The theory of need satisfaction was used to develop the IBS-QoL for irritable bowel syndrome[5].

*What concepts of HrQoL are relevant?*

The only assured way of knowing which aspects of HrQoL are pertinent to persons with CGID is to ask them directly. Few measures have been constructed with sufficient attention given to the concepts, concern, and language of persons with these disorders. Existing studies would suggest that many aspects of the lives of patients with CGID can be affected: work, leisure, travel, intimacy, emotional life, and relationships[6]. Concepts potentially relevant to the assessment of HrQoL for persons with CGID are shown in Table 1.

Time without symptoms and its quality[7] can be important in freeing the person from worry or the inconveniences of gastrointestinal symptoms. Symptoms themselves may have many consequences ranging from decreased functioning to worry about survival. One of the primary concerns of patients with IBD, for example, is worry about the future, such as the development of cancer or being a burden on others, in the presence of diarrhea and pain[8]. Physical, emotional, and social functioning are important in that gastrointestinal disorders may limit what persons want to do or have to do in their daily lives. Mobility, for example, may be limited unless there is assurance of a restroom nearby, one of the items frequently included in generic functional status measures such as the Sickness Impact Profile[9].

Perceptions of health and the ability to function and overall feelings of well-being are at the heart of assessments of "quality," which connotes a value placed on life with the disorder. These perceptions may be highly influenced by the psychological adaptation to the disorders, but are separate from anxiety or depressive symptoms in that they are global evaluations. As most clinicians know, individuals vary greatly in accommodation to symptoms and this individual response may affect treatment effectiveness. Finally, stigma is a major issue with most gastrointestinal disorders in that patients can feel shame about odors, about some treatments such as colostomies, and about the inability to control a central body function such as elimination.

Concepts of HRQoL potentially relevant to persons with chronic gastrointestinal disorders

| Concepts | Potential relevance and indicators |
|---|---|
| *Opportunity* | |
| • Resilience | • Ability to withstand stress |
| • Disadvantage | • Inability to achieve personal goals; stigma; shame over "visible" or "invisible" illness |
| *Perceptions* | |
| • Satisfaction | • Satisfaction with health and ability to function |
| • General | • Overall feelings of well-being; worries and concern |
| *Functional Status* | |
| • Physical | • Reduction in activity, mobility, sleep |
| • Psychological | • Cognitive and emotional restrictions in activity due to nervousness, sadness, or other psychological stress |
| *Impairments* | |
| • Symptoms | • Heartburn, dyspepsia, diarrhea, abdominal pain, nausea, vomiting, pelvic floor pain, incontinence; difficulty falling asleep |
| *Survival* | • Quality-adjusted life expectancy; time without symptoms |

Table 1

Conceptual clarity and conceptual distinctiveness are important in HrQoL assessments for gastrointestinal disorders. Symptoms are important to HrQoL, but they are not sufficient to assess the impact of different conditions. Table 2 illustrates the relationship of symptom bothersomeness for persons with IBS and scores on the IBS-QoL[5], a 34-item self-report measure specific to IBS organized into the eight subscales shown in Table 2.

IMPACT OF SYMPTOM BOTHERSOMENESS ON SPECIFIC MEASURE OF QUALITY OF LIFE FOR PERSONS WITH IRRITABLE BOWEL SYNDROME (IBS-QoL)

| Domain | Mild (N=51) | Moderate (N=49) | High (N=53) |
|---|---|---|---|
| Overall | 72.2 | 64.8 | 53.8 |
| Dysphoria | 71.9 | 63.0 | 55.5 |
| Interference with activity | 70.7 | 64.4 | 55.7 |
| Body image | 73.9 | 64.3 | 50.5 |
| Health worry | 70.0 | 64.1 | 45.3 |
| Food avoidance | 51.8 | 42.5 | 37.0 |
| Social reaction | 78.3 | 72.2 | 58.6 |
| Sexual | 84.1 | 77.3 | 60.9 |
| Relationship | 80.1 | 75.0 | 63.1 |

Table 2

Adapted from Patrick DL, Drossman DA, Frederick IO et al.[5].

This table suggests that symptoms, regardless of their level of bothersomeness, affect most profoundly the eating (food avoidance) and health worry domains of the IBS-QoL. The least affected domains are the sexual and relationship domains.

It is also important to distinguish between functional status or disability arising from gastrointestinal disorders and the perceptions of value placed on these impacts. Functional status is sometimes called "quality of life", although how a person functions in daily life, such as limitations in working or in mobility, may not be synonymous with how they view the quality of their life or how happy or unhappy they are with their restrictions or their opportunities. Functional status and perceptions can be highly related, but the best chance of sorting out the impact of disorders on the different components of HrQoL is to evaluate the domains separately.

In clinical and epidemiological studies, conceptual distinctiveness is important in assessing the impact of the correlates (cross-sectional) or determinants (longitudinal) of each domain controlling at minimum for type and severity of disorder, age, gender, ethnicity, and co-existing conditions. In clinical practice, symptom frequency and bothersomeness assessed separately from functional status and perceptions can help clinicians and patients decide on the type and intensity of treatment, the level of self care, or the frequency of consultation.

*What are the types of measures developed for CGID?*

Two basic approaches based on content are available: generic instruments that provide a summary of HrQoL and can be used across different conditions and populations; and specific instruments that focus on problems associated with a single disease state, syndrome, or patient group, such as IBS[10]. Generic profiles have been shown to be useful in patients with IBD, but are not as sensitive in applications to functional disorders[11]. Specific measures are more common for functional GI disorders, because the detection of small but important changes requires targeted assessment. Measures specific to individuals are at the frontier of HrQoL assessment. One such individual approach, the SEIQoL or Schedule for Evaluation of Individual Quality of Life, has been applied to gastrointestinal disorders[12].

Both generic and specific measures can be classified further by the types of scores available for analyses. Profiles are instruments that provide multiple measures on each domain of the measure. Indexes are single summary scores that can be derived from profiles, from single item measures, or from measures developed using economic and psychologic techniques of preference measurement called utility assessments. Utility measures reflect the preferences of patients for different health states in relation to each and are used in cost-utility analyses that combine duration and quality of life. One of these techniques - time trade off - has been used to measure the HrQoL value of patients with ileoanal pull-through (highest HrQoL), patients with a history of Barrett's esophagus who have undergone esophagectomy for adenocarcinoma, and patients with a history of esophageal disorders[13]. All values for these groups produced by this technique were extremely high (>0.95 on a 0-1 scale where 0 represents the value for death and 1 the value for perfect health). These results suggest that some patients do not perceive their condition as undesirable and that considerable difficulties can be encountered in applying preference-based or utility measures in this area.

Self - or interviewer-administered questionnaires exist for evaluating inflammatory bowel disorders such as ulcerative colitis and Crohn's disease and functional gastrointestinal disorders, such as IBS. Measures can be used to detect differences in HrQoL between patients at a point in time (discriminative instruments) or longitudinal changes within patients during a period of time (evaluative instruments)[10]. Instruments used to discriminate or evaluate must be valid (really measuring what they are supposed to measure) and have a high ratio of signal to noise. Instruments built as closely as possible from the point of view of persons who have the condition have greater validity. If a treatment results in a small but important difference in HrQoL, the clinician wants to be confident that he or she will detect that difference. Responsiveness will be related to the magnitude of the difference in score in patients who have improved or deteriorated, and the extent to which patients who have not changed provide more or less the same score. The instruments should be able to identify differences in scores that correspond to small, moderate, and large changes[14].

Drossman et al.[15] have reviewed the disease-specific measures of HrQoL for IBD and concluded that for most ambulatory patients, HrQoL is generally good and that functional impairment is greater in the psychological and social domains than in the physical domains. Disease severity clearly affects HrQoL, and patients with Crohn's disease report a lower quality of life, in general, than patients with ulcerative colitis. HrQoL measures have been shown to be strong predictors of health care visits and to be responsive to interventions such as surgery.

Specific HrQoL measures developed for IBS have been recently published or are under preparation[5,16-19] (Table 3). Most of these measures have only been tested cross-sectionally and results are awaited of their application in clinical trials and more generalizable clinical settings.

## Specific HrQoL instruments for irritable bowel syndrome

| Names | Scales | Comments |
|---|---|---|
| **Irritable bowel syndrome quality-of-life measure (IBS-QoL)[5]**<br>• 34 items; Likert scale<br>• Self-administered | Dysphoria, interference with activity, body image, health worry, food avoidance, social reaction, sexual relationships | Created using theoretical model; tested cross-sectionally; culturally adapted prior to validation |
| **Irritable bowel syndrome Quality-of-life questionnaire (IBS-QoL)[16]**<br>• 30 items; Likert scale<br>• Self-administered | Emotional, mental health, sleep, energy, physical functioning, diet, social role, role physical, sexual relations | Well-standardized; mix of symptoms, functional status, perceptions |
| **Quality of life questionnaire for functional digestive Disorders[17,18]**<br>• 43 items; Likert scale<br>• Self-administered | Impact on daily activities, anxiety, food, sleep, discomfort, coping, control of symptoms, stress | Includes dyspepsia, mix of symptoms, functional status, perceptions |
| **Quality of life questionnaire in irritable bowel syndrome[19]**<br>• 26 items; 7 graded scale | Bowel function, fatigue, emotional distress, activities | Mix of symptoms, functional status, perceptions |

Table 3

These instruments contain many comparable items, although the range of concepts, the type of response scales, and the psychometric properties differ between the instruments.

Criteria have been developed for evaluating the psychometric properties of HrQoL measures by the Scientific Advisory Committee of the Medical Outcomes Trust[20]. Eight criteria have been suggested on the conceptual and measurement model, reliability, validity, responsiveness, interpretability, burden, alternative forms, and cultural and language adaptations of instruments. Measurement model pertains to the conceptual domains of the instrument and the assignment of items to different domains. The underlying dimensionality of HrQoL instruments is an important measurement concern. Most HrQoL measures are multi-dimensional and some produce overall scores. Techniques for evaluating measurement models have evolved primarily from classical test theory[21] or from commonly used statistical methods such as principal components analyses. More recently, the item-response theory[22] has been applied to the development of HrQoL instruments to analyze respondent ability and item difficulty on the same metric and to understand the structure, order, and interrelations of items.

Internal consistency and test-retest reliability criteria suggest that high values (>0.70) are needed for group comparisons and even higher values (>0.90) for applications to individual patients. Few, if any, gastrointestinal-specific measures currently meet the criteria for application to individual patients, although most appear suitable for applications to groups. Validity of HrQoL measures is difficult because no gold standard exists and thus rigorous testing of hypothesized relationships between constructs is necessary to understand how an instrument behaves[1]. The construct validity of the IBDQ, a specific instrument for persons with inflammatory bowel disease, was evaluated by comparing predicted correlations with those that were observed[23]. For example, the prediction that physician rating of change in IBD should correlate approximately 0.40 with change in IBDQ bowel symptoms was tested with an observed correlation of measurements of these constructs of 0.38 indicating high validity. The validity of the IBS-QoL was evaluated by testing the ability of the measure to discriminate successfully between known groups, including severity of condition, number of IBS episodes per week, missed work days, and medical visits[5].

Statistically significant differences were observed between different groups according to disease severity, subjective severity, number of medical visits, and missed work days.

The most important psychometric criteria for HrQoL instruments used in clinical trials and assessments of treatment effectiveness are: validity for assessing change over time, or the responsiveness of the measure; and the interpretation of observed changes, i.e., are they small, medium, or large with significance to patients and clinicians. Interpretation of instrument scores over time requires that observed changes be related to clinically meaningful changes in symptoms or frequently used clinical measures[14]. Few studies on the measurement of change and relationship to changes in symptoms and clinical measures exist in gastroenterology. Irvine et al.[24,25] evaluated the observed responsiveness statistics and effect sizes of the IBDQ and found acceptable score differences among patients who had a relapse in their condition and mean changes that differentiated patients who remained stable from those who worsened.

Overall, existing measures for IBD and IBS meet many of the established minimal criteria for HrQoL assessments in cross-sectional application. A number of longitudinal investigations are underway that should provide information on the interpretation of observed changes in these measures, the most formidable challenge to HrQoL assessment and use of these measures by clinicians.

*What are the challenges in developing and using HrQoL measures in CGID?*

HrQoL measures for inflammatory bowel diseases and functional GI disorders have been used primarily in clinical trials to evaluate the efficacy of treatments. These clinical trial populations are not always comparable to populations seen in clinical practice. Use of these measures in clinical practice will require shortening the measures or finding the means for rapid assessment and studying their use in routine clinical practice. Computerized adaptive testing shows promise, although routine applications are years away[26]. Studies comparing the responsiveness and validity of shorter or rapid assessments will be necessary to see if it is appropriate to substitute the shorter instrument for the longer, research version. Even if a valid, responsive, and short instrument exists, assessments must be linked to treatment decisions and patient monitoring. Research indicates that feeding back HrQoL information to clinicians does not change their practice, or lead to improved patient outcomes[27].

The potential for use of HrQoL measures in communicating with patients about their disorder has not yet been tapped fully. Clinicians often obtain HrQoL information on an informal basis using questions such as "how are you?" Discussing actual measurement results to find out why patients rated individual items the way they did or to evaluate perceptions of change under different treatments might be useful to both patients and clinicians, particularly for the functional gastrointestinal disorders. Research will continue to outweigh practical applications, however, until evidence becomes available to support routine, formal assessments.

Cross-cultural use of HrQoL measures presents another challenge. Many measures show high agreement across cultures, such as energy, ability to conduct daily activities, but many cultures retain distinct ways of expressing what is good health and good quality of life. Taking measures developed solely within one culture and translating them to another culture without allowing for changes in the source measure is increasingly being replaced by rigorous cultural adaptation or simultaneous development[28].

HrQoL assessments have great potential to help unravel the "biopsychosocial" connections in gastrointestinal disorders. This work will proceed most rapidly when patterns of associations can be recognized between clinical and HrQoL measures, between measures obtained from clinicians and from patients and their relatives, and between different patient-reported domains such as symptoms and functional status. Treatment efficacy and effectiveness cannot be judged by changes in HrQoL measures alone, particularly without evidence from repeated tests of proposed relationships between different measures of outcome. Knowing the relationship between measures will also aid interpretation of observed changes so that clinicians and patients can identify minimally important changes and their significance.

From the more proximal measures of disease activity and symptoms to the more distal outcomes of lost productivity and reductions in perceived quality of life, there is an epidemiology of outcomes to discover in gastrointestinal disorders.

Determinants will be intrinsic to the individual - such as personality and prior bowel functioning-and extrinsic-such as social support and environmental demands. Little cumulative knowledge of this epidemiology exists to date. HrQoL measures add to the battery of assessments and provide evidence of outcomes that are perhaps most relevant to patients in their everyday lives.

Regardless of the challenges and shortcomings to HrQoL assessments, at present, there is little doubt these assessments will be part of treatment evaluations and will find their way increasingly into clinical settings. In some countries, organized systems of care and regulators will use HrQoL measures to evaluate populations and treatment effectiveness.

Potentially these measures can provide complementary information about the range and magnitude of treatment effects on patients, detect previously unrecognized adverse experiences, and improve adherence to treatments. Clinicians and clinical investigators, working with patients and with HrQoL experts, will facilitate the research and applications needed to make the assessments more widespread and useful.

## *References*

1. Patrick DL, Erickson P. *Health status and health policy: quality of life in health care evaluation and resource allocation.* New York: Oxford University Press; 1993.
2. Patrick DL, Bergner M. *Measurement of Health Status in the 1990s.* Annu Rev Public Health 1990;11:165-83.
3. McKenna SP. *A new theoretical approach to the measurement of quality of life.* Drug Inf J 1994;28:13-18.
4. Szabo S. *The World Health Organization Quality of Life (WHOQOL) Assessment Instrument.* In: Spilker, editor. *Quality of life and pharmacoeconomics in clinical trials.* 2nd ed. Philadelphia: Lippincott-Raven Publishers; 1995;355-62.
5. Patrick DL, Drossman DA, Frederick IO, et al. *Quality of life in persons with irritable bowel syndrome: Development and validation of a new measure.* Dig Dis Sci 1998;43:400-11.
6. Dancey CP, Backhouse S. *Towards a better understanding of patients with irritable bowel syndrome.* J Adv Nursing 1993;18:1443-50.

7. Gelber RD, Goldhirsch A, Cole BF. *Evaluation of effectiveness: Q-TWiST.* The International Breast Cancer Study Group. Cancer Treat Rev 1993;19(Suppl A):73-84.
8. Drossman DA, Patrick DL, Mitchell CM, Zagami EA. *Health-related quality of life in inflammatory bowel disease: functional status and patient worries and concerns.* Dig Dis Sci 1989;34:1379-86.
9. Bergner M, Bobbitt RA, Carter WB, Gilson BS. *The Sickness Impact Profile: development and final revision of a health status measure.* Medical Care 1981;19:787-805.
10. Guyatt GH, Feeny DH, Patrick DL. *Measuring health-related quality of life.* Ann Intern Med 1993;118:622-9.
11. Drossman DL, Creed FH, Fava GA, et al. *Psychosocial aspects of the functional gastrointestinal disorders.* Gastroenterol Int 1995;8:47-90.
12. McGee HM, O'Boyle CA, Hickey A, et al. *Assessing the quality of life of the individual: the SEIQoL with a healthy and a gastroenterology unit population.* Psychol Med 1991;21:749-59.
13. Provenzale D, Shearin M, Phillips-Bute BG, et al. *Health-related quality of life after ileoanal pull-though: evaluation and assessment of new health status measures.* Gastroenterology 1997;113:7-14.
14. Lydick E, Epstein RS. *Interpretation of quality of life changes.* Qual Life Res 1993;2:21-6.
15. Drossman DA. *Inflammatory Bowel Disease.* In: Spilker, editor. Quality of Life and Pharmacoeconomics in Clinical Trials. 2nd ed. New York: Lippincott-Raven; 1996; 925-35.
16. Hahn BA, Kirchdoerfer LJ, Fullerton S, Mayer E. *Evaluation of a new quality of life questionnaire for patients with irritable bowel syndrome.* Aliment Pharmacol Ther 1997;11:547-52.
17. Bergmann JF, Chassany O. *Quality of Life Questionnaire for Functional Digestive Disorders.* Hopital Lariboisiere, Institut de Recherche Jouveinal; Paris: 1995.
18. Marquis P. *Development and validation of a disease-specific quality of life instrument in functional digestive disorders* [Abstract]. J Econ Med 1996;14:41.
19. Mayer E, Fullerton S, FitzGerald L, Chang Lin. *Clinical Study Protocol: A comparison of outcome instruments in Irritable Bowel Syndrome.* Los Angeles: UCLA & VA Study Center; 1998.
20. Scientific Advisory Committee. *Instrument Review Criteria.* Medical Outcomes Trust; Boston: 1997.
21. Nunnally JC. *Psychometric Theory.* 2nd ed. New York: McGraw-Hill; 1978.
22. Hambleton RK, Swaminathan H. *Item response theory: principles and applications.* Boston: Kluwer Nijoff; 1985.

23. Irvine EJ. *Quality of life – rationale and methods for developing a disease-specific instrument for inflammatory bowel disease.* Scand J Gastroenterol 1993;199:22-7.
24. Irvine EJ, Feagan B, Rochon J, et al. *Quality of life: a valid and reliable measure of therapeutic efficacy in the treatment of inflammatory bowel disease.* Gastroenterology 1994;106:287-96.
25. Irvine EJ, Feagan BG, Wong CJ. *Does self-administration of a quality of life index for inflammatory bowel disease change the results?* J Clin Epidemiol 1996;49:1177-85.
26. McHorney C. *Generic health measurement: past accomplishments and a measurement paradigm for the 21st Century.* Ann Intern Med 1997;127:743-50.
27. Brook RH. *Using scientific information to improve quality of health care.* Ann NY Acad Sci 1993;703:74-84.
28. Patrick DL, Wild DJ, Johnson ES, et al. *Cross-cultural validation of quality-of-life measures.* In: Orley J, Kuyken W, editors. Quality of Life assessment: International perspectives. Berlin: Springer-Verlag; 1994;19-32.

## *Address for correspondence*

**PATRICK DL, PhD, MSPH**
Box 357660, University of Washington
Seattle, Washington 98195 - 7660 USA
Fax: +1 206 543 3964
E-mail: donald@u.washington.edu

# WHY STUDY CO-MORBIDITY IN CHRONIC GASTROINTESTINAL DISORDERS?

*RC Heading*

Recent studies of co-morbidity in chronic gastrointestinal conditions have been particularly directed at the functional disorders, trying to establish the groupings and associations of symptoms with the aim of clarifying disease concepts and nosology. Major progress is difficult, however, because of assumptions that must be made in interpreting the data. For example, if a significant association is found between the occurrence of two symptoms and only one of them also has significant association with a third, it is necessary to know something about the reliability of symptom detection and symptom recording before even beginning to consider whether the observed associations are cause and effect, reflections of a common underlying disease process or nothing more than consequences of some other common variable among the population studied. Much uncertainty therefore surrounds the interpretation of studies of co-morbidity, even when the raw data itself is comprehensive.

The difficulties of the undertaking should nevertheless be seen only as a reminder to perform and interpret studies with great care, not as reason to give up on the task. Any association of symptoms or diseases which occurs more often than predicted by chance invites a search for the linking factors. These may be relevant to underlying disease mechanisms, and offer opportunity for improved understanding of the disease process. In contrast, however, relatively little study has hitherto been directed to the significance of co-morbidity for impacts of disease. To establish the effects of disease co-morbidity on the individual and the additional demands imposed by this co-morbidity on health-care systems would both seem to be desirable in respect of diseases which are prevalent in the population. For example, it is well-recognised that gastro-oesophageal reflux disease affects many elderly individuals, including individuals who have other major diseases. The clinical management of these patients will be tailored to their overall circumstances but we have undertaken little study of the frequency or significance of clinical management modifications made because of co-morbidity.

It may therefore be helpful to consider in sequence the purpose of studying co-morbidity in terms of

- ✓ improving our understanding of disease concepts and classifications
- ✓ improving our understanding of disease mechanisms and
- ✓ enhancing our knowledge of the impact of disease, both for the individual sufferer and for society at large.

## Improving understanding of disease concepts and classifications

Epidemiological studies which establish that diseases occur together more frequently than by chance may serve to confirm predictions that follow logically from our understanding of those diseases, or alternatively may reveal a wholly unexplained association, for which an explanation must be sought. Table 1 gives some examples of linked diseases and disorders to illustrate the questions that such observed associations may provoke. For example, most gastroenterologists now accept that there is an association between Gastro-Oesophageal Reflux Disease (GORD) and bronchial asthma, and that the relationship is probably one of cause and effect[1]. The evidence supporting this hypothesis, particularly for adults, is not particularly robust however. Although there is experimental evidence supporting airway obstruction as a consequence of gastro-oesophageal reflux, and the sequence reflux - airway aspiration - airway obstruction is plausible, the likelihood of gastro-oesophageal reflux occurring as a *consequence* of airway obstruction and attendant breathing difficulty introduces significant doubt about the cause-effect relationship[2]. Only the disappearance of asthma following correction of gastro-oesophageal reflux would seem to offer a prospect of proving the point, but it appears that anti-reflux surgery may produce improvement rather than disappearance of co-existing asthma in many GORD patients[3].

Observed co-morbidities which may help understanding of disease concepts and classifications

| | |
|---|---|
| Linked diseases / disorders | Gastro-oesophageal reflux disease<br>• asthma |
| | Musculoskeletal pain - NSAID use<br>• dyspepsia /GI bleeding |
| | Inflammatory bowel disease<br>• primary sclerosing cholangitis |
| | Primary biliary cirrhosis<br>• coeliac disease |
| | Irritable bowel syndrome<br>• functional dyspepsia |
| Associated but unlinked (?) diseases / disorders | Ischaemic heart disease<br>• diverticular disease |
| | Duodenal ulcer<br>• chronic obstructive pulmonary disease |
| | Migraine<br>• irritable bowel syndrome |
| Linked diseases / disorders of uncertain significance | Diabetes mellitus<br>• constipation |
| | Irritable bowel syndrome<br>• previous enteric infection |
| | Irritable bowel syndrome<br>• quiescent colitis |

Table 1

Perhaps musculo-skeletal pains, NSAID use, dyspepsia and/or gastrointestinal bleeding is a more clear-cut sequence of co-morbidity, and one where good epidemological study has helped physicians by establishing the magnitude of the links. Given the frequency with which aspirin and other non-steroidal anti-inflammatory drugs are in therapeutic use, and recognising the variety of potential causes of upper gastro-intestinal bleeding, it is clearly ludicrous to suppose that every patient who has an upper GI bleed and is taking such medication has sustained their bleed as a consequence of the drug[4]. Nevertheless, young physicians have been taught to record patients' use of such medication as if it were a useful piece of information. Quite obviously, it is useful only when the magnitude of excess risk imposed by the medications has been established and a considered judgement of its significance (the risk benefit balance) can be made[5,6].

Some well-known associations reflect fundamental disease mechanisms and may be a useful stimulus to new lines of thought in considering the basic science of the diseases processes. The well-known association of inflammatory bowel disease and primary sclerosing cholangitis would be one such example, primary biliary cirrhosis with coeliac disease or with a CREST syndrome would be others. Is the association between irritable bowel syndrome and functional dyspepsia an analogous association? It may well be so, and this is discussed further below in the context of disease mechanisms in the functional gastrointestinal disorders.

The coincidence of some diseases may have a mundane explanation in a common underlying variable. For example, if the adult community at large is assessed, there is little doubt that raw data will show an association between ischaemic heart disease and diverticular disease. Age is the common variable and will be understood as such by most physicians. Observations such as this serve as a reminder that logistic regression and factor analyses are basic tools of epidemiological investigations and are the only way to convert raw empirical observations of supposed association into persuasive evidence of a link with significance.

There are still plenty such associations where it is the significance of the apparent link that remains obscure. Peptic ulceration has been said for many years to be associated with chronic obstructive pulmonary disease. Is this just an association through smoking, or is there more to it? Why does there appear to be co-morbidity of migraine and irritable bowel syndrome? Is it real or does it come about simply because sufferers from both conditions have lowered thresholds for distress from symptoms and an above-average likelihood of seeking medical attention for them? We do not really know.

Finally there are associations where levels of uncertainty are even greater. Constipation is very common in patients with diabetes mellitus, and may perhaps be attributed to subtle, unrecognised dysfunction of the intrinsic innervation of the colon, causing impaired motility. Both the link and the putative mechanisms are poorly defined. In contrast, the existence of irritable bowel syndrome as a consequence of previous enteric infection is widely accepted. The mechanism is still not clear, though the focus of ongoing research. Nevertheless, it is also clear that many patients with irritable bowel syndrome seem to lack any evidence of such an incident infection, so what is the link?

When considering the possibility of irritable bowel syndrome in patients with quiescent colitis, debate has swung backwards and forwards on grounds of definition alone. A strict definition of irritable bowel syndrome requires the absence of organic bowel disease, which might mean that no patient with an established diagnosis of inflammatory bowel disease could have an irritable bowel syndrome. Perhaps a more useful definition of irritable bowel syndrome requires the absence of organic disease to explain the symptoms, and in these circumstances a diagnosis of irritable bowel syndrome could be given to an individual with symptoms if the inflammatory bowel disease were completely quiescent. However, the physician's judgement is involved in determining whether or not the symptoms are to be attributed to a particular identified pathology, and substantial subjectivity is thereby introduced. What is not in doubt, however, is that some patients with quiescent colitis have symptoms which in all other respects fit with the criteria of the irritable bowel syndrome.

Now and again, an investigation is reported which challenges a cherished belief held by the gastroenterological community. One recent example is the study of Lagergren et al.[7], demonstrating that adenocarcinoma of the oesophagus is associated with severe heartburn, but has a less robust link with Barrett's oesophagus. Physicians brought up with a belief in the sequence gastro-oesophageal reflux - Barrett's metaplasia - dysplasia - adenocarcinoma as indisputable fact realised with shock that not only did Lagergren and colleagues report findings apparently at variance with this sequence, but indirectly drew attention to the fact that most (all?) the epidemiological evidence for the Barrett's oesophagus - adenocarcinoma association has failed to examine the role of heartburn as an independent variable. Is it conceivably possible that heartburn is the cause of adenocarcinoma and the observed link of Barrett's oesophagus and carcinoma is merely an incidental consequence of the relationship between gastro-oesophageal reflux and Barrett's? Quite clearly, this is a complex issue and epidemiological studies do not diminish the validity of other evidence, notably from cytology and molecular biology, supporting the metaplasia - dysplasia - carcinoma progression. Nevertheless, it is beyond dispute that epidemiological studies such as this can introduce new evidence which is both informative and intellectually challenging for our understanding of disease.

*Co-morbidity of functional gastrointestinal symptoms*

The term irritable bowel syndrome, now in common parlance, has actually replaced the more old-fashioned "irritable colon", representing recognition that although lower bowel symptoms are the principal problem for most sufferers, abnormality may affect the whole of the gastrointestinal tract. Simultaneous recognition of various overlaps and parallels between the irritable bowel syndrome and functional dyspepsia has led many physicians to think of the latter as little more than a proximal gastrointestinal form of irritable bowel. This is certainly a legitimate pragmatic belief, and may also have a deeper validity[8]. Much data supports links between the common gastrointestinal symptoms. The prevalence of irritable bowel syndrome in western societies appears to be in the range 10-15% and in one study reporting a 12% IBS prevalence, 57% of the IBS patients also had dyspeptic symptoms and 40% had frequent heartburn[9].

Observations of this sort raise questions about when symptoms should be regarded as distinct entities and, in turn, how we should classify these functional disorders. Agreus and colleagues[10] have argued that the symptoms of IBS and dyspepsia are neither distinctive nor stable, a view which would seem to support the contention that functional dyspepsia is a proximal gastrointestinal variant of irritable bowel. Other evidence suggests that lower and upper gastrointestinal tract symptoms are distinctive, and there is also a definable cohort of individuals describing both dyspeptic and IBS symptoms concurrently[9]. Thus for the moment at least, it is clear that there is certainly some instability of symptom pattern over time, and there is no doubt of the overlap between dyspeptic and irritable bowel symptoms, but it is premature to conclude that the two symptom presentations represent different manifestations of the same disorder.

In all studies of this sort on functional gastrointestinal disorders, care must be taken to guard against the possibility of misleading information being obtained as a result of variable data acquisition. In a study of gastro-oesophageal reflux symptoms in the community, 29% of individuals appeared to be sufferers[11]. Of these, 66% also had dyspeptic symptoms and 28% had irritable bowel syndrome. Interestingly, increased medical consultation was associated with co-existing dyspepsia, but not co-existing irritable bowel symptoms. If this pattern is generally true, it demonstrates that any study of patients, as distinct from sufferers, will record a stronger association of dyspepsia with gastro-oesophageal reflux than exists in the community at large.

*Heartburn and gastro-oesophageal reflux in studies of co-morbidity*

The relationship between a complaint of heartburn and the occurrence of gastro-oesophageal reflux disease remains a surprising difficulty and one that has caused much confusion in publications about co-morbidity in functional gastrointestinal disease. Unfortunately, the terms heartburn, reflux symptoms and reflux disease have often been used interchangeably and in the context of the functional gastrointestinal disorders, this may prove problematic.

It is generally agreed that classical reflux symptoms are a relatively specific indicator of gastro-oesophageal reflux disease[12]. The two cannot be equated, however, and many patients with reflux disease present with a less clear-cut symptom profile, which would not really justify the term "reflux symptoms"[13,14]. It is also generally agreed that pathological (abnormally increased) gastro-oesophageal acid reflux identified on ambulatory oesophageal pH monitoring justifies the term gastro-oesophageal reflux disease. There is less certainty, however, about the minority of individuals undergoing such tests in whom the magnitude of gastro-oesophageal acid reflux appears to be normal, but a convincing temporal association of reflux and symptoms is demonstrated (a high value of symptom index). This is usually regarded as acceptable proof that symptoms are attributable to the gastro-oesophageal acid reflux, thus meeting a widely accepted diagnostic criterion of gastro-oesophageal reflux disease. However, there is also good reason to regard such individuals as having "functional heartburn", if only because they appear to be perceiving a normal physiological event[15].

The terminology and the concepts relating to these patients are important both in respect of the heartburn or reflux symptoms they describe, and clarifying the nature of co-morbidity with other symptoms or disorders. Quantitatively, the issue is quite significant. Among individuals reporting heartburn who did not have oesophagitis, 37% were reported to have gastro-oesophageal acid reflux exposures within the normal range in one study[16]. It would seem that within this group, there will be some individuals who fulfil present definitions of gastro-oesophageal reflux disease while among the others, some forms of functional heartburn are associated with demonstrable gastro-oesophageal reflux events, and others are not. Studies of co-morbidity will need to disentangle these variants to interpret observations meaningfully.

Do patients identify heartburn reliably anyway? There is some evidence that within individual communities they do, but whether reliability would stand up comparing different populations in different countries is less clear. The wording of enquiry about heartburn is important. This is just another uncertainty with which investigators and journal readers have to contend.

## Understanding of disease mechanisms

Only brief mention of this important outcome of co-morbidity studies will be made here. As indicated above, valuable pointers to appropriate directions for basic science research may emerge from demonstrations of unexpected disease associations. The example of primary sclerosing cholangitis and inflammatory bowel disease was given above: many others can be cited. Even single anecdotal reports of the coincidence of rare conditions may be of interest. For example, consideration of the incidence of the respective disorders suggests that the development of achalasia in a 28 year old woman who had surgery for Hirschprung's disease in childhood hints at something linking these disorders, particularly when other anecdotal evidence may be added to suggest that there may even be a three-way link of achalasia (in adult life), infantile pyloric stenosis and Hirschprung's disease[17]. Is this a link? Quite what the mechanism could be remains to be seen, as it does not seem to be fully explained by our current knowledge of nitrergic nerve loss in the pathophysiology of these disorders.

So far as the functional gastrointestinal disorders are concerned, the links between the two common disorders, functional dyspepsia and irritable bowel syndrome, should help us to understand the underlying disease mechanisms. Causation, mechanism of symptom occurrence and the fundamental pathophysiology all require significant further investigation. Both the similarities and the differences between the disorders could be useful targets of research.

## Understanding of disease impact

It is necessary to distinguish the impact of disease co-morbidity on the individual from its impact on society as a whole. The former is probably adequately captured by conventional health-related quality of life assessment and may be relatively easy to achieve, though little study has attempted it so far. Economic and other impacts for society as a whole are less easily characterised, however, though they may be important and extend beyond simple summation of medications or other treatments for the co-existing disorders. For example the economic burden on the health-care system imposed by coeliac disease could be calculated. However comprehensive calculation might wish to take into account the additional costs that arise from other diseases which have an increased prevalence among coeliacs such as diabetes mellitus.

It is probably the impact of co-morbidity for the individual sufferer that justifies most original research at this time, however. As mentioned above, gastro-oesophageal reflux may be associated with the irritable bowel syndrome in some patients and with dyspepsia in others, and the GORD + dyspepsia group has a higher incidence of medical consultation. We do not know why, but one presumes that for some reason the combination is causing them greater distress.

Other aspects of co-morbidity have an obvious impact, though we rarely attempt its quantification or measure our ability to ameliorate the impact. How might we best assess the disease impact of diarrhoea in a diabetic who is also physically disabled with rheumatoid arthritis? What interventions are of greatest benefit for that individual?

## Conclusions

Studies of co-morbidity may produce information which will guide further epidemiological assessment, studies in basic or clinical science and appraisals of health economics and other health-care related research. In offering a judgement of where we are now, it is reasonable to claim that for functional disorders particularly, epidemiological studies of recent years have been of great help in establishing our definitions and our concepts of the disorders, as well as establishing numerical information about their frequency and distribution. Unfortunately, this progress has not been matched by comparable advancement in knowledge of their pathophysiology. This is now a real constraint on progress. It may be fruitful for physiological studies now to seek to identify differences between the functional gastrointestinal disorders, rather than further pursue the quest for similarities which distinguish these patients from the healthy asymptomatic population. For example, if there is a population with functional dyspepsia and the irritable bowel syndrome, it is of as much interest to know how they differ from individuals with either disorder alone as how they differ from the healthy population.

Additionally, too little is presently known about how and when common diseases and therapies summate to increase the impact of illness and how therapy - not drugs alone - affects all aspects of the lives of patients with more than one concurrent illness. This is also a subject worthy of substantial further attention.

## *References*


1. Harding SM, Richter JE, Guzzo MR, et al. *Asthma and gastroesophageal reflux: acid suppressive therapy improves asthma outcome.* Am J Med 1996;100:395-405.
2. Sontag SJ. *Pulmonary complications of gastroesophageal reflux.* In:. Castell DO, editor. *The Esophagus.* Boston: Little Brown & Co; 1995;555-70.
3. Larrain A, Carrasco E, Galleguillos F, et al. *Medical and surgical treatment of nonallergic asthma associated with gastroesophageal reflux.* Chest 1991;99:1330-5.
4. Coggon D, Langman MJS, Spiegelhalter D. *Aspirin, paracetamol, and haematemesis and melaena.* Gut 1982;23:34-44.
5. Slattery J, Warlow CP, Shorrock CJ, et al. *Risks of gastrointestinal bleeding during secondary prevention of vascular events with aspirin - analysis of gastrointestinal bleeding during the UK-TIA trial.* Gut 1995;37:509-11.
6. Dickinson JP, Prentice CRM. *Aspirin: benefit and risk in thromboprophylaxis.* Q J Med 1998;91:523-38.
7. Lagergren J, Bergstrom R, Lindgren A, et al. *Symptomatic gastroesophageal reflux as a risk factor for esophageal adenocarcinoma.* N Engl J Med 1999;340:825-31.
8. Caballero-Plasencia, AM, Sofos-Kontoyannis S, Valenzuela-Barranco M, et al. *Irritable bowel syndrome in patients with dyspepsia: a community-based study in southern Europe.* Eur J Gastroenterol Hepatol 1999;11:517-22.
9. Talley NJ, Boyce P, Jones M. *Identification of distinct upper and lower gastrointestinal symptom groupings in an urban population.* Gut 1998;42:690-5.
10. Agreus, L, Svardsudd K, Nyren O, et al. *Irritable bowel syndrome and dyspepsia in the general population: Overlap and lack of stability over time.* Gastroenterology 1995;109:671-80.
11. Kennedy T, Jones R. *Gastro-oesophageal reflux symptoms in the community.* Gut 1998;42 (Suppl 1):A64.
12. Klauser AG, Schindlbeck NE, Muller-Lissner SA. *Symptoms in gastro-oesophageal reflux disease.* Lancet 1990;335:205-8
13. Wienbeck M, Berges W. *Esophageal disorders in the etiology and pathophysiology of*

*dyspepsia.* Scand J Gastroenterol 1985; 20 (Suppl 109):133-7.
14. Rune SJ. *Heartburn and dyspepsia: the utility of symptom analysis.* Aliment Pharmacol Ther 1997;11 (Suppl 2):9-12.
15. Clouse R, Richter JE, Heading RC, et al. *Functional esophageal disorders.* Gut 1999;45(Suppl II):II31-II36.
16. Lind T, Havelund R, Carlsson O, et al. *Heartburn without oesophagitis: Efficacy of omeprazole therapy and features determining therapeutic response.* Scand J Gastroenterol 1997;32:974-9.
17. Castro A, Mearin F, Gil-Vernet JM, et al. *Infantile hypertrophic pyloric stenosis and achalasia: NO-related or non-related conditions?* Digestion 1997;58:596-8.

*ADDRESS FOR CORRESPONDENCE*

**HEADING RC, MD, FRCP**
Centre for Liver and Digestive Disorders
Royal Infirmary
Edinburgh EH3 9YW United Kingdom
Fax: +44 131 536 2197

# EXTRAGASTROINTESTINAL CO-MORBIDITY IN CHRONIC FUNCTIONAL GASTROINTESTINAL DISORDERS

*KW Olden*

Chronic Gastrointestinal (GI) disorders have been commonly associated with extraintestinal manifestations. Extraintestinal manifestations have been frequently seen in Inflammatory Bowel Disease (IBD) with its wide spectrum of dermatologic, ophthalmologic and hepatic complications. Likewise, chronic functional GI disorders have been frequently associated with a wide spectrum of nongastrointestinal symptoms. These extraintestinal symptoms can be conveniently categorized into comorbid psychiatric and non-psychiatric symptoms and/or syndromes.

To facilitate discussion of these comorbid conditions, this chapter will be divided into a review of psychiatric and non-psychiatric manifestations of chronic functional GI disorders as they manifest themselves outside the GI tract.

## Psychiatric comorbidity

In the last ten years, a number of studies have demonstrated a high prevalence of psychiatric comorbidity in patients presenting with functional GI disorders. Walker et al. in 1988[1] studied 25 women with recurrent abdominal pain determined to be of functional origin. The mean duration of pain in these patients was 12 months. These patients were compared to 30 women with known gynecologic problems, all of whom were also suffering from chronic abdominal and pelvic pain. In addition, all of the patients in both groups underwent diagnostic laparoscopy to rule out a structural cause of the patient's pain. The results of the laparoscopy were graded on a scale of 0 (normal) to 4 using criteria developed by the American Laparoscopic Society. In addition, the patients in both groups underwent detailed psychiatric evaluation which consisted of a structured psychiatric interview in the form of the Diagnostic Interview Schedule (DIS), a validated structured interview used to detect psychiatric disorders. Finally, the patients completed the Symptom Checklist 90 (SCL-90) to evaluate their overall emotional distress. The results of Walker's study were dramatic. The patients with current functional abdominal pain were 3 to 9 times more likely to have had a diagnosable psychiatric illness. The disorders most commonly seen were major depressive disorder, somatization disorder, panic disorder and phobias. In addition, the patients with chronic functional abdominal pain were much more likely to suffer a variety of sexually dysfunctional complaints, including dyspareunia, decreased libido or inhibited orgasm as compared to the patients with anatomically based pain (Table 1).

PSYCHIATRIC COMORBIDITY IN PATIENTS WITH RECURRENT ABDOMINAL PAIN

| | **Patients with recurrent abdominal pain** % | **Controls** % | **p** |
|---|---|---|---|
| Depression | 64 | 17 | <0.001 |
| Phobias | 32 | 10 | <0.05 |
| Dyspareunia | 52 | 7 | <0.001 |
| Decreased libido | 28 | 7 | <0.05 |
| Inhibited orgasm | 16 | 3 | <0.05 |

Table 1

Reproduced with permission from Walker EA, Katon WJ, Harrop-Griffiths J et al.[1]

When the SCL-90 was reviewed, all nine scales were significantly elevated in the patients with recurrent functional abdominal pain compared to the controls who had anatomically-based pain ($p<0.001$-$0.05$). This study demonstrated that patients with functional chronic abdominal pain differed in a number of ways from patients with similar, but structurally based pain. Most prominent was the fact that the functional patients, in addition to having a pain complaint, had a spectrum of psychological disturbance which differentiated them from the patients with structural lesions. Walker et al. also investigated the prevalence of sexual abuse in both populations. Patients were administered a structured interview inquiring whether they had experienced any sexual abuse either in childhood (prior to the age of 14 years) or as an adult. The results were startling. The patients with functional chronic abdominal pain were significantly more likely to have been sexually abused both in childhood as well as adulthood (Table 2).

PREVALENCE OF SEXUAL ABUSE IN PATIENTS WITH RECURRENT ABDOMINAL PAIN

| | **Patients with recurrent abdominal pain** % | **Controls** % | **p** |
|---|---|---|---|
| Sexual abuse (<14 y.o.) | 64 | 23 | <0.01 |
| Sexual abuse (>14 y.o.) | 48 | 13 | <0.01 |

Table 2

Reproduced with permission from Walker EA, Katon WJ, Harrop-Griffiths J et al.[1]

Caution must be taken, however, in ascribing these "extraintestinal manifestations" of a chronic functional GI disorder with a history of sexual abuse as being unique to Gastroenterology. Self-reported abuse itself is not uncommon. In one study of adults aged 30-49 years old, the age adjusted prevalence of self-reported abuse was 41% in women and 11% in men[2]. Studies have shown that patients who have been sexually abused tend to have a wide spectrum of medical complaints[3]. Moreover, recent studies have suggested that a history of abuse is an important factor in how patients experience illness. Drossman et al. evaluated 92 patients with functional GI disorders and 197 patients with chronic GI disorders which were organically based. They found

that both patients with functional and structural chronic GI disorders who had an abuse history experienced significantly more disability days ($p<0.0007$), pain ($p<0.001$) and psychological distress ($p<0.0001$)[4]. The spectrum of extraintestinal organ dysfunction in patients with functional GI disorders was demonstrated in studies by Whorwell et al.[5] and Arnold et al.[3]. Whorwell et al. described a wide spectrum of GI symptoms in a cohort of patients presenting for treatment of Irritable Bowel Syndrome (IBS). These symptoms included back pain, headaches, fatigue and sexual dysfunction[5].
Arnold et al. investigated intestinal and extraintestinal symptoms in a group of patients who reported a history of sexual abuse. In this study, the investigators were not looking at GI dysfunction per se. Rather, they attempted to determine the spectrum and prevalence of physical complaints in patients who had been abused. Although the patients in Arnold's study did not specifically present for treatment of bowel dysfunction, the prevalence of self reported GI symptoms was high. There was also a striking similarity in the spectrum of physical complaints seen in Whorwell's study of IBS patients (Table 3)[3,5].

EXTRAGASTROINTESTINAL ORGAN DYSFUNCTION IN PATIENTS WITH FUNCTIONAL GI DISORDERS

| **IBS patients**<br>Whorwell et al. 1986[5] | **Abused patients**<br>Arnold et al. 1990[3] |
|---|---|
| Back pain | Back pain |
| Headaches | Headaches |
| Pruritus | Chest pain |
| Fatigue | Dyspareunia |
| Unpleasant taste | Arthralgias |
| Sexual dysfunction | Sexual dysfunction |

Table 3

A logical question which arises from these data is whether patients who have endured physical or sexual abuse are more prone to experience complaints across a wide spectrum of organ systems in which the GI tract is only one of several organ systems affected. The work of Arnold and others would certainly support this conclusion. These data, in turn, need to be interpreted along with the research by Walker et al.[1] that demonstrated a high prevalence of psychiatric disorders, particularly major depressive disorder, sexual dysfunction and somatization disorder. Taken together, these findings may lead to the conclusion that patients with IBS who also complain of "extraintestinal manifestations" may actually be displaying multiorgan dysfunction as a result of a prior history of physical or sexual abuse.

## Specific organ dysfunction

Despite the findings cited above, the suggestion that a history of abuse, as opposed to IBS, may be the "primary" condition causing GI symptoms in patients presenting with IBS is not conclusive. It does appear that, in patients with IBS, there are certain organ systems that do seem to be selectively more likely to cause patients distress. These organ systems are the urinary, gynecologic and musculoskeletal systems.

## Urinary dysfunction

Patients with functional GI disorders, particularly IBS, tend to complain of a spectrum of symptoms. Several investigators have attempted to identify the prevalence of these symptoms in patients with functional GI disorders and to evaluate the differences between these patients and the population at large. Whorwell et al.[5] compared 100 patients with functional GI disorders to an age- and gender-matched control group who were not complaining of any bowel dysfunction. The IBS patients had a 7% - 33% prevalence of urinary symptoms. When compared to controls, patients with functional GI disorders were significantly more likely to have urinary symptoms[5]. Similar findings, reported by Terruzzi et al.[6] demonstrated a 33% prevalence of urinary symptoms in IBS patients. The prevalence of urinary symptoms was significantly greater in the

URINARY DYSFUNCTION IN PATIENTS WITH FUNCTIONAL GI DISORDERS

| Study, year ref | frequency % | dysuria % | urgency % | incontinence % | nocturia % |
|---|---|---|---|---|---|
| Whorwell et al. 1986[5] | 30 | 7 | 33 | 27 | 27 |
| Terruzzi et al. 1992[6] | 61 | - | 60 | 50 | 53 |
| Nyhlin et al. 1993[7] | 41 | - | - | - | - |

• Prevalence 33% (Terruzzi et al. 1992 and Whorwell et al. 1986)
• $p<0.05$ compared to controls in Whorwell et al. and Terruzzi et al. studies

Table 4

functional GI patients compared to the non-IBS controls ($p<0.02$) (Table 4)[6]. Nyhlin et al. also found a 41% prevalence of urinary frequency in his study population of IBS patients. However, this study did not ask about specific urinary symptoms but rather inquired about the presence or absence of any symptoms[7].

## Gynecologic and sexual dysfunction

In addition to urinary symptoms, patients with functional GI disorders frequently complain of sexual dysfunction. It is not clear what causes this dysfunction, but one possible mechanism may be dysfunction of the muscles of the pelvic floor. One other possibility is a lowered pain threshold and/or heightened visceral hypersensitivity which could affect the pelvic floor. Walker et al., in their study of patients with chronic functional abdominal pain, found a high prevalence of dyspareunia, decreased libido and inhibited orgasm[8]. Moreover, in a study of IBS patients who presented to a primary care clinic, Springs and Friedrich

found a significant increase in the prevalence of sexual dysfunction in patients who were abused[9], and also Springs found that the prevalence of gynecologic problems was significantly increased in the abused women ($p<0.004$). The study also showed that the prevalence of gynecologic problems increased as the severity of abuse increased.
These findings are consistent with those of others[5,7,8], all of whom found an increased prevalence of sexual dysfunction in patients with functional GI disorders when compared to controls (Table 5). It would seem reasonable to conclude that sexual dysfunction is a not an infrequent concomitant to a chronic GI disorder which may be influenced by a wide spectrum of factors, including abuse history, psychiatric comorbidity, and possible intrinsic dysfunction of the muscles of the pelvic floor.

SEXUAL DYSFUNCTION IN PATIENTS WITH FUNCTIONAL GI DISORDERS

| Study, year ref | Dyspareunia % | Dysmenorrhea % |
|---|---|---|
| Whorwell et al. 1986[5] | 42 | 68 |
| Walker et al. 1988[1] | 52 | - |
| Nyhlin et al. 1993[7] | 8 | 26 |

Table 5

## Fibromyalgia

In the last few years, there have been a number of interesting studies that have suggested an increased prevalence of fibromyalgia in patients with functional GI disorders. Fibromyalgia is a poorly understood rheumatologic condition characterized by aches and pains in multiple areas of the musculoskeletal system. It is not associated with classic markers of inflammatory disease of muscles, bones or joints, such as elevated erythrocyte sedimentation rate or C-reactive protein. The American College of Rheumatology has proposed symptom-based diagnostic criteria for fibromyalgia not unlike the symptom-based diagnostic criteria proposed for the various functional GI disorders. The variable course of this condition, the tendency of the pain site to migrate, and a diagnosis based on clinically empiric grounds makes fibromyalgia very similar to the chronic functional GI disorders. Thus, clinicians frequently encounter patients whose complaints are suggestive both of fibromyalgia as well as IBS. To clarify this relationship, Triadafilopoulos et al.[10] compared 123 patients with fibromyalgia and specifically screened them for IBS. These patients were compared to 54 patients presenting for treatment of degenerative joint disease and a control group of 46 patients with no rheumatologic complaint. Triadafilopoulos et al. found that 73% of the fibromyalgia patients complained of bowel dysfunction as compared to 37% of the degenerative joint disease patients and none of the controls ($p<0.001$). In addition, 81% of the fibromyalgia patients complained of a pattern of alternating constipation and diarrhea that was suggestive of IBS. Finally, 50% of the fibromyalgia patients reported that they experienced simultaneous flares of their bowel symptoms during flares in their rheumatologic disease. These results were significantly different from patients with degenerative joint disease or controls (Table 6)[10].

BOWEL SYMPTOMS IN PATIENTS WITH FIBROMYALGIA

| | Fibromyalgia patients % | Degenerative joint disease patients % | Controls % | p |
|---|---|---|---|---|
| • Bowel dysfunction | 73 | 37 | 0 | <0.001 |
| • Alternating constipation and diarrhea | 81 | 44 | 13 | <0.001 |
| • Bowel flares during joint disease | 50 | 28 | - | <0.05 |

Table 6

Reproduced with permission from Triadafilopoulos G, Simms RW, Goldenberg D[10].

These findings were similar to the findings of Veale et al.[11] who studied 20 patients with known IBS. The IBS patients were compared to 20 patients each with inflammatory arthritis and IBD. All of these groups were, in turn, compared to 20 normal controls. Veale et al. found that 65% of the IBS patients met the diagnostic criteria for fibromyalgia as compared to only 10% each of the IBD and arthritis patients, and 30% of the controls. The prevalence of IBS in the fibromyalgia, arthritis, IBD and control groups was then evaluated. Seventy percent of the fibromyalgia patients met the diagnostic criteria for IBS compared to only 10% in the IBD and 20% each in the arthritis patients and the controls[11]. A different study was performed by Sperber et al.[12]. They investigated 79 patients with IBS and specifically evaluated them for fibromyalgia using both their symptom reports as well as measuring muscle sensitivity with a dolorimeter, an instrument that measures muscle sensitivity to compression. These patients were then compared to 72 controls. In addition, Sperber et al. evaluated these patients' overall well being, measured by instances of sleep disturbance, patients' pain ratings, and the number of physician visits. Finally, both groups were administered an SCL-90 to evaluate their overall level of emotional distress. Sperber found that the IBS patients who presented simultaneously with fibromyalgia were significantly different from patients with IBS alone. The measures for global well-being, sleep disturbance, number of physician visits, pain ratings, and the global symptom index of the SCL-90 were all significantly different in the IBS patients with fibromyalgia compared to the IBS-only group (Table 7).

DYSFUNCTION IN IBS PATIENTS WITH FIBROMYALGIA COMPARED TO CONTROLS

| | p |
|---|---|
| Global well-being | <0.00001 |
| Sleep disturbance | <0.0003 |
| Physician visits | <0.003 |
| Pain rating | <0.0001 |
| Global symptom index (SCL-90R) | <0.0001 |

Table 7

Reproduced with permission from: Sperber A, Atzmon Y, Weitzman J et al.[12]

Sperber et al. concluded that IBS patients who presented with concomitant fibromyalgia represented a subset of particularly distressed patients compared to "pure" IBS patients and normal controls[12].

## Do extraintestinal manifestations represent the nonspecific stress of illness?

When considering the extraintestinal manifestations of a chronic functional GI disorder, it is important to consider the issue of the overall stress that the illness causes. In this concept, the discomfort and suffering induced by an illness can, in turn, create dysfunction, or at least discomfort, in other areas of the body. To evaluate this question, Fullerton et al.[13] evaluated 527 patients with IBS and compared them to 161 patients with known IBD. Both groups of patients suffered from abdominal pain, cramping, bloating and diarrhea. Patients in both groups were asked to complete the bowel disease questionnaire, a standardized instrument that measures bowel symptoms and the stress related to these symptoms. Fullerton et al. found no difference in the two groups along the following dimensions: presence of abnormal taste, weight change, appetite, sleep disturbance, sexual dysfunction, bladder dysfunction, mood changes, fatigue or low back pain[13]. These findings would suggest that the mere presence of a chronic bowel disorder can give rise to the sense of "asthenia" or not feeling well which, in turn, can lead to increased perception of discomfort in other organ systems.

## Conclusions

This review offers a discussion of an interesting and extremely poorly understood area of gastroenterology. What is clear is that patients with IBS and other chronic functional GI disorders commonly have extraintestinal dimensions to their bowel disorder. It is also clear at this point that these symptoms are most commonly referred to the musculoskeletal, gynecologic and genitourinary systems. However, the question still remains whether these symptoms are primary phenomena representing a true extraintestinal manifestation of the primary bowel disorder or whether they are secondary phenomena that are driven by a primary psychiatric disorder or an abuse history. Finally, one cannot rule out an effect from the stress of having any chronic GI disorder which may make symptoms perceivable in other organ systems more prominent or troublesome. Moreover, the issue of unrelated comorbidity has not been completely ruled out, with multiple organ systems interacting in independent but parallel ways such as the possible situation with fibromyalgia and IBS. All of these issues remain to be more fully investigated. It is also important to obtain a better understanding of how these organ system complaints interact to affect the patients' overall quality of life and overall prognosis. However, the preliminary work of Sperber et al. would suggest that these patients need particularly aggressive intervention to induce improvement not just in their bowel symptoms, but also in other organ systems along with their overall sense of well-being. One major goal for future research is to determine the prognostic significance and implications for treatment of these patients with extraintestinal manifestations of their functional GI disorders.

## *References*

1. Walker EA, Katon WJ, Harrop-Griffiths J, et al. *Relationship of chronic pelvic pain to psychiatric diagnoses and childhood sexual abuse.* Am J Psychiatry 1988;145:75-80.
2. Talley NJ, Fett SL, Zinsmeister AR, et al. *Gastrointestinal tract symptoms and self-reported abuse: a population-based study.* Gastroenterology 1994;107:1040-9.
3. Arnold R, Rogers D, Cook D. *Medical problems of adults who were sexually abused in childhood.* Br Med J 1990;300:705-8.
4. Drossman DA, Li Z, Leserman J, et al. *Health status by gastrointestinal diagnosis and abuse history.* Gastroenterology 1996;110:999-1007.
5. Whorwell PJ, McCallum M, Creed FH, et al. *Non-colonic features of irritable bowel syndrome.* Gut 1986;27:37-40.
6. Terruzzi V, Magatti F, Quadri G, et al. *Bladder dysfunction and irritable bowel syndrome* (letter). JAMA 1992;87:1231-2.
7. Nyhlin H, Ford MJ, Eastwood J, et al. *Non-alimentary aspects of the irritable bowel syndrome.* J Psychosom Res 1993;37:155-62.
8. Walker EA, Katon WJ, Hansom J, et al. *Psychiatric diagnoses and sexual victimization*

*in women with chronic pelvic pain.* Psychosomatics 1995;36:531-40.

9. Springs FE, Friedrich WN. *Health risk behaviors and medical sequelae of childhood sexual abuse.* Mayo Clin Proc 1992;67:527-32.
10. Triadafilopoulos G, Simms RW, Goldenberg D. *Bowel dysfunction in fibromyalgia syndrome.* Dig Dis Sci 1991;36:59-64.
11. Veale D, Kavanagh J, Fielding JF, et al. *Primary fibromyalgia and the irritable bowel syndrome: different expressions of a common pathogenetic process.* Br J Rheumatol 1991;30:220-2.
12. Sperber A, Atzmon Y, Weitzman I, et al. *A controlled study of fibromyalgia in IBS patients.* Gastroenterology 1998;114:A840.
13. Fullerton S, Anton PA, Chang L, et al. *Prevalence of extraintestinal symptoms in patients with irritable bowel syndrome and inflammatory bowel disease.* Gastroenterology 1998;114:A15.

*ADDRESS FOR CORRESPONDENCE*

**OLDEN KW, MD**
Division of Gastroenterology
Mayo Clinic Scottsdale
13400 East Shea Blvd
Scottsdale, Arizona 85259 USA
Fax: +1 480 391 9527
E-mail: olden.kevin@mayo.edu

# Alterations of eating behaviour
## Impact of biologic, psychologic and environmental factors and psychiatric disease

*G Stacher*

The relative importance of biologic, psychologic, environmental and sociocultural factors and of psychiatric disease in the development and course of eating disorders is, in contrast to many claims, not at all clear. There is even no general agreement as to which clinical entities have to be regarded as an eating disorder and as to whether the various eating disorders are clearly distinguishable from each other. By some investigators, they are rather viewed as lying on a continuum spread across a number of parameters which are partially independent of each other: undernutrition versus overnutrition, restriction versus indulgence, activity versus inactivity, abstinence behaviours such as dieting versus "purging behaviours" such as vomiting, and persistence of restraint eating versus intermittent reactive hyperphagia[1].

This review presents what is known about biologic, psychologic and environmental factors as well as psychiatric disease and the interactions of such factors, which may lead to and maintain a disordered eating behaviour.

### *Obesity*

Is obesity, the excess accumulation of body fat, an eating disorder? Against such a notion speak the facts that the obese typically have not become fat because of a particular eating behaviour, and that their maintenance of a given body weight cannot be accomplished by a normalisation of eating patterns, but rather by a sustained restriction of energy intake, in particular of energy-dense high-fat food[2], and an augmentation of energy expenditure[3]. Obesity not only is one of the most stigmatised physical attributes in the eyes of the general public, but also is regarded as a disorder greatly determined by psychological factors. The latter notion is held despite the lack of indications for a specific disturbance and the little evidence that obese individuals are psychologically more disturbed than others[4-6] or eat more in response to emotional distress[7]. The psychopathology encountered in obese individuals seems not to be a cause but rather a consequence of obesity, specifically a consequence of the prejudice and discrimination to which the overweight are subjected in our society[8]. By contrast, data are accumulating[9-14] to indicate that genetic factors play a major part in the development of obesity and this combined with the provocative environment in affluent societies. Genetic influences, however, are not so strong as to render dietary and behavioural treatments irrelevant[15]. The poor long-term results of dietary and behavioural treatments[16,17] may be attributable to the fact that many programmes of that type do not include teaching of weight maintenance behaviours. Patients discover that they are unable to reach their goal weight which reinforces their view that they are incapable of lowering their weight to any meaningful extent[18]. Of central importance for dietary/behavioural treatment approaches, therefore, is to help patients to adopt more realistic weight goals and to shift their focus from changing their appearance to improving their physical health[19].

*Binge-eating disorder*

Of obese individuals, 20% to 40% report significant problems with binge eating[20], that is, the eating of greater quantities than most people would eat during similar periods of time under similar circumstances[21, 22]. In a multisite field trial, about 30% of obese patients taking part in weight control programmes met the then proposed diagnostic criteria for binge-eating disorder[23]. These criteria in the meanwhile made their way into the Diagnostic and Statistical Manual of the American Psychiatric Association[24]. They define individuals who eat an amount of food definitively larger than most people would eat in a similar period of time under similar circumstances, have a sense of lack of control over eating during the episodes, but do not engage, in order to avoid weight gain, in compensatory activities such as purging, fasting or excessive exercise. Among obese subjects accepted into treatment programmes, bingeing was found to become significantly more prevalent with increasing degree of adiposity[25]. This was attributed to the facts that the excessive dieting associated with being overweight leads to eating binges and that the weight cycling resulting from repeated dieting and refeeding not only gives way to more rapid weight gain, but also to a greater propensity toward binge eating[26,27].

Obese binge eaters have been found to show more symptoms of affective disorders, i.e., depression, overall distress and anxiety, and also a greater life-time prevalence of psychiatric disorders than obese non-bingers[6,28-30]. In states of depressed mood, eating, especially the intake of simple carbohydrates, can yield a temporary lifting of mood[31-33] and energy levels[34]. Of grossly obese women with transient episodes of depression, 74% have been observed to crave carbohydrates in addition to their regular food intake[35]. A specific hunger for carbohydrate-rich foods and an inability to control carbohydrate consumption was suggested as being one factor promoting weight gain or hindering weight loss. The craving, furthermore, was regarded as being characteristic of seasonal affective disorders[36]. In some of the obese, by contrast, negative mood states may be overcome by the contrary of carbohydrate craving, i.e., the elimination of simple carbohydrates from the diet[37,38]. There is no evidence to suggest, however, that obesity, as such, is systematically related to depression. Obese girls were found to be discontent with their weight and figure but not depressed[39].

*Bulimia nervosa*

Binge eating can be encountered not only in the obese but in normal-weight individuals as well. Of the latter, many have a morbid fear of becoming fat and try to get rid of the unwanted calories they voraciously ingest using compensatory manoeuvres, such as self-induced vomiting, the use of laxatives or diuretics, strict dieting between the binges, or vigorous exercise. If the binge-eating episodes occur at a minimum average of two per week for at least 3 months, the over-concern with body shape and weight is persistent, and the affected individual has the feeling of a lack of control over her/his eating behaviour during the binges, the criteria for bulimia nervosa[24] are met. This disorder has been reported to become more and more prevalent among young women, especially on college campuses[40,41], although clinically significant bulimia seems to be rare[42, 43].

The duration of a binge-eating episode in a patient with bulimia may vary from a few minutes to 8 hours[44,45] and the ensuing energy intake from less than 100 kcal to several thousand kcal[46]. In patients having 24-hour access to food, a daily intake of up to 42694 kcal was observed[47]. Foods otherwise not eaten[31,46] or perceived, because of their high-fat and energy-dense nature, as forbidden[48] or dangerous[49] have been reported as being more likely to be consumed. Others, however, found that the macronutrient composition of a binge did not differ from that of the diet eaten by the general population[50]. Between their binges, patients with bulimia were observed to eat less at meal times than matched non-bulimics[51]. It is this self-control the patients are able to exert under normal conditions which leads them to consider a loss of control, and not having eaten too much, as the central feature of their disorder[52].

Upon the bulimic ingestion of large quantities of food, not only distension and pain[31,53,54], but also infarction and rupture of the stomach are encountered[55-57]. Distension may be due not only to acute overeating but to a stasis of ingesta as well: in no less than 9 out of 24 consecutive patients with bulimia, the gastric emptying of a semisolid standard meal of a nutrient content of 1168 kJ was found to be grossly delayed[58]. The emptying of liquids was found to be prolonged in 13 out of 23 and the emptying of solids in 7 out of 23 patients with bulimia[59]. In another study[60], the emptying of a liquid meal, which was ingested until the subjects felt extremely full and which contained 1.68 kJ/l, was significantly slower in its initial phase in 9 bulimic women than in matched healthy women. The fact that the bulimics also had a significantly greater capacity of the stomach led the authors to suggest that patients with bulimia felt satiated only after larger and larger quantities of food. This deficit in the mechanisms which normally serve to turn off eating and the increased gastric capacity have been suggested to give rise to a delayed gastric emptying and a blunted postprandial cholecystokinin release, leading to an impaired satiety response and thus a perpetuation of the disorder[61]. By contrast, other workers found normal gastric emptying to prevail in bulimic individuals[62-64]. In one of the latter studies[64], however, the gastric emptying data of 11 patients were compared to those of a very heterogenous group of 16 premenopausal females, which included individuals with morbid obesity and inflammatory bowel disease and whose gastric half-emptying times were highly scattered. Shih et al.[65] found the emptying of cream of wheat to be delayed in 12 of 20 bulimic patients, but to be rapid in the remaining eight. The latter finding contrasts sharply with the results of other studies[58,59,62-64], in which rapid emptying had not been encountered in any patient.

The factors contributing to an impaired gastric motor function in patients with bulimia have not been fully elucidated. Weakness and atrophy of gastric smooth muscle, caused by malnutrition and/or electrolyte depletion, primarily serum potassium[66,67] but also total potassium depletion[68], resulting from repetitive self-induced vomiting and/or an abuse of laxatives or diuretics, might play a crucial role. In one study [58], there was a significant inverse relationship between gastric half-emptying times and serum-potassium levels, which were below the normal range in 4 out of 24 patients studied and near the lower borderline of normal in another 8. As delayed emptying can readily be combatted by prokinetic agents, its detection is of great importance for the successful management and the outcome of patients. However, a normal eating behaviour cannot be attained by the normalisation of gastric emptying alone. The feeling of abdominal distension resulting from the large quantities eaten during a binge is terminated by self-induced vomiting, which allows either the continuation or termination of the binge. The recurrent vomiting gives rise to a progressive decalcification of tooth enamel. This leads to a loss of enamel and dentin mainly at the lingual surface of the teeth, an increased caries propensity and dental fracture rate, as well as an increased sensitivity to hot, cold and acidic substances[69]. Another feature frequently observed is an intermittent parotid swelling, occurring 2 to 6 days after the cessation of an overeating episode. The associated moderate elevation of serum amylase has been shown to be caused by an increased salivary-type amylase activity[70,71]. The habitual self-induced emesis may further cause oesophagitis, erosions, ulcers and strictures, and also lead to oesophageal perforation, mediastinitis and mediastinal emphysema[72,73]. Self-induced vomiting further may affect oropharyngeal swallowing. This is suggested by a videoradiographic study in 13 bulimic patients, all of whom were found to have abnormal oropharyngeal swallowing patterns[74]. In one study[58], four out of 32 consecutive patients diagnosed as having bulimia were revealed to have achalasia and one to have diffuse oesophageal spasms. All of the latter 5 patients reported experiencing two different types of vomiting: one self-induced, in which the vomited material tasted either acidic or non-acidic and like the preceding meal, and the other involuntary, in which the vomited material was always non-acidic and of the same taste as the preceding meal. Although the involuntary emesis occurred also in situations in which the patients did not intend to get rid of their ingesta, all of them thought that this vomiting, and their dysphagia and retrosternal pain, were consequences of the self-induced vomiting. This was the more plausible to them, as all had had no such symptoms prior to the onset of bulimia. Thus, the clinical evaluation of patients with bulimia should always include the taking of a thorough history with regard to swallowing and vomiting as well as to the nature and taste of the vomited materials. An important physiological consequence of binge eating is an increase in metabolic rate, which is partly due to an increased thyroid hormone activity[75].

For patients with bulimia nervosa, the bingeing and subsequent compensatory manoeuvres may provide relief from dysphoric moods[76] and feelings of anxiety. In one study, about three quarters of binge eaters stated that they were free of negative moods while eating[31]. However, eating may not only be precipitated but also maintained by negative mood states[77]. Mood has been observed to worsen[78] and depression ratings to increase after a binge[79,80]. Some authors suggested that bulimia was a variant expression of a primary affective disorder[81]. This concept seemed supported by reports that many patients, at least those presenting for treatment, were depressed[82-87] or differed from control subjects in a significantly higher prevalence of personal and familial major mood disorders[88]. The morbid risk for major depressive disorder was found to be significantly greater among first-degree relatives of patients with bulimia than among non-psychiatric control subjects[85] and similar to the risk in families of patients with bipolar disorder[89]. However, many of the features generally regarded as being at the core of classic melancholia, that is, anhedonia, irritability, decreased concentration, lack of reactivity to the environment, diurnal variation in mood, marked motor retardation, fatigability and diminished libido, were found to be conspicuously absent in most patients with bulimia[90]. Moreover, such symptoms may be attributable to starvation[91]: the nutritional status of patients with bulimia tends to be, despite a regular body weight, quite abnormal. In fact, a series of authors reported depression to be secondary to bulimia and/or malnutrition[92-94]. Against the concept that bulimia is a variant expression of a primary affective disorder are also the results of other studies. In first- and second-degree relatives of bulimic women, no higher rates of affective disorders were detected than in relatives of women with no history of an eating disorder[95].

A close relationship between bulimia and affective disorders seemed to be suggested by therapeutic successes obtained with the short-term medication of antidepressant drugs; with continued medication, however, only limited beneficial effects and a considerable relapse rate were observed[96,97]. Treatment with imipramine yielded results inferior to those of structured intensive group therapy and psychotherapy plus imipramine had no better effect than psychotherapy alone[98]. By contrast, two double-blind studies in 382[99] and 398[100] bulimic patients showed that 60 mg per day of the selective serotonin-reuptake inhibitor fluoxetine administered over 8 and 16 weeks, respectively, resulted in a significantly greater reduction of binge eating and vomiting than did placebo. An argument against the interpretation of bulimia as a variant of an affective disorder is provided by the fact that the sleep disturbances characteristic of patients with major depressive illness were found not to prevail in bulimic patients, who, by contrast, exhibited sleep patterns remarkably similar to those of healthy individuals[101]. A link between bulimia and affective disorders seemed to be indicated by the failure of about half of the patients studied to suppress their cortisol secretion in response to dexamethasone normally[81,102]. In the meanwhile, dexamethasone non-suppression has been shown to occur in a variety of physical and psychiatric disorders and not to be specific for patients with depression[103]. By contrast, the test proved to be highly sensitive to weight loss[104,105]. This is demonstrated also by the results of a study in bulimic patients, in whom the sole clinical correlate of dexamethasone non-suppression was a history of weight loss and/or anorexia nervosa[106]. To conclude the discussion about whether or not bulimia is associated with affective disorders, the preponderance of evidence suggests that the two entities are distinct from each other. In one patient, a depressed mood or depression may result from an eating disorder, whereas in another depression may be an antecedent to abnormal eating behaviour. A series of studies suggested an association of bulimia nervosa with personality disorders. In one investigation[107], 19 out of 91 and in another[108] 15 out of 39 patients with bulimia fulfilled the diagnostic criteria for at least one personality disorder, most often a borderline disorder. A strong association between bulimia and a borderline disorder was also reported by two further studies[109,110]. By contrast, Pope et al.[111] found the criteria for a borderline disorder to be met by only one out of 52 patients with bulimia. The latter finding, as well as the results of seven further studies[112], speak against a relationship between the two types of disorders.

A number of authors have suggested that experiences of childhood sexual abuse may contribute to the development of bulimia nervosa in adolescence or early adulthood. However, controlled studies, on the whole, did not support this hypothesis[113]. Sexual abuse was found to be a risk factor for the development of a psychiatric disorder in general, but not specifically for bulimia nervosa[114].

A genetic predisposition for bulimia nervosa is suggested by a report that 5 out of 6 monozygotic and 4 out of 15 dizygotic female twin pairs were concordant for the eating disorder[115].

*Anorexia nervosa*

The diagnostic criteria for anorexia nervosa[24] include a refusal to maintain body weight at or above a minimum weight for age and height, an intense fear of gaining weight or becoming fat even though underweight, a disturbance in the way in which body weight, size or shape are experienced, and the absence of at least three consecutive menstrual cycles when otherwise expected to occur. The term anorexia nervosa is a misnomer, as there is no loss of appetite. By contrast, affected individuals are engaged in a relentless pursuit of thinness and display a phobic avoidance of being fat[116]. The most important primary drive system, which yields pleasure or positive reinforcement with eating and negative reinforcement by hunger, is perverted: although hunger may still cause discomfort, the consequence of sustained hunger, that is weight loss, causes pleasure. Food stimuli become something to be abhorred although they, at the same time, dominate the patients' mind[117]. An increased physical activity of patients with anorexia has consistently been commented on, but also has been found in a controlled study[118]. Clinical[119,120] and cognitive studies[121,122] showed that anorexic women chiefly rejected foods rich in fat. However, patients with anorexia nervosa also avoid other calorie-rich foods such as meats, milk products and sweets[119], although their perceptions and preferences for a sweet taste do not differ from healthy control subjects[122].

In the course of food restriction, at first glycogen stores are depleted. Then, muscle tissue is consumed and the necessary substrate for gluconeogenesis is provided by aminoacids. At last, primary fat is mobilised and free fatty acids serve as energy supply. As free fatty acids cannot pass the blood-brain barrier, the brain becomes dependent on the metabolites of the free fatty acids, the ketone bodies. Upon renutrition, these changes rapidly subside. The same applies to abnormalities in hypothalamic-pituitary-adrenal function[123], elevated growth hormone levels[124], impaired or absent responses in plasma growth hormone and cortisol levels to insulin-induced hypoglycaemia[125], reduced hypothalamic serotoninergic responsiveness[126], impaired reproductive function[127] and raised levels of serum sex-hormone-binding globulin[128]. Thus, the available data suggest that the afore-mentioned neurobiologic changes represent adaptive responses to starvation and weight loss, whereas there is no evidence for a role of a primary hypothalamic or a neuroendocrine disorder in the development of anorexia.

In contrast to subjects affected by other disorders associated with severe malnutrition, patients with anorexia nervosa do not have an increased infection propensity[129]. This may be due to the maintenance of a normal number of T-lymphocytes of the CD4+ phenotype despite marked weight loss[130].

The emaciation associated with anorexia nervosa leads also to a reduced skin thickness and skin collagen content[131]. These processes may be triggered by the oestrogen deficiency accompanying emaciation. The same seems to be true for the genesis of osteoporosis and the reduced bone mass encountered in nearly all patients with anorexia[132,133]. The reduced bone density may persist despite nutritional repletion[134].

On primary evaluation of young females, vomiting and weight loss may be mistaken as indicating anorexia. The physician may be biased not only by the patients' emaciation but also by their young age and female sex, which may lead her/him to view certain aspects of history and behaviour as suggesting a pathological attitude towards eating. Another factor liable to contribute to misdiagnosis is that patients who are, or have been, in psychiatric or psychosomatically oriented treatment tend to learn "their" psychiatric or psychosomatic history. They thus may not only misinterpret their own sensations but also mislead their physicians. Symptoms such as epigastric distension and bloating are often overlooked or misinterpreted and one of the most renown researchers in the field, Hilde Bruch[135], stated: "Anorexics will complain of feeling full after a few bites ... One gains the impression that this sense of fullness is a phantom phenomenon, projection of formerly experienced sensations". Sensations of that type, which were found to be significantly more intense than in healthy subjects[136-139], are by no means phantom phenomena: a series of studies demonstrated that gastric emptying is markedly delayed in a high proportion of patients[66,140-147].

The mechanisms underlying disordered gastric motor function are still unclear, although malnutrition seems to play a crucial role. In depleted patients with anorexia, not only type 2-muscle fiber atrophy[148-150], which is characteristic for cachexia, but also significant changes in muscle contraction-relaxation characteristics and fatigability properties have been observed[151]. These features all disappeared with refeeding and the restoration of muscle electrolytes[151,152]. Muscular atrophy has also been observed to affect the heart, in particular the left ventricle[153-156]. Rhythm disturbances, mitral valve prolapse and diminished exercise capacity may ensue[157]. Large U-waves in the electrocardiogramme may be due to low serum-potassium levels[158]. As to the effects of malnutrition on gastric smooth muscle, atrophies to the point that stomach and intestine appeared as "tissue paper thin" have been observed in Indians with mixed deficiency diseases[159]. Muscular decompensation may underlie the acute gastric distension observed upon refeeding of patients with anorexia[160-162]. Acute distension has also been found to develop upon the ingestion of large quantities of food in chronically starved prisoners of war[163], neglected children[164,165], and healthy volunteers participating in starvation experiments[91]. With progressing gastric distension, venous occlusion, infarction and rupture may occur[60, 166,167]. The delayed gastric emptying in patients with anorexia can readily be combatted by prokinetic agents[142,143,168-170]. Their administration over prolonged periods of time may, by accelerating emptying, not only contribute to an amelioration of the nutrional status, but also help in the rehabilitation of patients[136]. The ultimate goal of therapy, however, i.e., the resumption of a normal eating behaviour enabling the patients' social reintegration and restoration to an appearance acceptable to the social environment, can not be achieved by a normalisation of gastric emptying alone.

Malnutrition may not only affect the stomach but also more aboral parts of the intestine. Ten out of 20 patients with anorexia were found, upon barium-meal examination, to have proximal duodenal dilatation[161]. A marked dilatation of the duodenum and an absence of the, under normal conditions, regularly recurring activity fronts of the interdigestive migrating motor complex as well as a prolonged intestinal transit were observed in a young female, in whom these abnormalities vanished with renutrition[171]. In a further study, about one third of the patients were found to have moderate dilatation of small bowel loops[172]. The jejunum, which is exposed to high nutrient concentrations under physiological conditions, is much more at risk to undergo hypoplastic changes in states of starvation than is the ileum, which normally has to deal with nutrient-rich chyme. The colon, interestingly, is also very sensitive to withdrawal of food. Constipation associated with slow colonic transit[173] and abuse of laxatives[174] is frequent in anorexic patients.

A series of papers reported an increased prevalence of anorexia in the higher socio-economic classes[175-179]. In 100 consecutive patients presenting to an outpatient clinic in London, there was a definite skew of prevalence towards the upper classes; the skew, however, was less marked than in a survey carried out in the same institution 10 years earlier[180]. A study in women taking part in bingo tournaments in Massachusetts suggested that anorexia may be at least as common amongst the more humble classes[181]. Thus, the assumption of an increased incidence in the higher classes may have arisen as a result of referral practices.

Much more under constant pressure than females of the upper social strata, to diet relentlessly, are professional dancers and athletes. A study in 183 professional dancers revealed that no less than 12 of them fulfilled the diagnostic criteria for anorexia nervosa[182]. However, a behaviour directed at inducing weight loss or maintaining a low body weight may promote unusual eating patterns, ritualised eating and obsessive food thoughts resembling those encountered in patients with anorexia[91]. A close relationship has been suggested to exist between anorexia nervosa and psychiatric disease. An association with affective disorders was hypothesised on the basis of a 5-year study showing that 18 out of 26 patients with anorexia had persistent dysphoric mood states and often a maternal history of depression[183]. A controlled 10-year follow-up study in 62 women with anorexia revealed a high life-time prevalence of major depressive disorders and a significant comorbidity of anxiety disorders[184]. Among these patients' first-degree relatives, the total number of psychiatric diagnoses as well as the prevalence of alcoholism were significantly higher than among age- and sex-matched individuals. Moreover, two of the patients' mothers had had bulimia and each two of other first-degree relatives, anorexia and bulimia, respectively. Of the control subjects' first-degree relatives, by contrast, none had an eating disorder[184]. Others found that 46 out of 82 outpatients with anorexia fulfilled the diagnostic criteria for major depressive disorder[82]. One argument brought forward as supporting a close relationship between anorexia and affective disorders was based on the observation that a number of anorexic patients showed an inadequate suppression of cortisol secretion in response to dexamethasone[185]. However, this test is highly sensitive for weight loss[104,105] and normalises with relatively small weight gain.

Against an association of anorexia nervosa with affective disorders stand the results of a study[82] in which the onset of an affective disorder post-dated, in the great majority of patients, the onset of the eating disorder by at least 1 year. This led the authors to conclude that the depression was secondary. Such an interpretation seems also to be supported by the fact that there is less than meager evidence that antidepressant drugs are of benefit to the majority of patients with anorexia[97,186]. Notwithstanding, comorbid mood and anxiety disorders must be diagnosed and treated.

An association of anorexia nervosa with personality disorders has been suggested in view of the overlap between the phenomenologies of the two disorders, i.e., the rigid dietary routine and rumination about food as well as the repeated weighing and calorie counting. Premorbid obsessional personality traits may be over-represented in patients with anorexia, and the process of the illness may serve to exaggerate such traits[187]. In 20 patients having recovered from anorexia nervosa, characteristics such as a need for order and precision were found to be significantly more accentuated than in healthy women[188]. Of 31 patients, seven were found to fulfill the criteria for at least one personality disorder[107]. A previous history of anorexia was found in 12 out of 105 patients with an obsessive-compulsive disorder[189]; in these 12 patients, the two diseases had a similar time of onset, which may point to common vulnerability factors.

A genetic predisposition may play a role in the development of anorexia nervosa. Holland et al.[190] found that 14 out of 25 monozygotic and 1 out of 20 dizygotic female twin pairs were concordant for anorexia. Of the female first-degree relatives of these twins, nearly 5% also had a history of anorexia. This led the investigators to conclude that up to 80% of the variance in liability to develop anorexia may be accounted for by genetic factors. In a study in the family members of 97 patients, it was found that two out of the 98 sisters had anorexia and four had bulimia nervosa[191]. These prevalence rates were significantly higher than those occurring in families with no eating disorder and also significantly higher than the prevalence rates for anorexia in the families of 66 patients with primary affective disorder and 117 patients with various non-affective disorders. Against a genetic predisposition for anorexia nervosa stand the results of a study which revealed that none of the same-sex co-twins of 11 patients with anorexia was concordant for the eating disorder[192]. Another contra argument is provided by the finding that 58 mothers of girls with anorexia and 204 mothers of healthy girls of similar age and socio-economic status did not differ in their weight history and their attitudes towards weight-related matters[193]. Furthermore, no differences, in terms of attitudes to weight control and dieting, were found between the parents of another group of patients with anorexia and matched healthy individuals[194].

In conclusion, there is no clear-cut evidence to suggest that distinct biologic, environmental, psychologic, or psychiatric factors are of primary aetiological importance for binge-eating disorder bulimia nervosa and anorexia nervosa. The development and course of an eating disorder, however, should be seen as determined by an interplay of forces at the biologic, psychologic, familial and sociocultural levels of organisation[179]. The thorough evaluation of these forces and their interaction may not only yield insight into the origin and course of the eating disorder in an individual patient, but also provide the basis for a successful therapy.

## Summary

The relative importance of biologic, psychologic and environmental factors and psychiatric disease in the development and course of eating disorders is unclear. Obesity is widely regarded as being determined psychologically, although the psychopathology encountered appears rather as a consequence of the disorder. There is no evidence that obesity is related to affective or personality disorders, but genetic factors seem to be crucial. Obese patients with binge-eating disorder showed more symptoms of depression and anxiety, and a greater lifetime prevalence of psychiatric disorders than obese patients without binge-eating disorder. In bulimia nervosa, binge-eating and subsequent compensatory activities, such as self-induced vomiting and purging, may yield relief from dysphoric moods, but evidence for an interrelation with affective or personality disorders is meager. The bulimic behaviour and electrolyte depletion resulting from repetitive vomiting may impair oesophageal and gastric motility. Anorexia nervosa is associated with neurobiologic changes adaptive to starvation, but there is no evidence for a primary neuroendocrine disorder or an association with affective or personality disorders. By contrast, a genetic predisposition may play a role. Delayed gastric emptying develops secondary to malnutrition and subsides with refeeding. The development and course of eating disorders seems not to be determined primarily by psychological or psychiatric factors but by the interplay of such factors with forces at the biological and sociocultural levels, the evaluation of which may provide the basis for a successful therapy.

*REFERENCES*


1. Beumont PJV. *Bulimia: is it an illness entity?* Int J Eating Dis 1988;7:167-76.
2. Gibney MJ. *Epidemiology of obesity in relation to nutrient intake.* Int J Obesity 1995;19(Suppl 5):S1-3.
3. Wardle J. *Obesity and behaviour change: matching problems to practice.* Int J Obesity 1996;20(Suppl 1):S1-8.
4. Crisp AH, Queenan M, Sittanmpaln Y, Harris G. *"Jolly fat" revisited.* J Psychosom Res 1980;24:233-41.
5. McRenolds WT. *Toward a psychology of obesity: review of research on the role of personality and level of adjustment.* Int J Eating Dis 1982;2:37-57.
6. Kuehnel RH, Wadden TA. *Binge eating disorder, weight cycling, and psychopathology.* Int J Eating Dis 1994;15:321-9.
7. Allison DB, Heshka S. *Emotion and eating in obesity? A critical analysis.* Int J Eating Dis 1993;13:289-95.
8. Wadden TA, Stunkard AJ. *Psychosocial consequences of obesity and dieting: research and clinical findings.* In: Stunkard AJ, Wadden TA, editors. Obesity: theory and therapy. 2nd ed. New York: Raven; 1993;163-77.
9. Stunkard AJ, Sørensen TIA, Hanis C, et al. *An adoption study of human obesity.* N Engl J Med 1986;314:193-8.
10. Stunkard AJ, Foch TT, Hrubec Z. *A twin study of human obesity.* JAMA 1986;256:51-4.
11. Stunkard AJ, Harris JR, Pedersen NL, McClearn GE. *The body-mass index of twins who have been reared apart.* N Engl J Med 1990;322:1483-7.
12. Bouchard C, Tremblay A, Després J-P, et al. *The response to long-term overfeeding in identical twins.* N Engl J Med 1990;322:1477-82.
13. Bouchard C. *The genetics of obesity in humans.* Curr Opin Endocrinol Diabet 1996;3:29-35.
14. Burguera B, Jensen MD. *Obesity: is the brain responsible?* Curr Opin Gastroenterol 1998;14:147-50.
15. Carek PJ, Sherer JT, Carson DS. *Management of obesity: medical treatment options.* Am Fam Physician 1997;55:551-8.
16. Wadden TA, Sternberg JA, Letizia KA, et al. *Treatment of obesity by very low calorie diet, behavior therapy and their combination: a five-year perspective.* Int J Obesity 1989;13:39-46.
17. Wadden TA. *Treatment of obesity by moderate and severe caloric restriction: results of clinical research trials.* Ann Intern Med 1993;119:688-93.

18. Wolfe BL. *Long-term maintenance following attainment of goal weight: a preliminary investigation.* Addict Behav 1992;17:469-77.
19. Fairburn CG, Cooper Z. *New perspectives on dietary and behavioural treatments for obesity.* Int J Obesity 1996;20(Suppl 1):S9-13.
20. Stunkard AJ. *Eating patterns and obesity.* Psychiatr Q 1959;33:284-95.
21. Loro AD, Orleans CS. *Binge eating in obesity: preliminary findings and guidelines for behavioral analysis and treatment.* Addict Behav 1981;6:155-66.
22. Marcus MD, Wing RR, Lamparski DM. *Binge eating and dietary restraint among obese patients.* Addict Behav 1985;10:163-8.
23. Spitzer RL, Yanovski S, Wadden T, et al. *Binge eating disorder: its further validation in a multisite study.* Int J Eating Dis 1993;13:137-53.
24. American Psychiatric Association. *Diagnostic and statistical manual of mental disorders.* 4th ed. Washington, DC: American Psychiatric Association; 1994.
25. Telch CF, Agras WS, Rossiter EM. *Binge eating increases with increasing adiposity.* Int J Eating Dis 1988;7:115-59.
26. Polivy J, Herman CP. *Dieting and bingeing: a causal analysis.* Am Psychol 1985;40:193-201.
27. Brownell KD, Greenwood MR, Stellar E, Shrager EE. *The effects of repeated cycles of weight loss and regain in rats.* Physiol Behav 1986;38:459-64.
28. Marcus MD, Wing RR, Ewing L. *Psychiatric disorders among obese binge eaters.* Int J Eating Dis 1990;9:69-77.
29. Wadden TA, Foster GD, Letizia KA, Wilk JE. *Metabolic, anthropometric, and psychological characteristics of obese binge eaters.* Int J Eating Dis 1993;14:17-25.
30. Yanovski SZ, Nelson JE, Dubbert BK, Spitzer RL. *Association of binge eating disorder and psychiatric comorbidity in obese subjects.* Am J Psychiatry 1993;150:1472-9.
31. Abraham SF, Beumont PJV. *How patients describe bulimia or binge eating.* Psychol Med 1982;12:625-35.
32. Lieberman HR, Wurtman JJ, Chew B. *Changes in mood after carbohydrate consumption among obese individuals.* Am J Clin Nutr 1986;44:772-8.
33. Wurtman JJ, Brzezinski A, Wurtman RJ, Laferrere B. *Effect of nutrient intake on premenstrual depression.* Am J Obstet Gynecol 1989;161:1228-35.
34. Thayer RE. *Energy, tiredness, and tension effects of a sugar snack versus moderate exercise.* J Pers Soc Psychol 1987;52:119-25.
35. Hopkinson G, Bland RC. *Depressive symptoms in grossly obese women.* Can J Psychiatry 1982;27:213-5.
36. Wurtman JJ. *The involvement of brain serotonin in excessive carbohydrate snacking by obese carbohydrate cravers.* J Am Diet Assoc 1984;84:1004-7.
37. Christensen L, Krietsch K, White B, Stagner B. *Impact of a dietary change on emotional*

*distress.* J Abnorm Psychol 1985;94:565-79.

38. Christensen L, Burrows R. *Dietary treatment of depression.* Behav Res Ther 1990;21:183-93.
39. Wadden TA, Foster GD, Stunkard AJ, Linowitz JR. *Dissatisfaction with weight and figure in obese girls: discontent but not depression.* Int J Obes 1989;13:89-97.
40. Halmi KA, Falk JR, Schwarz E. *Binge eating and vomiting: a survey of a college population.* Psychol Med 1981;11:697-706.
41. Pyle RL, Halvorson PA, Neuman PA, Mitchell JE. *The increasing prevalence of bulimia in freshman college students.* Int J Eating Dis 1986;5:631-47.
42. Connors ME, Johnson CL. *Epidemiology of bulimia and bulimic behaviors.* Addict Behav 1987;12:165-79.
43. Schotte DE, Stunkard AJ. *Bulimia vs bulimic behaviors on a college campus.* JAMA 1987;258:1213-5.
44. Mitchell JE, Pyle RL, Eckert ED. *Binge eating behavior in patients with bulimia.* Am J Psychiatry 1981;138:835-6.
45. Pyle RL, Mitchell JE, Eckert ED. *Bulimia: a report of 34 cases.* J Clin Psychiatry 1981;42:60-4.
46. Rosen JC, Leitenberg H, Fisher C, Khazam C. *Binge-eating in bulimia nervosa: the amount and type of food consumed.* Int J Eating Dis 1986;5:255-67.
47. Kaye WH, Weltzin TE, McKee M, et al. *Laboratory assessment of feeding behavior in bulimia nervosa and healthy women: methods for developing a human-feeding laboratory.* Am J Clin Nutr 1992;55:372-80.
48. Kales EF. *Macronutrient analysis of binge eating in bulimia.* Physiol Behav 1990;48:837-40.
49. Sunday SR, Einhorn A, Halmi KA. *Relationship of perceived macronutrient and caloric content to affective cognition about food in eating-disordered, restrained, and unrestrained subjects.* Am J Clin Nutr 1992;55:362-71.
50. Kissileff HR, Walsh BT, Kral JG, Cassidy SM. *Laboratory studies of eating behavior in women and bulimia.* Physiol Behav 1986;38:563-70.
51. Rosen JC, Leitenberg H. *Eating behavior in bulimia nervosa.* In: Walsh BT, editor. Eating behavior in eating disorders. Washington, DC: American Psychiatric Press; 1988;161-73.
52. Beglin SJ, Fairburn CG. *What is meant by the term "binge"?* Am J Psychiatry 1992;149:123-4.
53. Chami TN, Andersen AE, Crowell MD, et al. *Gastrointestinal symptoms in bulimia nervosa: effects of treatment.* Gastroenterology 1991;100:A427.
54. Mitchell JE, Hatsukami D, Eckert ED, Pyle RL. *Characteristics of 275 patients with bulimia.* Am J Psychiatry 1985;142:482-5.

55. Mitchell JE, Pyle RL, Miner RA. *Gastric dilatation as a complication of bulimia.* Psychosomatics 1982;23:96-7.
56. Abdu RA, Garritano D, Culver O. *Acute gastric necrosis in anorexia nervosa and bulimia.* Arch Surg 1987;122:830-2.
57. Petrin C, Tacchetti G, Preciso G, et al. *Distension aigue suivie de rupture gastrique après un accès de boulimie. A propos d'un cas.* J Chir (Paris) 1990;127:213-35.
58. Kiss A, Bergmann H, Abatzi Th-A, et al. *Oesophageal and gastric motor activity in patients with bulimia nervosa.* Gut 1990;31:259-65.
59. Block GD, Van Thiel DH, Brouillette D, et al. *Gastrointestinal dysmotility in bulimic non-pregnant females.* Gastroenterology 1990;98:A22.
60. Geliebter A, Melton PM, McCray RS, et al. *Gastric capacity, gastric emptying, and test meal intake in normal and bulimic women.* Am J Clin Nutr 1992;56:656-61.
61. Devlin MJ, Walsh BT, Guss JL, et al. *Postprandial cholecystokinin release and gastric emptying in patients with bulimia nervosa.* Am J Clin Nutr 1997;65:114-20.
62. Robinson PH, Clarke M, Barrett J. *Determinants of delayed gastric emptying in anorexia nervosa and bulimia nervosa.* Gut 1988;29:458-64.
63. Leventhal RI, Brouillette D, Cuellar R, et al. *Gastric emptying in bulimia.* Gastroenterology 1989;96:A297.
64. Hutson W, Wald A. *Gastric emptying in patients with bulimia nervosa and anorexia nervosa.* Am J Gastroenterol 1990;85:41-6.
65. Shih W-J, Humphries L, Digenis GA, et al. *Tc-99m labeled tri-ethylene tetra-amine polysterene resin gastric emptying studies in bulimia patients.* Eur J Nucl Med 1987;13:192-6.
66. Crow SJ, Salisbury JJ, Crosby RD, Mitchell JE. *Serum electrolytes as markers of vomiting in bulimia nervosa.* Int J Eating Dis 1997;21:95-8.
67. Greenfeld D, Mickley D, Quinlan DM, Roloff P. *Hypokalemia in outpatients with eating disorders.* Am J Psychiatry 1995;152:60-3.
68. Powers PS, Tyson IB, Stevens BA, Heal AV. *Total body potassium and serum potassium among eating disorder patients.* Int J Eating Dis 1995;18:269-76.
69. Spigset O. *Oral symptoms in bulimia nervosa. A survey of 34 cases.* Acta Odontol Scand 1991;49:335-9.
70. Humphries LL, Adams LJ, Eckfeldt JH, et al. *Hyperamylasemia in patients with eating disorders.* Ann Intern Med 1987;106:50-2.
71. Kaplan AS. *Hyperamylasemia and bulimia: a clinical review.* Int J Eating Dis 1987;4:537-43.
72. Fergusson RJ, Shaw TRD, Turnbull CM. *Spontaneous pneumomediastinum: a complication of anorexia nervosa?* Postgrad Med J 1985;61:815-7.

73. Overby KJ, Litt IF. *Mediastinal emphysema in an adolescent with anorexia nervosa and self-induced emesis.* Pediatrics 1988; 81:134-6.
74. Roberts MW, Tylenda CA, Sonies BC, Elin RJ. *Dysphagia in bulimia nervosa.* Dysphagia 1989;4:106-11.
75. Altemus M, Hetherington MM, Flood M, et al. *Decrease in resting metabolic rate during abstinence from bulimic behavior.* Am J Psychiatry 1991;148:1071-2.
76. Christensen L. *Effects of eating behavior on mood: a review of the literature.* Int J Eating 1993;14:171-83.
77. Johnson C, Larson R. *Bulimia: an analysis of moods and behavior.* Psychosom Med 1982;44:431-51.
78. Davis R, Freeman R, Solyom L. *Mood and food: an analysis of bulimic episodes.* J Psychiatr Res 1985;19:331-5.
79. Chiodo J, Latimer PR. *Hunger perception and satiety responses among normal-weight bulimics and normals to a high-calorie, carbohydrate rich food.* Psychol Med 1986;16:343-9.
80. Elmore DK, Castro JM. *Self-rated moods and hunger in relation to spontaneous eating behavior in bulimics, recovered bulimics, and normals.* Int J Eating Dis 1990;9:179-90.
81. Hudson JI, Laffer PS, Pope HG Jr. *Bulimia related to affective disorder by family history and response to dexamethasone suppression test.* Am J Psychiatry 1982;139:685-7.
82. Herzog DB. *Are anorexic and bulimic patients depressed?* Am J Psychiatry 1984;141:1594-7.
83. Lee NF, Rush AJ, Mitchell JE. *Bulimia and depression.* J Affect Disord 1985;9:231-8.
84. Piran N, Kennedy SH, Garfinkel PE, Owens M. *Affective disturbance in eating disorders.* J Nerv Ment Dis 1985;173:395-400.
85. Hudson JI, Pope HG Jr, Jonas JM, et al. *A controlled family history study of bulimia.* Psychol Med 1987;17:883-90.
86. Hudson JI, Pope HG Jr, Yurgelun-Todd D, et al. *A controlled study of life-time prevalence of affective and other psychiatric disorders in bulimic outpatients.* Am J Psychiatry 1987;144:1283-7.
87. Simpson SG, Al-Mufti R, Andersen AE, DePaulo JR Jr. *Bipolar II affective disorder in eating disorder inpatients.* J Nerv Ment Dis 1992;180:719-22.
88. Keck PE Jr, Pope HG Jr, Hudson JI, et al. *A controlled study of phenomenology and family history in outpatients with bulimia nervosa.* Compr Psychiatry 1990;31:275-83.
89. Hudson JI, Pope HG Jr, Jonas JM, Yurgelun-Todd D. *Family history study of anorexia nervosa and bulimia.* Br J Psychiatry 1983;142:133-8; Erratum, 142:428-9.
90. Katz JL. *Eating disorder and affective disorder: relatives or merely chance acquaintances?* Compr Psychiatry 1987;28:220-8.

91. Keys A, Brozek J, Henschel A, et al. *The biology of human starvation.* Minneapolis: University of Minnesota Press; 1950;587-600.
92. Halmi K. *Relationship of the eating disorders to depression: biological similarities and differences.* Int J Eating Dis 1985;4:669-80.
93. Cooper PJ, Fairburn CG. *The depressive symptoms of bulimia nervosa.* Br J Psychiatry 1986;148:268-74.
94. Laessle RG, Kittl S, Fichter MM, et al. *Major affective disorder in anorexia nervosa and bulimia. A descriptive diagnostic study.* Br J Psychiatry 1987;151:785-9.
95. Stern SL, Dixon KN, Nemzer E, et al. *Affective disorder in the families of women with normal weight bulimia.* Am J Psychiatry 1984;141:1224-7.
96. Walsh BT, Hadigan CM, Devlin MJ, et al. *Long-term outcome of antidepressant treatment for bulimia nervosa.* Am J Psychiatry 1991;148:1206-12.
97. Walsh BT, Devlin MJ. *The pharmacologic treatment of eating disorders.* Psychiatr Clin North Am 1992;15:149-60.
98. Mitchell JE, Pyle RL, Eckert ED, et al. *A comparison study of antidepressants and structured group psychotherapy in the treatment of bulimia nervosa.* Arch Gen Psychiatry 1990;47:149-57.
99. Fluoxetine Bulimia Nervosa Collaborative Study Group. *Fluoxetine in the treatment of bulimia nervosa: a multicenter placebo-controlled double-blind trial.* Arch Gen Psychiatry 1992;49:139-47.
100. Goldstein DJ, Wilson MG, Thompson VL, et al. *Long-term fluoxetine treatment of bulimia nervosa.* Fluoxetine Bulimia Nervosa Research Group. Br J Psychiatry 1995;166:660-6.
101. Walsh BT, Goetz R, Roose SP, et al. *EEG-monitored sleep in anorexia nervosa and bulimia.* Biol Psychiatry 1985;20:947-56.
102. Mitchell JE, Bantle JP. *Metabolic and endocrine investigations in women of normal weight with the bulimia syndrome.* Biol Psychiatry 1983;18:355-65.
103. Coppen A, Abou-Saleh M, Harmood J, Bailey J. *Dexamethasone suppression in depression and other psychiatric illness.* Br J Psychiatry 1983;142:498-504.
104. Berger M, Pirke KM, Doerr P, et al. *Influence of weight loss on the dexamethasone suppression test.* Arch Gen Psychiatry 1983;40:585-6.
105. Kline MD, Beeber AR. *Weight loss and the dexamethasone suppression test.* Arch Gen Psychiatry 1983;40:1034-5.
106. O'Brien G, Hassanyeh F, Leake A, et al. *The dexamethasone suppression test in bulimia nervosa.* Br J Psychiatry 1988;152:654-6.
107. Herzog DB, Keller MB, Lavori PW, et al. *The prevalence of personality disorders in 210 women with eating-disorders.* J Clin Psychiatry 1992;53:147-52.

108. Fahy TA, Eisler I, Russell GFM. *Personality disorder and treatment response in bulimia nervosa.* Br J Psychiatry 1993;162:765-70.
109. Ames-Frankel J, Devlin MJ, Walsh BT, et al. *Personality disorder diagnoses in patients with bulimia nervosa: clinical correlates and changes with treatment.* J Clin Psychiatry 1992;53:90-6.
110. Skodol AE, Oldham JM, Hyler SE, et al. *Comorbidity of DSM-III-R eating disorders and personality disorders.* Int J Eating Dis 1993;14:403-16.
111. Pope HG Jr, Frankenburg FR, Hudson JI, et al. *Is bulimia associated with borderline personality disorder? A controlled study.* J Clin Psychiatry 1987;48:181-4.
112. Pope HG Jr, Hudson JI. *Are eating disorders associated with borderline personality disorder? A critical review.* Int J Eating Dis 1989;8:1-9.
113. Pope HG Jr, Hudson JI. *Is childhood sexual abuse a risk factor for bulimia nervosa?* Am J Psychiatry 1992;149:455-63.
114. Welch SL, Fairburn CG. *Sexual abuse and bulimia nervosa: three integrated case control comparisons.* Am J Psychiatry 1994;151:402-7.
115. Fichter MM, Noegel R. *Concordance for bulimia nervosa in twins.* Int J Eating Dis 1990;9:255-63.
116. Bruch H. *The golden cage.* New York: Vintage Books; 1978.
117. Ploog DW, Pirke KM. *Psychobiology of anorexia nervosa.* Psychol Med 1987;17:843-59.
118. Casper RC, Schoeller DA, Kushner R, et al. *Total daily energy expenditure and activity level in anorexia nervosa.* Am J Clin Nutr 1991;53:1143-50.
119. Beumont PJV, Chambers TL, Rouse L, Abraham SF. *The diet composition and nutritional knowledge of patients with anorexia nervosa.* J Hum Nutr 1981; 35:265-73.
120. Drewnowski A, Halmi KA, Pierce B, et al. *Taste and eating disorders.* Am J Clin Nutr 1987;46:442-50.
121. Drewnowski A, Pierce B, Halmi KA. *Fat aversion in eating disorders.* Appetite 1988;10:119-31.
122. Simon Y, Bellisle F, Monneuse M-O, et al. *Taste responsiveness in anorexia nervosa.* Br J Psychiatry 1993;162:244-6.
123. Gold PW, Gwirtsman H, Avgerinos PC, et al. *Abnormal hypothalamic-pituitary-adrenal function in anorexia nervosa. Pathophysiologic mechanisms in underweight and weight-corrected patients.* N Engl J Med 1986;314:1335-42.
124. Casper RC, Davis JM, Pandey GM. *The effect of nutritional status and weight changes on hypothalamic function tests in anorexia nervosa.* In: Vigersky RA, editor. Anorexia nervosa. New York: Raven; 1977;137-48.
125. Nakai Y, Koh T, Kinoshita F, et al. *The prolactin, growth hormone, and cortisol responses to insulin-induced hypoglycemia in anorexia nervosa.* Int J Eating Dis 1987;6:357-65.

126. Jimerson DC, Lesem MD, Kaye WH, et al. *Eating disorders and depression: is there a serotonin connection?* Biol Psychiatry 1990;28:443-54.
127. Treasure JL, Wheeler M, King EA, et al. *Weight gain and reproductive function: ultrasonographic and endocrine features in anorexia nervosa.* Clin Endocrinol 1988;29:607-16.
128. Barbe P, Bennet A, Stebenet M, et al. *Sex-hormone-binding globulin and protein-energy malnutrition indexes as indicators of nutritional status in women with anorexia nervosa.* Am J Clin Nutr 1993;57:319-22.
129. Bowers TK, Eckert E. *Leukopenia in anorexia nervosa. Lack of increased risk of infection.* Arch Intern Med 1978;138:1520-3.
130. Fink S, Eckert E, Mitchell J, et al. *T-lymphocyte subsets in patients with abnormal body weight: longitudinal studies in anorexia nervosa and obesity.* Int J Eating Dis 1996;20:295-305.
131. Savvas M, Treasure J, Brincat M, et al. *The effects of anorexia nervosa on skin thickness, skin collagen content and bone density* [Abstract]. Br J Obstet Gynaecol 1988;95:1210.
132. Rigotti NA, Nussbaum SR, Herzog DB, Neer RM. *Osteoporosis in women with anorexia nervosa.* N Engl J Med 1984;311:1601-6.
133. Treasure J, Fogelman I, Russell GF. *Osteopaenia of the lumbar spine and femoral neck in anorexia nervosa.* Scott Med J 1986;31:206-7.
134. Iketani T, Kiriike N, Nakanishi S, Nakasuji T. *Effects of weight gain and resumption of menses on reduced bone density in patients with anorexia nervosa.* Biol Psychiatry 1995;37:521-7.
135. Bruch H. *Anorexia nervosa.* In: Lindner AE, editor. Emotional factors in gastro-intestinal illness. Amsterdam: Excerpta Medica; 1973;1-15.
136. Robinson RG, Tortosa M, Sullivan J, et al. *Quantitative assessment of psychologic state of patients with anorexia nervosa or bulimia: response to caloric stimulus.* Psychosom Med 1983;45:283-92.
137. Halmi KA, Sunday S, Puglisi A, Marchi P. *Hunger and satiety in anorexia and bulimia nervosa.* Ann NY Acad Sci 1989;575:431-44.
138. Halmi KA, Sunday S. *Temporal patterns of hunger and fullness ratings and related cognitions in anorexia and bulimia.* Appetite 1991;16:219-37.
139. Hetherington MM, Rolls BJ. *Eating behavior in eating disorders: response to preloads.* Physiol Behav 1991;50:101-8.
140. Dubois A, Gross HA, Ebert MH, Castell DO. *Altered gastric emptying and secretion in primary anorexia nervosa.* Gastroenterology 1979;77:319-23.
141. Holt S, Ford MJ, Grant S, Heading RC. *Abnormal gastric emptying in primary*

*anorexia nervosa.* Br J Psychiatry 1981;39:550-2.

142. McCallum RW, Grill BB, Lange R, et al. *Definition of a gastric emptying abnormality in patients with anorexia nervosa.* Dig Dis Sci 1985;30:713-22.
143. Stacher G, Kiss A, Wiesnagrotzki S, et al. *Oesophageal and gastric motility disorders in patients categorised as having primary anorexia nervosa.* Gut 1986;27:1120-6.
144. Stacher G, Bergmann H, Wiesnagrotzki S, et al. *Intravenous cisapride accelerates delayed gastric emptying and increases antral contraction amplitude in patients with primary anorexia nervosa.* Gastroenterology 1987;92:1000-6.
145. Abell TL, Malagelada J-R, Lucas AR, et al. *Gastric electromechanical and neurohormonal function in anorexia nervosa.* Gastroenterology 1987;93:958-65.
146. Rigaud D, Bedig G, Merrouche M, et al. *Delayed gastric emptying in anorexia nervosa is improved by completion of renutrition program.* Dig Dis Sci 1988;33:919-25.
147. Stacher G, Bergmann H, Wiesnagrotzki S, et al. *Primary anorexia nervosa: gastric emptying and antral motor activity in 53 patients.* Int J Eating Dis 1992;11:163-72.
148. Lindboe CF, Askevold F, Sletterbø M. *Changes in skeletal muscles of young women with anorexia nervosa. An enzyme histochemical study.* Acta Neuropathol (Berlin) 1982;56:299-302.
149. Sletterbø M, Lindboe CF, Askevold F. *The neuromuscular system in patients with anorexia nervosa: electrophysiological and histologic studies.* Clin Neuropathol 1984;3:217-24.
150. Alloway R, Reynolds EH, Spargo E, Russell GFM. *Neuropathy and myopathy in two patients with anorexia and bulimia nervosa.* J Neurol Psychiatry 1985;48:1015-20.
151. Lopes J, Russell DMcR, Whitwell J, Jeejeebhoy KN. *Skeletal muscle function in malnutrition.* Am J Clin Nutr 1982;36:602-10.
152. Russell DMcR, Prendergast PJ, Darby PL, et al. *A comparison between muscle function and body composition in anorexia nervosa: the effect of refeeding.* Am J Clin Nutr 1983;38:229-37.
153. Gottdiener JS, Gross HA, Henry WL, et al. *Effects of self-induced starvation on cardiac size and function in anorexia nervosa.* Circulation 1978;58:425-33.
154. Moodie DS, Salcedo E. *Cardiac function in adolescents and young adults with anorexia nervosa.* J Adolesc Health Care 1983;4:9-14.
155. Moodie DS. *Anorexia and the heart. Results of studies to assess effects.* Postgrad Med 1987;81:46-48, 51-52, 55.
156. Powers PS, Schocken DD, Feld J, et al. *Cardiac function during weight restoration in anorexia nervosa.* Int J Eating Dis 1991;10:521-30.
157. Schocken DD, Holloway JD, Powers PS. *Weight loss and the heart. Effects of anorexia nervosa and starvation.* Arch Intern Med 1989;149:877-81.

158. Kay GN, Hoffman GW, Boswick J, et al. *The electrocardiogram in anorexia nervosa.* Int J Eating Dis 1988;7:791-5.
159. Passmore R. *Mixed deficiency diseases in India: a clinical description.* Trans R Soc Trop Med Hyg 1947;41:189-206.
160. Russell GFM. *Acute dilatation of the stomach in a patient with anorexia nervosa.* Br J Psychiatry 1966;112:203-7.
161. Scobie BA. *Acute gastric dilatation and duodenal ileus in anorexia nervosa.* Med J Aust 1973;2:932-4.
162. Jennings KP, Klidjian AM. *Acute gastric dilatation in anorexia nervosa.* Br Med J 1974;2:477-8.
163. Markowski B. *Acute dilation of the stomach.* Br Med J 1947;2:128-30.
164. Gloebl HJ, Capitano MA, Kirkpatrick JA. *Radiographic findings in children with psychosocial dwarfism.* Pediatr Radiol 1976;4:83-6.
165. Franken EA, Fox M, Smith JA, Smith WL. *Acute gastric dilatation in neglected children.* Am J Roentgen 1978;130:297-9.
166. Evans DS. *Acute dilatation and spontaneous rupture of the stomach.* Br J Surg 1968;55:940-2.
167. Saul SH, Dekker A, Watson CG. *Acute gastric dilatation with infarction and perforation.* Gut 1981;22:978-83.
168. Stacher G, Bergmann H, Granser-Vacariu GV, et al. *Lack of systematic effects of the 5-hydroxytryptamine$_3$ receptor antagonist ICS 205-930 on gastric emptying and antral motor activity in patients with primary anorexia nervosa.* Br J Clin Pharmacol 1991;32:685-90.
169. Stacher G, Peeters TL, Bergmann H, et al. *Erythromycin effects on gastric emptying, antral motility and pancreatic polypeptide concentrations in anorexia nervosa.* Gut 1993;34:166-72.
170. Stacher G, Abatzi-Wenzel Th-A, Wiesnagrotzki S, et al. *Gastric emptying, body weight and symptoms in primary anorexia nervosa: long-term effects of cisapride.* Br J Psychiatry 1993;162:398-402.
171. Buchman AL, Ament ME, Weiner M, et al. *Reversal of megaduodenum and duodenal dysmotility associated with improvement in nutritional status in primary anorexia nervosa.* Dig Dis Sci 1994;39:433-40.
172. Haller JO, Slovis TL, Baker DH, et al. *Anorexia nervosa-the paucity of radiologic findings in more than fifty patients.* Pediatr Radiol 1977;5:145-7.
173. Kamal N, Chami T, Andersen A, et al. *Delayed gastrointestinal transit times in anorexia nervosa.* Gastroenterology 1991;101:1320-4.
174. Pryor T, Wiederman MW, McGilley B. *Laxative abuse among women with eating*

*disorders: an indication of psychopathology?* Int J Eating Dis 1996;20:13-8.

175. Morgan HG, Russell GFM. *Value of family background and clinical features as prediction of long term outcome in anorexia nervosa.* Psychol Med 1975;5:355-72.
176. Crisp AH, Palmer RL, Kalucy RS. *How common is anorexia nervosa? A prevalence study.* Br J Psychiatry 1976;128:549-54.
177. Crisp AH. *Anorexia nervosa: let me be.* New York: Grune & Stratton; 1980.
178. Jones DJ, Fox MM, Babigian HM, Hutton HE. *Epidemiology of anorexia nervosa in Monroe County, New York: 1960-1976.* Psychosom Med 1980;42:551-8.
179. Garfinkel PE, Garner DM. *Anorexia nervosa: a multidimensional perspective.* New York: Brunner/Mazel; 1982.
180. Gowers S, McMahon JB. *Social class and prognosis in anorexia nervosa.* Int J Eating Dis 1989;8:105-9.
181. Pope HG Jr, Champoux RF, Hudson JI. *Eating disorder and socioeconomic class. Anorexia nervosa in nine communities.* J Nerv Ment Dis 1987;175:620-3.
182. Garner DM, Garfinkel PE. *Socio-cultural factors in the development of anorexia nervosa.* Psychol Med 1980;10:647-56.
183. Cantwell DP, Sturzenberger S, Burroughs J, et al. *Anorexia nervosa: an affective disorder?* Arch Gen Psychiatry 1977;34:1087-93.
184. Halmi KA, Eckert E, Marchi P, et al. *Comorbidity of psychiatric diagnoses in anorexia nervosa.* Arch Gen Psychiatry 1991;48:712-8.
185. Walsh BT, Gladis M, Roose SP. *Food intake and mood in anorexia nervosa and bulimia.* Ann NY Acad Sci 1987;499:231-8.
186. Kennedy SH, Goldbloom DS. *Current perspectives on drug therapies for anorexia nervosa and bulimia nervosa.* Drugs 1991;41:367-77.
187. Holden NL. *Is anorexia nervosa an obsessive-compulsive disorder?* Br J Psychiatry 1990;157:1-5.
188. Srinivasagam NM, Kaye WH, Plotnicov KH, et al. *Persistent perfectionism, symmetry, and exactness after long-term recovery from anorexia nervosa.* Am J Psychiatry 1995;152:1630-4.
189. Fahy TA, Osacar A, Marks I. *History of eating disorders in female patients with obsessive-compulsive disorder.* Int J Eating Dis 1993;14:439-43.
190. Holland AJ, Sicotte N, Treasure J. *Anorexia nervosa: evidence for a genetic basis.* J Psychosom Res 1988;32:561-71.
191. Strober M, Lampert C, Morrell W, et al. *A controlled family study of anorexia nervosa: evidence of familial aggregation and lack of shared transmission with affective disorders.* Int J Eating Dis 1990;9:239-53.
192. Waters BGH, Beumont PJV, Touyz S, Kennedy M. *Behavioural differences between*

*twin and non-twin sibling pairs discordant for anorexia nervosa.* Int J Eating Dis 1990;9:265-73.

193. Hall A, Leibrich J, Walkey FH, Welch G. *Investigation of "weight pathology" of 58 mothers of anorexia nervosa patients and 204 mothers of schoolgirls.* Psychol Med 1986;16:71-6.
194. Garfinkel PE, Garner DM, Rose J, et al. *A comparison of characteristics in the families of patients with anorexia nervosa and normal controls.* Psychol Med 1983;13:821-8.

*ADDRESS FOR CORRESPONDENCE*

**STACHER G, MD**
Psychophysiology Unit
University of Vienna
Waehringer Guertel 18-20
1090 Wien Austria
Fax: +43 1 40400 3478
E-mail: georg.stacher@akh-wien.ac.at

# ALTERATIONS OF DEFECATORY BEHAVIOR ATTRIBUTABLE TO PSYCHOSOCIAL AND ENVIRONMENTAL MECHANISMS

*WE Whitehead*

This chapter will address the impact of psychological, life-style, and environmental factors on the etiology and course of diarrhea, constipation, and fecal incontinence. It is appropriate that the title refers to these as defecatory "behaviors" rather than symptoms because this chapter will emphasize the psychosocial factors which influence their etiology and treatment.

## Diarrhea

### *Definition and epidemiology*

Chronic or recurrent diarrhea may arise from many causes including inflammatory bowel disease, resection of a part of the gastrointestinal tract, and carbohydrate malabsorption. However, the most common causes of recurrent problems with frequent loose stools are functional diarrhea and Irritable Bowel Syndrome (IBS).

Functional diarrhea is defined by the following symptoms occurring at least 12 weeks (not necessarily consecutive weeks) in the last 12 months[1]:

1. unformed (mushy or watery) stools three-fourths of the time
2. absence of abdominal pain

These symptoms are often accompanied by a strong urge to defecate and may be accompanied by fecal incontinence. Urgency and incontinence are not among the diagnostic criteria for functional diarrhea, but they may cause more subjective distress than frequent loose stools and may be responsible for the patient's decision to consult a physician.

When diarrhea is accompanied by abdominal pain, the patient will usually meet diagnostic criteria for IBS. This requires that the patient have one or more of three symptoms: abdominal pain or discomfort which is relieved by defecation, looser stools with the onset of pain, and/or more frequent stools with the onset of pain[1].

The prevalence of chronic diarrhea is estimated to be 4% of the population[2], but may be greater than this. The reported prevalence of IBS ranges from 9%[3] to 22%[4], and the majority of people with irritable bowel experience frequent episodes of loose stools, often alternating with periods of constipation[5].

*Life-style and habits*

A few life-style variables are recognized to cause or exacerbate diarrhea. "Runner's diarrhea" affects an estimated 47% of people who regularly engage in vigorous exercise, and it is associated with occasional fecal incontinence in 12% of runners[6]. One study suggests that vigorous exercise alters the motility of the colon in ways which are conducive to diarrhea[7]. Another common life-style variable contributing to recurrent diarrhea is milk ingestion in people who are lactase deficient. An estimated 17% of the USA population are lactose intolerant[8], and the prevalence is higher in some other parts of the world.

*Psychosocial factors*

Diarrhea frequently occurs as a response to acute stress or anxiety. Sandler et al.[9] classified 566 young adults as having IBS-like symptoms vs those having no chronic bowel symptoms, and then asked both groups whether psychological stress affected their bowel habits: 85% of people with IBS and 66% of people without chronic bowel symptoms reported altered bowel habits in response to stress. It is reported anecdotally that stress or anxiety may trigger or exacerbate postprandial diarrhea. Lydiard et al.[10] have drawn attention to the association between panic attacks and IBS symptoms including diarrhea.

*Response to psychological treatment*

In studies which have examined the effectiveness of psychological treatments for IBS, the symptoms which have consistently shown the greatest improvement are diarrhea and abdominal pain: IBS-associated diarrhea is decreased by interpersonal psychotherapy[11], hypnosis[12], cognitive behavior therapy[13], and tricyclic antidepressants[14]. Despite these positive outcomes, however, when the primary complaint is functional or idiopathic chronic diarrhea, the first choice of treatment is not psychotherapy but an antidiarrheal drug. The most specific and effective antidiarrheal agents are loperamide and diphenoxylate, but anticholinergics such as hyoscyamine and dicyclomine may also reduce diarrhea in patients with IBS. Bile salt binders such as cholestyramine have also been reported to help some patients with functional causes of diarrhea. Antidiarrheal agents may be used in conjunction with psychotherapy for patients with stress or anxiety-related diarrhea.

## Constipation

### *Definition and epidemiology*

Functional constipation is defined[1] by the presence of two or more of the following six symptoms on at least 12 weeks, which need to be consecutive, in the preceding 12 months:

1. straining with more than 1/4 of defecations
2. lumpy or hard stools with more than 1/4 of defecations
3. sensation of incomplete evacuation with more than 1/4 of defecations
4. sensation of anorectal obstruction/blockage with more than 1/4 of defecations
5. manual maneuvres to facilitate defecation with more than 1/4 of defecations
6. fewer than 3 bowel movements per week.

When pain accompanies constipation, the patient will usually meet criteria for a diagnosis of IBS.

Organic causes of constipation including mechanical obstruction and drug side-effects should be excluded before diagnosing functional constipation.

The prevalence of constipation has been estimated to be 2-9%[3,15-17]; the differences appear to be due to variations in the methods used to define constipation. Most epidemiologic studies have simply asked patients whether they are constipated, whatever constipation may mean to them. Epidemiological studies consistently show that constipation is more common in women than in men[3,15-17] except in children, where boys outnumber girls[18]. The frequency of self-reported constipation also increases with age, especially past age 60 years[3,15-17]. However, the self-reported frequency of bowel movements does not appear to decrease significantly with advancing age[17]. This seeming paradox, in combination with other evidence[19,20], suggests that pelvic floor dyssynergia and associated symptoms of straining and incomplete evacuation are responsible for the increasing frequency of self-reported constipation among elderly people.

*Life-style and habits*

Life-style variables such as diet and exercise are believed to play a greater role in the etiology of constipation than of diarrhea. Epidemiologic studies show that more physically active individuals are much less likely to report constipation[17], although experimental studies in which the acute effects of physical conditioning on whole gut transit time are studied, have yielded mixed results[21,22]. Constipated subjects consume less dietary fiber and liquids[17], and increases in fiber improve the symptoms of constipation. The effects of diet on constipation may help to explain the epidemiologic observations that constipation is more common among the poor than among the wealthy segments of society and also more prevalent in African Americans than among Caucasian Americans[17].

Medication side-effects are very common causes of constipation. Many of the drugs prescribed for pain (narcotic analgesics), hypertension, and depression are constipating.

*Psychosocial factors*

Healthy controls are able to inhibit defecation and to delay whole gut transit time significantly when they are motivated to do so by monetary incentives[23,24]. This has led to the speculation that learning to inhibit defecation to avoid pain (frequently seen in children) or habitually ignoring the urge to defecate may contribute to the development of functional constipation. It has also been reported that women with a history of sexual abuse are at greater risk for developing pelvic floor dyssynergia type constipation[25]; this may also represent a type of learning.

When psychological tests are administered to people with constipation, they are found to have mild to moderate degrees of anxiety and depression[26]. Although an early report[27] suggested that symptoms of psychological distress might be more common in patients whose constipation was associated with normal whole gut transit times, subsequent studies showed that patients with objectively documented slow transit constipation[28] and pelvic floor dyssynergia also score higher on tests of psychological distress.

The psychological symptom most commonly found in patients with constipation is anxiety. The explanation for this association may relate to the fact that anxiety is often accompanied by increased levels of skeletal muscle tension throughout the body including the muscles of the pelvic floor, and this increased muscle tension may make it more difficult for patients to relax the external anal sphincter during attempts to defecate. Although patients with constipation often appear to be anxious, there is no published evidence that acute stressors make constipation worse; acute stress is more frequently associated with diarrhea.

However, the failure of patients to detect a link between stress and constipation may be due to the difficulty of detecting a relationship between "not" having a bowel movement and what is going on in the environment. There is anecdotal evidence to support this view: many patients report that they are more constipated when they travel, and others report that being under time pressure makes it more difficult for them to pass stool.

Many patients with severe constipation correctly report that they rarely or never have bowel movements without laxatives. However, a subgroup of patients mistakenly hold this belief and are afraid to omit taking laxatives on a daily basis for fear of developing an impaction. These patients often have daily watery bowel movements. The psychological mechanism responsible for these mistaken beliefs have not been described. Anorexia and bulimia are frequently associated with subjective complaints of constipation[29,30] and with laxative abuse or laxative dependency. Whole gut transit time does, in fact, slow down with food restriction in patients with eating disorders[29]. However, there is also a psychological basis for some of the symptoms of constipation since these symptoms are correlated with scores on a depression inventory, and improvements in constipation are correlated with improvements in depression following treatment[30]. In these patients, laxative abuse may be motivated less by a fear of fecal impaction than by a fear of looking fat.

Another psychological disorder which may lead patients to consult for constipation is an obsessive-compulsive ritual around the need to defecate. These patients often spend many hours in the toilet each day and take multiple enemas or suppositories to rid themselves of any sensation of stool in the anal canal or rectum. On rare occasions these patients are found to have a pathophysiological basis for these symptoms consisting of a rectocele which retains fecal material and gives rise to the sensation of incomplete evacuation, or an enterocele with loops of small intestine pressing on the pelvic floor. In most cases, however, this is simply an obsessive-compulsive disorder.

*Psychological treatment*

Functional constipation is less likely than diarrhea to improve in response to psychotherapy or other psychological interventions directed at the relief of anxiety and depression[26]. This may be due to the poor correlation between stress and exacerbations of constipation in most patients. Constipation is also less responsive to pharmacological treatment with antidepressants or $5HT_3$ antagonists than is diarrhea.

On the other hand, a growing body of literature suggests that biofeedback training to teach patients to relax the pelvic floor when straining to defecate may be the treatment of choice for pelvic floor dyssynergia. A large number of uncontrolled trials have been reported which suggest that two-thirds of patients may expect to benefit from this form of treatment[31]. However, no studies have been published which compared biofeedback to a placebo treatment or to standard medical therapy in adults.

For the patient with laxative dependency due to fear of impaction, an approach which is often successful is to persuade the patient to abstain from laxatives for 6 days while measuring whole gut transit time to document the severity of constipation. A normal whole gut transit time and the occurrence of bowel movements while off laxatives, confirms the diagnosis and provides a bridge to persuade the patient to forego laxatives.

Patients with obsessive-compulsive toilet rituals cannot be treated medically; they require psychological treatment for the obsessive-compulsive disorder and/or clomipramine, a drug which is specifically effective for obsessive-compulsive disorders[32].

## Fecal incontinence

Fecal incontinence is defined[2] as frequent uncontrolled passage of stool in an individual over four years of age. The most common causes are:

- constipation with accumulation of a fecal mass in the rectum and subsequent leakage, and
- diarrhea which overwhelms the sphincter mechanism for continence.

However, chronic fecal incontinence may also occur in response to weakness of the external anal sphincter secondary to muscle injury (usually obstetrical trauma), weakness of the external anal sphincter secondary to neurological injury (often seen in diabetes mellitus), impaired ability to perceive rectal filling with fecal material (frequently seen in diabetes mellitus and spinal cord injury), or decreased compliance of the rectum (often seen in radiation proctitis, ischemic bowel disease, or inflammatory bowel disease).

Fecal incontinence is more prevalent than is frequently appreciated. Surveys in the USA[3], France[33], and Germany[34] show that 6-7% of the population report fecal soiling, although the frequency of large volume fecal incontinence appears to be closer to 0.3% in adults[3]. The prevalence of fecal incontinence is related to age, with children and also elderly people reporting a much higher incidence than young and middle-aged adults[3,18]. Among children[18] and possibly also among the elderly[3], males outnumber females, but among young and middle-aged people, fecal incontinence appears to be more common in women because obstetrical injuries are a frequent cause of fecal incontinence in these age groups[35].

### *Life-style and habits*

Constipation and diarrhea are the most common causes of fecal incontinence. Approximately 96% of children with fecal incontinence are constipated[18], and constipation is a frequent cause or exacerbating factor in the fecal incontinence seen in adults. This association is believed to be due to fecal impaction of the rectum which:

- dilates the internal anal sphincter allowing liquid stool to seep out, and
- reduces the patient's ability to perceive the movement of new fecal material into the rectum.

Diarrhea is also frequently associated with fecal incontinence. An estimated 20% of IBS patients experience fecal incontinence[5], and an estimated 12% of long-distance runners report fecal incontinence[6]. The prevalence of fecal incontinence in other forms of chronic or recurrent diarrhea is not known. The mechanism by which diarrhea contributes to fecal incontinence has not been studied in detail, but it is believed that the consistency of the stools (loose to watery) and the type of motility (increased frequency of high amplitude propagated contractions) are contributing factors.

Other risk factors for fecal incontinence include mobility impairment or dexterity impairment in the elderly, and dementia or other causes of cognitive impairment[36]. Willful soiling in order to manipulate caregivers or to gain their attention have been described, but they appear to be rare.

Additional life-style variables believed to contribute to fecal incontinence because they trigger diarrhea include lactose ingestion in patients with lactase deficiency[9], other types of food intolerance, and stress in patients with IBS[8].

*Psychosocial factors*

Psychological factors rarely play any significant role in the etiology of fecal incontinence. Among children, fecal incontinence is often associated with behavior problems or symptoms of anxiety[37], but effective treatment of the fecal soiling frequently leads to disappearance of the psychological symptoms. On the other hand, although fecal incontinence is not caused by psychological symptoms, it appears to cause significant psychological distress and impaired quality of life[38]. The psychological consequences of fecal incontinence may include lowered self-esteem, social isolation, anxiety, and depression. Anecdotal experience suggests that the psychological impact of fecal incontinence is related to the developmental stage of the patient. Preadolescent children generally deal with their incontinence through denial – they report that their friends are unaware of the incontinence. Adolescents and young adults who have had fecal incontinence while going through puberty, tend to develop and to retain a negative image of themselves as dirty and socially unacceptable individuals. People whose fecal incontinence begins during adulthood tend to view their incontinence as an illness or injury which happened to them, and they may react to it by embarrassment.

*Psychological treatment*

When fecal incontinence is associated with stress-related or post-prandial diarrhea, cognitive or behavioral therapy techniques directed at the control of stress may be effective. Similarly, patients who develop a phobia of eating in public because of a fear of developing diarrhea and incontinence may benefit from cognitive and behavioral techniques.

Habit training is a behavioral training technique developed for the treatment of fecal incontinence secondary to constipation in children. It involves an initial evacuation of the colon with laxatives followed by having the child attempt a bowel movement at a scheduled time each day, usually immediately after a meal. Parents may be encouraged to remind the child to attempt defecation and to reward successful bowel movements with small gifts or special privileges. Habit training may be combined with laxatives to keep the stools soft and easier to pass. Habit training leads to the achievement of continence in approximately 80% of fecally incontinent children short-term and in approximately 50% long-term[39]. It may also be effective in adults with constipation-related fecal incontinence[40].

When constipation is due to inappropriate contraction of the external anal sphincter and/or puborectalis muscles during attempts to defecate, whether voluntary or involuntary, biofeedback may be effective at teaching the patient to relax these striated muscles enough to allow defecation to occur. Biofeedback is associated with more rapid elimination of fecal incontinence in children[41], but at follow-up assessment 6 months or more after treatment, biofeedback may be no more effective than laxative therapy[42] in children with fecal incontinence.

A different type of biofeedback has been used to treat fecal incontinence associated with weakness of the external anal sphincter. Here patients are provided with visual and/or auditory feedback and instructions to help them learn how to contract the sphincter muscles appropriately, and they are encouraged to perform daily exercises (Kegal exercises) to improve the strength of the muscles. There are no large scale controlled trials to prove that this type of treatment is effective, but in multiple uncontrolled trials, it has been found to be effective in approximately 70% of patients with fecal incontinence associated with sphincter weakness[31].

A third type of biofeedback training has been developed for patients whose fecal incontinence is associated with inability to perceive rectal distention due to peripheral nerve injury[43,44]. This type of biofeedback takes the form of discrimination training. The patient is instructed to respond to rectal distention by contracting the external anal sphincter, and the rectum is first distended with a volume large enough to be perceived. The volume of distention is progressively decreased on successive trials until the patient begins to make mistakes (i.e., to miss some distentions), and at this point, the volume of distention is varied above and below the perception threshold in an effort to teach the patient to recognize and respond to weaker and weaker distentions. Two research teams[43,44] have reported that this type of biofeedback training is associated with improved continence in the majority of patients tested.

Acknowledgements
Preparation of manuscript was supported by grants K05 MH00133 and R01 DK31369.

## *REFERENCES*

1. Thompson WG, Longstreth GF, Drossman DA, Heaton KW, Irvine EJ, Müller-Lissner SA. *Functional bowel disorders and functional abdominal pain.* Gut 1999;45(Suppl II):II43-47.
2. Whitehead WE. *Functional anorectal disorders.* Semin Dig Dis 1996;7:230-6.
3. Drossman DA, Li Z, Andruzzi E, et al. *U.S. householder survey of functional GI disorders: Prevalence, sociodemography, and health impact.* Dig Dis Sci 1993;38:1569-80.

4. Jones R, Lydeard S. *Irritable bowel syndrome in the general population.* Br Med J 1992;102:1962-7.
5. Drossman DA, Sandler RS, Broom CM, McKee DC. *Urgency and fecal soiling in people with bowel dysfunction.* Dig Dis Sci 1986;31:1221-5.
6. Sullivan SN, Wong C. *Runners' diarrhea. Different patterns and associated factors.* J Clin Gastroenterol 1992;14:101-4.
7. Cheskin LJ, Crowell MD, Kamal N, et al. *The effects of acute exercise on colonic motility.* J Gastrointest Mot 1992;4:173-7.
8. Johnson JD. *Regional and ethnic distribution of lactose malabsorption: Adaptive and genetic hypothesis.* In: Paige DM, Bayless TM, editors. *Lactose digestion: Clinical and nutritional implications.* Baltimore: Johns Hopkins University Press; 1981;11-22.
9. Sandler RS, Drossman DA, Nathan HP, McKee DC. *Symptom complaints and health care seeking behavior in subjects with bowel dysfunction.* Gastroenterology 1984;87:314-8.
10. Lydiard RB, Laraia MT, Howell EF, Ballenger JC. *Can panic disorder present as irritable bowel syndrome?* J Clin Psychiatry 1986;47:470-3.
11. Guthrie EA, Creed F, Dawson D, Tomenson B. *A controlled trial of psychological treatment for the irritable bowel syndrome.* Gastroenterology 1991;100:450-7.
12. Whorwell PJ, Prior A, Colgan SM. *Hypnotherapy in severe irritable bowel syndrome: further experience.* Gut 1987;28:423-5.
13. Payne A, Blanchard EB. *A controlled comparison of cognitive therapy and self-help support groups in the treatment of irritable bowel syndrome.* J Consult Clin Psychol 1995;63:779-86.
14. Greenbaum DS, Mayle JE, Vanegeren LE, et al. *The effects of desipramine on IBS compared with atropine and placebo.* Dig Dis Sci 1987;32:257-66.
15. Sonnenberg A, Koch TR. *Epidemiology of constipation in the United States.* Dis Colon Rectum 1989;32:1-8.
16. Probert CSJ, Emmett PM, Cripps HA, Heaton KW. *Evidence for the ambiguity of the term constipation: the role of irritable bowel syndrome.* Gut 1994;35:1455-8.
17. Everhart JE, Go VL, Johannes RS, et al. *A longitudinal survey of self-reported bowel habits in the United States.* Dig Dis Sci 1989;34:1153-62.
18. Loening-Baucke V. *Chronic constipation in children.* Gastroenterology 1993;105:1557-64.
19. Cheskin LJ, Kamal N, Crowell MD, et al. Mechanisms of constipation in older persons and effects of fiber compared with placebo. J Am Geriatr Soc 1995;43:666-9.
20. Whitehead WE, Drinkwater D, Cheskin LJ, et al. *Constipation in the elderly living at home: Definition, prevalence, and relationship to lifestyle and health status.* J Am Geriatric Soc 1989;37:423-9.
21. Koffler KH, Menkes A, Redmond RA, et al. *Strength training accelerates gastrointestinal transit time in middle-aged and older men.* Medicine Science Sports, Exercise 1992;24:415-9.

22. Kayaleh RA, Meshkinpour H, Avinashi A, Tamadon A. *Effect of exercise on mouth-to-cecum transit in trained athletes: a case against the role of runners' abdominal bouncing.* J Sports Med Physical Fitness 1996;36:271-4.
23. Klauser AG, Voderholzer WA, Heinrich CA, et al. *Behavioural modification of colonic function: can constipation be learned?* Dig Dis Sci 1990;35:1271-5.
24. Enck P, Bielefeld K, Legler T, et al. *Kann man Verstopfung lernen? Eine experimentelle Untersuchung bei gesunden Probanden.* Z Med Psychol 1991;1:31-7.
25. Leroi AM, Berkelmans I, Denis P, et al. *Anismus as a marker of sexual abuse. Consequences of abuse on anorectal motility.* Dig Dis Sci 1995;40:1411-6.
26. Whitehead WE. *Illness behaviour.* In: Kamm MA, Lennard-Jones JE, editors. Constipation. Petersfield, UK: Wrightson Biomedical Publishing; 1993;95-100.
27. Wald A, Burgio K, Holeva K, Locher J. *Psychological evaluation of patients with severe idiopathic constipation: which instrument to use.* Am J Gastroenterol 1992;87:977-80.
28. Devroede G, Girard G, Bouchoucha M, et al. *Idiopathic constipation by colonic dysfunction: relationship with personality and anxiety.* Dig Dis Sci 1989;34:1428-33.
29. Kamal N, Chami T, Andersen A, et al. *Delayed gastrointestinal transit times in anorexia nervosa and bulimia nervosa.* Gastroenterology 1991;86:599-602.
30. Chami TN, Andersen AE, Crowell MD, et al. *Gastrointestinal symptoms in bulimia nervosa: Effects of treatment.* Am J Gastroenterol 1995;90:88-92.
31. Enck P. *Biofeedback training in disordered defecation: A critical review.* Dig Dis Sci 1993;38:1953-60.
32. Flament MF, Biserbe JC. *Pharmacologic treatment of obsessive-compulsive disorder: comparative studies.* J Clin Psychiatry 1997;58(Suppl 12):18-22.
33. (Anonymous). *Incontinence fecale: enquete après de la population generale.* Paris: IPSOS Marketing; 1989.
34. Enck P, Gabor S, von Ferber L, et al. *Haufigkeit der Stuhlinkontinenz und informationsgrad von Hausarzten und Krankenkassen.* Z Gastroenterol 1991;29:538-40.
35. Nelson R, Norton N, Cautley E, Furner S. *Community-based prevalence of anal incontinence.* JAMA 1995;274:559-61.
36. Johansonn JF, Irizarry F, Doughty A. *Risk factors for fecal incontinence in a nursing home population.* J Clin Gastroenterol 1997;24:156-60.
37. Bellman, MM. *Studies on encopresis.* Acta Paed Scand 1966;56(Suppl 170):1-151.
38. Burnett CK, Palsson O, Whitehead WE, Drossman D. *Psychological distress and impaired quality of life in patients with functional anorectal disorders.* Gastroenterology 1998;114:A729.
39. Lowery SP, Srour JW, Whitehead WE, Schuster MM. *Habit training as treatment of encopresis secondary to chronic constipation.* J Ped Gastroenterol Nutr 1985;4:397-401.

40. Whitehead WE, Burgio KL, Engel BT. *Biofeedback treatment of fecal incontinence in geriatric patients.* J Am Geriatr Soc 1985;4:397-401.
41. Loening-Baucke V. *Modulation of abnormal defecation dynamics by biofeedback treatment in chronically constipated children with encopresis.* J Pediatr 1990;116:214-22.
42. Loening-Baucke V. *Biofeedback treatment for chronic constipation and encopresis in childhood: long-term outcome.* Pediatrics 1995;96:105-10.
43. Wald A, Tunuguntla AK. *Anorectal sensorimotor dysfunction in fecal incontinence and diabetes mellitus: modification with biofeedback therapy.* N Engl J Med 1984;310:1282-7.
44. Buser WD, Miner PB Jr. *Delayed rectal sensation with fecal incontinence. Successful treatment using anorectal manometry.* Gastroenterology 1986;91:1186-91


*ADDRESS FOR CORRESPONDENCE*


**WHITEHEAD WE, PhD**

Division of Digestive Diseases, CB #7080
University of North Carolina at Chapel Hill
Chapel Hill, North Carolina 27599-7080 USA
Fax: +1 919 966 0285
E-mail: william.whitehead@med.unc.edu

PART TWO

# BIOPSYCHOSOCIAL MODEL AND PATIENT EVALUATION

# THE BIOPSYCHOSOCIAL MODEL AND CHRONIC GASTROINTESTINAL DISEASE

*DA Drossman*

This presentation addresses the application of the biopsychosocial model in the understanding and care of patients with chronic Gastrointestinal (GI) disorders[1]. As you may know, within the field of gastroenterology, technology has flourished. Using endoscopy, Computerized Tomography (CT) scan, ultrasound, and Magnetic Resonance Imaging (MRI), we can visualize subtle morphologic abnormalities throughout the GI tract. With manometric techniques, we can evaluate disturbed motility, and with surgical and histologic evaluation, we can identify pathology. Yet, even the most sophisticated diagnostic techniques are not sufficient to explain the degree, variability or even the presence of chronic GI symptoms, or the patient's experience and behavior related to them.

Consider the following clinical examples:

*1. GERD* Two patients having gastroesophageal reflux disease (GERD): Mr. H. has severe heartburn that limits his ability to work. But, a 24 hour pH study shows only "mild" reflux, and endoscopy is normal. In contrast, Mr. L. has occasional mild heartburn and is hospitalized for dysphagia. Yet, a pH study indicates severe reflux, and endoscopy shows a 5 mm peptic stricture and Barrett's esophagus, a premalignant condition.

*2. Chronic functional abdominal pain* Ms. S. visits the emergency room with chronic, severe abdominal pain. Despite negative diagnostic evaluations in the past, the pain led to several surgeries for appendectomy, hysterectomy, and cholecystectomy. She takes narcotics for symptom relief. There is a history of sexual and physical abuse beginning in childhood. She is forgetful, feels helpless and out of control with her symptoms, and with life in general, and urges her physician to make a diagnosis. Previously, a psychiatrist diagnosed a dissociative disorder with somatization. The current diagnostic studies are negative. However, her severe symptoms lead to an exploratory laparotomy where only flimsy adhesions are lysed. Several weeks after the operation, the pain returns.

These cases challenge certain biomedical assumptions. For the two men with GERD, we see a very poor correlation between the symptom experience and the associated physiology and pathology. The patient with severe symptoms had no esophagitis, and the patient with esophageal stricture and Barrett's esophagus had minimal heartburn symptoms. In addition, Ms. S. with chronic abdominal pain had "no" medical findings to explain her disabling symptoms. Furthermore, despite the psychosocial difficulties, she received another operation with insignificant findings, and then the pain returned. So, she had severe illness, without evident "disease".

At this point, we need to make a distinction between disease and illness. I will define "disease" as the externally verifiable evidence of a pathologic state. Evidence would include X-rays, laboratory and endoscopic findings and histopathology. "Illness" is defined as the patient's perception of ill health which is evident from the person's symptom reports, perceptions and behavior[2]. Using these definitions, we see that these clinical examples challenge existing assumptions that illness and disease are closely related.

## Biomedical and biopsychosocial models

To understand why illness and disease do not always correlate, we should recognize that the "Biomedical" model is traditional and dominant within Western medical education and research[3]. This model has two assumptions:

1. ***Reductionism*** - that all conditions can be linearly reduced to a single etiology,
   and
2. ***Dualism*** - where illness and disease are dichotomized either to an "organic" disorder having an objectively defined etiology, or a "functional" disorder, with no specific etiology or pathophysiology.

So, from a biomedical perspective, an etiologic factor would lead, in a linear and unidirectional fashion, to the development of a medical disease, and the disease fully explains the illness and the clinical

outcome. In other words, the etiologic factor is both necessary and sufficient for disease, including its diagnosis and cure. But, as illustrated in these cases, the patient with disease experienced little illness and those with severe symptoms (illness) had little or no disease.
From an epidemiologic perspective, finding a specific disease for most medical illnesses is the exception rather than the rule. In one clinic study[4], the authors identified the most common medical symptoms seen among 1000 ambulatory internal medicine patients, and after 3 years' follow-up, only 16% of 567 new complaints, and 10% of abdominal pain eventually related to a specific etiology.
Also, we recognize that a clinical condition can range from disease without illness (e.g., asymptomatic ulcer or hypertension), to illness without disease (e.g., chronic abdominal pain or fatigue). From a biomedical perspective, this may produce certain values:

1. no illness and no disease is health
2. disease with illness is understood as "rightful" suffering
3. disease without illness may even be considered "coping"
   but what about
4. illness without disease?

From the biomedical perspective, this illegitimate condition does not exit, and may be labeled as "psychosomatic", a pejorative term that questions the credibility of the symptoms, even though they are very real to the patient.
By now, it is evident that I should like to propose an alternative understanding. The "Biopsychosocial" model of illness and disease[3] improves upon the biomedical model, and addresses its limitations. It proposes that illness and disease result from simultaneously interacting systems at the cellular, tissue, organismal, interpersonal and environmental level. It integrates biologic science with the unique features of the individual, and determines the degree to which biologic and psychosocial factors interact to explain the disease, illness and outcome.
In this manner, both biologic "and" psychologic predispositions contribute to the expression of disease and illness. Environmental exposures and psychosocial modifiers also affect the clinical expression

of the condition, and ultimately, the outcome, and they do so in a reciprocal fashion. Thus, a biological event such as HIV infection can affect organ function, the person, the family and society, and reciprocally, a change at the psychosocial level, such as the death of a spouse or other psychosocial trauma, can affect psychologic status and clinical outcome, or even have biological effects on cellular immunity resulting in disease activation[5]. This model also accepts the reciprocal influences of disease and illness, and the clinical variability among individuals for a given medical condition.

## A paradigm shift

For some, understanding this biopsychosocial model requires a "paradigm shift"[6]: a break from the constraints of biomedical reductionism, in order to "see" these medical conditions in another more integrated way. It is much like the shifts in perception that occur when first seeing two faces and then a vase in the well-known optical illusion. But seeing health and illness from a biomedical perspective was not always the case. Societal beliefs on how psychosocial factors interact with biology in explaining human illness have vacillated throughout Western history depending on the existing explanatory ("folk") models of the time[7]. These explanatory models strongly influence the nature of scientific inquiry and the conclusions drawn from the data.

## An historical perspective

About 3,000 years ago, in Western society, the ancient Greeks[8] proposed the concept of "Holos", that medical disease involves the whole person rather than just the diseased part, and this view is still held in many non-Western societies. However, in 1637 the writings of Rene Descartes led to a major "paradigm shift"[9] in Europe, by proposing the separation of the thinking mind (res cogitans) from the machine-like body (res extensa). Cartesian dualism harmonized with existing social and political influences relating to the separation of Church (the spirit) and State (the body). Within medicine, dualism allowed for the dissection of human cadavers, a process previously discouraged by the church, and it led to a clinical distinction between medical and psychiatric disorders, the former being amenable to scientific inquiry including dissection, and the latter being relegated to the asylums.

Over the next 300 years, dualism held ground, but was occasionally disputed by medical physicians and scientists. At the beginning of the 19th Century, Dr. Benjamin Rush[10] in the United States, tried to develop a medical curriculum that would integrate psychologic and biologic information in diagnosis and treatment. However, the impact of Pasteur's discovery of microorganisms, and Koch's development of the germ theory of disease moved medicine more in the direction of biomedical reductionism. For the GI disorders, a link between mind and gut were proposed by notables such as Sir William Beaumont, Ivan Pavlov, Walter Cannon, Tom Almy, and Stewart Wolf, but their views were not fully accepted by mainstream medical investigators.

Within psychiatry, Franz Alexander in the 1940's and 1950's[11] proposed a psychosomatic model for several diseases including ulcerative colitis and peptic ulcer, that attempted to counter early reductionistic views that medical illness was purely psychogenic[8]. He proposed that certain unconscious conflicts engendered chronic emotional tensions, which, when combined with a "biologically predisposing factor (Factor X)", could lead to physiological dysfunction, and ultimately development of the disease. Although his ideas were an advancement over the psychogenic theories, the concepts are now considered too simplistic:

1. small sample sizes
2. uncontrolled psychologic assessment
3. poor disease validation
4. use of a research model that did not consider psychosocial modifiers such as coping and social support.

Furthermore, it led to "bad press", as many medical physicians incorrectly assumed this to be a psychogenic model. Resultingly, the next few decades were associated with a decline in interest in the psychosocial investigation of medical conditions within gastroenterology.

By the 1960's, purely biological research flourished, leading to dramatic increases in understanding the mechanisms of medical and psychiatric disease. However, this was associated with relatively little research support (until recently) for a more integrated multidisciplinary investigation or

for those conditions not fitting a biomedical understanding.
Only within the last two decades has biomedical reductionism been challenged by newer studies that uncovered its limitations. How can we reconcile mounting evidence that infectious disorders like TB and HIV are merely conditional factors in the etiology of disease, rather than the cause? Host resistance and the social environment also contribute to their clinical expression. How can we accept the concept of unicausality when evidence for biologic and psychologic heterogeneity exists in disorders like inflammatory bowel disease, diabetes and cancer? How can we understand, as with Ms. S. the many clinical disorders where the patient suffers from their illness condition, yet the work up is negative for disease?
By the late 1970's, these dilemmas provided the basis for another "paradigm shift". At that time, George Engel began publishing a series of articles where he coined the term: "Biopsychosocial Model"[3,12,13]. He offered a modern exposition of holistic theory, proposing that illness is the product of biologic, psychologic and social subsystems interacting at multiple levels. Rather than consider any one factor as etiologic, Engel proposed that it is the "interaction" of these subsystems that determine the illness in any given individual.
This model provided the framework to reconcile the emerging data that could not be explained by biomedicine. It allowed for the heterogeneity of medical disorders and the uniqueness of its clinical expression in each individual. It also provided the stimulus and justification for collaborative multidisciplinary research and for research groups like the FBGRG (Functional Brain Gut Research Group) in the United States and ANEMGI (Associazione per la NeUroGastroenterologia e la Motilità Gastrointestinale) in Italy.
So what has emerged in the last twenty years has been the rapid growth of multidisciplinary research, newer investigative methods, and even new disciplines that embrace the biopsychosocial concept[7]. Some examples include:

1. development of symptom-based criteria in psychiatry (DSM-IV) and the functional GI disorders (Rome Criteria) to standardize patient selection and permit biopsychosocial investigation of the individual (rather than the organ system)

2 development of standardized questionnaires to evaluate the modulating effects: life stress, social support, sexual/physical abuse and coping in medical illness

3 emergence of health related quality of life as a research discipline, and the development of generic and disease-specific questionnaires for various medical conditions

4 emphasis on "outcome" research which is providing evidence that psychosocial factors are predictors of outcome independent of disease type and severity

5 development of newer areas of basic investigation (e.g., psychoneuroimmunology, psychoendocrinology, neurogastroenterology, brain-gut peptides) which are providing the tools to understand the clinical observation

6 development of more sophisticated techniques in GI physiology (e.g., ambulatory monitoring, visceral sensitivity testing, brain imaging with Photon Emission Tomography [PET], fMRI, and cortical evoked potentials) in order to elaborate on physiological correlates in the brain to chronic GI conditions.

## A model for the gastrointestinal disorders

Figure 1 portrays the biopsychosocial model for functional GI illness. The symptom experience and clinical outcome result from certain interacting subsystems. Early life factors, either biologic or behaviorally conditioned, affect later psychosocial experiences, physiologic functioning or susceptibility to a pathological condition. The medical condition, either functional or structural, in turn, will be influenced by one's psychosocial milieu leading to unique and varying effects on the symptom experience and clinical outcome. With the functional GI disorders, this may be mediated through the Central Nervous System/Enteric Nervous System (CNS/ENS) axis, and for immune or inflammatory disorders, possibly through the hypothalamic-pituitary-adrenal-immune axis[14].

Furthermore, the symptom experience itself or the outcome may have reciprocal effects on its determinants.

Figure 1

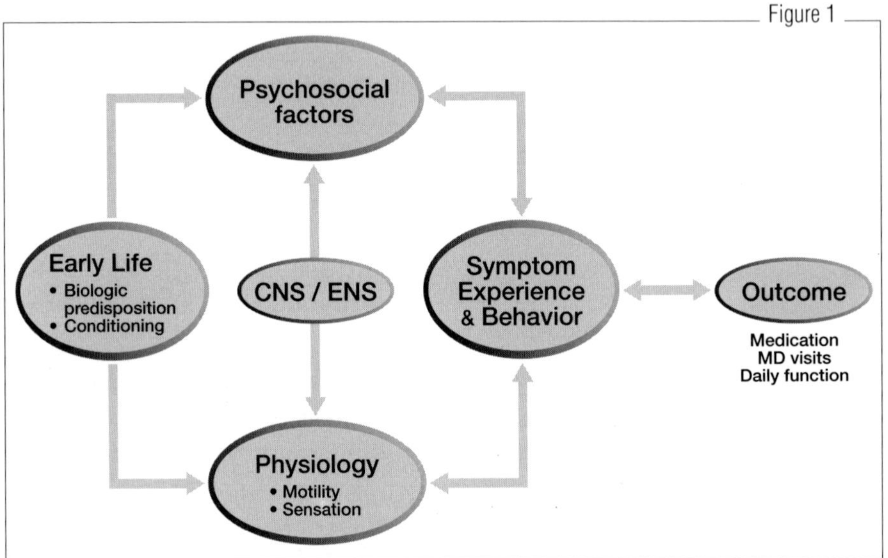


Biopsychosocial model for functional GI illness - see text for details.

So, biopsychosocial research considers not the cause of a condition, but the degree to which these interacting factors explain a given illness condition. So for irritable bowel syndrome (IBS), we recognize that:

1. it is not "caused" by intestinal dysmotility, but rather, it may reflect dysregulation of CNS-ENS linkages
2. enhanced visceral sensitivity may amplify even normal regulatory GI input to the brain
3. cortical processes may regulate symptom perception either intrinsically or through descending influences on the spinal cord
4. psychosocial factors do not define the disorder, but uniquely influence one's illness experience and behavior.

For the structural disorders, the issues are similar, though biological factors contribute more (though not exclusively) to the clinical condition. For example, identifying Helicobacter pylori (H. pylori) has revolutionized our understanding of the biology of peptic ulcer disease, and has refuted earlier theories of psychogenesis. However, its existence does not eliminate the contribution of psychosocial factors. It does not explain why some individuals are more or less susceptible to developing ulcers. Perhaps psychoneuroendocrine (e.g., via hypothalamic Thyrotropine Releasing Hormone [TRH] expression) or psychoimmune factors will be shown to affect host resistance for this condition as has occurred with other infectious diseases[15].

Finally, for gastroenterologists and other clinicians in practice the task is to determine how the contributing biologic and psychosocial factors affect the individual, and using this information, develop rational diagnostic and treatment strategies. So one individual with abdominal pain may become distressed from the pain and seek medical assistance if he/she recently lost a family member to intestinal cancer, and has a history of receiving attention and security when ill. Conversely, another individual, with the same degree of nociceptive input, may ignore the symptom if he/she has learned to consider such pain to be of little consequence, or has been taught that complaining is a "weakness". Given the acquisition of this knowledge, clearly, the clinical approach to these individuals will be different and more satisfying to the patient if properly addressed.

## The future

Given the historical perspective, it is hard to know whether future social, cultural or political forces will lead to another "paradigm shift". For the time being, the biopsychosocial model harmonizes well with what we do, and the products of this research model are new and important. Another benefit is that the collaborative efforts of basic scientists, medical investigators and behaviorists are beginning to yield far more than any discipline alone. I believe that future multidisciplinary research will help advance our understanding of chronic GI illnesses in several directions[1]:

1. the areas of psychoimmunology, neurophysiology and brain-gut associations will help us understand the hardwiring and communication between brain and gut
2. basic and clinical pharmacological studies targeted at GI and brain receptor sites will lead to more specific treatments for GI pain, dysmotility, and inflammatory effects on the gut

3 clinical research of psychosocial and outcome assessment (including health related quality of life) will clarify the importance of psychosocial factors such as abuse, life stress, psychiatric diagnosis, social support and coping on the onset and clinical expression of the GI disorders

4 research on gender-specific factors and sociocultural influences on GI illness will lead to more psychological treatments that are consistent with the patient's explanatory model of their illness

5 ongoing and future research involving behavioral treatments including cognitive-behavioral therapy, relaxation, interpersonal psychotherapy, and hypnosis, will prove to be more lasting than pharmacologic treatments

6 finally, research on the medical interview and the patient-doctor relationship will show the importance of patient-centered medical care in improving adherence to treatment, patient satisfaction, the outcome, and possibly the clinical course of the disease.

So to conclude, the interaction of psychosocial factors with illness and disease has been recognized for a long time. But as investigators involved in multidisciplinary research in these chronic GI disorders, we have a responsibility to improve this understanding through high quality research, and an obligation to communicate our work to the rest of the world. I believe we are doing this.

## *REFERENCES*

1. Drossman DA. *Presidential address: gastrointestinal illness and biopsychosocial model.* Psychosom Med 1998;60:258-67.
2. Reading A. *Illness and disease.* Med Clin N Am 1977;61:703-6.
3. Engel GL. *The need for a new medical model: a challenge for biomedicine.* Science 1977;196:129-36.
4. Kroenke K, Mangelsdorff AD. *Common symptoms in ambulatory care: incidence, evaluation, therapy, and outcome.* Am J Med 1989;86:262-6.

5. Kiecolt-Glaser JK, Glaser R. *Psychoneuroimmunology and health consequences: data and shared mechanisms.* [Review]. Psychosom Med 1995;57:269-74.
6. Kuhn TS. *The structure of scientific revolutions.* Chicago: Unversity of Chicago Press; 1970.
7. Drossman DA. *Psychosocial and psychophysiologic mechanisms in GI illness.* In: Kirsner JB, editor. The growth of gastroenterologic knowledge in the 20th Century. Philadelphia: Lea & Febiger; 1993;419-32.
8. Lipowski ZJ. *Psychosomatic medicine: past and present. Part 1, historical background.* Can J Psychiatry 1986;31:2-7.
9. Descartes R. *Discourse on method.* Translated by J.Veitch. La Salle: Open Court; 1946.
10. Rush B. *Sixteen introductory lectures.* Philadelphia: Bradford and Innskeep; 1811;256.
11. Alexander F. *Psychosomatic medicine: its principles and applications.* New York: W.W. Norton;1950.
12. Engel GL. *The clinical application of the biopsychosocial model.* Am J Psychiatry 1980;137:535-44.
13. Engel GL. *The biopsychosocial model and medical education.* N Engl J Med 1981;306:802-5.
14. Drossman DA. *Psychosocial factors in the care of patients with gastrointestinal disorders.* In: Yamada T, editor. Textbook of gastroenterology. 2nd ed. Philadelphia: JB Lippincott Co.; 1995; 620-37.
15. Levenstein S. *Stress and peptic ulcer: life beyond Helicobacter.* Br Med J 1998;316:538-41.

*Address for correspondence*

**DROSSMAN DA, MD**

Division of Digestive Diseases

726 Burnett-Womack

CB #7080, University of North Carolina

Chapel Hill, North Carolina 27599-7080 USA

Fax: +1 919 9668929

E-mail: drossman@med.unc.edu

# PATIENTS' ILLNESSES AND DOCTORS' BEHAVIOURS
# ARE PATIENTS WITH IRRITABLE BOWEL SYNDROME IDENTICAL TO THOSE WITH CHRONIC PELVIC PAIN - AND WHAT DETERMINES THE FINAL DIAGNOSIS?

*J Kruse, P Enck*

Clinically, patients with the Irritable Bowel Syndrome (IBS) as seen in gastroenterology are difficult to distinguish from patients with Chronic Pelvic Pain (CPP) as seen in gynaecological practice, but it is unknown why a part of the (female) patients with bowel symptoms will consult a family physician or an internist, while others will go to their gynaecologist. It is also unknown why many of the people affected by bowel symptoms will not go to a doctor at all, but some will excessively utilize the health care system. This immediately raises the question of whether IBS and CCP are two seperate disease entities with mutually high comorbidity, or whether they are the same syndrome in which different subgroups utilize the health care system in specific ways? While each assumption implies that the symptoms of the patients determine the final diagnosis and the clinical management, an alternative interpretation may be that clinical management depends more on the doctors' subspecialty (training, referral and reimbursement practice etc.). With this paper, we will review the evidence from the published literature of the basic hypothesis that IBS and CPP represent the same disorders rather than different entities. It will cover epidemiology and psychosocial aspects of the disease such as personality, stress, and illness behaviour.

## Epidemiology

### *Irritable Bowel Syndrome*

Functional bowel disorders of the IBS type are very common in the general population, but in older epidemiologic studies the estimate of their prevalence is critical due to patient selection. Only in recent years large-scale questionnaire studies from the US and England allowed a more precise judgement of the prevalence in the general population as well as in specific patient groups[1,2] despite the fact that the entry criteria for such studies have not been standardized until recently: The initially so-called "Manning criteria"[3] were subsequently redefined as "Rome criteria"[4]. According to this set of criteria, the diagnosis IBS is based on the continuous or recurrent presence of 2 or more symptoms over at least 3 months which cannot be explained by organic abnormalities. Symptoms include abdominal pain, relieved by a bowel movement or associated with altered stool frequency and/or consistency, bloating, or feeling of incomplete evacuation.

According to new data, the prevalence of functional bowel disorders in the general population can be estimated to be in the range of 14 to 21%[1,5-7], with women having a 3.2 times higher prevalence than men[8]. A large survey by Jones and Lydeard[1] reported the male:female ratio to be 1:1.38 with an overall prevalence of 20%. These data are somewhat at variance with data from Heaton et al.[9] according to which 13% of women but only 5% of men in a British community were diagnosed IBS. Even in older age groups, IBS is quite common: IBS symptoms were found in up to 20% of the people above 80 years[10].

These rather low estimates, in contrast to earlier studies, are probably due to better patient selection and more representative sample sizes. This is further supported by the notion that only a minority of people suffering from functional bowel symptoms will consult a doctor[9,11,12]. A survey in private practice showed a consultation rate of only 1%[13] which is comparable to German data[14].

Talley et al.[2] were able to show that an IBS population is not stable: of 582 subjects without symptoms at a first survey, 9% would report symptoms 2 years later, while 38% of initially IBS labelled patients were no longer fulfilling the diagnostic criteria at follow-up. A Scandinavian study reported similar results[15].

### *Chronic Pelvic Pain syndrome*

Despite the fact that CPP is quite common among women, reliable epidemiologic data are rare. Earlier studies included only patients utilizing

health care institutions. They imply that up to 25% of patients in gynaecological practice suffer from CPP[16,17]. Five to 10% of all laparoscopies and 20% of all hysterectomies are performed because of chronic lower abdominal complaints[18].
Mathias et al.[19] surveyed a representative sample of 5263 US American women for 3 months and found an overall prevalence of 14.7%. The reported prevalence of CPP is nearly identical to the percentage of IBS women patients (14.5%) in the US householder survey by Drossman et al.[6] which was similar in size and approach.

*Coincidence of CPP and IBS*
It is evident from the above cited literature that there must be at least a significant overlap between CPP and IBS: Longstreth[20] noted that almost half of the patients who had undergone laparoscopy because of CPP and 40% of patients who had had an elective hysterectomy had symptoms compatible with the diagnosis IBS. Most gynaecologists were unaware of the bowel symptoms so that they could not establish this diagnosis. Walker et al.[21] found 35% of IBS patients to also demonstrate CPP complaints; this group, however, showed significantly higher rates of affective disorders, anxiety, somatization disorders, sexual abuse in early childhood, and a history of hysterectomy than those patients with IBS symptoms alone. This raises the question whether IBS and CCP are two separate disease entities with mutually high comorbidity, or whether they are the same syndrome.

## Psychosocial aspects in IBS and CPP

Patients with CPP and IBS have been reported to show similarities with respect to psychosocial aspects of their disease; these are discussed with regard to:

1. personality profiles and psychometric characteristics
2. recent or acute stressful life events in association with illness onset or course, more specifically
3. a history of sexual of physical abuse, and
4. illness behaviour and health care utilization.

*Personality and emotions*

Standardized psychiatric interviews were used to study whether IBS patients would show an increased incidence of emotional disturbances. Hislop[22] found depression in 73% and anxiety in 69% of his IBS patients in contrast to 18 and 22%, respectively, in a control group. A lower incidence of depression (22%) in patients was reported by Hill and Blendis[23]. According to studies using diagnostics criteria, in up to 72% of IBS patients[24] a psychiatric diagnosis could be assigned, mainly hysteria, anxiety, and depression. Young et al.[25] classified 72% of 29 IBS patients as psychiatrically disturbed as compared to 18% of a control group. Latimer et al.[26] found all of his 16 IBS patients to fit into psychiatric diagnostic groups as compared to 47% of healthy controls.

Besides interviews, standardized psychometric tests have also been used to answer this question: Wise et al.[27] reported increases on all clinical subscales except paranoia und phobia of the Hopkins Symptom Check List (SCL-90-R). Other authors using the same test[28-31] found IBS patients to score higher for somatization, depression, anxiety, and hostility. Depression was also shown to be elevated in 50 out of 100 patients with gastrointestinal complaints of different origin using the Beck Depression Inventory; in 64% of depressive patients no organic intestinal disease could be found[32], but depression scores of IBS patients were lower than in psychiatric patients with a main diagnosis of depression[33].

Various attempts were made to identify a specific IBS personality profile. West[34] used the Multiphasic Personality Inventory (MMPI) in IBS patients and demonstrated significantly higher scores for hysteria, hypochondriasis, and depression, a profile often referred to as the "psychosomatic triade" since it is frequently found in patients with psychosomatic disorders. Bergeron and Monto[35] described 4 subtypes of personality patterns in IBS patients: inadequate dependency (28%), somatization of emotions (16%), reactive depression (16%) as well as anger and denial (8%).

Talley et al.[36] found IBS patients to be similar to patients with functional dyspepsia or organic gastrointestinal diseases with respect to MMPI test scores for hypochondria, depression, conversion neurosis, ego strength, and schizophrenia, but all patient groups had elevated scores as compared to healthy control subjects. Richter et al.[37] showed IBS patients to be similar to patients with nutcracker oesophagus with respect to most

MMPI scales, but with higher depression and anxiety scores. When the Eysenck Personality Inventory (EPI) was used, IBS patients showed higher than normal neuroticism scores[23,32,38,39].

Patients with CPP were also found to demonstrate increased levels of depression, anxiety disorders, borderline disturbances, and a tendency for somatization[40,41]. They also showed disturbances in sexuality and relationship to their partner[42,43], and reported more pregnancy related complications[44]. Pevler et al.[45] compared patients with endometriosis to those with CPP without such potential explanation for their symptoms and found no differences in affective symptoms and personality characteristics, but patients with endometriosis reported significantly higher pain scores and were more often affected by symptoms in their daily social life. Hodgkis and Watson[46] also found no differences in personality profiles and illness behaviour between patients with lower abdominal pain with and without endometriosis. One has to keep in mind, however, that only a fraction of patients with endometriosis will experience pain[47], which implies that the presence of an endometriosis alone is not sufficient to explain the symptoms.

In "summary", these data show that overall IBS patients show more psychologic or psychiatric disturbances than the normal population. For patients with CPP, this question has not yet been sufficiently addressed. Most of these studies have, however, been performed in health care utilizers within medical institutions; since only a minority of people suffering from IBS and CPP symptoms will go to a doctor, this raises the question as to whether the psychological disturbances determine the health care utilization and illness behaviour rather than the abdominal symptoms themselves.

*Stressful life events and symptoms*

A significant correlation between stressful life events and symptom detoriation was noted very early in 50 to 85% of IBS patients[48,49]. Chaudhary and Truelove[50] found the most frequently increased life events of IBS patients to be concerns regarding profession (in men) and family (in women). Hill and Blendis[23] reported that specifically professional concerns bothered IBS patients, but altogether 33% also reported death of a parent as the event preceding the symptom onset.

Early childhood social deprivation seems to play a major aetiological role since 31% of 333 IBS patients had lost parents before age 15 through death, divorce, or separation[51]. Unfortunately, these studies all lack appropriate control groups.

Mendeloff et al.[52] compared self-reported life-events in 102 IBS patients, 227 patients with chronic inflammatory bowel diseases, and in 735 healthy adults. A life-event scale demonstrated that IBS patients were more exposed to life stressors than the control groups. Fava and Pavan[53] repeated this study with another scale: their 20 IBS patients also reported more such events than 20 patients with ulcerative colitis and 20 patients with appendicitis.

Drossman et al.[54] found also normal subjects without IBS symptoms to attribute changes in stool frequency to life stressors, and 45% reported abdominal pain in response to stressful social or personal events. Abdominal responses to stressful events are, therefore, not specific to IBS patients, and no direct association between experienced daily-life stress and symptom severity could be observed when this was evaluated prospectively[29]. However, IBS patients reported overall more life events in the three months preceding the investigation, and were more susceptible to stressors than the control counterparts[55]. In agreement with a study by Ford et al.[56], life events alone seem not to be specific for functional bowel disorders, but tend to elicit feelings of anxiety and helplessness. Stress coping strategies may be of more relevance for distinguishing IBS patients from controls.

At onset of CPP symptoms, stressful life events have also been reported to be increased, but here specifically the onset of sexual relationships, marriage or closer personal bondage, and the first pregnancy have been named[57] besides more general psychosocial factors[58]. Data are, however, rare.

In "summary", both patients with CPP as well as those with IBS reported increased incidences of stressful life events with disease onset. Interpersonal relationship and sexual conflicts are predominant in CPP while IBS patients report more professional and social conflicts. It is likely that the presence and severity of these events as well as the subsequent coping determine how the patient will perceive the symptoms, whether he/she wants to consult a doctor and if so, which doctor will be the final choice.

*Physical and sexual abuse*

A more specific stressful life event such as physical and sexual abuse during childhood or as an adult was recently found to be present in up to 40% of patients with IBS and with organic bowel disorders. In these initial studies "sexual abuse" was defined as involuntary presentation of sexuality during childhood or sexual acts against one's own will during adulthood[59-61]. When the same instrument was used in the general population, a high prevalence of up to 40% reported such events[61], and a significant association of symptoms of functional bowel disorders and abuse history were noted. Comparable data are reported from European countries, e.g. France[62].

In CPP patients, a similar high incidence of sexual and violent physical abuse both during childhood and in later life phases was noted. Toomey et al.[63] recorded in 58% of patients with lower abdominal pain, a history of sexual abuse as a child or as an adult, Peters et al.[64] reported in 20% of CPP patients of a gynaecological university hospital an early childhood sexual abuse, and Walker et al.[65] described an increased prevalence of adult CPP patients - as compared to a group of patients without pelvic pain - to have experienced childhood or adult-life sexual abuse. In these cases, increased rates of somatization and affective disorders are found as well. Walling et al.[66,67] compared 3 patient groups (patients with CPP, patients without pain symptoms, and patients with pain symptoms other than pelvic) and found specific relationships between sexual abuse and CPP as well as a general association between a violent abuse and chronic pain in general. Even with high plausibility of an association between abuse and pelvic pain syndrome, empirical evidence is rather poor[68]. Rapkin et al.[69] could not find any differences between any abuse history in patients with CPP, patients with pain in other regions, and patients without pain symptoms.

*Illness behaviour and health care utilization*

Sandler et al.[70] investigated subjects with abdominal dysfunctions who had not consulted a doctor for these and found that focusing on such symptoms is the major factor leading IBS patients to search for medical help. Greenbaum et al.[71] was the first to show that subjects with symptoms suggestive of IBS which had not consulted a doctor for these symptoms, were significantly less psychologically disturbed than their clinical counterparts. They had, however, still more psychopathological traits than patients without any symptoms. Whitehead et al.[29] and Drossman et al.[54] in the US and Heaton et al.[9] in England noted further that psychosocial factors such as those discussed above are associated with the patient status rather than with the disease per se. The main difference between consulters and nonconsulters is symptom severity[9], more experience with stressful life events[54,72] and self-reported psychological stress[29]. While some authors noted significant differences between first-time consulters and chronic health care users[73], others could not find any group differences[74]. Latimer et al.[26] finally reported that psychoneurotic control subjects showed a similar colonic myoelectrical motor pattern irrespective of pain symptoms and concluded[75] that symptom reports, nonverbal and observable behaviours, and psychological responses can be quite independent from each other, and that clinical IBS patients represent a subgroup of patients with bowel complaints, who misperceive symptoms arising from the gut or misinterpret them and cope inadequately, e.g. by consulting a physician[76]. Psychopathology may be independent from stool behaviours and abdominal symptoms, but does co-determine who will utilize the health care system. This is further supported by the fact that IBS patients more frequently consult alternative medicine remedies than patients with organic gastrointestinal disorders[77], will consult more frequently gynaecologists[78], and will undergo more laparoscopic and gynaecologic operations[79,80]. For patients with CPP the study by Mathias et al.[19] implies similar problems to those described for IBS. Of the 773 patients of a representative sample in the general population who suffered from symptoms suggestive of CPP, in 61% of cases, the diagnosis was unknown since they had not consulted a doctor. In less than 10% an endometriosis had been diagnosed. Only 25% of the patients had consulted a doctor because of this symptom during the last 3 months. Most of the patients (86%) used non-prescribed pain relievers, while 23% had prescription for pain medication and 12% used prescribed oral contraceptives.

## Conclusions

It is evident from the above referenced literature that IBS and CPP are most likely the same, rather than different, clinical entities, since similarities outnumber differences by far. If this holds true, the question why some patients go to their gynaecologist while other consult a family physician or internist cannot be attributed to symptoms and symptom characteristics alone. The fact that illness behaviours and health care utilization also show remarkable agreement between both diagnoses make the concept of individual behavioural patterns as the major factor for the choice of a medical subspecialty also highly unlikely. The fact, finally, that the diagnosis CPP does not exist in some countries, indicates that the role of the health care system itself in distributing patients to subspecialties and attributing final - and different - diagnoses to patients with similar symptoms has to be re-evaluated. Very little data exist on the contributing role of medical training, referral and reimbursement policy, health plans, and other factors on medical decision making, especially in such large populations as in patients with IBS and CPP.

Acknowledgement
This work was supported by a grant from the Deutsche Forschungsgemeinschaft, Kr 1933/1.

## *References*

1. Jones R, Lydeard S. *Irritable bowel syndrome in the general population.* Br Med J 1992;304:87-90.
2. Talley NJ, Weaver AL, Zinsmeister AR, Melton LJ III. *Onset and disappearance of gastrointestinal symptoms and functional gastrointestinal disorders.* Am J Epidemiol 1992;136:165-77.
3. Manning AP, Thompson WG, Heaton KW, Morris AF. *Towards a positive diagnosis of the irritable bowel.* Br Med J 1978;2:653-4.
4. Drossman DA, Richter JE, Talley NJ et al., editors. *The functional gastrointestinal disorders. Diagnosis, pathophysiology, and treatment. A multinational consensus.* Boston: Little Brown; 1994.
5. Talley NJ, Zinsmeister AR, Van Dyke C, Melton LJ III. *Epidemiology of colonic symptoms and the irritable bowel syndrome.* Gastroenterology 1991;101:927-34.
6. Drossman DA, Li Z, Andreuzzi E et al. *U.S. householder survey on functional gastrointestinal disorders.* Dig Dis Sci 1993;38:1569-80.

7. Kay L, Jorgensen T, Jensen KH. *The epidemiology of irritable bowel syndrome in a random population: prevalence, incidence, natural history and risk factors.* J Int Med 1994;236:23-30.
8. Sandler RS. *Epidemiology of irritable bowel syndrome in the United States.* Gastroenterology 1990;99:409-15.
9. Heaton KW, O'Donnell LJD, Braddon FEM, et al. *Symptoms of irritable bowel syndrome in a British urban community: consulters and nonconsulters.* Gastroenterology 1992;102:1962-7.
10. Talley NJ, O'Keefe EA, Zinsmeister AR, Melton LJ III. *Prevalence of gastrointestinal symptoms in the elderly: a population-based study.* Gastroenterology 1992;102:895-901.
11. Drossman DA, Sandler RS, McKee DC, Lovitz AJ. *Bowel patterns among subjects not seeking health care. Use of a questionnaire to identify a population with bowel dysfunction.* Gastroenterology 1982;83:529-34.
12. Thompson WG, Heaton KW. *Functional bowel disorders in apparently healthy people.* Gastroenterology 1980;79:283-8.
13. Everhardt JE, Renault PF. *Irritable bowel syndrome in office-based practice in the United States.* Gastroenterology 1991;100:998-1005.
14. Rathmann W, Haastern B, Giani G. *Arzneimittelverordnungen und Kosten bei Patienten mit Colon irritabile in algemeinärztlichen und internistischen Praxen in Deutschland: eine Pilotstudie* (unveröffentlichtes Manuskript); 1998.
15. Agreus L, Svärdsudd K, Nyren O, Tibblin G. *Irritable bowel syndrome and dyspepsia in the general population: overlap and lack of stability over time.* Gastroenterology 1995;109:671-80.
16. Reiter RC. *A profile of women with chronic pelvic pain.* Clin Obstet Gynecol 1990;33:130-6.
17. Vercellini P, Fedele P, Molteni P, et al. *Laparoscopy in the diagnosis of gynecologic pelvic pain.* Int J Gyn Obstet 1990;32:261-5.
18. Reiter RC, Gambone JC. *Nongynecologic somatic pathology in women with chronic pelvic pain and negative laparoscopy.* J Reprod Med 1991;36:253-9.
19. Mathias SD, Kuppermann M, Liberman RF, et al. *Chronic pelvic pain: prevalence, health-related quality of life, and economic correlates.* Obstet Gynecol 1996;87:321-7.
20. Longstreth GF. *Irritable bowel syndrome and chronic pelvic pain.* Obstet Gynecol Surv 1994;49:505-7.
21. Walker EA, Gelfand AN, Gelfand MD, et al. *Chronic pelvic pain and gynecological symptoms in women with irritable bowel syndrome.* J Psychosom Obstet Gynaecol 1996;17:39-46.

22. Hislop IG. *Psychological significance of the irritable colon syndrome.* Gut 1971;12:452-7.
23. Hill DW, Blendis L. *Physical and psychological evaluation of 'non-organic' abdominal pain.* Gut 1967;8:221-9.
24. Liss JL, Alpers D, Woodruff RA. *The irritable colon syndrome and psychiatric illness.* Dis Nervous System 1973;34:151-7.
25. Young SJ, Alpers DH, Norland CC, Woodruff RA. *Psychiatric illness and the irritable bowel syndrome: practical implications for the primary physician.* Gastroenterology 1976;70:162-6.
26. Latimer P, Sarna S, Campbell D, et al. *Colonic motor and myoelectrical activity: a comparative study of normal subjects, psychoneurotic patients, and patients with irritable bowel syndrome.* Gastroenterology 1981;80:893-901.
27. Wise TM, Cooper JN, Ahmed S. *The efficacy of group therapy for patients with irritable bowel syndrome.* Psychosomatics 1982;23:465-9.
28. Whitehead WE, Engel BT, Schuster MM. *Irritable bowel syndrome: physiological and psychological differences between diarrhea-predominant and constipation-predominant patients.* Dig Dis Sci 1980;25:404-13.
29. Whitehead WE, Bosmajian L, Zonderman AB, et al. *Symptoms of psychologic distress associated with irritable bowel syndrome.* Gastroenterology 1988;95:709-14.
30. Enck P, Whitehead WE, Schuster MM, Wienbeck M. *Psychosomatik des Reizdarms. Spezifität klinischer Symptome, psychopathologischer Merkmale und motorischer Aktivität im Rektosigmoid.* Dtsch Med Wschr 1988;113:459-62.
31. Enck P, Whitehead WE, Schuster MM, Wienbeck M. *Klinische Symptomatik, Psychopathologie und Darmmotilität bei Patienten mit "irritablem Darm".* Z Gastroenterol 1989;27:357-61.
32. Rose JDR, Throughton AH, Harvey JS, Smith PM. *Depression and functional bowel disorders in gastrointestinal outpatients.* Gut 1986;27:1025-8.
33. Toner BB, Garfinkel PE, Jeejeebhoy KN, et al. *Self-schema in irritable bowel syndrome and depression.* Psychosom Med 1990;52:149-55.
34. West KL. *MMPI correlates of ulcerative colitis.* J Clin Psychol 1970;26:214-9.
35. Bergeron CM, Monto GL. *Personality patterns seen in irritable bowel syndrome patients.* Am J Gastroenterol 1985;80:448-51.
36. Talley NJ, Phillips SF, Bruce B, et al. *Relation among personality and symptoms in nonulcer dyspepsia and irritable bowel syndrome.* Gastroenterology 1990;99:327-3.
37. Richter JE, Obrecht WF, Bradley LA, et al. *Psychological comparison of patients with nutcracker esophagus and irritable bowel syndrome.* Dig Dis Sci 1988;31:131-8.
38. Esler MD, Gouldston KJ. *Levels of anxiety in colonic disorders.* N Engl J Med 1973;288:16-20.

39. Palmer RL, Stonehill E, Crisp AH, et al. *Psychological characteristics of patients with the irritable bowel syndrome.* Postgrad Med J 1974;50:416-9.
40. Walker FA, Katon WJ, Hansom J et al. *Medical and psychiatric symptoms in women with childhood sexual abuse.* Psychosom Med 1992;54:658-64.
41. Gross RJ, Doerr H, Caldirola D, et al. *Borderline syndrome and incest in chronic pelvic pain patients.* Int J Psychiat Med 1980-81;10:79-98.
42. Wurm B, Heel G, Karpellus, et al. *Der chronische Beckenschmerz bei Frauen - eine soziopsychosomatische Verlaufsuntersuchung.* In: Söllner W, Wesiack W, Wurm B, editors. Sozio-psycho-somatik. Gesellschaftliche Entwicklung und psychosomatische Medizin. Berlin, New York: Springer; 1989;229-37.
43. Kantner J, Söllner W, Rumplmair W, et al. *Schmerzen im Unterleib.* Sexualmedizin 1992;21:256-65.
44. Gidro-Frank L, Gordon Th, Taylor H. *Pelvic pain and female identity: a survey of emotional factors in forty patients.* Am J Obstet Gynecol 1960;79:1184-202.
45. Pevler R, Edwards J, Daddow J, Thomas E. *Psychosocial factors and chronic pelvic pain: a comparison of women with endometriosis and with unexplained pain.* J Psychosom Res 1996;40:305-15.
46. Hodgkis AD, Watson JP. *Psychiatric morbidity and illness behaviour in women with chronic pelvic pain.* J Psychosom Res 1994;38:3-9.
47. Renaer M. *Chronic pelvic pain without obvious pathology in women.* Eur J Obstet Gynecol Reprod Biol 1980;10:415-63.
48. Bockus HL, Bank J, Wilkinson SA. *Neurogenic mucous colitis.* Am J Med Sci 1928;176:813-29.
49. White BV, Jones CM. *Mucous colitis: a delineation of the syndrome with certain observations on its mechanism and on the role of emotional tension as a precipitating factor.* Ann Int Med 1940;14:854-72.
50. Chaudhary NA, Truelove SC. *The irritable colon syndrome: a study of the clinical features, predisposing causes and prognosis in 130 cases.* Quart J Med 1962;31:307-23.
51. Hislop IG. *Childhood deprivation: an antecedent of the irritable bowel syndrome.* Med J Aust 1979;1:372-4.
52. Mendeloff AI, Monk M, Siegel CI, Lilienfeld A. *Illness experience and life stresses in patients with irritable colon and with ulcerative colitis. An epidemiologic study of ulcerative colitis and regional enteritis in Baltimore, 1960-1964.* N Engl J Med 1970;282:14-7.
53. Fava GA, Pavan L. *Large bowel disorders I. Illness configuration and life events.* Psychother Psychosom 1976;27:93-9.
54. Drossman D, McKee DC, Sandler RS, et al. *Psychosocial factors in the irritable bowel syndrome. A multivariate study of patients and nonpatients with irritable bowel syndrome.* Gastroenterology 1988;95:701-8.

55. Whitehead WE, Crowell MD, Robinson JC, et al. *Effects of stressful life events on bowel symptoms: subjects with irritable bowel syndrome compared with subjects without bowel dysfunction.* Gut 1992;33:825-30.
56. Ford MJ, Miller PMC, Eastwood J, Eastwood MA. *Life events, psychiatric illness and the irritable bowel syndrome.* Gut 1987;28:160-5.
57. Castelnuovo-Tedesco P, Krout BM. *Psychosomatic aspects of chronic pelvic pain.* Psychosom Med 1970;1:109-26.
58. Beard R, Reginald PH, Pearce SH. *Psychological and somatic factors in women with pain due to pelvic congestion.* Adv Exp Med Biol 1988;245:413-21.
59. Drossman DA, Leserman J, Nachman G, et al. *Sexual and physical abuse in women with functional or organic gastrointestinal disorders.* Ann Int Med 1990;113:828-33.
60. Longstreth GF, Shragg GP. *Irritable bowel syndrome and childhood abuse in HMO health examinees.* Gastroenterology 1992;102:A477.
61. Talley NJ, Fett SL, Zinsmeister AR, Melton LJ.III. *Gastrointestinal tract symptoms and self-reported abuse: a population-based study.* Gastroenterology 1994;107:1040-9.
62. Delvaux M, Denis P, Allemand H, et al. *Sexual abuse is more frequently reported by IBS patients than by patients with organic digestive diseases or controls. Results of a multicentre inquiry.* Eur J Gastroenterol Hepatol 1997;9:345-52.
63. Toomey TC, Seville JL, Mann JD, et al. *Relationship of sexual and physical abuse to pain description, coping, psychological distress, and health-care utilization in a chronic pain sample.* Clin J Pain 1995;11:307-15.
64. Peters AA, Van Dorst E, Jellis B et al. *A randomized clinical trial to compare two different approaches in women with chronic pelvic pain.* Obstet Gynecol 1991;77:740-4.
65. Walker EA, Katon WJ, Hansom J et al. *Psychiatric diagnoses and sexual victimization in women with chronic pelvic pain.* Psychosomatics 1995;36:531-40.
66. Walling MK, O'Hara MW, Reiter RC, et al. *Abuse history and chronic pain in women: I. Prevalences of sexual abuse and physical abuse.* Obstet Gynecol 1994;84:193-9.
67. Walling MK, Reiter RC, O'Hara MW, et al. *Abuse history and chronic pain in women: II. A multivariate analysis of abuse and psychological morbidity.* Obstet Gynecol 1994;84:200-6.
68. Howard FM. *Abuse history and chronic pain in women: I. Prevalences of sexual abuse and physical abuse.* [letter]Obstet Gynecol 1995;85:158-9.
69. Rapkin AJ, Kames L, Darke L, et al. *History of physical and sexual abuse in women with chronic pelvic pain.* Obstet Gynecol 1990;76:92-6.
70. Sandler RS, Drossman DA, Nathan HP, McKee DC. *Symptom complaints and health care seeking behavior in subjects with bowel dysfunction.* Gastroenterology 1984;87:314-8.
71. Greenbaum D, Abitz L, VanEgeren L, et al. *Irritable bowel syndrome prevalence, rectosigmoid motility, and psychosomatics in symptomatic subjects not seeing physicians.* Gastroenterology 1984;86:1174.

72. Smith RC, Greenbaum DS, Vancouver JB, et al. *Psychosocial factors are associated with health care seeking rather than diagnosis in irritable bowel syndrome.* Gastroenterology 1990;98:293-301.
73. Guthrie E, Creed FH, Whorwell PJ, Tomenson B. *Outpatients with irritable bowel syndrome: a comparison of first time and chronic attenders.* Gut 1992;33:361-3.
74. Welch GW, Hillman LC, Pomare EW. *Psychoneurotic symptomatology in the irritable bowel syndrome: a study of reporters and non-reporters.* Br Med J 1985;291:1382-4.
75. Latimer P. *Colonic psychophysiology. Implications for functional bowel disorders.* In: Hoelzl R, Whitehead WE, editors. Psychophysiology of the gastrointestinal tract. New York: Plenum Press; 1983;263-88.
76. Whitehead WE, Winget C, Fedoravicius AS, et al. *Learned illness behavior in patients with irritable bowel syndrome and peptic ulcer.* Dig Dis Sci 1982;79:283-8.
77. Smart HL, Mayberry JF, Atkinson M. *Alternative medicine consultations and remedies in patients with the irritable bowel syndrome.* Gut 1986;27:826-8.
78. Prior A, Whorwell PJ. *Gynaecological consultation in patients with the irritable bowel syndrome.* Gut 1989;30:996-8.
79. Longstreth GF, Preskill DB, Youkeles L. *Irritable bowel syndrome in women having diagnostic laparoscopy or hysterectomy.* Dig Dis Sci 1990;35:1285-90.
80. Prior A, Stanley KM, Smith ARB, Read NW. *Relation between hysterectomy and the irritable bowel: a prospective study.* Gut 1992;33:814-7.

*ADDRESS FOR CORRESPONDENCE*

**ENCK P, PhD**
Universitätsklinikum Tübingen
Abt. Allg. Chirurgie - Forschungsbereich
Zentrum Medizinische Forschung (ZMF)
Waldhörnlestr. 22
72072 Tübingen Germany
Fax: +49 7071 29 5142
E-mail: paul.enck@uni-tuebingen.de

# PSYCHOSOCIAL ASSESSMENT OF CHRONIC GASTROINTESTINAL DISORDERS

*FH Creed*

The psychosocial assessment of patients with chronic gastrointestinal (GI) disorders will be illustrated by reference to patients with chronic Irritable Bowel Syndrome (IBS). These patients may be compared with patients who have a) more typical IBS, and b) Inflammatory Bowel Disease (IBD) with concurrent psychiatric disorder. Such patients may prove difficult to manage in clinical practice; they illustrate some of the processes which may be active in patients of all types with chronic GI disorders.

### *Chronic IBS*

In their original description of irritable colon syndrome, Chaudhury and Truelove[1] observed that patients whose IBS symptoms persisted (over two years) were less likely to have had a dysenteric illness at the onset of the IBS and they experienced psychological difficulties. Harvey et al.[2] found that a chronic disorder was associated with a long history when first seen, female sex, absence of an infective illness at onset and to experience diarrhoea more than constipation. A comparison of persistent clinic attenders and recent attending IBS patients[3] indicated differences between the two groups in the following dimensions: severity of bowel and non-colonic symptoms, type of pain, degree and duration of disability.

Psychosocial assessment is, therefore, aimed at identifying the psychological factors which may contribute to this chronic illness pattern.

### *Organic GI disorders and psychiatric disorder*

To illustrate the importance of psychosocial factors in chronic disorders of organic origin, reference will be made to patients with IBD, who also have concurrent psychiatric disorder. Compared to IBD patients without a psychiatric disorder, those with anxiety/depression had a greater number of psychiatric symptoms, more GI and non-GI symptoms, were more likely to be female. They were also much more likely to have experienced childhood abuse, show fear and dissociation as personality traits. Treatment of the depression led to an improvement in several aspects of disability[4].

This chapter will review these dimensions, which distinguish chronic from more short-lived bowel disorders and explore psychosocial dimensions which may help to explain these differences. There are three central concepts: numerous medically unexplained symptoms, disability, somatic presentation of anxiety/depression and hypochondriacal illness worry. Each of these will be considered in turn.

## Number and characteristics of symptoms

By comparison with recent attenders with IBS, chronic clinic attenders had a pattern of illness that was "severe over many years" in 24% of patients and "constantly severe for many months" in 16% compared to corresponding figures of 8% and 5% for recent clinic attenders[3].

The GI symptoms were described as severe or very severe by the chronic attenders (compared to recent attenders) as follows: abdominal pain (61.5% vs 10%), abdominal distension (63.5% vs 2%), constipation (54% vs 1%).

Non-GI symptoms were also reported as severe or very severe: backache (34.5% vs 4%), headaches (23.5% vs 1%), premenstrual tension (31% vs 10%) and lethargy (55.7% vs 6.2%).

By contrast, there were no significant differences in type and severity of bowel symptoms: number of bowel actions per day, consistency of stool, site of abdominal pain. Similar findings were reported in the comparison of IBD patients with and without psychiatric disorder: medically unexplained symptoms were significantly more common (6.5 vs 2.5) in the IBD patients with psychiatric disorder. This difference held for GI and non-GI symptoms (2.6 vs 0.7 and 5.5 vs 2.1, respectively)[4]. Such differences indicate a marked difference in symptom reporting style; this may reflect comorbid anxiety/depression and/or may be regarded as one aspect of illness behaviour (see below).

## Psychiatric disorder-Anxiety and depression

In the Guthrie et al. study, there was no significant difference in the overall prevalence of psychiatric disorder between recent and chronic attenders with IBS (45.4% vs 49%, respectively). However, chronic attenders were more likely to have depression, indicating a more severe psychiatric disorder. This is a very important finding as depression is a treatable disorder.

By definition, IBD patients with a current psychiatric disorder reported a greater number of anxiety symptoms (13.7 vs 6.7) and the presence of the psychiatric disorder was associated with increased disability and certain personality features (see below).

The symptoms of anxiety and depressive disorders are well known to most doctors. The diagnostic criteria have been published in the Diagnostic and Statistical Manual of Mental Disorders: DSM IV[5].

*Somatising and factitious disorders*

In addition to anxiety and depressive disorders, the gastroenterologist should be aware of a diagnostic category "somatoform disorders". The somatoform disorders are characterized by a number of abnormal illness behaviours:

- disability disproportionate to detectable disease
- a relentless search for causes and cures
- adoption of lifestyle around the sick role, with a repertoire of passive plus aggressive behaviours to sustain the sick role, and avoidance of healthy roles due to lack of skills or fear of failure
- reinforcement of sick role by family, disability payments and, possibly, health care providers.

There are a number of factors which lead to such behaviours. Firstly, the patient may have marked personality problems and there may also be current relationship difficulties. There may have been a history of prolonged illness during childhood (either in the patient themselves or their parents) and/or a history of lack of parental care during childhood[6]. There may also be current depressive illnesses which exacerbate the somatizing syndrome.

## Disability

Chronic attenders with IBS had dramatically different patterns of disability from recent attenders[3]. The proportion who reported severe

limitations in each domain (compared to recent attenders) were: work/housework (38.5% vs 2.1%), social life (25% vs 1%), housebound (27% vs 0%), mood state (21 vs 2%), and irritability (17.5% vs 2%).
In the Walker et al. study, patients with IBD with current psychiatric disorder showed significantly lower scores (i.e., more disabled) in terms of physical, role and emotional function as well as reduced vitality and health perception. Vitality and role function changed significantly with antidepressant treatment; physical and emotional function also improved[4].

## Personality

IBD patients with psychiatric disorder were noted to have significantly different responses to a personality questionnaire indicating fear and avoidance of harm, but also a tendency to develop somatic symptoms when under stress, without awareness of the psychological disturbance (dissociation)[4]. This personality pattern may be related to difficult circumstances during childhood, including abuse, which has been associated with severe IBS[7,8].
The psychological measures used in patients with chronic GI disorders can be classified into the following areas:

1. personality traits
2. psychiatric symptoms
3. illness attitudes and beliefs.

*Personality traits*
Personality measures in chronic GI disorders include the Minnesota Multiphasic Personality Inventory (MMPI) and Eysenck Personality Inventory (EPI). The former can be profoundly distorted by a disabling illness because items such as inability to work and sleep loss are interpreted as symptoms of depression when they may equally be due to the disabling effect of a physical illness[9]. A number of studies have demonstrated that IBS clinic patients are more neurotic and anxious in their personality than people without health problems or a non-clinical population with organic bowel disorders (for details see Drossman et al.[10]). A raised neuroticism score on the EPI is common in chronic GI

disorders but may simply reflect chronic symptoms, which limits the usefulness of measuring personality in chronic GI disorders.

*Psychiatric symptoms*

Scores on scales such as Speilberger State Anxiety Inventory and Middlesex Hospital Questionnaire demonstrate higher scores in chronic GI disorder patients but these findings are not confined to this patient group - other medical patient groups show elevated levels of depression, anxiety and somatisation, which may reflect the distress associated with many disorders[11].

The common scales used in chronic GI disorders include the General Health Questionnaire (GHQ)[12], which provides a measure of psychiatric symptoms as a whole and the Hospital Anxiety and Depression Scale (HADS) which provides a score for anxiety and depression separately; it may be particularly useful in this population as it specifically excludes items concerning bodily symptoms - it was designed for use in medical populations. The Beck Depression Inventory (BDI) is a measure of severity of depression alone. Each of these scales has an accepted "cut-off" score above which the patient has probably anxiety or depression. Such scales are very useful in clinical practice as they help the clinician to identify patients with anxiety and/or depression, which may improve with specific treatment.

*Abnormal illness attitudes and beliefs*

The way that a person responds to his/her functional bowel symptoms, especially in relation to medical treatment-seeking is determined primarily by the patient's attitude towards their symptoms. It is well recognised that patients attending a pain clinic may show abnormal illness behaviours. Two scales have been developed in the pain clinic and used in other patient groups-the Illness Behaviour Questionnaire (IBQ)[13] and Illness Attitude Scale (IAS)[14].

Examples of the items that make up the hypochondriacal beliefs, disease phobia and bodily pre-occupation scales of the IAS are: "Do you believe that you have a physical disease but the doctors have not diagnosed it correctly?" "When your doctor tells you that you have no physical disease, do you refuse to believe him?" "Are you afraid that you have cancer/another serious illness?" "If you feel unwell and someone tells you that you are looking well do you get annoyed?".

Patients with chronic gastro-intestinal disorders may have abnormal scores on the IBQ as a result of comorbid anxiety and depressive disorders[15]. This is important because it indicates that patients who have anxiety/depressive disorders worry more about their illness, are more convinced that there is an organic cause and see it in somatic (rather than psychological) terms compared to patients who have organic GI disorders.

The clinician should always ask patients with chronic GI disorders what they think their illness is due to and what they fear the symptoms represent - i.e., explore illness beliefs. Normal investigation results may not reassure patients - open discussion between doctor and patient is much more likely to be successful in correcting hypochondriacal beliefs, disease phobia and bodily pre-occupation.

## Rationale for a psychosocial assessment in the gastroenterology clinic

Owens et al.[16] assessed the quality of the physician/patient interaction at the first appointment with functional bowel disorder and noted fewer return visits in those patients for whom the doctor had documented in the notes:

1. the patient's psychosocial history
2. notation of a factor or factors that precipitated the patients seeking medical help
3. notation of discussion with the patient about test results and diagnosis.

Following a satisfactory consultation with a gastroenterologist, Van Dulmen et al.[17] found a significant reduction in the patient's:

- overall state anxiety
- fear of having cancer
- pre-occupation and helplessness in relation to the pain.

These should be the aims of the consultation with the doctor of patients with chronic GI disorders.

*Response to antidepressants and psychological treatment*

Lydiard et al.[18] and Noyes et al.[19] showed a significant improvement in bowel symptoms concurrent with improved anxiety when patients were treated with psychotropic medication. Greenbaum et al.[20] had found that reduction of depression was associated with improvement of diarrhoea. Studies using psychological treatments[21,22] have illustrated that improved anxiety and depression is highly correlated with improved bowel symptoms, suggesting that anxiety and depression are very closely linked to the bowel symptoms. For these reasons, the gastroenterologist must search hard for clues of a treatable psychiatric disorder in chronic GI patients.

In the GI clinic, patients with chronic GI disorders need to be assessed along the following dimensions:

- number of non-GI symptoms
- psychological distress, including the possible presence of an anxiety or depressive disorder
- personality dimensions - a possible life-long tendency to worry including long-standing excessive concerns about the significance of the gut and other bodily symptoms, and habitual response to stress
- abnormal illness attitudes and behaviours.

Each of these requires assessment in its own right as well as assessment of the bowel symptoms. This can be achieved briefly if the patient is asked:

1. "When did you last feel quite well?"
2. "What do you think your symptoms are due to?"
3. "Do you worry a lot about them?"
4. "Have you had pain or discomfort in other parts of your body?"
5. "Have you been very worried or down recently?"

These questions will demonstrate to the patient that the gastroenterologist is as interested in psychological aspects of the patient's disorder as well as the bowel symptomatology.

They will also help the gastroenterologist to decide if referral to a psychologist or psychiatrist is required. This is usually indicated when the gastroenterologist:

- believes that the patient has a psychiatric disorder which requires assessment and treatment
- discovers that the patient is seriously depressed and/or has suicidal ideas
- needs advice regarding the use of psychotropic drugs (e.g., antidepressants in chronic pain)
- finds serious impairment of social functioning that cannot be explained by the functional gut disorder
- believes the patient shows chronic somatization with multiple referrals to many different departments
- uncovers a history of sexual abuse, or other major trauma, which requires more specialized psychological treatment than the gastroenterologist and GP can offer[23].

## Conclusions

The patient with a GI disorder provides the gastroenterologist with a special problem[24]. The form of assessment outlined above

- provides a framework for assessment of a possible anxiety/depressive disorder, which commonly accompany chronic symptoms
- acknowledges (repeatedly if necessary) the reality of the pain
- assesses excessive illness behaviour.

Following such assessment, management of the psychological aspects of the person's problems can complement the treatment for the GI symptoms to optimise outcome.

### *REFERENCES*

1. Chaudhury NA, Truelove SC. *Irritable colon syndrome. A study of the clinical features. Predisposing causes, and prognosis in 130 cases.* Quart J Med 1962;31:307-22.

2. Harvey RF, Manad EC, Brown AM. *Prognosis in the irritable bowel syndrome: a 5 year prospective study.* Lancet 1987;i:963-5.
3. Guthrie E, Creed FH, Whorwell PK. *Outpatients with irritable bowel syndrome: a comparison of first time and chronic attenders.* Gut 1992;33:361-3.
4. Walker EA, Gelfand MD, Gelfand AN, et al. *The relationship of current psychiatric disorder to functional disability and distress in patients with inflammatory bowel disease.* Gen Hosp Psychiatry 1996;18:220-9.
5. *Diagnostic and Statistical Manual of Mental Disorders*: DSM IV, 4th Ed. Washington; American Psychiatric Association, 1994.
6. Craig TK, Boardman AP, Mills K, et al. *The South London somatisation study. I: Longitudinal course and the influence of early life experiences.* Br J Psychiatry 1993; 163:579-88.
7. Longstreth GF, Wolde-Tsadik G. *Irritable bowel-type symptoms in HMO Examinees. Prevalence, demographics and clinical correlates.* Dig Dis Sci 1993;38:1581-9.
8. Drossman DD, Zhiming L, Leserman J, et al. *Health status by gastrointestinal diagnosis and abuse history.* Gastroenterology 1996;110:999-1007.
9. Pincus T, Callahan LF, Bradley LA, et al. *Elevated MMPI scores for hypochondriasis, depression, and hysteria in patients with rheumatoid arthritis reflect disease rather than psychological status.* Arthr Rheum 1986;29:1456-66.
10. Drossman DA, Creed FH, Fava GA, et al. *Psychosocial aspects of the functional gastrointestinal disorders.* Gastroenterol Int 1995;8(2):47-90.
11. Palmer RL, Stonehill E, Crisp AH, et al. *Psychological characteristics of patients with the irritable bowel syndrome.* Postgrad Med J 1974;50:416-9.
12. Goldberg D. *Use of the general health questionnaire in clinical work.* Br Med J 1986;293:1188-9.
13. Pilowsky I, Spence ND. *Manual for the illness behaviour questionnaire (IBQ).* 2nd ed. Adelaide: University Adelaide; 1983.
14. Kellner R. *Abridged manual of the illness attitude scale.* Albuquerque: University of New Mexico; 1983.
15. Colgan S, Creed FH, Klass H. *Symptom complaints, psychiatric disorder and abnormal illness behaviour in patients with upper abdominal pain.* Psychol Med 1988;18:887-92.
16. Owens DM, Nelson DK, Talley NJ. *The irritable bowel syndrome: long-term prognosis and the physician-patient interaction.* Ann Int Med 1995;122:107-12.
17. Van Dulmen AM, Fennis JFM, Mokkink HGA, et al. *Doctor-dependent changes in complaint-related cognitions and anxiety during medical consultations in functional abdominal complaints.* Psychol Med 1995;25:1011-8.

18. Lydiard RB, Laraia MT, Howell EF, et al. *Can panic disorder present as irritable bowel syndrome?* J Clin Psychiatry 1986;57:470-3.
19. Noyes R, Cook B, Garvey M, et al. *Reduction of gastrointestinal symptoms with treatment for panic disorder.* Psychosomatics 1990;31:75-9.
20. Greenbaum D, Mayle JE, Vanegeran LE, et al. *Effects of desipramine on irritable bowel syndrome compared with atropine and placebo.* Dig Dis Sci 1987;32:257-66.
21. Guthrie E, Creed FH, Dawson D, Tomenson B. *A controlled trial of psychological treatment for the irritable bowel syndrome.* Gastroenterology 1991;100:450-7.
22. Rumsey N. *Group stress management versus pharmacological treatment in the irritable bowel syndrome.* In: Heaton K, Creed F, Goeting N, editors. Towards confident management of irritable bowel syndrome. Duphas Laboratories Ltd; 1991.
23. Goldberg DP, Benjamin S, Creed F. *Psychiatry in medical practice.* 2nd ed. London and New York: Routledge; 1994.
24. Drossman DA, Thompson WG. *The irritable bowel syndrome: review and a graduated, multicomponent treatment approach.* Ann Int Med 1992;116:1009-16.

### *ADDRESS FOR CORRESPONDENCE*

**CREED FH, MD, FRCP, FRCPsych**
Rawnsley Building, Manchester Royal Infirmary
Oxford RD
Manchester M13 9WL United Kingdom
Fax: +44 161 273 2135

# THE PHYSICIAN-PATIENT RELATIONSHIP

*DA Drossman*

Most of us involved with investigating the chronic or functional Gastrointestinal (GI) disorders, are also responsible for caring for patients with these conditions. At times, physicians feel "at odds" with this relationship, because of time constraints, dissatisfaction with the course of treatment, or merely the sense that they are not "connecting"[1,2]. This may relate to difficulties in establishing an effective physician-patient relationship. I would like to offer a few suggestions that may help improve this relationship and possibly lead to greater satisfaction, and a better clinical outcome. My comments, directed primarily to gastroenterologists and other medical physicians, could also apply to psychiatrists, psychologists and other health personnel. Additional information relating to building a more effective physician-patient relationship can be found elsewhere[2-7].

It is helpful to consider that certain comments made to reassure patients with functional GI disorders (e.g., "Don't worry, its nothing serious", or "Your problem is due to stress"), can "backfire" simply because the patient perceives his/her illness differently. Patients see that it is serious, and do not consider it to be caused by stress. Also, the physicians' comments may be viewed by patients as diminishing what they see as "real" problems.

The solution to these occurrences is not accomplished by trying harder to convince the patient what is "right" (or, alternatively, by dismissing the patient as "difficult"). Rather, the effort involves clarifying and accepting the patient's perspective on each issue, and engaging in a dialog to reach a common understanding and set of goals. This has been called the "patient-centered" approach[4,8]. Listed below are suggestions to implement this approach.

***Listen actively*** Clinical data are obtained not by a passive transfer of information, but through an active process of listening, observing and facilitating. Patients do not always tell us what they mean, and physicians do not always hear what they tell us. All of us can remember the student presenting a clinical case, and then when personally obtaining the history, getting a completely different story. While it is easy to assume that the patient is a "bad historian", the problem may exist more in how the information is obtained. Understanding the patient's story also involves integrating features such as the tone of voice, facial expressions, body movements and postural changes as well as the content itself. When in doubt, it helps to restate the information obtained back to the patient for clarification, and this reaffirms the physician's commitment to hear the patient.

*Be aware of questioning style and non-verbal messages* It has been said: "It's not what you say, but how you say it that makes the difference", and that certainly applies in communicating with patients. Table 1 gives examples of several behaviors that either facilitate or inhibit the acquisition of data from the patient. In general, the physician wants to communicate nonjudgmental interest in an environment of comfort, support and security.

*Identify the agenda(s)* Patients may have concerns and expectations that are different from that of their health care providers. They may be coming to the doctor for fear of cancer, because of less ability to function or manage the symptoms, or fear of a psychiatric diagnosis ("Am I crazy?"). The doctor may be approaching the issue of diagnosis and treatment or whether to refer the patient. So, in addition to the important issues of diagnosis and treatment, the doctor must also:

- elicit the patient's agenda
- communicate his or her agenda
- work toward a mutually specified set of goals.

When the problem relates to a GI bleed or acute diarrhea, the issues are usually clear, but with chronic functional disorders, negotiation becomes more important. For example, even with years of chronic pain, patients may expect the physician to diagnose a specific disease and effect a cure. But the doctor's agenda should be to help the patient accept and cope with the pain.

## Behaviors influencing accurate data collection

| **Behavior** | **Facilitates** | **Inhibits** |
|---|---|---|
| **Nonverbal** | | |
| • Clinical environment | • Private, comfortable | • Noisy, physical barriers |
| • Eye contact | • Frequent | • Infrequent or constant |
| • Body posture | • Direct, open, relaxed | • Body turned, arms folded |
| • Head nodding | • Helpful if well timed | • Infrequent, excessive |
| • Body proximity | • Close enough to touch | • Too close or too distant |
| • Facial expression | • Interest, empathy, understanding | • Preoccupation, boredom, disapproval |
| • Touching | • Helpful when used to communicate empathy | • Insincere if not appropriate or properly timed |
| **Verbal** | | |
| • Question forms | • Open ended to generate hypotheses | • Rigid or stereotyped style |
| | • Closed ended to test hypotheses | • Multiple choice or leading questions (*"You didn't...?"*) |
| • Question style | • Use of patient's words | • Use of unfamiliar words |
| | • Fewer questions and interruptions | • More |
| | • Nonjudgmental | • Judgmental |
| | • Follows lead of patient's earlier responses | • Follows preset agenda or style |
| | • Use a narrative thread | • HPI → PMH → ROS → Psych |
| | • Appropriate use of silence | • Frequent interruptions |
| | • Appropriate reassurance | • Premature or unwarranted reassurance |
| | • Elicits pertinent psychosocial data in a sensitive and skillful manner | • Ignores psychosocial data or uses "probes" |

**HPI** History of Present Illness **PMH** Past Medical History **ROS** Review Of Systems **Psych** Psychosocial history

Table 1

*Acknowledge the pain-Empathy* The physician provides empathy by demonstrating an understanding of the patients pain and distress, while maintaining an objective and observant stance. An empathic statement would be: "I can see how difficult it has been for you to manage with your pain". Providing empathy improves patient satisfaction and adherence to treatment.

*Validate the patients feelings* When patients disclose personally meaningful information, they may experience shame or embarrassment. So, the physician needs to validate the patient's feelings, rather than make personal judgments or close the communication by a quick reassurance or solution.

*Do not overreact* Circumstances may lead some patients to interact in ways that are perceived as dependent, demanding or adversarial. Frequent phone calls or visits for narcotics, disability, or diagnostic studies are examples. Physicians may "overreact" by getting angry, doing unnecessary studies or overmedicating. It helps to address these behaviors as ineffective communications rather than patient problems, and to "tune in" on inner thoughts and feelings (e.g., "What is it about this patient's behavior that makes me feel frustrated?") before acting impulsively.

*Educate* Rather than just giving information, education involves several steps:

- eliciting the patient's understanding;
- addressing misunderstandings,
- providing information that is consistent with the patient's frame of reference or knowledge base, and
- checking the patient's understanding of what was discussed.

For example, with functional GI disorders, it helps to explain that the symptoms are real, and are caused by abnormal or increased responses in gut motility and/or gut sensitivity to dietary or hormonal (e.g., menses) factors, or stresses that can occur in everyone. A diagram of the gate control mechanism, can be used to illustrate how the brain can modify pain. So, intense concentration like playing sports can "close the gate" and decrease pain, while psychological distress (e.g., hassles at work, losing a loved one) "opens the gate", and increases pain. This approach provides an acceptable framework for using antidepressants or psychological treatments.

***Reassure*** Patients also need to be reassured: they fear serious disease or surgery, and may feel helpless with their condition. To reassure, the physician should:

1. identify the patient's worries and concerns
2. acknowledge or validate them
3. respond to their specific concerns, and
4. avoid "false" reassurances (e.g., "Don't worry, everything's fine") particularly before the medical evaluation is complete, since the patient may view this as a doctor's lack of commitment.

For example, for the patient with IBS who is worried about an underlying cancer, the physician might say: "I can understand your concern about the possibility of cancer. However, the symptoms you have, and the results of the studies are typical for irritable bowel syndrome, and this does not turn into cancer. If new symptoms develop we'll address them, and when you turn 50 (even if you don't have symptoms), we'll also begin the recommended screening program for polyps and early cancer".

***Negotiate*** The patient and physician must mutually agree on the treatment. This is done after an adequate evaluation is performed, and with the patient's full understanding of the condition. The physician should then ask about the patient's personal experience, understanding and interests in various treatments, and then provide choices (rather than directives) that are consistent with the patient's beliefs. Simply stated, if the patient doesn't believe that stress causes symptom exacerbation, then stress reduction techniques won't work. However, if the treatment options can be related to the patient's symptom experience, then the patient will be more accepting. Negotiation is particularly important in certain situations such as recommending an antidepressant (which may be viewed as a "psychiatric" drug rather than a centrally acting analgesic), or when referring to a psychologist for pain management techniques.

*Help the patient take responsibility* Patients need to actively participate in their health care, and this can be communicated in several ways. For example, rather than asking the patient: "How is your pain?", one might say: "How are you managing with your symptoms?". The former question tends to leave the responsibility for dealing with the pain with the physician, while the latter acknowledges the patient's role. Other methods include using a diary, so the patient can identify exacerbating factors in an effort to deal with them, or to offer any of several treatment approaches with a discussion of their risks, so the patient can make the choice. If the treatment doesn't work, then both patient and doctor can consider other options.

*Establish boundaries* In the care of some patients, maintaining "boundaries" in terms of frequent phone calls, unexpected visits, a tendency toward lengthy visits, or unrealistic expectations for care need to be addressed. Physicians who want to help, may extend their care beyond what feels right in order to "help", but then feel trapped when these circumstances are repeated. Physicians have a right to assert their needs in terms of time and availability, and to not do so, poses the risk of developing feelings of anger or helplessness which is countertherapeutic. The task is to present the physician's needs in a way that is not perceived as rejecting or belittling to the patient. For example, setting limits on time can be accomplished by scheduling brief but regular appointments of a fixed duration, rather than attempting to extend the time of a particular visit. With frequent unnecessary phone calls, once it is established that the problem does not require an immediate intervention, the physician should politely reduce the length of the discussion, and refer the issue to the next scheduled appointment.

It has been said that physician's, in all specialties, spend most of their time speaking with patients. The above suggestions will hopefully aid the clinician not only in improving this process, but in making it more enjoyable and clinically rewarding.

## *References*

1. Quill TE. *Recognizing and adjusting to barriers in doctor-patient communication.* Ann Intern Med 1989;111:51-7.
2. Drossman DA. *Psychosocial sound bites: exercises in the patient-doctor relationship.* Am J Gastroenterol 1997;92:1418-23.
3. Morgan WLJ, Engel GL. *The approach to the medical interview.* In: Morgan WLJ, Engel GL, editors. The clinical approach to the patient. Philadelphia: W.B. Saunders; 1969; 26-79.
4. Lipkin MJ, Putnam SM, Lazare A. *The medical interview: clinical care, education, and research.* New York: Springer-Verlag; 1995;1-643.
5. Drossman DA. *Struggling with the "controlling" patient.* Am J Gastroenterol 1994;89:1441-6.
6. Drossman DA. *Psychosocial factors in the care of patients with gastrointestinal disorders.* In: Yamada T, editor. Textbook of gastroenterology. 3rd ed. Philadelphia: Lippincott-Raven; 1998;638-59.
7. Drossman DA. *Diagnosing and treating patients with refractory functional gastrointestinal disorders.* Ann Intern Med 1995;123:688-97.
8. Kaplan SH, Greenfield S, Gandek B, et al. *Characteristics of physicians with participatory decision-making styles.* Ann Intern Med 1996;124:497-504.

## *Address for correspondence:*

**DROSSMAN DA, MD**

Division of Digestive Diseases
726 Burnett-Womack
CB #7080, University of North Carolina
Chapel Hill, North Carolina 27599-7080 USA
Fax: +1 919 9668929
E-mail: drossman@med.unc.edu

# PART THREE

# MECHANISMS OF GASTROINTESTINAL PAIN AND DISCOMFORT

# NEUROANATOMY AND NEUROPHYSIOLOGY OF THE GASTROINTESTINAL TRACT AND OF CHRONIC GUT PAIN

*DG Thompson*

This chapter introduces the reader to some of the most basic concepts of the neuroanatomy and neurophysiology of the human Gastrointestinal (GI) tract.

It is not intended to be a comprehensive review but merely to serve as a general introduction to the subject. For further more detailed information[1] readers are requested to turn to more detailed texts.

In addition to the basic concepts, the chapter also deals with a description of the newer techniques which are being employed to study the pathways between the brain and the gut for the first time in intact man and finally, the chapter provides a conceptual basis for the development of chronic pain arising from the gut.

## BASIC CONCEPTS

The GI tract has both an intrinsic and an extrinsic nervous system.

### Intrinsic nervous system

The intrinsic nervous system comprises a complex network of neurones which encircle the entire GI tract from the mid-oesophagus to the anorectum. This enteric nervous system is an essential component of the normal, day-to-day control function of the GI tract. The nerve cells are situated both in the sub-mucous ganglia and, more importantly, in the myenteric ganglia (Auerbach's plexus). There are more neurones present in the myenteric plexus than in the spinal cord.

The myenteric plexus comprises sensory nerves, inter-neurones, and motor nerves which are together 'programmed' to provide simply, local reflexes such as the migrating motor complex and the peristaltic reflex.

*The migrating motor complex*

In the stomach and upper intestine the myenteric plexus runs a cyclic pattern of motility during the fasted state with an approximately ninety-minute periodicity. Periods of complete motor quiescence alternate with periods of irregular activity and culminate with a period of intense regular contractile activity which starts in the distal stomach and migrates slowly through the entire small intestine. This Migrating Motor Complex (MMC) is a function of the intrinsic nervous system and requires no extrinsic control. The passage of contractions down the gut appears to serve to maintain the intestinal lumen free of food debris and undigested material during the fasted state, hence the term 'inter-digestive housekeeper'.

After the ingestion of food, particularly foodstuffs containing lipid or protein, this inter-digestive pattern is disrupted and replaced by a seemingly irregular pattern of intestinal motility.

This interruption of the MMC appears to require an intact vagus nerve pathway since the switch from the fasted to the fed state is disrupted following truncal vagotomy in man. This failure to initiate a fed pattern probably contributes to the poor digestion and diarrhoea suffered post vagotomy.

*Peristaltic reflex*

A further programme of the myenteric plexus is the peristaltic reflex. This reflex has been known for over one hundred years since it was first discovered by Bayliss and Starling.

In response to localised distension of the lumen of the gut, a specific pattern of motor responses is induced. Above the level of the distension, neural excitatory activity increases whilst below the level of the distension, neural inhibitory activity occurs. Together, these two responses serve to propel the distending material through the gut in an aboral direction and hence clear the gut of distending material. Abnormalities of the myenteric plexus such as in intestinal neuropathies may be identified by the absence of a normal peristaltic reflex and MMC pattern.

## Extrinsic nervous system

The innervation of the gut by the extrinsic nervous system is through two pathways, the vagal/sacral, and the spinal/sympathetic pathways.

*Vagal/sacral pathways*
The vagal/sacral pathways appear to be largely involved in the Central Nervous System (CNS) control of the vegetative functions of the upper and lower gut, respectively.
***The vagus*** This important neural conduit innervates the major portion of the GI tract to the mid-colon. The vagus is largely a sensory nerve (90%). Its major function is to sample the intestinal milieu and to 'inform' the brain stem and higher centres of the presence of food, motor activity, and distension. The nerve bodies of the vagal afferents are located in the nodose ganglion, which is situated on the vagus nerve, just outside the skull. Distally, nerve endings innervate the sub-mucosal area sending projections between villi where they are able to respond to neurotransmitters such as cholecystokinin (CCK) and 5HT released from the epithelium. Centrally, projections from the vagus synapse with the Nucleus of the Tractus Solitarius (NTS). Neurones synapsing with these endings project both to higher centres, e.g. hypothalamic areas or more locally to the motor neurones of the vagus to form long reflexes. Motor neurones travelling in the vagus influence the pattern of motility in the gut, in particular in response to food. Vagal efferent nerves do not directly influence motor or secretory function but influence the myenteric plexus. This explains why relatively few motor nerves can influence such a large organ as the gut.

***Sacral nerves*** Sacral nerves have their cell bodies located in the sacral region of the spinal cord with efferent fibre projecting to the lower colon and rectum.

*Spinal/sympathetic pathways*
***Spinal afferent nerves*** The major pathway for perception appears to be via the spinal cord as, in the conduction of sensation from the somatic tissue and skin, information travels from the gut via spinal afferent nerves

to the spinal cord. These nerves largely innervate the outer layers of the gut and serosa and have cell bodies located in the dorsal root ganglia. Their central connections are with dorsal horn neurones, which then project to the CNS via spinal thalamic pathways.
Spinal afferent neurones, as in the skin, are of several types; major types being C-fibres, which are unmyelinated, and A-fibres which are rapidly conducting myelinated fibres.
Sensations travelling via spinal afferents are largely interpreted as being uncomfortable and painful, e.g. gut distension.
Motor fibres from the spinal cord to the gut comprise the efferent 'sympathetic' pathways, which synapse in the pre-vertebral ganglia from which adrenergic fibres innervate the myenteric plexus. In general, sympathetic neurones serve an inhibitory function reducing secretion and inhibiting motor activity.
Activation of the spinal reflexes appears to be the major mechanism for ileus seen after gut injury or surgery.

## METHODS FOR STUDYING NEUROANATOMY AND NEUROPHYSIOLOGY OF BRAIN-GUT PATHWAYS IN MAN

In recent years, our understanding of brain-gut pathways has been revolutionised by the development of a series of novel techniques.

### Gut to brain pathways

A series of techniques are now available to study pathways from the gut to the brain.

*Cortical evoked potentials* This technique is a development of basic electroencephalography (EEG). Stimulations of the gut, either by electrical or mechanical means, are detected by electrodes placed at strategic points on the surface of the scalp and recorded as variable waveforms. By 'triggering' the recording apparatus precisely at the time of the stimulus delivery and averaging the responses over many repetitions, extraneous information is removed and the information of interest becomes more apparent.

Using this technique, areas of the brain which are activated in response to gut stimulation can be identified and a temporal sequence of activations determined.

The advantage of this technique is that it is relatively simple and inexpensive. The disadvantage is that its spatial resolution is poor so that areas of activation can be localised only to within several centimetres.

*Magnetoencephalography (MEG)* This technique is a development of EEG. Instead of the detection of electrical signals from the brain, magnetic signals are detected using highly sensitive magnetometers. Since magnetic signals pass through the tissues of the skull without deflexion, unlike electrical signals, their detection allows a much more clearly localised source to be identified.

The advantage of this technique is, therefore, that it can provide much better resolution than EEG. The disadvantage of the technique, however, is that it is expensive, currently restricted to a few centres in Western Europe and, in general, its utility is restricted to acquiring information from the brain surface.

*Positron Emission Tomography (PET)* This technique is currently regarded as the gold standard for detecting areas of the brain activated by peripheral stimulation including the gut. The technique relies upon the principle that areas of brain, which are activated by afferent signals, have a higher blood flow than quiescent areas. When a radioactive emitter of positrons is delivered into the circulation, the flow through the active brain area increases compared to the inactivated condition. By using sensitive detectors of positron emission, the areas of increased blood flow can be accurately localised. Current 'state of the art' machines provide resolution down to a few millimetres. The advantage of this technique is high spatial resolution.

The disadvantage of the technique, however, is that signal acquisition is relatively slow so that sequences of brain activation cannot be obtained. Furthermore, the technique requires radioisotope exposure so that it is not possible to perform repeated studies on the same individual.

*Functional Magnetic Resonance Imaging (FMRI)* This newest technique is still in its developmental phase.
Like PET, it detects alterations in blood flow between states of brain activation and states of quiescence. Unlike PET, it requires no addition of isotope but uses changes in the relationship between oxygenated and deoxygenated haemoglobin as the marker for brain observation.
With further development of analytical paradigms, this technique promises to be the method of choice for future studies. Its advantage is that it provides good spatial resolution and is repeatable in the same individual. Its disadvantage is that it is still largely in a developmental phase and has not yet been applied to diseased states.

*Advances in the brain-gut axis using these techniques* In the last four to five years, these above techniques have begun to be used both in healthy volunteers and in patients.
In healthy volunteers, it has been found that non-painful distension activates the primary somatosensory cortex with specific areas of the sensory cortex responding to different gut organs. A crude viscerotopic representation of the gut, therefore, exists on the brain.
When painful stimulation is applied to the gut, additional areas of the brain are activated, including the insular cortex and the cingulate cortex, the latter being an area known to be involved in the autonomic responses of the body to pain.
These techniques, therefore, provide, for the first time, an approach to an understanding of brain processing of gut signals and promise a method for measuring responsive, independently of subjective, reporting by the individual.
So far their use in clinical conditions has been limited but already a number of interesting differences between patients with functional GI disorders and healthy volunteers have been made.

## Brain to gut pathways

A further interesting development, in recent years, has been the ability to stimulate the brain of healthy volunteers in a non-invasive manner and detect signals from the human gut.
The most commonly used technique involves magnetic stimulation of

the brain by discharging a magneto-electric coil in close proximity to the scalp. A magnetic flux induced by this discharge travels through the skull without deflection and induces an electrical charge in the underlying neurones, which, in turn, initiates neural activity.
By moving the stimulating coil over the motor cortex, areas of the motor cortex can be identified which are able to initiate oropharyngeal and oesophageal EMG responses and also areas which initiate anal and pelvic floor responses. So far, this technique has been restricted to the striated muscle parts of the GI tract. It has not been possible to detect any motor signals from smooth muscle areas of the gut.

*Swallowing pathways* Using this technique, it has now been discovered that swallowing is represented in two distinct areas of the brain, one on each hemisphere, with, in most people, significant asymmetry of representation, independent of handedness. These cortical 'command' centres appear to modulate the brain stem swallowing centre rather than to control swallowing themselves. Damage to one of the hemispheric centres, e.g. in stroke, can cause severe dysphagic symptoms, especially if the centre dominant for swallowing is involved. Interestingly, recovery of swallowing after a dysphagic stroke is accompanied by an increase in the size of the representation on the undamaged hemisphere indicating a degree of neuroplasticity in the swallowing system and offering exciting possibilities for developing therapy for dysphagia.

*Anorectal pathways* As with swallowing, a cortical control of pelvic floor and anorectal function exists on both cerebral hemispheres. In some individuals, asymmetry has also been noted although this is more difficult than for the swallowing centre because the control centres are medially located and, therefore, difficult to resolve. Abnormalities of brain to gut control of the anorectum seem likely but await further study.

## Putative mechanisms for chronic gut pain

With steadily increasing understanding of the physiology and anatomy of the gut, brain pathways should come a better understanding both of the cause and treatment of chronic pain. So far, however, our

understanding of the pathophysiology of chronic pain has not been advanced by these techniques so that mechanisms remain speculative. In future, however, application of the new techniques outlined above will undoubtedly make a major impact on the field.
Chronic pain referred to the GI tract could arise from disordered function at a series of levels:

1. *Gut dysfunction* One plausible hypothesis for chronic pain is chronic changes in the mucosal function induced by inflammation. It is known that 5HT release by the gut mucosa can stimulate spinal afferent nerves and induce pain. It remains to be proven, however, whether chronic disorder of 5HT production release by the gut mucosa is responsible for chronic pain.
2. *Afferent nerves* A disorder of the spinal nerves could also theoretically account for chronic pain. Hyperstimulation by the mucosa might, in turn, leads to hyper-reactivity of the spinal nerve. Again evidence for this mechanism remains speculative.
3. *Spinal cord* It is known that chronic stimulation of spinal afferents can sensitise the neurones of the dorsal horn and induce hyperalgesia. Such long-term changes present a plausible mechanism for visceral pain. So far, however, its mechanism has not been well explored and its relationship to chronic pain remains uncertain.
4. *Higher cortical centres* It must be recognised that, in many cases of chronic pain reporting, abnormalities of cortical recognition are as likely as GI hyper-reactiveness. Chronic psychological disturbance, e.g. somatisation, depression, anxiety are all known to induce states of 'hypervigilance' and to alter pain perception.

## Conclusions

Our increased knowledge of neuroanatomy and physiology of the GI tract together with the newer techniques for the direct study of brain-gut pathways now provides a major opportunity to explore pathophysiology in patients.

The time is now right for a major investment of time and energy in this field, exciting new advances are to be expected within the next few years.

## *Further reading*

1. Aziz Q, Thompson DG. *The Brain-Gut Axis.* Gastroenterology 1998;114:559-78.
2. Bayliss WM, Starling EH. *The movements and innervation of the small intestine.* J Physiol 1899;24:99-145.

## *Address for correspondence*

**THOMPSON DG, MD, FRCP**
GI Science, University of Manchester
Clinical Science Building, Hope Hospital
Salford M68HD United Kingdom
Fax: +44 161 787 4364

# CHEST PAIN OF OESOPHAGEAL ORIGIN

*JF Tack*

Angina-like chest pain is an alarming symptom, not only for the patient who is frightened by its cardiac connotations, but also for the physician who has to decide whether or not he is dealing with a life-threatening condition. One third to half of patients presenting with chest pain sufficiently severe to perform more invasive examinations have no evidence of coronary artery disease[1-4]. On the basis of the number of cardiac catheterizations, it has been estimated that more than 100,000 new cases of non-cardiac chest pain are identified yearly in the U.S.[5]. The clinical relevance of the problem may well be underestimated, because not all patients with chest pain will undergo coronary arteriography. The vital prognosis of patients with angina-like chest pain and normal coronary angiograms is favourable[6-8]. However, many of these patients continue to see a physician, remain or become unemployed, remain on cardiac medications, and regard their lives as significantly disabled after having been told that their coronaries were normal[9-12].

It has been known for a long time that oesophageal symptoms can mimic cardiac symptoms. A positive diagnosis, establishing the oesophageal origin of the non-cardiac chest pain, may result in a significant reduction in the need for medical facilities[13-15] and may increase the number of patients able to keep their job[14]. Therefore, a good understanding of the causes of recurrent non-cardiac chest pain is of major importance to the quality of life of many patients.

## Clinical characteristics of oesophageal chest pain

The clinical history often does not distinguish between cardiac and oesophageal causes of chest pain[4]. Chest pain of oesophageal origin is usually located retrosternally and may irradiate to the arms, neck, jaw or back. In patients with non-cardiac chest pain, careful evaluation of oesophageal symptoms, especially the presence of dysphagia, may increase the likelihood of an underlying oesophageal disorder[16].

Unfortunately, as many as 50% of patients with a cardiac cause of chest pain may have one or more symptoms of oesophageal pain, such as heartburn, regurgitation or dysphagia[17]. Hence, the existence of underlying cardiac or oesophageal disease cannot be precluded on the basis of history and clinical presentation alone.

## Mechanisms of oesophageal chest pain

Chest pain of oesophageal origin may arise either from stimulation of acid-sensitive receptors, or from stimulation of oesophageal mechanoreceptors during abnormal motility. In addition, hypersensitivity to oesophageal balloon distention has been found in a subset of patients with noncardiac chest pain, although studies have shown inconsistent results[18,19].

### *Reflux-related oesophageal chest pain*

Both acid perfusion tests and ambulatory pH- and pressure monitoring in patients with non-cardiac chest pain have confirmed that intra-oesophageal acid may trigger chest pain. The mechanism by which chest pain occurs after exposure of the oesophageal mucosa to acid remains largely unknown. Although structures acting as oesophageal chemoreceptors have not formally been identified, it seems likely that intra-epithelial free nerve endings may act as acid-sensitive nociceptors[20]. It has been shown that intra-oesophageal acid infusion is able to trigger myocardial ischaemia in patients with coronary disease or with microvascular angina[21,22]. However, there is no convincing evidence that coronary ischaemia underlies acid-induced pain in patients with non-cardiac chest pain. In these patients, episodes of symptomatic acid reflux are not associated with changes in the electrocardiogram[23].

### *Motility-related oesophageal chest pain*

It is well known that patients with symptomatic diffuse oesophageal spasm may have retrosternal angina-like pain[24]. In many patients with non-cardiac chest pain, high-amplitude contractions of prolonged duration and with impaired peristaltic progression can be observed during oesophageal manometry. The most frequent findings are non-specific motor disorders, followed by nutcracker oesophagus and diffuse oesophageal spasm[19,25]. Initially, a causal link between these abnormal patterns of contraction and the patient's symptoms seemed obvious. The relationship, however, between the manometric findings and the chest pain has remained complex and incompletely understood. Patients are generally asymptomatic at the time when the motor disorders are identified. It has been assumed that these abnormal contractions might be a marker for even more severe motor disturbances during spontaneous episodes of chest pain. However, prolonged oesophageal pressure monitoring studies have demonstrated that this is only rarely the case[19,26]. Moreover, the reduction of the amplitude of contractions by pharmacotherapy does not correlate with a symptomatic improvement[27]. Recent data suggest that psychological factors may contribute to the phenomenon. Psychological stress alone is able to increase the amplitude of oesophageal contractions, and this is more marked in patients with a nutcracker oesophagus[28].

*Visceral hypersensitivity*

Patients with non-cardiac chest pain have significantly higher pain sensation scores during intra-oesophageal balloon distension than healthy control subjects[18]. This abnormal sensory perception appears to be independent of oesophageal contractions or oesophageal wall tone. In contrast to healthy subjects or patients with non-structural dysphagia, patients with non-cardiac chest pain report increasing pain sensation scores during repeated balloon distensions[29]. These data suggest that patients with non-cardiac chest pain exhibit a conditioning phenomenon during repeated distensions. The level at which this conditioning occurs is unknown.

A belching disorder may be the mechanism responsible for chest pain in some patients with abnormal sensitivity to intra-oesophageal balloon distention[30,31]. Oesophageal wall distension, mimicked during balloon distension, may occur spontaneously during eructation against a closed upper oesophageal sphincter[31].

*Irritable oesophagus*

The irritable oesophagus concept was derived from the observation that some patients with non-cardiac chest pain, when studied by 24-hour pH and pressure measurements, sometimes developed pain associated with reflux alone (without motor disorders), and, on other occasions, during the same study experienced the same pain together with motility disorders alone (without acid reflux)[32]. The oesophagus of these patients appears to be hypersensitive to a variety of stimuli. The diagnosis of irritable oesophagus is, therefore, based on the demonstration that the patient's familiar chest pain can be elicited by both mechanical and chemical stimuli. The mechanism underlying this irritability is unclear. Mutual sensitization of acid sensitive and mechanosensitive mechanisms may contribute to the development of irritability in the oesophagus.

## Diagnostic tools in chest pain of oesophageal origin

Gastrointestinal work-up is aimed at demonstrating symptomatic gastro-oesophageal reflux, oesophageal motor abnormalities or hypersensitivity of the oesophagus to balloon distention. The examination sequence may consist of endoscopy, stationary oesophageal manometry, oesophageal provocation tests using acid infusion, balloon distention and edrophonium chloride iv, and 24-hour oesophageal pH and manometry recording. Alternatively, the physician may embark on a therapeutic trial.

*Endoscopy and manometry*

Gastrointestinal endoscopy reveals reflux oesophagitis in up to 31% of the patients with non-cardiac chest pain[33-35]. Stationary manometry in patients with non-cardiac chest pain is able to demonstrate abnormalities in up to 29% of the patients[19,25]. As oesophageal motor disorders and low-grade reflux oesophagitis are a common finding in many patients, the mere presence of these disorders cannot be accepted as proof for the oesophageal origin of the chest pain. The best way to accept the oesophagus as the likely cause of non-cardiac angina-like chest pain is to show a temporal correlation between the occurrence of chest pain and an abnormal oesophageal event. To increase the chance of recording a pain episode during oesophageal testing, one can use provocation tests, or one can extend the recording period.

*Provocation tests*

The acid perfusion test was first described by Bernstein and Baker[36]. When 0.1 N hydrochloric acid, infused into the middle third of the oesophagus, is able to induce the familiar chest pain, the test is called positive related. When acid induces only a retrosternal burning sensation, or another unfamiliar sensation, the test is called positive unrelated, and is not accepted as proof that the chest pain has an oesophageal origin. The Bernstein test is positive related in 10 to 38% of the patients with non-cardiac chest pain (Table 1).[4,19,26,32,37-46]

DIAGNOSTIC ACCURACY OF OESOPHAGEAL PROVOCATION TESTS IN PATIENTS WITH NON-CARDIAC CHEST PAIN

| | Accuracy | | |
|---|---|---|---|
| **Study** ref | **Bernstein** | **Edrophonium** | **Balloon** |
| Vantrappen et al.[32] | 11/33 | 6/12 | - |
| De Caestecker et al.[39] | 21/60 | 12/60 | - |
| Peters et al.[26] | 7/20 | 9/18 | - |
| Soffer et al.[37] | 2/20 | 0/20 | - |
| Hewson et al.[38] | 15/45 | 24/44 | - |
| Ghillebert et al.[19] | 18/50 | 16/50 | 1/20 |
| Humeau et al.[41] | 4/40 | 6/40 | 13/34 |
| Nevens et al.[4] | 14/37 | 7/37 | 3/37 |
| Goudot-Pernot et al.[42] | - | 19/78 | 33/78 |
| Hewson et al.[43] | 18/95 | 15/78 | - |
| Rokkas et al.[40] | 29/110 | 26/110 | - |
| Mehta et al.[44] | 3/25 | 10/25 | - |
| Ghillebert et al.[45] | 106/270 | 58/220 | 26/182 |
| Frøbert et al.[46] | 10/63 | 9/63 | - |

Table 1

The cholinesterase inhibitor edrophonium has been shown to be the most reliable and safest pharmacological agent for routine provocative testing in the clinical setting[47]. Administration of edrophonium increases oesophageal contraction amplitude and the number of repetitive waves after wet swallows in both age-matched control subjects and patients with non-cardiac chest pain. Inclusion of a placebo iv injection when using edrophonium is advisable. The test is positive if slow intravenous injection of 80 μg/kg edrophonium, but not placebo, induces the familiar chest pain within 5 minutes of administration of the drug. The test has been reported to be positive in 0-55% of the patients with non-cardiac chest pain (Table 1)[4,19,26,32,37-46].
In 1955, Bayliss et al., proposed intra-oesophageal balloon distension as a diagnostic test to distinguish oesophageal from cardiac chest pain[48]. In 1986, the test was resurrected as a provocative test in the evaluation of patients with non-cardiac chest pain[18]. A small balloon is placed 10 cm above the lower oesophageal sphincter and inflated with 1 ml increments to a total volume of 10 ml. Richter et al. observed that balloon distension with a volume of 8 ml reproduced chest pain in 15 out of 30 patients and had no effect in controls[18]. In other studies, the sensitivity of the test has been reported to vary between 5 and 50% (Table 1)[4,19,40-46]. The reasons for this discrepancy are not completely understood. When increasing balloon volumes are used as a stimulus to activate tension receptors in the oesophagus, the variable oesophageal diameter in different persons may result in a highly variable tension stimulus. Using isobaric distensions, and simultaneously assessing the oesophageal diameter, allows us to calculate the wall tension that elicits typical sensations[49].

*Prolonged oesophageal pH and pressure recordings*

Ambulatory pH and pressure recordings allow us to demonstrate a temporal relationship between chest pain, signalled on the record by the patient, and the occurrence of an abnormal oesophageal event such as reflux or motor abnormalities, or both. Since the original development of prolonged oesophageal pH and pressure recordings[50], several studies have reported the reproducibility of this technique[51,52]. The diagnostic accuracy of 24-hour pH and pressure recordings in the diagnosis of an oesophageal cause for chest pain ranges from 10 to 56% in several published studies (Table 2).

DIAGNOSTIC ACCURACY OF 24 h ph AND PRESSURE RECORDINGS IN PATIENTS WITH NON-CARDIAC CHEST PAIN

| **Study** ref | **No. patients** | **No. patients with chest pain related to** | | | |
|---|---|---|---|---|---|
| | | Dysmotility | Acid | Both | **Global** |
| Janssens et al.[50] | 60 | 8 | 4 | 9 | **21** |
| Peters et al.[26] | 24 | 3 | 5 | 5 | **13** |
| Soffer et al.[37] | 20 | 0 | 6 | 4 | **10** |
| Ghillebert et al.[19] | 50 | 4 | 12 | 3 | **19** |
| Hewson et al.[43] | 45 | 6 | 11 | 4 | **21** |
| Breumelhof et al.[53] | 44 | 2 | 2 | 4 | **8** |
| Nevens et al.[4] | 37 | 1 | 4 | 1 | **6** |
| Lam et al.[54] | 41 | 10 | 13 | - | **23** |
| Lux et al.[55] | 30 | 4 | 5 | 1 | **10** |

Table 2

The optimal time window in symptom analysis of 24-hour oesophageal pressure and pH data begins at 2 minutes before the onset of the pain and ends at the onset of the pain [56]. However, many uncertainties exist concerning the way 24-hour pH and pressure measurements should be analyzed. The definition of abnormal motility or abnormal pH to be used in the analysis of the data is controversial. Oesophageal pH monitoring is able to demonstrate pathological gastro-oesophageal reflux in up to 62% of the patients with non-cardiac chest pain[4,26,37,38,41,43,50,53,57-62]. However, even in the absence of pathological reflux, reflux can still be the cause of a patient's symptoms of chest pain. A group of patients have a normal acid exposure, but still have a significant temporal relationship between reflux episodes and chest pain events. These patients are considered to have an acid-hypersensitive oesophagus[63]. To quantify a temporal relationship between symptoms and episodes of gastro-oesophageal reflux, several indices have been developed. The most frequently used is the symptom index, defined as the percentage of reflux-related symptom episodes[64]. To overcome several drawbacks of the symptom index, more complex methods were proposed, such as the symptom sensitivity index, the binomial symptom index, a mathematical approach based on the Kolmogorov-Smirnov test and the symptom-association probability[19, 65-67]. However, most of these methods can only be applied to oesophageal pH, and not to pressure events.

### *Diagnostic impact of provocation tests versus 24-hour pH and pressure measurements*

A number of studies performed edrophonium and Bernstein provocation tests and also prolonged ambulatory pH and pressure recording in patients with non-cardiac chest pain (Table 3).

DIAGNOSTIC ACCURACY OF PROVOCATION TESTS COMPARED TO 24 h pH AND PRESSURE RECORDINGS IN PATIENTS WITH NON-CARDIAC CHEST PAIN

| Study ref | No. patients | Positive provocation tests | Positive 24 h recording | Positive 24 h and negative provocation | Positive provocation and negative 24 h |
|---|---|---|---|---|---|
| Peters et al.[26] | 18 | 13 | 8 | 3 | 7 |
| Soffer et al.[37] | 20 | 2 | 10 | 8 | 0 |
| Ghillebert et al.[19] | 50 | 24 | 19 | 5 | 11 |
| Hewson et al.[43] | 44 | 30 | 20 | 5 | 15 |
| Nevens et al.[4] | 37 | 17 | 6 | 1 | 6 |
| Ghillebert et al.[45] | 190 | 94 | 48 | 14 | 60 |

Table 3

In 50% of the patients, at least one provocation test was positive. Twenty-four-hour recording revealed an oesophageal origin in 31% of the patients (Table 3).

A combination of the acid perfusion test and the edrophonium test revealed the oesophageal origin of the chest pain in 105 patients who did not have painful abnormalities during prolonged monitoring (gain 29%). In contrast, the diagnostic gain of ambulatory pH and pressure monitoring in patients found to have positive provocation tests was only 10%. Hence, it seems logical to perform an acid perfusion and an edrophonium test first. However, if these provocation tests are negative, the chance to establish the oesophageal origin by performing an ambulatory pH and pressure monitoring is still 20%. Prolonged ambulatory pH and pressure recordings remain the only method to demonstrate the mechanism underlying spontaneous pain attacks.

## Psychological factors

Patients with non-cardiac chest pain and patients with the nutcracker oesophagus have significantly higher scores of gastrointestinal susceptibility and somatic anxiety than controls[68]. Several studies found a high incidence of psychiatric diagnoses, such as panic disorder, generalized anxiety disorder or depression and somatization disorder in patients with non-cardiac chest pain[69-72]. However, a subset of up to 50% of patients with non-cardiac chest pain have no active psychiatric syndrome at the time of evaluation[70,73]. Anxiety is an important factor that contributes to symptom perception in patients with chest pain. The multiple interactions between psychological factors and chest pain may also explain why patients with contraction abnormalities and symptoms benefit from psychotropic drugs[74,75], even though the drugs do not influence the manometric parameters.

## Diagnostic evaluation

The existence of coronary artery disease cannot be ruled out on the basis of the history and the clinical presentation only[4]. As this is a potentially life-threatening disorder, evaluation of patients with chest pain should always start with the exclusion of cardiac disease. Gastrointestinal work-up is aimed at demonstrating symptomatic gastro-oesophageal reflux, oesophageal motor abnormalities or hypersensitivity of the oesophagus to balloon distention. Endoscopy is the examination of choice to start with. If this shows oesophagitis, or an unusual cause of chest pain such as an ulcer, appropriate treatment can be started. As reflux is the most common oesophageal cause of chest pain, an empiric trial of acid suppression with a high dose of a proton pump inhibitor can be considered if the endoscopy was negative. Alternatively, one may proceed to perform stationary oesophageal manometry with provocation tests. In the case of uncertain results of provocative tests, 24-hour ambulatory oesophageal pH and pressure monitoring can be performed in the attempt to identify the factors that trigger spontaneously occurring episodes of chest pain. Finally, a psychiatric work-up may identify underlying psychological disorders that require appropriate treatment.

## Treatment

The medical therapy of angina-like chest pain of oesophageal origin remains controversial. Many patients may improve with confident reassurance alone, although it seems important for many patients to establish a definite cause for the symptoms to avoid ongoing concern[2]. Nitroglycerin and long-acting nitrates have been shown to be beneficial in patients with symptomatic diffuse oesophageal spasm[76,77], but no data have been published on the effect of these agents in patients with motility-related non-cardiac chest pain without a manometric picture of diffuse spasm. Several studies have examined the effect of the calcium channel blocker diltiazem on non-cardiac chest pain, but the results are conflicting with regard to symptom relief as well as the effect on oesophageal contraction amplitude[78-80]. Nifedipine was shown to decrease the amplitude of oesophageal contractions in patients with nutcracker oesophagus, but it was no better than placebo in symptom relief after 6 weeks' treatment[27,81]. A beneficial effect on symptom relief was obtained with a low dose of the antidepressant trazodone in symptomatic patients with oesophageal contraction abnormalities[75]. A thoracoscopic longitudinal myotomy has been reported to give symptomatic relief in some patients with chest pain due to oesophageal motor alterations[82]. However, we feel that surgical management of oesophageal chest pain is very rarely indicated.

In patients with non-cardiac chest pain and proven gastro-oesophageal reflux, intensive anti-reflux therapy with high doses of $H_2$-blockers or with proton pump inhibitors, is able to improve symptoms[83,84]. It is unclear whether acid suppression may improve symptoms in patients with coexisting motor disorders and pathologic acid reflux.

The treatment of patients with an irritable or a hypersensitive oesophagus is even more difficult. Acid blocking agents will, at best, only partially relieve symptoms, while motor inhibitory drugs may aggravate reflux. Drugs which interfere with pain perception may well be indicated in these patients. Such a mechanism could explain the beneficial effect on symptom relief obtained with a low dose of the antidepressant trazodone in symptomatic patients with oesophageal contraction abnormalities[75]. Imipramine, a tricyclic antidepressant helpful in the management of patients with chronic pain syndromes, was evaluated in the treatment of patients with chest pain and normal coronary angiograms[74]. Imipramine reduced by approximately 50% the number of chest pain episodes, and it also reduced the sensitivity to cardiac pain during electrical stimulation. Oesophageal motility testing did not identify patients who were likely to respond to imipramine.

## Follow-up

The long-term follow-up of patients with non-cardiac chest pain has been inadequately studied. The use of oesophageal testing has been controversial. It has been reported that oesophageal testing in subjects with non-cardiac chest pain decreased the number of emergency room visits and increased the patients' resumption of their normal activity[85]. However, some patients did not fully comprehend the results of oesophageal testing, and more than half of the patients who were found to have an oesophageal abnormality still did not consider the oesophagus as the source of the pain[85].

## *References*

1. Kemp HG, Vokonas PS, Cohn PF, Gorlin R. *The anginal syndromes associated with normal coronary arteriograms: Report of a six year experience.* Am J Med 1973;54:735-42.

2. Ockene IS, Shay MJ, Alpart JA, et al. *Unexplained chest pain in patients with normal coronary arteriograms. A follow-up study of functional status.* N Engl J Med 1980;303:1249.
3. Wilcox RG, Roland JM, Hampton JR. *Prognosis of patients with "chest pain? cause".* Br Med J 1981;282:431-3.
4. Nevens F, Janssens J, Piessens J, et al. *Prospective study on the prevalence of esophageal chest pain in patients referred on an elective basis to a cardiac unit for suspected myocardial ischemia.* Dig Dis Sci 1991;36:228-35.
5. Richter JE, Bradley LA, Castell DO. *Esophageal chest pain: current controversies in pathogenesis, diagnosis and therapy.* Ann Intern Med 1989;110:66-78.
6. Bemiler CR, Pepine CJ, Rogers AK. *Long term observation in patients with angina and normal coronary arteries.* Circulation 1973;47:36-43.
7. Day LJ, Sowton E. *Clinical features and follow-up of patients with angina and normal coronary arteries.* Lancet 1976;ii:334-7.
8. Marchandise B, Bourassa MG, Chaitman BR, Lesperance J. *Angiographic evaluation of the natural history of normal coronary arteries and mild coronary atherosclerosis.* Am J Cardiol 1978;41:216-20.
9. Lavey EB, Winkle RA. *Continuing disability of patients with chest pain and normal coronary arteriograms.* J Chron Dis 1979;32:191-6.
10. Faxon DP, McCabe CH, Kreigel DE, Ryan TJ. *Therapeutic and economic value of a normal coronary angiogram.* Am J Med 1982;73:500-5.
11. Bass C, Wade C, Hand D, Jackson G. *Patients with angina with normal and near normal coronary arteries: clinical and psychosocial state 12 months after angiography.* Br Med J 1983;287:1505-8.
12. Lantinga LJ, Sprafkin RP, McCroskery JH, et al. *One-year psychosocial follow-up of patients with chest pain and angiographically normal coronary arteries.* Am J Cardiol 1988;62:209-13.
13. Ward B, Wu WC, Richter JE, et al. *Long term follow-up of patients with non cardiac chest pain: is diagnosis of esophageal etiology helpful?* Am J Gastroenterol 1987;82:215-8.
14. Schofield PM. *Follow-up study of morbidity in patients with angina pectoris and normal coronary angiograms and the value of investigation for esophageal dysfunction.* Angiology 1990;41:286-96.
15. Swift GL, Alban-Davies N, McKirdy H, et al. *A long term clinical review of patients with esophageal pain.* Q J Med 1991;295: 937-44.
16. Bak YT, Lorang M, Evans PR, et al. *Predictive values of symptoms profiles in patients with suspected esophageal dysmotility.* Scand J Gastroenterol 1994;29: 392-7.
17. Alban-Davies H, Page Z, Rush EM, et al. *Oesophageal stimulation lowers exertional angina threshold.* Lancet 1985;i:1011-4.

18. Richter JE, Barish CF, Castell DO. *Abnormal sensory perception in patients with esophageal chest pain.* Gastroenterology 1986;91:845-52.
19. Ghillebert G, Janssens J, Vantrappen G, et al. *Ambulatory 24 hour intraoesophageal pH and pressure recordings vs provocation tests in the diagnosis of chest pain of oesophageal origin.* Gut 1990;31:738-44.
20. Lynn RB. *Mechanisms of esophageal pain.* Am J Med 1992;92:11-9.
21. Mellow MH, Simpson AG, Watt L, et al. *Oesophageal acid perfusion in coronary artery disease: induction of myocardial ischemia.* Gastroenterology 1983;85:306-12.
22. Chauhan A, Petch MC, Schofield PM. *Effect of oesophageal acid instillation on coronary blood flow.* Lancet 1993;341:1309-10.
23. Wani M, Hishon S. *ECG record during changes in oesophageal pH.* Gut 1990;31:127-8.
24. Vantrappen G, Hellemans J. *Diffuse muscle spasm of the oesophagus and hypertensive oesophageal sphincter.* Clin Gastroenterol 1976;5:59-72.
25. Benjamin SB, Gerhardt DC, Castell DO. *High amplitude, peristaltic esophageal contractions associated with chest pain and/or dysphagia.* Gastroenterology 1979;77:478-83.
26. Peters L, Maas L, Petty D, et al. *Spontaneous non-cardiac chest pain. Evaluation by 24-hour ambulatory esophageal motility and pH monitoring.* Gastroenterology 1988;94:878-86.
27. Richter JE, Dalton CB, Bradley LA, Castell DO. *Oral nifedipine in the treatment of non-cardiac chest pain in patients with the nutcracker esophagus.* Gastroenterology 1987;93:21-8.
28. Anderson, KO, Dalton CB, Bradley LA, Richter JE. *Stress induced alteration of esophageal pressures in healthy volunteers and non-cardiac chest pain patients.* Dig Dis Sci 1989;34:89-91.
29. Patterson WG, Wang H, Vanner SJ. *Increasing pain sensation to repeated esophageal balloon distension in patients with chest pain of undetermined etiology.* Dig Dis Sci 1995;40:1325-31.
30. Kahrilas PJ, Dodds WJ, Hogan WJ. *Dysfunction of the belch reflex. A cause of incapacitating chest pain.* Gastroenterology 1987;93:818-22.
31. Gignoux C, Bost R, Hostein J, et al. *Role of upper esophageal reflex and belch reflex dysfunctions in non-cardiac chest pain.* Dig Dis Sci 1993; 38:1909-14.
32. Vantrappen G, Janssens J, Ghillebert G. *The irritable esophagus - a frequent cause of angina-like pain.* Lancet 1987;i:1232-4.
33. Voskuil JH, Cramer MJ, Breumelhof R, et al. *Prevalence of esophageal disorders in patients with chest pain newly referred to the cardiologist.* Chest 1996;109:1210-4.
34. Hsia PC, Maher KA, Lewis JH, et al. *Utility of upper endoscopy in the evaluation of noncardiac chest pain.* Gastrointest Endosc 1991;37:22-6.
35. Frøbert O, Funch-Jensen P, Jacobsen NO, et al. *Upper endoscopy in patients with*

*angina and normal coronary angiograms.* Endoscopy 1995;27:365-70.

36. Bernstein LM, Baker LA. *A clinical test for esophagitis.* Gastroenterology 1958;34:760-81.
37. Soffer EE, Scalabrini P, Wingate DL. *Spontaneous non-cardiac chest pain: value of ambulatory esophageal pH and motility monitoring.* Dig Dis Sci 1989;24:1651-5.
38. Hewson EG, Dalton CB, Richter JE. *Comparison of esophageal manometry, provocative testing and ambulatory monitoring in patients with unexplained chest pain.* Dig Dis Sci 1990;35:302-9.
39. De Caestecker JA, Pryde A, Heading RC. *Comparison of intravenous edrophonium and esophageal acid perfusion during esophageal manometry in patients with non-cardiac chest pain.* Gut 1988;29:1029-34.
40. Rokkas T, Tanggiansah A, McCullagh M, Owen W. *Acid perfusion and edrophonium provocation tests in patients with chest pain of undetermined etiology.* Dig Dis Sci 1992;27:1212-6.
41. Humeau B, Cloarec D, Simon J, et al. *Angina-like chest pain of esophageal origin. Results of functional tests and value of balloon distension.* Gastroenterol Clin Biol 1990;14:334-41.
42. Goudot-Pernot C, Champignuelle B, Bigard MA, et al. *Prospective study comparing the edrophonium test and the intra-esophageal balloon distension test in 78 non-cardiac chest pain patients and 12 healthy controls.* Ann Gastroenterol Hepatol 1991;27:41-8.
43. Hewson EG, Sinclair JW, Dalton CB, Richter JE. *Twenty-four-hour esophageal pH monitoring: the most useful test for evaluating non-cardiac chest pain.* Am J Med 1991;90:576-83.
44. Mehta AJ, De Caestecker JS, Camm AJ, Northfield TC. *Sensitisation to painful distension and abnormal sensory perception in the esophagus.* Gastroenterology 1995;108:311-9.
45. Ghillebert G, Janssens J. *Provocation tests versus 24-hour pH and pressure measurements.* Eur J Gastroenterol Hepatol 1995;7:1141-6.
46. Frøbert O, Funch-Jensen P, Bagger JP. *Diagnostic value of esophageal studies in patients with angina-like chest pain and normal coronary angiograms.* Ann Intern Med 1996;124:959-69.
47. Richter JE, Hackshaw BT, Wu WC, Castell DO. *Edrophonium: a useful provocative test for esophageal chest pain.* Ann Intern Med 1985;103:14-21.
48. Bayliss JH, Komitz R, Trounce JR. *Observation on distension of the lower end of the esophagus.* Q J Med 1955;94:143-54.
49. Rao SSC, Gregersen H, Hayek B, et al. *Unexplained chest pain: the hypersensitive, hyperreactive, and poorly compliant esophagus.* Ann Intern Med 1996;124:950-8.
50. Janssens J, Vantrappen G, Ghillebert G. *24-hour recording of esophageal pressure and pH in patients with non-cardiac chest pain.* Gastroenterology 1986;90:1978-84.

51. Emde C, Armstrong D, Castiglione F, et al. *Reproducibility of long term ambulatory esophageal combined pH/manometry.* Gastroenterology 1990;100:1630-7.
52. Wang H, Beck IT, Paterson WG. *Reproducibility and physiological characteristics of 24-hour ambulatory esophageal manometry/pH-metry.* Am J Gastroenterol 1996;91:492-7.
53. Breumelhof R, Nadorp JHSM, Akkermans LMA, Smout AJPM. *Analysis of 24-hour esophageal pH and pressure data in unselected patients with non-cardiac chest pain.* Gastroenterology 1990;99:1257-64.
54. Lam HGTH, Breumelhof R, Van Berge Henegouwen GP, Smout AJPM. *Temporal relationships between episodes of non-cardiac chest pain and abnormal oesophageal function.* Gut 1994;35:733-6.
55. Lux G, Van Els J, The GS, et al. *Ambulatory esophageal pressure, pH and ECG recording in patients with normal and pathological coronary angiography and intermittent chest pain.* Neurogastroenterol Motil 1995;7:23-30.
56. Lam HGT, Breumelhof R, Roelofs JMM, et al. *What is the optimal time window in symptom analysis of 24-hour esophageal pressure and pH data?* Dig Dis Sci 1994;39:402-9.
57. DeMeester TR, O'Sullivan GC, Bermudez G, et al. *Esophageal function in patients with angina-type chest pain and normal coronary angiograms.* Ann Surg 1982;196:488-98.
58. Cherian P, Smith LF, Bardhan DK, et al. *Esophageal tests in the evaluation of non-cardiac chest pain.* Dis Esophagus 1995;8:129-33.
59. Voskuil JH, Cramer MJ, Breumelhof R, Heading RC. *Prevalence of esophageal disorders in patients with chest pain newly referred to the cardiologist.* Chest 1996;109:1210-4.
60. De Caestecker JS, Blackwell JN, Brown J, et al. *The oesophagus as a cause of recurrent chest pain: which patients should be investigated and which tests should be used?* Lancet 1985;ii:1143.
61. Schofield PM, Bennett DH, Whorwell PJ, et al. *Exertional gastroesophageal reflux: a mechanism for symptoms in patients with angina pectoris and normal coronary angiograms.* Br Med J 1987;294:1459-61.
62. Lam HGT, Dekker W, Kan G, et al. *Acute non-cardiac chest pain in a coronary care unit.* Gastroenterology 1992;102:453-60.
63. Shi G, Bruley des Varannes S, Scarpignato C, et al. *Reflux-related symptoms in patients with normal oesophageal exposure to acid. The acid hypersensitive oesophagus.* Gut 1995;37:457-64.
64. Wiener GJ, Richter JE, Copper JB, et al. *The symptom index: a clinically important parameter of ambulatory 24-hour esophageal pH monitoring.* Am J Gastroenterol 1988;83: 358-61.
65. Breumelhof R, Smout AJPM. *The symptom sensitivity index: a valuable additional parameter in 24 hour esophageal pH recording.* Am J Gastroenterol 1991;86:160-4.

66. Emde C, Armstrong D, Blum AL. *Chest pain due to gastroesophageal reflux: presentation of a mathematical procedure to assess its significance.* J Gastrointest Motil 1990;2:140.
67. Weusten BLAM, Roelofs JMM, Akkermans LMA, et al. *The symptom association probability: an improved method for symptom analysis of 24 h esophageal pH data.* Gastroenterology 1994;107:1741-5.
68. Richter JE, Obrecht WF, Bradley LA, et al. *Psychological similarities between patients with the nutcracker esophagus and irritable bowel syndrome.* Dig Dis Sci 1986;31:131-8.
69. Cornier LE, Katon W, Russo J, et al. *Chest pain with negative cardiac diagnostic studies. Relationship to psychiatric illness.* J Nerv Mental Dis 1988;176:351-8.
70. Katon W, Hall HL, Russo J, et al. *Chest pain: relationship of psychiatric illness to coronary arteriography results.* Am J Med 1988;84:1-9.
71. Ayuso Mateos JL, Bayon Perez C, Santo-Domingo Carrasco J, Olivares D. *Atypical chest pain and panic disorder.* Psychother Psychosom 1989;52:92-5.
72. Beitman BD, Lamberti JW, Mukerji, et al. *Panic disorder in patients with chest pain and angiographically normal coronary arteries.* Am J Cardiol 1989;63:1399-403.
73. Clouse RE, Lustman PJ. *Psychiatric illnesses and contraction abnormalities of the esophagus* N Engl J Med 1982;309:1337-42.
74. Cannon RO, Quyyumi AA, Mincemoyer R, et al. *Imipramine in patients with chest pain despite normal coronary angiograms.* N Engl J Med 1994;19:1411-7.
75. Clouse RE, Lustman PJ, Eckert TC, et al. *Low dose trazodone for symptomatic patients with esophageal contraction abnormalities.* Gastroenterology 1987;92:1027-36.
76. Orlando RC, Bozymski EM. *Clinical and manometric effects of nitroglycerin in diffuse esophageal spasm.* N Engl J Med 1973;289:23.
77. Swamy N. *Esophageal spasm: clinical and manometric responses to nitroglycerin and long acting nitrites.* Gastroenterology 1977;72:23.
78. Frachtman RL, Botoman VA, Pope CE. *A double blind crossover trial of diltiazem shows no benefit in patients with dysphagia and/or chest pain of esophageal origin.* Gastroenterology 1986;90:1420.
79. Richter JE, Spurling TJ, Cordova CM, Castell DO. *Effects of oral calcium blocker, diltiazem, on esophageal contractions. Studies in volunteers and patients with nutcracker esophagus.* Dig Dis Sci 1984;29:649-56.
80. Cattau EL Jr, Castell DO, Johnson DA, Spurling TJ, et al. *Diltiazem therapy for symptoms associated with nutcracker esophagus.* Am J Gastroenterol 1991;86:272-6.
81. Richter JE, Dalton CB, Castell DO. *Nifedipine: a potent inhibitor of esophageal contractions. Is it effective in the treatment of non cardiac chest pain?* Dig Dis Sci 1985;30:790.
82. Cuschieri A. *Endoscopic esophageal myotomy for specific motility disorders and non-cardiac chest pain.* Endosc Surg Allied Technol 1993;1:280-7.

83. Singh S, Richter JE, Hewson EG, et al. *The contribution of gastro-esophageal reflux to chest pain in patients with coronary artery disease.* Ann Intern Med 1992;117:824-30.
84. Stahl WG, Beton R, Johnson CS, et al. *Diagnosis and treatment of patients with gastroesophageal reflux and non-cardiac chest pain.* South Med J 1994;87:739-42.
85. Rose S, Achkar E, Easly KA. *Follow-up of patients with non-cardiac chest pain: value of esophageal testing.* Dig Dis Sci 1994;39:2069-73.

*ADDRESS FOR CORRESPONDENCE*

**TACK JF, MD, PhD**
Department of Internal Medicine, Division of Gastroenterology
University Hospitals Leuven
Herestraat 49
3000 Leuven Belgium
Fax: +32 16 344419
E-mail: jan.tack@med.kuleuven.ac.be

# UNEXPLAINED NAUSEA AND VOMITING

*KL Koch*

Nausea and vomiting are very common human symptoms. While vomiting is rather easy to describe in objective terms, the symptom of nausea may be difficult for patients to describe. Nausea may be reported as a "sick to the stomach" sensation, a "queasiness", and as an urge to vomit and may range from mild to severe in intensity. Nausea may be briefly experienced, come in "waves" or may be chronic and persistent. Finally, nausea is a noxious, debilitating and depressing symptom, whereas vomiting is often associated with relief of nausea and a general feeling of improvement after the vomiting episode.

The differential diagnosis of nausea and vomiting is extensive[1]. Causes range from Central Nervous System (CNS) disorders to a variety of gastrointestinal, metabolic and idiopathic disorders. In addition, epidemiologic studies of the general population indicated that abdominal symptoms clustered into three categories that could be categorized as irritable bowel syndrome-like, gastroesophageal reflux and nausea and vomiting[2]. Thus, nausea and vomiting occurs as a distinct symptom entity in the general population.

Patients with unexplained nausea and vomiting who present to the primary care physician, to the subspecialist in gastroenterology or to the tertiary referral center can represent challenging diagnostic and therapeutic problems. When diseases and disorders which are associated with nausea or vomiting are eliminated, then the symptoms may be referred to as idiopathic or functional nausea and vomiting. Many of these patients have subtle neuromuscular abnormalities of the stomach or visceral hypersensitivities which are associated with nausea symptoms. These disorders range from abnormalities in gastric tone to gastric dysrhythmias and idiopathic gastroparesis.

The purpose of the present review is to explore approaches to the patient with chronic unexplained nausea and vomiting.

## Differential diagnosis of nausea and vomiting

When the patient is seen by the gastroenterologist, the nausea and vomiting are usually chronic problems. A detailed history and physical examination should be performed. The diagnostic possibilities listed in Table 1 should be reviewed[1]. Most of these disorders can be excluded on the basis of a good history and physical examination. Routine laboratory tests such as a complete blood count, erythrocyte sedimentation rate, liver function tests and urinalysis should be performed.

The physician needs to consider common causes of nausea symptoms that often occur in the postprandial period. Postprandial nausea often occurs with other symptoms such as early satiety, bloating and vague, diffuse upper abdominal discomfort. These rather non-specific symptoms are referred to as dysmotility-like dyspepsia or meal-related symptoms or simply idiopathic or functional nausea, idiopathic bloating, etc. if no cause for the symptoms is found[3,4].

These post-prandial dyspeptic symptoms should be contrasted with symptoms more typical for peptic ulcer disease. Classical peptic ulcer symptoms are burning epigastric pain that is worse during fasting and is relieved (not worsened) by food. The use of Non-Steroidal Anti-Inflammatory Drugs (NSAIDs) or previously documented peptic ulcer disease increase the likelihood of peptic ulcer disease. Helicobacter pylori (H. pylori) remains a controversial cause of nausea and dyspepsia symptoms[5], but is a causative agent of duodenal ulcers. In the absence of mucosal ulceration, antibiotic therapy for H. pylori results in symptom improvement in only 10-20% of patients with functional dyspepsia.

Extra-gastric and common conditions that may present with predominantly nausea include gastroesophageal reflux disease, chronic cholecystitis, pancreatitis, and the irritable bowel syndrome. Other common and uncommon causes of nausea and vomiting are listed in Table 1.

Empiric trials of proton pump inhibitors, prokinetic drugs, or fiber therapy for irritable bowel syndrome may be tried in the absence of alarm symptoms[6]. However, if alarm symptoms occur in addition to nausea, then the pace of formal diagnostic investigations should be accelerated[6,7]. Alarm symptoms include dysphagia, frequent vomiting, hematemesis or hematochezia, anemia, weight loss, and age over 50 years with new onset symptoms. The standard diagnostic tests described below should be obtained in patients with alarm symptoms or in patients who have failed empiric drug therapy.

## Diseases and disorders associated with nausea and vomiting

**Mechanical obstruction**
- Stomach, duodenum
- Small bowel, colon
- Hepatobiliary disease
- Pancreatic duct diseases

**Peptic disease**
- Esophagus - GERD
- Stomach - gastritis, ulcer, H. pylori
- Duodenum - duodenitis, ulcer

**Peritoneal irritation (peritonitis, cancer, irradiation)**

**Carcinoma**
- Gastric, ovarian
- Hypernephroma
- Paraneoplastic syndrome

**Metabolic-hormonal**
- Diabetes mellitus
- Uremia, hypercalcemia
- Addison's disease
- Hyperthyroidism, hypothyroidism
- Pregnancy, progesterone/estrogen

**Drugs**
- Levodopa, digitalis, phenytoin, cardiac anti-arrhythmias, NSAIDs, antibiotics, chemotherapy agents, morphine, nicotine, progesterone, estrogen

**Ischemic gastroparesis**

**Postoperative** (with gastroparesis or dumping syndrome)
- Vagotomy
- Partial/total gastrectomy
- Fundoplication, fundic resection

**Intestinal pseudo-obstruction (visceral neuropathy/myopathy)**
- Scleroderma, amyloidosis
- Idiopathic

**CNS disease**
- Migraine
- Infections
- Tumors
- Vestibular nerve-brain stem lesions
- Parkinson's disease

**Psychologic/psychiatric disorders**
- Anorexia nervosa
- Bulimia nervosa
- Rumination, psychogenic nausea (vomiting)

**Idiopathic nausea and vomiting**
- With gastroparesis (idiopathic)
- Without gastroparesis
- Gastric dysrhythmias
- Cyclic vomiting syndrome

Table 1

## Standard diagnostic tests for chronic, unexplained nausea and vomiting

Standard diagnostic tests for the evaluation of unexplained nausea and vomiting should include evaluation of the mucosa of the esophagus, stomach, and duodenum. Barium X-ray studies of esophagus, stomach and duodenum and ultrasound studies of gallbladder and pancreas may have already been performed and are normal (Figure 1).

Figure 1

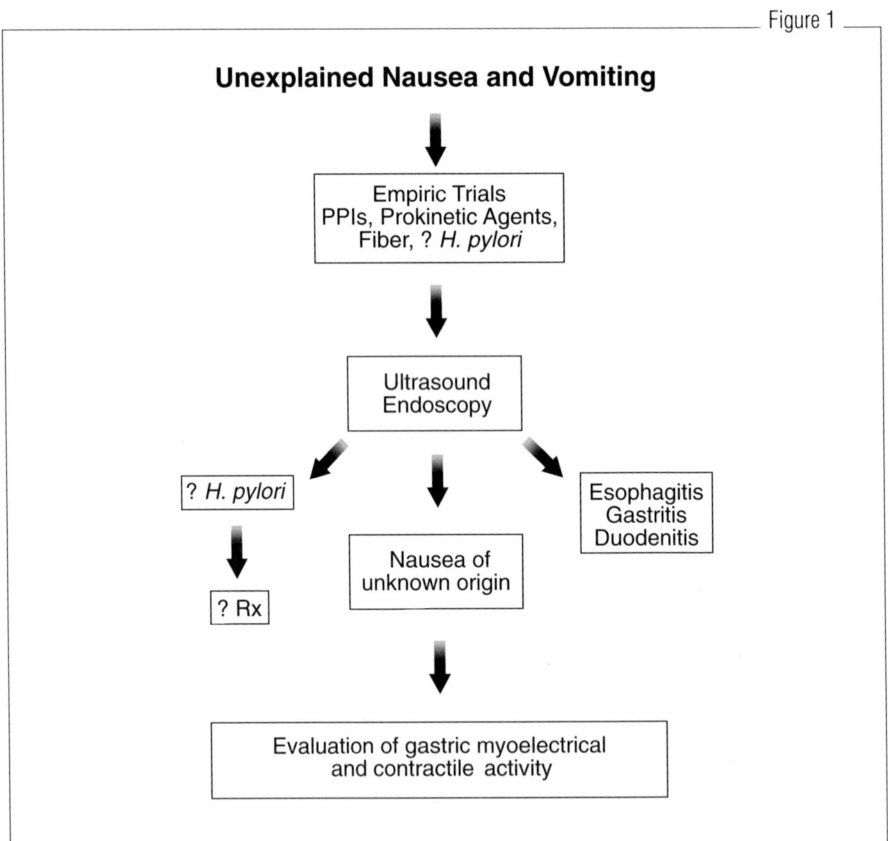


Approach to unexplained nausea and vomiting with standard tests to exclude common gastric, duodenal, gallbladder and pancreas diseases and disorders. When laboratory tests, empiric drug trials and these diagnostic tests are normal, chronic nausea is of unknown origin. The tests to consider "beyond endoscopy" are investigations of gastric myoelectrical and contractile activity.

The gastroenterologist will perform an upper endoscopy to diagnose subtle esophagitis, gastritis, or duodenitis[3]. Evidence for an infiltrative disease of the stomach, such as adenocarcinoma, may also be found at this time. A biopsy for H. pylori can be obtained during the endoscopy. A Computerized Axial Tomography (CAT) scan of the abdomen may be indicated. The gastroenterologist should also consider CNS diseases and disorders in the differential diagnosis of patients with nausea and vomiting[8]. With CNS diseases, headache, blurred vision or vertigo/instability are often present. Morning nausea and nausea and vomiting after movement are reported with CNS disorders. If these studies are normal, a CAT scan or Magnetic Resonance Imaging (MRI) of the head and neurology consultation may be indicated.

In many patients, these diagnostic studies are all normal, but nausea and vomiting persist. Gastric myoelectrical and contractile disorders should be considered in such patients[1,6]. The diagnostic tests to be considered when mucosal and mechanical abnormalities of the GI tract are excluded are tests "beyond endoscopy" that reveal neuromuscular disorders of the stomach and duodenum. These disorders alter the functions of the stomach (i.e., functional disorders), particularly in the postprandial period when sustained gastric neuromuscular activity is required for mixing and emptying ingested food.

In the section below, electrogastrography and gastric emptying tests, non-invasive tests of gastric neuromuscular activity, are briefly described. The pattern of results from these two tests provide four diagnostic categories that may lead to different treatment approaches for the patient with unexplained nausea and vomiting.

## Electrogastrography

Electrogastrography (EGG) is the method used to measure myoelectrical activity of the stomach with cutaneous electrodes positioned on the epigastrium[9,10]. This technique is much like an electrocardiogram or EKG in that the surface electrodes detect rhythmic or cyclical electrical changes from internal organs beneath the recording electrodes. Careful attention to recording techniques will allow visual interpretation of the EGG signal, but computer analysis is helpful in detecting the variety of frequencies and frequency changes that may be present during the EGG recording[9]. The normal EGG signal ranges in frequency from 2.5-3.75 cycles per minute (cpm)[9,11]. The EGG frequencies can be displayed as pseudo 3-D plots or expressed as a percentage distribution of the total power in the EGG signal.

Abnormally fast gastric rhythms are 3.75-10.0 cpm and are termed tachygastrias[9,11]. Slower frequency EGG waves (1.0-2.5 cpm) are present normally, but predominant 1.0-2.5 cpm EGG activity is termed bradygastria[11]. Gastric dysrhythmias are present in patients with gastroparesis from diabetes[12-15], post-surgical[16], renal failure[17] or idiopathic causes[15,18,19]. Obstruction of the stomach is associated with nausea and vomiting, and robust 3 cpm activity[19]. Gastric dysrhythmias are frequently present in functional dyspepsia[3,6,20].

## Gastric emptying studies

Solid-phase gastric emptying studies using a standard meal assesses the global work of emptying performed by the contractions of the stomach musculature. In Nuclear Medicine departments, technetium-labeled scrambled eggs or liver are frequently used for test meals[21,22]. The percentage of the meal emptied over a 2 hour period of time is calculated by identifying the region of interest (the stomach) and calculating the percentage of isotope retained in the stomach during a defined period of time. Usually, a one minute scan is performed every 15 minutes for the duration of the study. When compared with control values, patients with gastroparesis or rapid gastric emptying (dumping) are identified. Dumping syndrome may also cause post-prandial nausea, bloating, and uncomfortable abdominal distention. In the future, gastric emptying studies may be more accessible in the office as a variety of $C^{13}$ labeled meals[23,24] will be available to measure gastric emptying rates.

The rate of emptying of solid food reflects the overall contractile efficiency of the stomach in emptying a standard meal and the EGG measures gastric myoelectrical activity before and after ingestion of a provocative water load test. The non-invasive tests, gastric emptying and EGG, are useful for measuring gastric neuromuscular activity. By careful review of the history and physical and by considering the gastric emptying and EGG results, the diagnosis and management of patients with unexplained nausea and vomiting (and normal standard test results) can be advanced as discussed below.

## Gastric emptying and electrogastrogram patterns in patients with unexplained nausea and vomiting

When the gastric emptying and EGG results are interpreted together, four diagnostic categories become apparent[6].
The four categories (Figure 2) suggest different pathophysiologies for the symptoms of nausea and vomiting and suggest different approaches for further diagnoses and/or treatments:

Figure 2

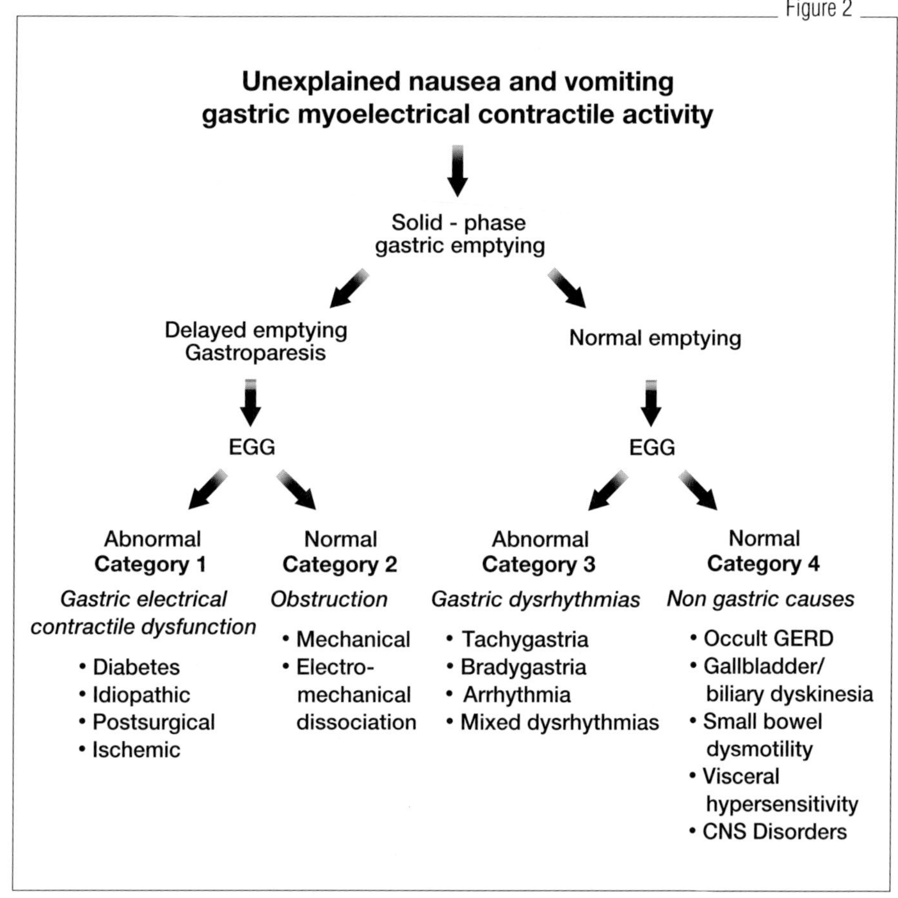


Evaluation of gastric myoelectrical and contractile activity utilizing solid-phase gastric emptying and electrogastrograms (EGGs). See text for details.

*Category 1. Delayed gastric emptying and gastric dysrhythmias*
The most severe electrocontractile or neuromuscular disorders are diabetic gastroparesis, post-surgical gastroparesis, and idiopathic gastroparesis. A specific cause of gastroparesis should be sought. Ischemic gastroparesis is an uncommon but important and reversible electrocontractile disorder of the stomach[25]. The gastric dysrhythmias are generally classified as tachygastrias, bradygastrias, arrhythmias or mixed dysrhythmias (Figure 3).

Figure 3

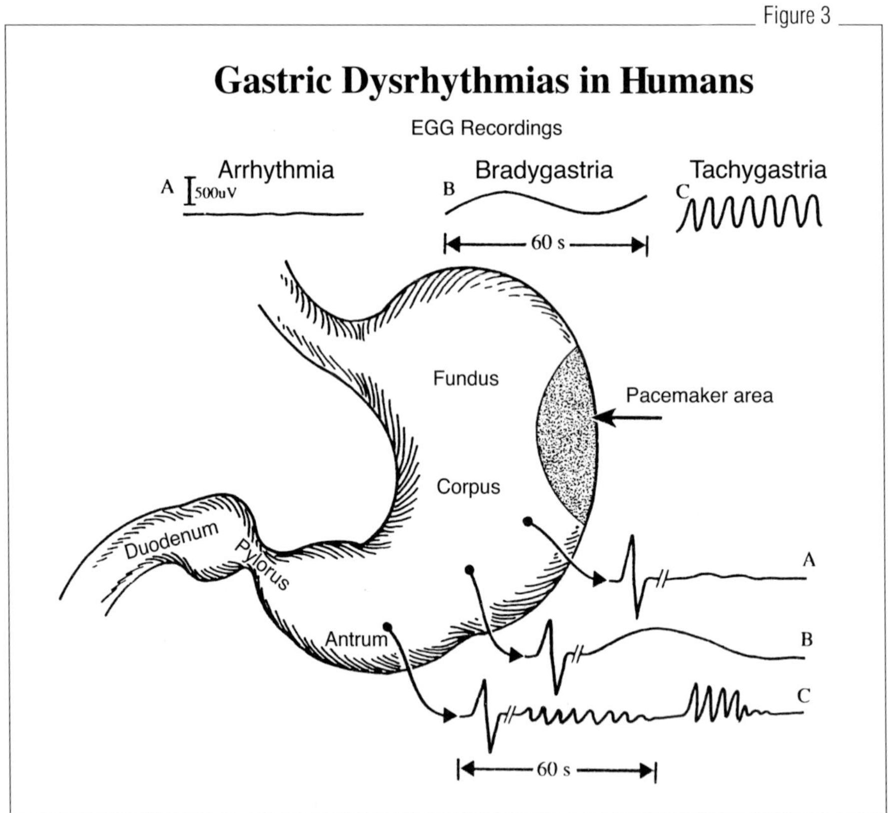


Illustrations of gastric dysrhythmias recorded in humans. Three major categories of dysrhythmias are the arrhythmia or flatline pattern, 1.0-2.5 cpm bradygastrias and 3.5-10.0 cpm tachygastrias. These dysrhythmias originate in the corpus and antrum and are recorded with serosal or cutaneous electrodes.
Reproduced with permission from Koch KL, Stern RM[3].

In tertiary medical centers, up to 50% of patients with chronic nausea and vomiting have gastroparesis[7]. These patients represent the most severe spectrum of abnormalities of gastric neuromuscular dysfunction.

*Category 2. Delayed gastric emptying and eugastria*

A normal 3 cpm EGG rhythm (eugastria) is not expected in patients with nausea and gastroparesis. This combination was found in patients with mechanical obstructions of the stomach, such pyloric stenosis or postbulbar strictures (Figure 4)[26].

Figure 4

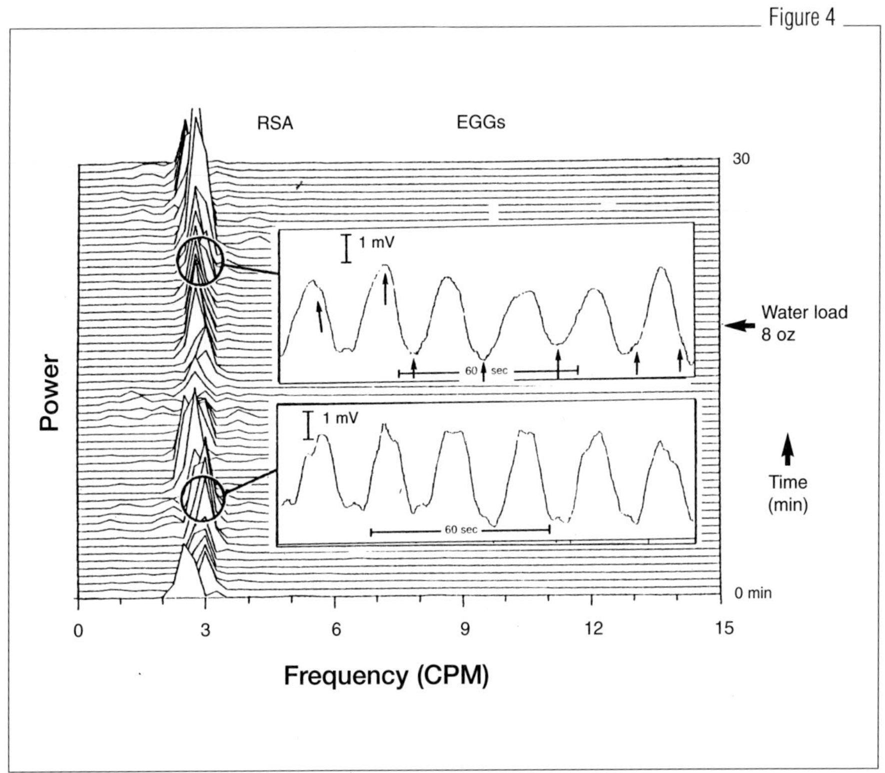


Electrogastrograms (EGGs, inserts) and running spectral analysis (RSA) of an EGG from a patient with mechanical obstruction of the stomach. The EGG recording shows high amplitude 3 cpm electrical waves before and after a water load. Arrows in insert refer to visible peristalses observed in patient's epigastrium. Note persistent and unvarying 3 cpm peaks in the RSA. Reproduced wiht permission from Brzana RJ, Koch KL, Bingaman S et al[26].

In obstruction, the 3 cpm EGG waves have prominent amplitude at baseline and do not change after a water load. This pattern suggests the possibility of mechanical obstruction should be considered or re-evaluated. A second pattern in this category has normal 3 cpm EGG activity at baseline but decreased 3 cpm activity after the water load test or ingestion of food. This pattern suggests electromechanical dissociation, wherein the myoelectrical rhythm is maintained but appropriate contractile responses of the gastric smooth muscle are absent or decreased in response to a water load or food challenge.

*Category 3. Normal gastric emptying and gastric dysrhythmias*

The causes of gastric dysrhythmias in these patients are unknown. Potential causes of the dysrhythmias include increased sympathetic and/or decreased parasympathetic nerve activity, injury to the smooth muscle, enteric nerves, or interstitial cells of Cajal. Injury to and dysfunction of one or more of these structures may play a role in producing gastric dysrhythmias and reducing normal 3 cpm gastric myoelectrical activity in patients with nausea. In the spectrum of abnormalities, these patients have milder neuromuscular dysfunction of the stomach in that emptying of the standard meal is normal. However, symptoms may still be significant. Several studies have shown that treatment with prokinetic agents abolish the gastric dysrhythmias and improve symptoms[12,15,18]. More studies on this group of patients are needed.

*Category 4. Normal gastric emptying and eugastria*

In the patient with normal gastric emptying and a normal EGG pattern (Figure 5), the symptoms of nausea and vomiting may originate from non-gastric causes. For example, occult gastroesophageal reflux disease was detected with 24 hour esophageal pH studies; nausea resolved with aggressive acid suppression therapy (Figure 5)[27]. Central nervous system abnormalities should be excluded in these patients[1,8]. It is also possible that patients who have normal gastric emptying and normal EGG patterns have a form of gastric visceral hypersensitivity with vagal or splanchnic afferent nerve dysfunction.

Figure 5

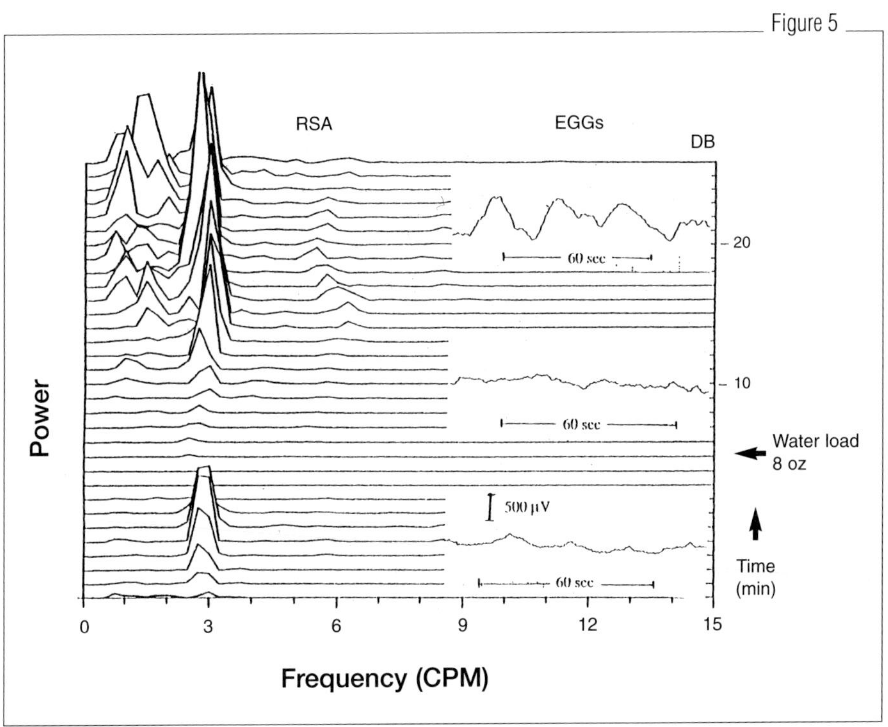


Normal electrogastrogram (EGG, insert) recordings from a patient with unexplained nausea and normal gastric emptying. The baseline EGG shows low amplitude 3 cpm waves. After the water load (8.5 oz. ingested), there is temporary suppression of the 3 cpm activity, but it returns approximately 10 min later. The running spectral analysis RSA shows peaks at 3 cpm, at baseline and after the water load.

Some of these patients may have abnormal gastric tone, sphincter of Oddi dysfunction or small bowel dysmotility, and intraluminal pressure recordings or barostatography may detect other gastrointestinal neuromuscular abnormalities.

## Therapeutic concepts and considerations

When the pathophysiology of nausea and vomiting is related to gastric neuromuscular dysfunction described above, then therapeutic approaches can be conceptualized in terms of cardiac diseases/disorders and therapies (Tables 2, 3)[28].

SIMILARITIES BETWEEN GASTRIC AND CARDIAC ELECTRICAL ACTIVITY AND EMPTYING

| **Cardiac** | **Gastric** |
|---|---|
| Cardiac dysrhythmias | Gastric dysrhythmias |
| Dilated ventricle | Dilated antrum |
| Ventricular hypomotility | Antral hypomotility |
| Delayed ventricular emptying | Delayed gastric emptying |
| (Chronic heart failure) | (Chronic gastric failure) |

Table 2

Modified from Liberski SM, Koch KP, Atnip RG, Stern RM[25].

Dysrhythmias, decreased contractility, decreased emptying and functional organ failure occur in cardiac and gastric diseases and disorders and the similarities in the two organs are shown in Table 2.
To continue the cardiac analogies, current and new therapies can be described as:

1. gastric anti-arrhythmic drug based receptors such as $5HT_3$, $5HT_4$,or dopamine receptors
2. gastric prokinetic agents, drugs designed to increase corpus-antral contractility
3. drugs to alter fundic or antral tone;
4. non-drug treatment such as acustimulation and gastric electrical stimulation (pacemakers)
5. revascularization procedures for mesenteric artery occlusions; and
6. removal of fixed obstructions with Billroth I and II operations. A review of individual drugs and non-drug therapies is beyond the scope of this review.

SIMILARITIES BETWEEN TREATMENTS FOR GASTRIC AND CARDIAC NEUROMUSCULAR DYSFUNCTION

| Cardiac therapies | Gastric therapies |
| --- | --- |
| • Antiarrhythmic agents<br>Class I-IV | • Antiarrhythmic agents<br>receptor-based<br>metoclopramide<br>domperidone<br>cisapride |
| • Inotropic agents | • Prokinetic agents<br>metoclopramide<br>domperidone<br>cisapride<br>erythromycin |
| • Electrical stimulation<br>(pacing) | • Electrical stimulation<br>pacing<br>electrical stimulation |
| • Coronary artery bypass operation | • Mesenteric Artery Bypass operation |
| • Aortic stenosis<br>Relieve obstruction-AVR | • Gastric outlet obstruction<br>Relieve obstruction-BI, BII |

Table 3

Modified from Liberski SM, Koch KL, Atnip RG et al[25].

Dietary counseling should be provided for patients with neuromuscular dysfunctions of the stomach. Food represents the substrate upon which the stomach must exert muscular work in order to mix and empty nutrient suspensions into the duodenum. An outline of a three step diet for patients with nausea and vomiting is shown in Table 4[1]. The proper diet requires a minimum amount of gastric work, but provides enough nutrients to maintain weight and minimize symptoms.

## NAUSEA/VOMITING (GASTROPARESIS) DIET

STEP 1. GATORADE AND BOUILLON

**Diet:** Patients with severe nausea and vomiting should sip small volumes of salty liquids such as gatorade or bouillon in order to avoid dehydration. These liquids include salt and sugar in addition to water. Any liquid to be ingested should have some caloric content.

**Goal:** To ingest 1,000 to 1,500 ml per day in multiple servings, e.g. twelve 4 oz. servings over the course of 12 - 14 hours. 1 - 2 oz at a time may be sipped to reach approximately 4 oz per hour.

**Avoid:** Citrus drinks of all kinds and highly sweetened drinks.

STEP 2. SOUPS

**Diet:** If Gatorade or bouillon is tolerated, the diet may be advanced to include a variety of soups with noodles or rice and crackers. Peanut butter, cheese and crackers may be tolerated in small amounts. Caramels or other chewy confections may be tried. These foods should be given in at least six divided meals per day.

**Goal:** To ingest approximately 1,500 calories per day. Patients who can accomplish this will avoid dehydration and will hopefully ingest enough calories to maintain their weight. In many patients, maintenance of their present weight, not weight gain, is the realistic goal.

**Avoid:** Creamy, milk-based liquids.

STEP 3. SOLID FOOD: STARCHES, CHICKEN AND FISH

**Diet:** Starches such as noodles, pastas, potatoes and rice are easily mixed and emptied by the stomach. Thus, soups, mashed or baked potatoes, pasta dishes, rice and baked chicken breast and fish are usually well tolerated sources of carbohydrate and protein. These solids should also be ingested in six divided meals per day. A one-a-day vitamin should be prescribed.

**Goal:** To find a diet of common foods that the patient finds interesting, satisfying and that evoke minimal nausea/vomiting symptoms. As the patient learns what liquids and solids are tolerated, the variety and number of foods that can be enjoyed will increase.

**Avoid:** Fatty foods which delay gastric emptying and red meats and fresh vegetables which require considerable trituration. Avoid pulpy fibrous foods like celery, cabbage, orange pulp that promote formation of bezoars.

Table 4

Modified from Koch KL[1].

## Conclusions

Nausea and vomiting are often times chronic, disabling and depressing symptoms. A large differential diagnosis of the causes of nausea and vomiting, ranging from central nervous system lesions to gastrointestinal motility disorders, must be considered. If no alarm symptoms are present, empiric therapy for nausea and vomiting is reasonable for a short period of time. A battery of standard tests which include laboratory tests, radiographic studies and endoscopy are suggested to diagnose relatively common gastrointestinal causes of nausea and vomiting. If the standard tests are normal, then gastric neuromuscular disorders should be considered as causes of chronic nausea and vomiting syndromes. Gastric emptying tests and electrogastrography are non-invasive tests for measuring global gastric muscle function and gastric myoelectrical rhythms, respectively. Gastroparesis and gastric dysrhythmias are frequently found in patients with chronic, unexplained nausea and vomiting. More drug therapies, specific diet counseling and non-drug therapies for nausea and vomiting are needed to help patients with chronic nausea and vomiting.

Acknowledgements
The author wishes to acknowledge the excellent assistance of Mrs. Pamela Petito in preparing this manuscript.

### *References*

1. Koch KL. *Approach to the patient with nausea and vomiting.* In: Yamada T, editor. Textbook of Gastroenterology. Philadelphia: J.B. Lippincott; 1995;731-49.
2. Kay L, Jorgensen T. *Redefining abdominal syndromes. Results of a population based study.* Scand J Gastroenterol 1996;31:469-75.
3. Koch KL, Stern RM. *Functional disorders of the stomach.* Semirr Gastrointest Dis 1996;4:185-95.
4. Talley NJ, Collin Jones D, Koch KJ, et al. *Functional dyspepsia: A classification with guidelines for diagnosis and management.* Gastroenterol Int 1991;4:145-60.

5. NIH Consensus Development Panel. *Helicobacter pylori in peptic disease.* JAMA 1994;272:65-9.
6. Koch KL. *Dyspepsia of unknown origin: Pathophysiology, diagnosis, and treatment.* Dig Dis 1997;15:316-29.
7. Lin HC, Hasler WL. *Disorders of gastric emptying.* In: Yamada T, editor. Textbook of Gastroenterology. Philadelphia: J.B. Lippincott Company; 1995;1318-46.
8. Camilleri M. *Disorders of gastrointestinal motility in neurologic diseases.* Mayo Clin Proc 1990;65:825-46.
9. Koch KL, Stern RM. In: *Electrogastrography. Illustrated Guide to Gastrointestinal Motility.* Kumar D, Wingate D, editors. London: Churchhill Livingstone; 1993; 290-307.
10. Koch KL. *The stomach.* In: Schuster MM, editor. Atlas of Gastrointestinal Motility in Health and Disease. Baltimore: Williams & Wilkins; 1993;158-76.
11. Stern RM, Koch KL, Stewart WR, Vasey MW. *Electrogastrography: Current issues in validation and methodology.* Psychophysiology 1987;24:55-64.
12. Koch KL, Stern RM, Stewart WR, et al. *Gastric emptying and gastric myoelectrical activity in patients with symptomatic diabetic gastroparesis: Effect of long-term domperidone treatment.* Am J Gastroenterol 1989;84:1069-75.
13. Jebbink HJA, Bruijs PPM, Bravenboer B, et al. *Gastric myoelectrical activity in patients with Type I diabetes mellitus and autonomic neuropathy.* Dig Dis Sci 1994;39:2376-83.
14. Abell TL, Camilleri M, Hench VS, Malagelada J-R. *Gastric electromechanical function and gastric emptying in diabetic gastroparesis.* Europ J Gastroenterol Hepatol 1991;3:163-7.
15. Rothstein RD, Alavi A, Reynolds J. *Electrogastrography in patients with gastroparesis. Effect of long term cisapride.* Dig Dis Sci 1993;38:1518-24.
16. Stoddard CJ, Smallwood RH, Duthie HL. *Electrical arrhythmias in the human stomach.* Gut 1981;22:705-12.
17. Ravelli AM, Ladermann SE, Bisset WM, et al. *Foregut motor function in chronic renal failure.* Arch Dis Child 1992;67:1343-7.
18. Cucchiara S, Minella R, Riezzo G, et al. *Reversal of gastric electrical dysrhythmias by cisapride in children with functional dyspepsia: report of three cases.* Dig Dis Sci 1992;37:1136-40.
19. Koch KL, Bingaman S, Sperry N, Stern RM. *Electrogastrography differentiates mechanical vs idiopathic gastroparesis in patients with nausea and vomiting.* Gastroenterology 1991;100:A99.
20. Koch KL, Medina M, Bingaman S, Stern RM. *Gastric dysrhythmias and visceral sensations in patients with functional dyspepsia.* Gastroenterology 1992;102:A469.

21. Akkermans LMA, Jacobs F, Smout AJPM, et al. *Radionuclide measurement of normal and disturbed gastric motility.* Scand J Gastroenterol 1984 (Suppl 96);19:19-26.
22. Collins PJ, Horowitz M, Cook DJ, et al. *Gastric emptying in normal subjects - a reproducible technique using a single scintillation camera and computer system.* Gut 1983;24:1117-25.
23. Braden B, Adams S, Duan LP, et al. *The C13 acetate breath test accurately reflects gastric emptying of liquids in both liquid and semilsolid test meals.* Gastroenterology 1995;108:1048-55.
24. Choi MG, Camilleri M, Burton DD, et al. *(C13) octanoic acid breath test for gastric emptying of solids: accuracy, reproducibility, and comparison with scintigraphy.* Gastroenterology 1997;112:1155-62.
25. Liberski SM, Koch KL, Atnip RG, Stern RM. *Ischemic gastroparesis: Resolution of nausea, vomiting and gastroparesis after mesenteric artery revascularization.* Gastroenterology 1990;99:252-57.
26. Brzana, RJ, Koch KL, Bingaman S. *Gastric myoelectrical activity in patients with gastric outlet obstruction and idiopathic gastroparesis in patients with nausea and vomiting.* Am J Gastroenterol 1998;93:1083-89.
27. Brzana RJ, Koch KL. *Gastroesophageal reflux disease presenting with intractable nausea.* Ann Intern Med 1997;126:704-7.
28. Koch KL. *Clinical approaches to unexplained nausea and vomiting.* Adv Gastroenterol Hepatol Clin Nutr 1998;3:163-178.

## *Address for correspondence*

**KOCH KL, MD**
Division of Gastroenterology and Hepatology, H045
Hershey Medical Center
500 University Drive
Hershey, Pennsylvania 17033 USA
Fax: +1 717 531 6770

# Chronic abdominal pain and discomfort

## Relevance of intestinal gas dynamics

*J-R Malagelada*

At the present time we do not have a unifying hypothesis to explain the mechanism of chronic abdominal pain and discomfort in functional gut disorders. A number of partial hypotheses have been developed based on experimental and clinical observations. However, each of these hypotheses postulates a different physiological disturbance and it is difficult to accept that so many altered mechanisms would coexist in the same patient. Thus, we are left with various putative explanations:

- different mechanisms are interlinked in an, as yet, unidentified way
- different patients have similar symptoms based on different disease mechanisms
- none of the mechanisms identified so far are relevant and the true cause of abdominal symptoms remains to be discovered.

Mechanisms identified so far include gut dysmotility, minimal inflammation, visceral hypersensitivity and psychological disturbances. In this review, I will update and analyze the supporting evidence for each of these postulated mechanisms. At the same time, I will introduce the concept of intestinal gas dynamics and provide preliminary information concerning its relevance to the pathogenesis of abdominal symptoms in patients with functional gut disorders.

### Gut dysmotility in patients with chronic abdominal pain

Regional disturbances of motility in the gastrointestinal tract have been detected in some patients with functional gut disorders and, hence, proposed as likely pathogenetic mechanisms. Unfortunately, not all symptomatic patients exhibit dysmotility. If we considered functional disorders as a single condition, symptoms would correlate poorly with abnormal motility, be it delayed gastric emptying, antral hypomotility or intestinal dysmotility.

However, motor events may be undetectable in some patients with concurrent symptoms simply because our current measuring devices are not sensitive enough. Conversely, abnormal motor events recorded during physiological studies may not be temporarily associated with symptoms but, at other times, and in conjunction with other mechanisms (? central) disturbances in motility may, indeed, turn into uncomfortable sensations. The concept that functional gastrointestinal symptoms are derived from abnormal gut motility has also obtained some support from the therapeutic use of prokinetic agents. It must be admitted, however, than even when there is a statistically significant drug response, it is often difficult to establish a causal relation between drug-induced changes in motility and relief of symptoms in individual patients. Finally, we should consider the possibility that certain subgroups of patients may show a stronger association between dysmotility and symptoms than unselected patient populations.

Perhaps the best evidence that abnormal gut motility is a potential inductor of pain comes from oesophageal data. First of all, various oesophageal motor disorders are associated with pain. This is usually described by patients as chest pain, with or without associated dysphagia. Among painful oesophageal conditions, diffuse oesophageal spasm is best characterized[1] but other oesophageal dysmotilities such as nutcracker oesophagus, hypertensive lower oesophageal sphincter and non-specific motor disorders may be associated with sporadic pain[2]. As always, however, the difficulty lies in proving that the motor abnormalities are directly causing the pain. There are two lines of evidence: temporal association and provocative tests. The former evidence is derived primarily from manometric studies, stationary or ambulatory, that show concurrence between abnormal motor events and pain. Unfortunately, such data provide only indirect and rather soft support. For instance, in one study[3] only 18% of patients showed temporary association between chest pain and abnormal oesophageal motility. Provocative studies go one step beyond and they are based on the idea that certain stimuli would induce simultaneously motor abnormalities and chest pain in predisposed patients. Edrophonium, bethanechol or ergonovine are pharmacological stimuli that have been used for test purposes. Again, however, temporal association provides only indirect evidence. In the study conducted by Lee et al.[4], abnormal manometry could be induced by edrophonium in about 1/3 of patients but it was not always associated with chest pain. In another study employing ergonovine stimulation, oesophageal motor abnormalities could be detected in the majority of individuals who experienced chest pain[5] but other origins of the pain (i.e., cardiac) could not be unequivocally excluded.

It is apparent from the above data that a causal relation between oesophageal dysmotility (spontaneous or induced) and pain is plausible but cannot be conclusively established. However, in some individuals, and, on some occasions, it seems quite evident suggesting, as indicated above, that other interacting mechanisms are important. Mucosal sensitivity to acid reflux has been excluded in some studies by concomitant oesophageal pH measurements but not in others. Visceral hypersensitivity may also play a determinant role and some patients may, indeed, share a hyperkinetic oesophagus and visceral hyperalgesia. It is even conceivable that, in some patients, both motor and sensory abnormalities would be mediated by a central mechanism activated either spontaneously or provoked by certain stimuli or environmental situations.

Elsewhere in the gastrointestinal tract, it is even more difficult than in the oesophagus to prove an association between dysmotility and pain, not to speak of a causal relation. In the stomach, distension (and the consequent increased wall tension) appears to be definitely associated with pain[6]. However, it is not known whether motor abnormalities can, by themselves, induce sufficient distension to induce pain, even in hypersensitive subjects. The closest that it may come to spontaneously-induced distension pain in the stomach is the clinical situation usually referred to as postsurgical gastroparesis that may develop in patients who have undergone distal gastric resection with gastroenteric anastomosis. These patients accumulate mostly solid debris in their residual stomach and very often complain of gastric pain. We have shown that their gastric wall is rather inelastic, and therefore, painful tension easily develops[7]. At the other end of the clinical spectrum, in patients with functional dyspepsia, antral hypomotility seems, in itself, unlikely to cause pain. Except, as it appears to be sometimes the case, when maldistribution of gastric postcibal content occurs with resulting antral accumulation and uncomfortable distension.

Intestinal dysmotility has been recognized rather unequivocally by clinical manometry in some conditions such as advanced diabetes, other autonomic neuropathies and in gut neuromuscular disorders associated with the clinical syndrome of chronic pseudo-obstruction[8]. Nevertheless, it has not been possible to prove that intestinal dysmotility is a direct cause of abdominal pain, and it seems more likely that "neuropathic pain" from a coexisting sensory neuropathy or pain secondary to local stasis and wall distension are responsible for the symptoms. In some individuals with irritable bowel syndrome, there is an exaggerated "minute rhythm" and/or the presence of either spontaneous or induced giant waves, particularly in the ileum, that have also been associated with pain[9,10].

Evidence in favour of colonic dysmotility as a cause of abdominal pain is somewhat more compelling. Early studies focused on the association between sigmoid colon dysmotility and different bowel movement patterns as well as changes in myoelectric rhythms. However, these observations did not prove subsequently too credible[11]. Distension pain (as opposed to spasm) was also investigated by distending balloons in various colonic sites and recording the symptomatic response. Evidence for heightened perception in patients with the irritable bowel syndrome was obtained but this feature probably relates more to sensory than motor abnormalities. These bowel distension studies led to the concept that visceral hypersensitivity to mechanical, and perhaps also to other gut luminal stimuli, is responsible for symptoms as opposed to, or in conjunction with, altered contractile patterns. Indeed, the results of recent research suggest that visceral hypersensitivity plays a significant pathogenic role in functional gut disorders. However, the issue is extremely complex since it must take into account the interactions that occur between neural control of gut motility, conscious perception of gut signals and modulation at spinal and brain centres. Thus, although sensory perception hypersensitivity has been well documented in several functional abdominal disorders, the precise mechanism or even the "site" of the abnormality (gut wall, central nervous system) remains unknown. In functional gut disorders, region specificity is not, by any means, absolute. For instance, patients with irritable bowel syndrome whose pain is conventionally attributed to a colonic source may manifest hypersensitivity both to distension of the jejunum[12] and the sigmoid colon, suggesting that the sensory disorder is widespread along the gut (Figure 1). These observations have led some investigators to embrace the concept of an "irritable gut" implying also that the faulty mechanism responsible for the hypersensitivity is located at a "central" site (either the brain or the spinal cord) rather than peripherally.

In disease, the gut may become hypersensitive to different forms of stimulation, as described above. The implication is that hypersensitivity determines symptoms either by making patients aware of normal motor events or by exaggerating perception of abnormal events, or both.

Figure 1

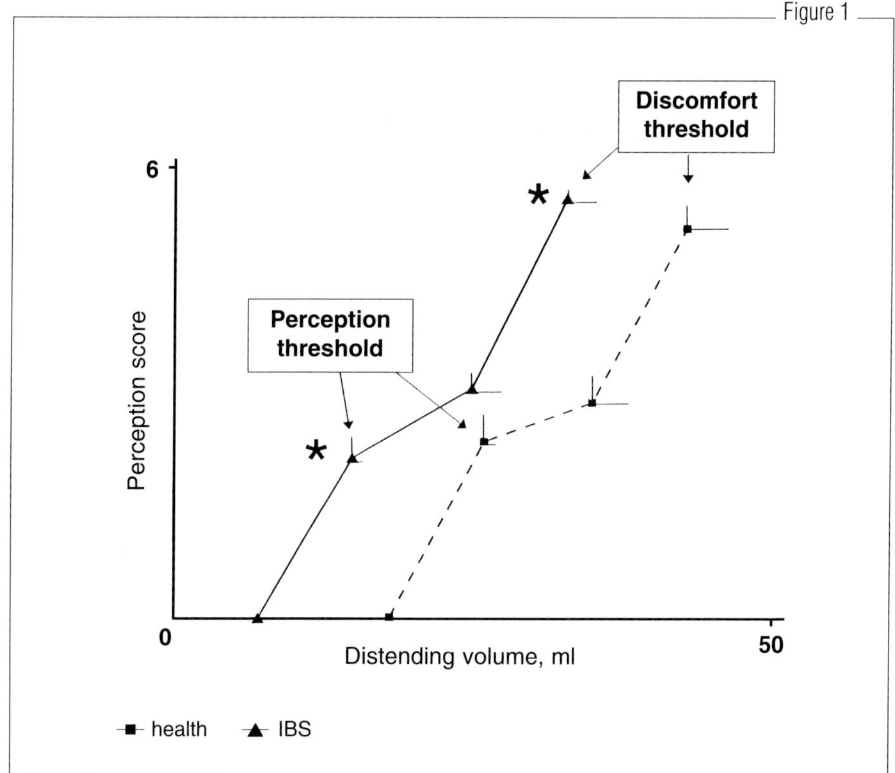


Gut hypersensitivity to mechanical stimuli in the irritable bowel syndrome. Note (★) the lower perception and discomfort thresholds shown by patients with irritable bowel syndrome (▲) versus healthy subjects (■).Reproduced with permission from Accarino A, Azpiroz F, Malagelada J-R[12].

Furthermore, visceral hypersensitivity is not a concept restricted to functional gut disorders. It has been recognized, for instance, in the inflamed rectum of ulcerative colitis, and there are other examples of organic conditions that exhibit gut hypersensitivity to diverse luminal stimuli.

Nevertheless, a significant problem remains on how to integrate motility and sensory disturbances. Do they coexist? Are they linked by common central control? Impaired reflex activity (for instance, a decreased gastric relaxatory response to duodenal distension) has been demonstrated in some patients with functional disorders, who are also hypersensitive to gut distension. This kind of observation suggests that not only conscious sensory systems, but also motor control systems, may be simultaneously impaired in certain patients. Although, so far, it has not been possible to establish a direct link between impaired sensitivity and disturbed motility, the latter clearly being a feature of some, but not all, patients with functional gut syndromes. The paucity of pharmacological agents to modulate visceral sensitivity constitutes a major obstacle to progress, because we cannot evaluate the hypersensitivity hypothesis by selectively blocking afferent sensory signals.

## Gas in the gut

Recently, we have developed a complementary and, we believe, important concept. Abnormal motility and visceral hypersensitivity manifest both by an alteration of the dynamics of intestinal gas and by enhancing the symptomatic response to regional gas distension. Thus, it emerges that some of the best evidence linking bowel dysmotility to abdominal discomfort/pain comes, rather indirectly, from studies of gas dynamics in the bowel.

There is gas in the normal gut that originates, in part, from swallowing and, in part, from a series of chemical reactions of the foodstuffs within the gut[13]. The resulting intestinal gas load is normally unperceived. Most of it is transported along the bowel and evacuated per anus without excess accumulation[14]. Abdominal complaints such as bloating, borborygmi, cramps and, sometimes, frank distension are, at times, attributable to altered dynamics of intestinal gas. In fact, patients themselves intuitively ascribe many of these symptoms to a gas problem. But, in most cases, it remains uncertain whether the symptoms are due to a gas overload, an impaired intestinal handling of gas or a poor tolerance and increased perception[15,16].

Based on the knowledge that gas is an important component of digestive tract content, we hypothesized that abnormal handling of normal or excessive intestinal gas loads might represent a, heretofore, unrecognized mechanism of functional gut distress. Thus, we established and validated a method for quantifying gas transit in the human gut while simultaneously assessing symptomatic responses and physiological effects, such as abdominal distension. In the course of our studies, we observed that a subgroup of healthy individuals and a significantly larger proportion of individuals with functional abdominal symptoms retain large quantities of gas, develop abdominal distension and discomfort. Gas retention and symptoms do not appear to be due to impaired anal relaxation because they remain unmodified during intrarectal gas collection. Further studies compared the effects of pharmacological gut motor inhibition and restrained voluntary evacuation on gas dynamics. Our results suggest that abdominal distension depends on the volume of gas retention, whereas symptom perception depends on gut motor activity and the mechanism of retention.

Our method for measuring intestinal gas dynamics is based on proximal jejunal infusion at a constant rate of a poorly diffusible gas mixture, with simultaneous quantification of anal expulsion rates[17]. We use an intestinal polyvinyl tube assembly that incorporates a gas infusion channel with multiple distal side holes over the 1 cm distal segment, an orad latex balloon with a separate inflation channel to prevent gaseous backflow and a drainage channel with multiple side holes orad to the balloon to remove accumulating secretions. In the initial studies, we also used a separate gastric polyvinyl tube, that incorporated a venting channel with multiple side holes to aspirate refluxed gas, but, in subsequent studies, we eliminated this component since there is virtually no backflow of infused jejunal gas into the stomach.

The gas mixture infused contains 88% nitrogen, 6.5% carbon dioxide and 5.5% oxygen bubbled into water for saturation. This gas mixture is designed to mimic the partial pressures of the gases in venous blood, and

hence, to minimize diffusion across the intestinal blood barrier[18].
The volume of gas passed per anus is controlled by a barostat, which is an electronic pressure clamp, that drives an air pump based on a strain gauge input[19,20]. The barostat provides a low resistance collection line since a minimal pressure increment produced by gas evacuation, immediately activates the pump (< 5 ms lag) and displaces the volume along the line. Anal gas is collected by a low resistance external cannula that fits hermetically in between the buttocks, with the concavity lining the perineal midline, the tip ventral to the coccyx, the collection port facing the anus, and the collecting line emerging ventrally between the thighs. The open end of the anal cannula is connected via separate channels to the air pump and to the strain gauge of the barostat.
We normally intubate participants in the morning after an 8-hour fast. The intestinal tube assembly is introduced through the mouth into the intestine and we position, under fluoroscopic control, the tip of the infusion tube about 5 cm caudad to the angle of Treitz. During the study, participants lay supine in the bed at an angle of 30° to the horizontal. Once they are positioned, a non-distensible, flaccid belt is placed around their abdomen at the level of the flanks and umbilical region. The overlapping ends of the belt are adjusted by means of two elastic bands, so that the belt constantly follows changes in girth by adapting to the abdominal wall. During the study, we use a graded questionnaire to measure the intensity and the type of sensations perceived, and an anatomical questionnaire to measure the location and extension of the perceived sensations. Each sensation is independently scored on a graphic rating scale that combines verbal descriptors on a visual analog scale graded from 0 to 6[22].
During the test, we calculate, at various time periods, the volume of gas retained within the gut as the difference between the volume of gas infused and the volume of gas recovered. We have performed validation studies using an inert gaseous marker, $SF_6$, that is neither produced nor absorbed by the gut[23].
In most normal individuals, gas loads, within a very broad range (1 to 30 ml/min), are appropriately handled by the gut so that evacuation rates parallel infusion rates with no apparent gas retention within the gut (Figure 2). Thus, in our studies greater volumes of gas infused were associated with both an increased number of evacuations and larger gas volumes per evacuation.

Figure 2

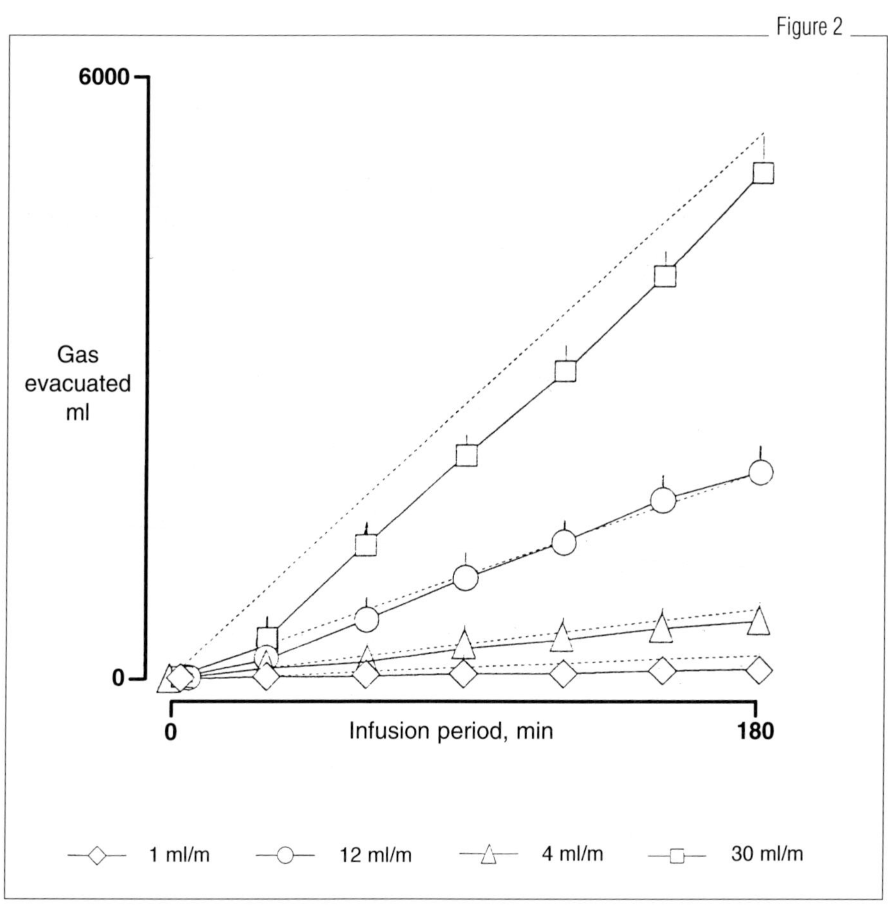


Gas evacuation during continuous intestinal infusion of gas; dose response study in different groups of healthy subjects. Note the close approximation between gas infusion and evacuation rates. Reproduced with permission from Serra J, Azpiroz F, Malagelada J-R[17].

In most of our normal study subjects, gas retention within the gut was in the range between +400 ml and –400 ml; some subjects that evacuated more gas than infused had a negative balance of retention. There is, however, no noticeable interindividual variability in the dynamics of intestinal gas. Six out of 46 normal volunteers in our initial studies retained gas above the 400 ml. Furthermore, in contrast to the remainder of the subjects who promptly equilibrated evacuation and infusion rates, these 6 subjects progressively retained gas during the study (Figure 3).

Figure 3

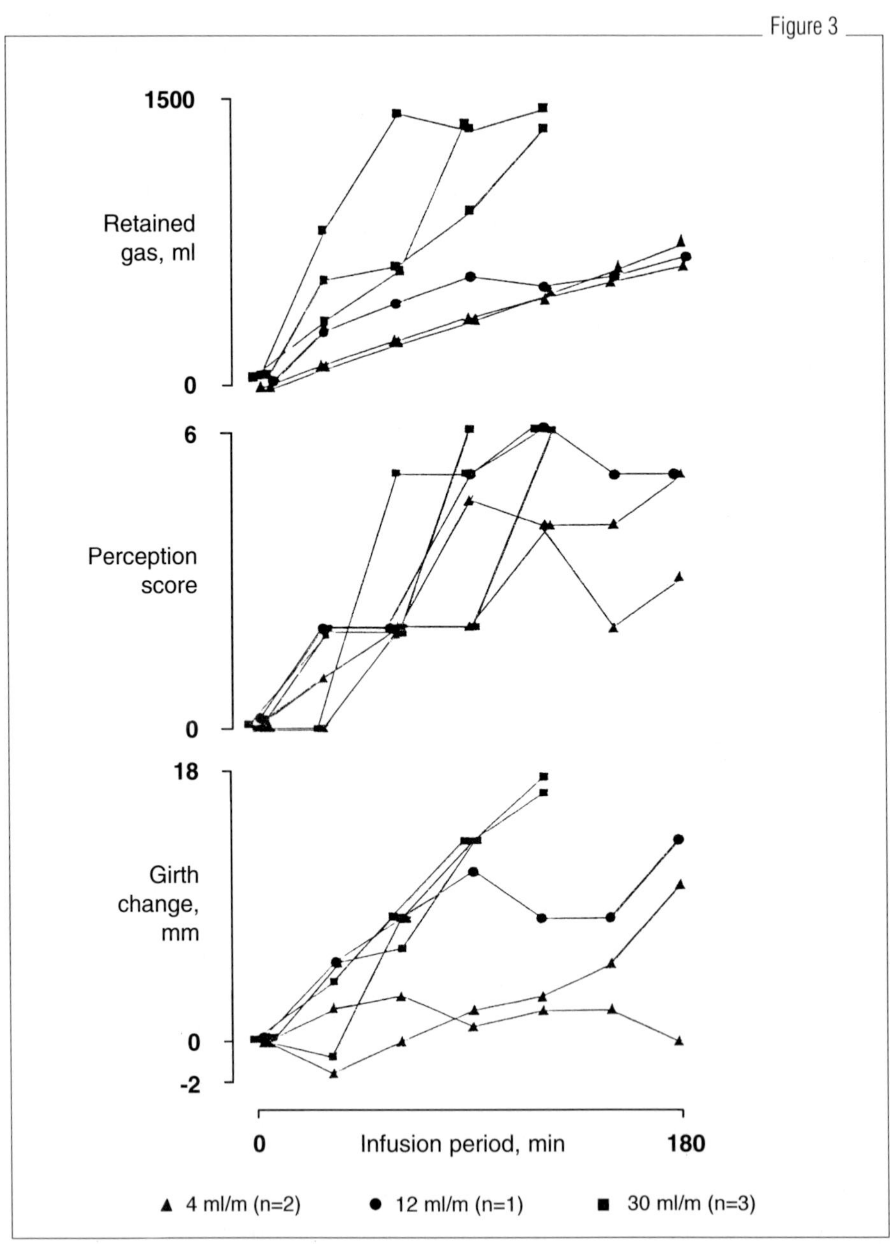


Gas transit, symptoms and abdominal distension in 6 subjects with >400 ml of gas retention during a gas challenge test. Reproduced with permission from Serra J, Azpiroz F, Malagelada J-R[17].

We observed that the intensity of perception was related to the volume of gas retained within the gut. Neither the rate of infusion, nor the amount of gas propelled through the gut, appear to influence perception. Therefore, the dynamics of intestinal gas play a key role in determining perception of gas in the bowel. If the gas moves normally, it is expelled without retention or symptoms. By contrast, if relatively small volumes exceeding 400 ml accumulate, then symptoms develop.

Interestingly the type of abdominal sensations produced by gas accumulation is similar regardless of the volume of gas retained and the intensity of perception. Thus, subjects who retained more gas reported the same sensations as the others, and, even more remarkable, they did not report any difficulty expelling gas per anus. Normal individuals who were not gas retainers did not develop any significant abdominal distension. However, in subjects who retained more than 400 ml gas, there was a concomitant and progressive increase in girth (Figure 3).

The mechanisms that produce displacement of gas within the gut are not well known. Our data demonstrate a distinctive gas and chyme discrimination within the gut, since, at high infusion rates, gas transit was expeditious, but despite the large volumes of gas evacuated per anus no subject reported a call for stools. Previous investigators have shown that intestinal propulsive activity for solids and liquids depends on different patterns of phasic motor activity[24,25] but the role of this type of motor activity in moving gas is conceivably small. High amplitude propagated contractions in the colon have been related to faecal mass movements[26]. Again, the role of these known contractile patterns in moving gas is unknown and further research will have to be undertaken to characterize the specific motility pattern responsible for gas propulsion.

An intriguing issue addressed by our studies is the quantity of intestinal gas that would trigger symptoms. Our data indicate that gas volumes above the 400 ml range may induce conscious perception, predominantly sensation of abdominal bloating. It is interesting that the subjects who retained gas did not report any difficulty in evacuating gas which suggests that the retention site is located proximal to the rectum. The mechanisms involved in gas have not been well characterized but presumably depend on bowel distension. It has been shown that a small amount of gas may induce symptoms when the intraluminal pressure and the tension on the gut wall reach a certain level.

However, the presence of another gas bubble, even at a distant site in the gut, considerably increases the intensity of perception[27,28]. Likewise, a given amount of gas, when distributed along a large segment of intestine, induces symptoms at a lower wall tension that may be required in a shorter loop because of summation effects. Along these lines, it is remarkable that, as shown by a recent study in our laboratory, a volume of only about 200 ml air contained in a 36 cm tubular bag within the jejunum, induced discomfort (Figure 4a and 4b)[28].

Figure 4a

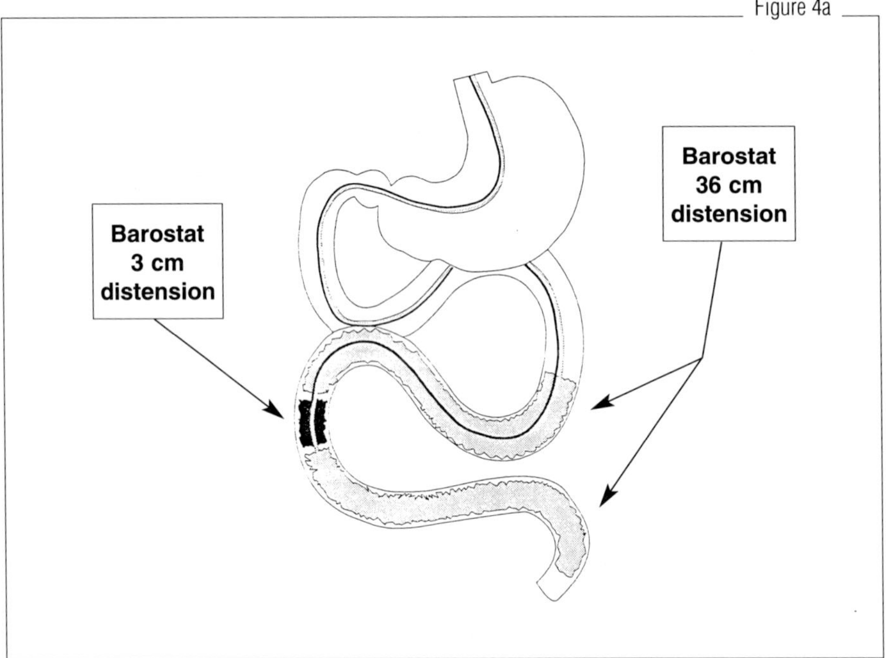


Experimental method. Isobaric intestinal distensions were applied over a short (3 cm) and a long segment (36 cm) by means of two separate barostats in healthy individuals. The long bag was divided into two compartments sharing pressure and volume connections, and the short bag was located in-between.

More recently, we have studied a group of patients with non-specific functional gut disorders (unexplained abdominal pain and/or bloating) and observed that gas infusion was well tolerated by healthy subjects, but induced abdominal discomfort and substantial gas retention in many.

Figure 4b

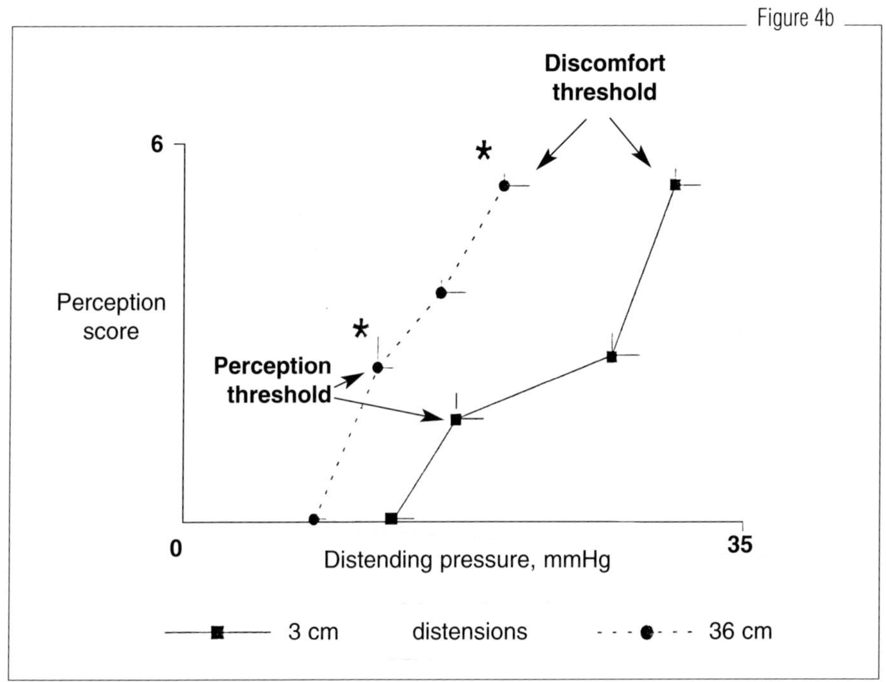


Experimental results. Perception of fixed-pressure intestinal distensions applied over the short segment and the long segment of small bowel. Reproduced with permission from Serra J, Azpiroz F, Malagelada J-R[28].

Gas retention and symptoms were not attributable to impaired anal evacuation, because they were unmodified during intrarectal gas collection. Thus, a significant proportion of patients with functional gut disorders have impaired handling of intestinal gas loads, and exhibit gas retention and/or symptoms.

## Biliary dysmotility in patients with chronic abdominal pain

Evidence that functional type biliary motor disturbances can give rise to abdominal pain is fairly compelling, although not overwhelming. Sphincter of Oddi dysfunction has been proposed as a cause of postcholecystectomy pain in the absence of calculi. Such patients often describe their pain as being identical to that experienced prior to removal of the gallbladder. However, pain may not be limited to the epigastrium or right upper quadrant, and atypical referral patterns do occur. Sphincter of Oddi dysfunction may have either a structural or physiological basis, or both. Structural abnormalities may consist in narrowing and irregularity of the intraduodenal segment of the distal choledocus (papillary stenosis), whereas physiological abnormalities relate primarily to abnormal contractile activity whether or not associated with actual hypertrophy of the sphincteric muscle. Sphincter of Oddi dysfunction is, therefore, a condition that may be diagnosed either by imaging techniques (anatomy or anatomy and physiology) or motility recording techniques (physiology), or a combination of both. An indirect diagnosis of sphincter of Oddi dysfunction may be obtained from point elevation of liver enzymes coinciding with an episode of pain. In fact, such an event remains one of the most reliable clinical clues, with a much higher predicting value than pain which, even when described by the patient in a highly persuasive manner can be rather non-specific.

There are three recognizable forms of sphincter of Oddi dysfunction based on the presence of ductal dilatation, elevated liver enzymes or delayed drainage of the common bile duct at the time of endoscopic retrograde cholangiography or hepatobiliary scintigraphy ($^{99m}$TC-HIDA) scan. Patients with suggestive pain and all three of the findings are classified as having type I sphincter of Oddi dysfunction. The majority of these patients are found to have elevated basal sphincter pressures during biliary manometry and tend to respond to endoscopic sphincterotomy. Patients with two of the three associated findings, or type II sphincter of Oddi dysfunction show elevated basal pressures at sphincter of Oddi manometry about 50% of the time. In turn, the majority of those patients with elevated pressures experience significant pain relief after endoscopic sphincterotomy. Patients who have pain but lack any of the associated findings, or type III sphincter of Oddi dysfunction, are less predictable both in the frequency of elevated basal sphincter pressures and positive response to sphincterotomy[29].

## Conclusions

It is, to some extent, surprising that a common symptom such as abdominal pain, in the absence of evident organic disease, remains, much of a mystery as to its origin and mechanism. Nevertheless, considerable progress has been made in recent years. We now recognize that there are common pathogenetic features in pain arising from various segments of the digestive tract including the oesophagus, the colon and the biliary tract.

The most relevant link appears to be disturbed regulation of motility and visceral hypersensitivity, both perhaps arising from spinal or brain dysfunctions since the central nervous system plays a major role in the regulation of digestive tract physiology. But there are other, perhaps less esoteric, factors involved. One of these is gas. Recent studies conducted by our laboratory indicate that the dynamics of intestinal gas are the key to preventing accumulation of gas inside the bowel. Some normal individuals and a substantial fraction of patients with the irritable bowel syndrome are incapable of moving gas inside the bowel with the consequent pooling and distension of segments of bowel.

It seems logical to conclude from this information that motility disturbances may impair intestinal gas transit and that conscious perception of bowel distension by gas may be amplified by visceral hypersensitivity phenomena, resulting in significant abdominal pain and other symptoms. Thus, at this point, we put forward the hypothesis that functional type gut pain may be generated by various "local" mechanisms: spasm, perhaps most relevant in the oesophagus, distension, by gas in the bowel, by impaired bile flow in the biliary tract, etc.

For these local mechanisms to elicit pain or discomfort, however, visceral hypersensitivity either from amplified wall afferent signals or by anomalous central nervous system modulatory and reception symptoms would be important, since similar stimuli in normal people may go unperceived.

In any event, only further observations and a better understanding of basic mechanisms will provide a clue.

## References

1. Richter JE. *Motility disorders of the esophagus.* In: Yamada T, Alpers DH, Owyang C, Powell DW and Silverstein FE, editors. Textbook of Gastroenterology. Philadelphia: Lippincott; 1991;1083-122.
2. Kahrilas PJ. *Nutcracker esophagus: an idea whose time has gone?* Am J Gastroenterol 1993;88:167-9.

3. Breumelhof R, Nadorp JHSM, Akkermans LMA, Smout AJPM. *Analysis of 24-hour esophageal pressure and pH data in unselected patients with non cardiac chest pain.* Gastroenterology 1990;99:1257-64.
4. Lee CA, Reynolds JC, Ouyang A, et al. *Esophageal chest pain: value of manometries.* Dig Dis Sci 1987;32:682-8.
5. Alban Davies H, Kaye MD, Rhodes J, et al. *Diagnosis of esophageal spasm by ergometrine provocation.* Gut 1982;23:89-97.
6. Mearin F, Cucala M, Azpiroz F, Malagelada J-R. *The origin of symptoms on the brain-gut axis in functional dyspepsia.* Gastroenterology 1991;100:999-1006.
7. Azpiroz F, Malagelada J-R. *Gastric tone measured by an electronic barostat in health and postsurgical gastroparesis.* Gastroenterology 1987;92:934-43.
8. Camilleri M, Malagelada J-R, Stanghellini V, et al. *Gastrointestinal motility disturbance in patients with orthostatic hypotension.* Gastroenterology 1985;88:1852-9.
9. Kellow JE, Eckeerskey GM, Jones MP. *Enhanced perception of physiological intestinal motility in the irritable bowel syndrome.* Gastroenterology 1991;101:1621-7.
10. Thompson DG, Laidlow JM, Wingate DL. *Abnormal small-bowel motility demonstrated by radiotelemetry in a patient with irritable colon.* Lancet 1979;22/29:1321-3.
11. Latimer P, et al. *Colonic motor and myoelectric activity: a comparative study of normal subjects, psychoneurotic patients and patients with the irritable bowel syndrome.* Gastroenterology 1981;80:893-901.
12. Accarino A, Azpiroz F, Malagelada J-R. *Selective dysfunction of mechanosensitive intestinal afferents in the irritable bowel syndrome.* Gastroenterology 1995;108:636-43.
13. Levitt MD, Bond JH. *Volume, composition, and source of intestinal gas.* Gastroenterology 1970;59:921-9.
14. Levitt MD. *Volume and composition of human intestinal gas determined by means of an intestinal washout technic.* N Engl J Med 1971;284:1394-8.
15. Poynard T, Hernandez M, Xu P, et al. and Cooperative Study Group. *Visible abdominal distension and gas surface: description of an automatic method of evaluation and application to patients with irritable bowel syndrome and dyspepsia.* Eur J Gastroenterol Hepatol 1992;4:831-6.
16. Maxton DG, Martin DF, Whorwell PJ, Godprey M. *Abdominal distension in female patients with irritable bowel syndrome: exploration of possible mechanisms.* Gut 1991;32:662-4.
17. Serra J, Azpiroz F, Malagelada J-R. *Intestinal gas dynamics and tolerance in humans.* Gastroenterology 1998; 115:542-50.
18. Foster RE. *Physiological basis of gas exchange in the gut.* Ann NY Acad Sci 1968;150:4-12.

19. Azpiroz F, Malagelada J-R. *Physiologic variations in canine gastric tone measured by an electronic barostat.* Am J Physiol 1985;247:G265-G272.
20. Azpiroz F, Malagelada J-R. *Gastric tone measured by an electronic barostat in health and postsurgical gastroparesis.* Gastroenterology 1987;92:934-43.
21. Azpiroz F. *Sensitivity of the stomach and small bowel: human research and clinical relevance.* In: Gebhart GF, editor. Progress in pain research and management. Vol. 5, Visceral pain. Seattle: IASP;1995;391-428.
22. Gracely RH. *Studies of pain in normal man.* In: Wall PD, Melzac R, editors. Textbook of pain. 3rd ed. Edinburgh: Churchill Livingstone; 1994;315-36.
23. Jonmarker C, Castor R, Drefeldt B, Werner O. *An analyzer for in-line measurement of expiratory sulfur hexafluoride concentration.* Anesthesiology 1985;63:84-8.
24. Bueno L, Fioramonti J, Ruckebusch Y. *Rate of flow of digesta and electrical activity of the small intestine in dogs and sheep.* J Physiol (Lond) 1975;249:69-85.
25. Ehrlein HJ, Schemann M, Siegle ML. *Motor patterns of small intestine determined by closely spaced extraluminal force transducers and videofluoroscopy.* Am J Physiol 1987;253: G259-G267.
26. Christensen J. *The motility of the colon.* In: Johnson LR, editors. Physiology of the gastrointestinal tract. Vol. 1. 3rd ed. New York: Raven; 1994;991-1024.
27. Serra J, Azpiroz F, Malagelada J-R. *Perception and reflex responses to intestinal distention in humans are modified by simultaneous or previous stimulation.* Gastroenterology 1995;109:1742-9.
28. Serra J, Azpiroz F, Malagelada J-R. *Modulation of gut perception in humans by spatial summation phenomena.* J Physiol (Lond) 1998;506:579-87.
29. Geenen JE, Hogan WJ, Dodds WJ, et al. *The efficacy of endoscopic sphincterotomy after cholecystectomy in patients with sphincter of Oddi dysfunction.* N Engl J Med 1989;320: 82-7.


*Address for correrspondence*


**MALAGELADA J-R, Prof, MD**

Hospital General Vall D'Hebron, Digestive Diseases Dept.
Pg. Vall d'Hebron, 119-129
08035 Barcelona Spain
Fax: +34 93 209 62 05

# Chronic pelvic pain

*M Delvaux, Y Aggadi, J Frexinos*

Chronic Pelvic Pain (CPP) can be defined as painful sensations originating from the pelvic area and present in the same location for at least 6 months[1]. It is a common clinical problem, and leads to a large number of consultations and care procedures.

The pelvis is characterized by the close relationship of organs belonging to various physiological systems. All may be responsible for pain and consequently patients complaining of CPP will be referred to several specialists including urologists, gastroenterologists, neurologists and gynaecologists. Moreover, CPP is frequently observed in patients with psychological disturbances and psychiatric disorders may be contributing factors, the majority of which can be treated medically. Frequently, the work-up of the patients by different physicians and the constant care seeking of the patients results in repeated or unnecessary investigations, which often fail to reveal an identifiable organic cause.

No study has, so far, been performed that provides an accurate estimate of the prevalence of CPP. A rate of 39% was reported in women undergoing laparoscopy for sterilisation or investigation of infertility in the only study from the United Kingdom investigating CPP unrelated to menstruation or sexual intercourse[2]. In the USA, 10% of outpatient gynaecological consultations, 20% of laparoscopies and 12% of hysterectomies were performed for CPP[3]. By contrast, little is known about the prevalence of CPP in the practice of other specialties like gastroenterology. In gastroenterology consultations, one of the most common causes of CPP is the "levator ani syndrome" (see below) which could be as frequent as 6.6% in the general population and be observed more frequently in women (up to 80%)[4]. But this syndrome is often associated with other causes of CPP, like dyschezia[5] and proctalgia fugax[6] and the diagnosis remains mainly based on clinical examination and exclusion of other causes of pain.

## Chronic pelvic pain of gynaecologic origin

Chronic pelvic pain occurs more frequently in women and is often spontaneously referred, by the patient herself, to gynaecological origin.

Pain may be isolated or associated with changes in frequency of menses and in menstrual cycle. CPP may be continuous or related to sexual intercourse or other life events. It frequently threatens the daily life of the patient. Laparoscopy has become routine in the investigation of CPP so far as history and physical examination are often inaccurate in excluding other organic causes of pain. Studies on laparoscopic findings in women with CPP revealed that approximately one-third have endometriosis, one-third, adhesions and one-third had no obvious pathology[7]. After thorough physical and psychological evaluation of 122 women with negative findings at laparoscopy presenting to a tertiary referral interdisciplinary CPP clinic, occult somatic pathology was further diagnosed in 47%[8]. Myofascial pain was the most common diagnosis and was caused by scars of the lower abdominal wall, followed by atypical cyclic pain (dysmenorrhea), gastrointestinal causes (constipation, Irritable Bowel Syndrome [IBS]), urological causes (urethral syndrome, cystitis), sciatic hernia[9] and pelvic vascular congestion[10].

## Chronic pelvic pain of gastrointestinal origin

Chronic pelvic pain is frequently reported by patients consulting for various functional gastrointestinal disorders. It is frequently reported together with constipation responsible for straining at stool and with IBS. However, two forms of functional ano-rectal pain syndromes have been recognized in the Rome classification of functional digestive disorders[11]: the "levator ani syndrome" and "proctalgia fugax". They are distinguished on the basis of the duration (hours of constant or frequent pain for "levator ani syndrome" versus seconds to minutes for "proctalgia fugax") and characteristics of pain (dull pain for levator ani syndrome or sharp pain for "proctalgia fugax").

The ***levator ani syndrome*** was described for the first time in the 60's . It is mainly characterized by a spasm involving the levator muscles and has also been termed puborectalis syndrome, chronic proctalgia, pyriformis syndrome and pelvic tension myalgia. The pathophysiology remains unclear, although some aetiological factors have been evoked such as repeated pelvic injury, multiparity, pelvic or rectal surgery. Psychological factors are also often recognized. It is observed mainly (75% of cases) in women between 40 and 60 years of age[12]. Pain is often related to position, triggered by long periods in a standing position or by movements. Walking and the supine position often relieve it. Most of the time pain is perceived at the level of the anus and rectum but it may project to gynaecological organs, the buttocks and thighs. Physical examination reveals overly contracted levator ani muscles and tenderness on palpation of the pelvic floor. Clinical signs are often unilateral and may, for unknown reasons, predominate on the left[6]. The differential diagnosis includes peripheral nerve syndromes like spinal stenosis, spinal tumour or injury[13] and coccygodynia. In the latter condition, tenderness of the levator muscles is absent and pain can be reproduced by mobilization of the coccyx. Several studies have shown an increased resting pressure in the anal canal[5,14].

***Proctalgia fugax*** is estimated to be as frequent as 15% of the general population. It is defined by the occurrence of sudden, severe pain in the anal area, lasting a few seconds to minutes and occurring more frequently during the night[15]. Some attacks are accompanied by neurovegetative signs. Males report it more frequently than females and it seems to be associated with sexual intercourse in only 6% of cases but constipation and straining at stool is present in more than one third of them[16]. Proctalgia fugax is often seen in young adults and tends to disappear with increasing age. The aetiology remains unknown. It might be related to a contraction of the levator ani. Diagnosis is made mainly from the patient history and the physical examination, which is normal between attacks. In some privileged observations, high pressure contractions of the sigmoid were reported but there appeared to be no relationship between occurrence of motor events and pain attacks[17,18].

***Neuralgia of the pudendal nerve*** or ***Syndrome of the Alcock canal*** is due to a compression of the pudendal nerve, arising from second, third and fourth sacral nerve roots. The pudendal nerve is compressed when it passes through a canal made on one side from a bony limit (the ischio-pubis branch) and, on the other, the internal obturator muscle and its fascia (Figure 1). Compression is due to fibrosis which is primary in most cases, although its can be secondary to a number of general conditions, like diabetes, hypothyroidism, ethylism and general inflammatory diseases.

Figure 1

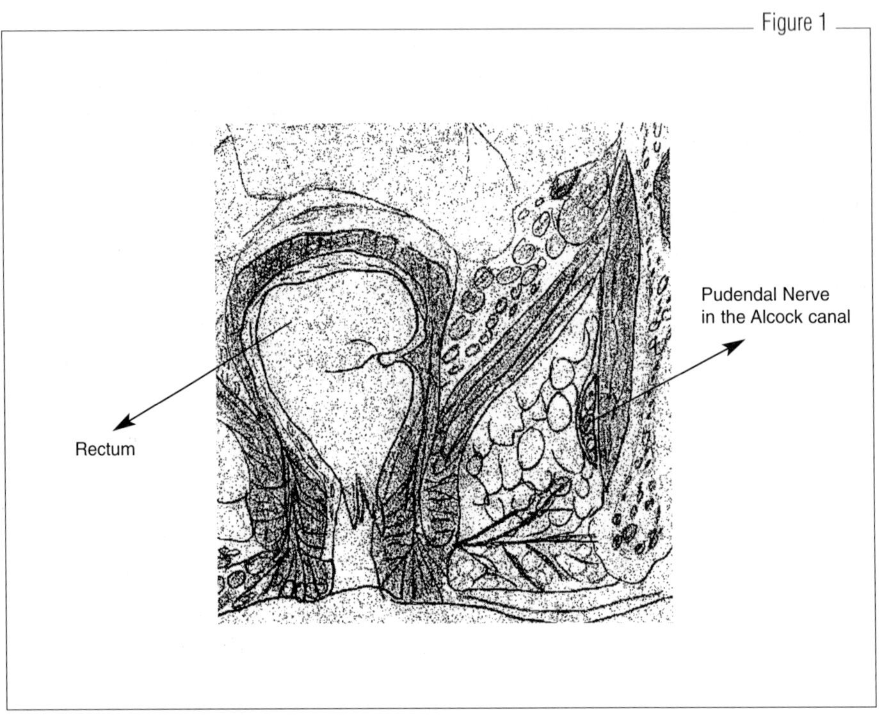


Anatomical location of the Alcock canal.

This syndrome is more frequently observed in women, after 50 years of age. Pain is elicited by a prolonged standing-up position, walking or a supine position. It involves the pelvis but frequently starts from the perineum. Clinical examination is essential. Palpation of the area of the ischion may trigger pain. Diagnosis may be supported by electrophysiological studies of the pudendal nerve. Treatment consists in local anaesthesia of the nerve. If the result is not satisfactory, infiltration may be repeated using local corticosteroids, every two to three weeks. In refractory cases, surgical decompression of the pudendal nerve may be proposed[19].

Patients with "disorders of pelvic statics and idiopathic rectal pain" describe, more specifically, the pain originating from the rectum itself and apparently not originating from the perineum nor caused by perineal dysfunction. However, like patients with CPP, these patients frequently present a particular psychological profile. Much more uncommon are causes of pelvic pain like the "cavernous haemangioma of the rectum"[20]. IBS is one of the most common functional bowel disorders in the community. It is defined by the association of several symptoms, the primary ones including abdominal pain and bowel disturbances[21]. However, as constipation-prone IBS is the most frequent situation, patients may also complain of pelvic pain, which they relate to straining at stool and feeling of incomplete evacuation. Interrelationship with gynaecological disorders is also common since about 80% of patients are women, symptoms worsen during menstruation and/or are associated with various premenstrual symptoms. Psychosocial factors including depression, somatization, substance abuse and sexual abuse are similarly encountered in patients with IBS and CPP. IBS predisposes women to undergo hysterectomy and negatively influences postoperative pain relief. Therefore, IBS should be considered in the differential diagnosis of CPP[22].

## Therapeutic approach

CPP frequently requires a multidisciplinary approach both for establishing a reliable diagnosis and proposing a successful management. It may require medical, surgical or combined treatments as well as a psychological work-up of the patient (Figure 2). When endometriosis is demonstrated, treatment may be either surgical or medical. Medical therapy includes Non-Steroidal Anti-Inflammatory Drugs (NSAIDs), danazol, an androgenic steroid, and gonadotropin releasing hormone analogs. Surgical therapy includes laparoscopic laser ablation of deposits, total abdominal hysterectomy and bilateral salpingo-oophorectomy. More recently, laparoscopic uterine nerve ablation and pre-sacral neurectomy have been proposed. When adhesions were found, laparoscopic adhesiolysis has been successful in many cases but relief of pain may be transient and the surgical procedure may by itself cause further adhesions[23]. Treatment which has been of benefit in patients with pelvic congestion include daily medroxy-progesterone acetate coupled with psychotherapy the latter leading to a more lasting effect[24]. Surgical treatment includes bilateral oophorectomy and hysterectomy, ovarian venous ligation and ovarian vein embolization[25].

In patients with pelvic pain presumably originating from the gastrointestinal tract (mainly the ano-rectum), various treatments have been proposed, including: massage of the levator ani muscle, and electrical stimulation of this muscle which results in 80% of improvement[26]. NSAIDs, antalgics and myorelaxants may help.

Figure 2

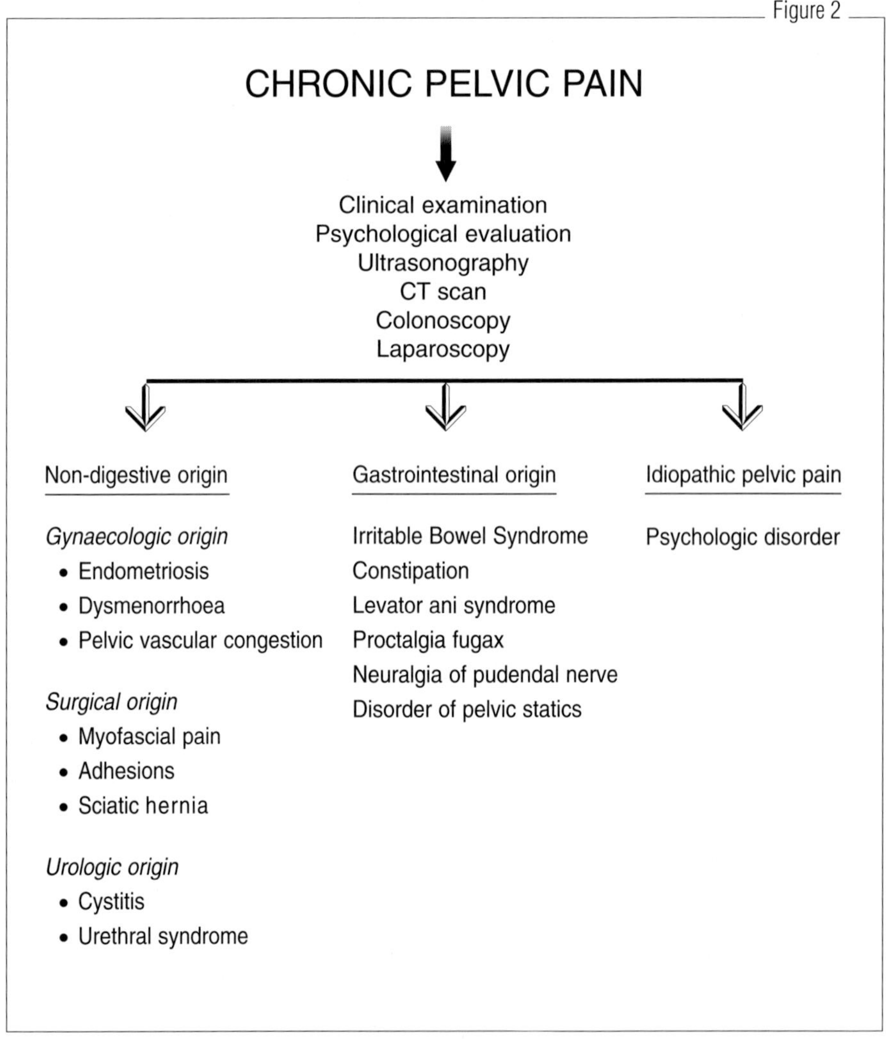


Diagram of the various causes of pelvic pain.

Psychotherapy is frequently beneficial and can be accompanied by prescription of anxiolytics and/or antidepressants. In cases of failure, local injection of corticosteroids or anaesthetics can be tried. In some patients, biofeedback was reported to be effective[5]. In most cases, treatment should be as conservative as possible. In the case of proctalgia fugax, cold sitz baths, self administered rectal massage and some drugs are regularly efficient: calcium channel inhibitors, nitrate derivatives. Psychological and behavioural therapies should also be considered.
Whatever the condition, it seems important to consider in a global approach the numerous aetiological factors often simultaneously present in patients with CPP. In a study evaluating a multispecialty work-up of patients with CPP, 67% of patients treated in an out-patient facility experienced more than 40% improvement in pain which was maintained at least 6 months[27].

## Conclusions

Chronic pelvic pain is a very frequent complaint of patients, more frequently women than men. A fair work-up of these patients is most of the time multidisciplinary but as the condition is benign in most cases, treatment should avoid unnecessary surgical attempts. As for any functional disorder the psychological component is important to recognize and specific management will frequently be required.

### *References*

1. Campbell F, Collett BJ. *Chronic pelvic pain.* Br J Anaesth 1994;73:571-3.
2. Zondervan KT, Yudkin PL, Vessey PL, et al. *The prevalence of chronic pelvic pain in women in the United Kingdom: a systematic review.* Br J Obstet Gynaecol 1998;105:93-9.
3. Reiter RC. *Chronic pelvic pain.* Clin Obstet Gynec 1990;33:117-8.
4. Drossman DA, Li Z, Andreuzzi E, et al. *US Householder survey of functional GI disorders: prevalence, sociodemography and health impact.* Dig Dis Sci 1993;38:1569-80.
5. Grimaud JC, Bouvier M, Naudy-Bguien C, Salducci J. *Manometric and radiologic investigations and biofeedback treatment of chronic idiopathic anal pain.* Dis Colon Rectum 1991;34:690-5.

6. Grant SR, Salvati EP, Rubin RJ. *Levator syndrome: an analysis of 316 cases.* Dis Colon Rectum 1975;18:161-3.
7. Raokins AJ. *Adhesions and pelvic pain: a retrospective study.* Obstet Gynecol 1986;68:13.
8. Reiter RC, Gambone JC. *Nongynaecologic somatic pathology in women with chronic pelvic pain and negative laparoscopy.* J Reprod Med 1991;36:253-9.
9. Miklos JR, O'Reilly MJ, Saye WB. *Sciatic hernia as a cause of chronic pelvic pain in women.* Obstet Gynecol 1998;91:998-1001.
10. Charles G. *Syndromes congestifs pelviens.* Rev Fr Gynecol Obstet 1995;90:84-90.
11. Whitehead WE. *Functional disorders of the anus and rectum.* In: Drossman DA, Richter JE, Talley NJ, Thompson WG, Corazziari E, Whitehead WE, editors. The functional gastrointestinal disorders. Boston: Little Brown Co; 1994;217-63.
12. Salvati EP. *The levator syndrome and its variants.* Gastroenterol Clin N Am 1987;16:71-8.
13. Schuster MM. *Rectal pain.* In: Bayless T, editor. Current therapy in gastrointestinal and liver diseases. Toronto: Decker;1990;378-9.
14. West L, Abell TL, Cutts T. *Long-term results of pelvic floor muscle rehabilitation of constipation.* Gastroenterology 1992;102:A533.
15. Thompson WG. *Proctalgia fugax.* Dig Dis Sci 1981;26:1121-4.
16. Thompson WG. *Proctalgia fugax in patients with the irritable bowel, peptic ulcer or inflammatory bowel disease.* Am J Gastroenterol 1984;79:450-2.
17. Harvey RF. *Colonic motility in proctalgia fugax.* Lancet 1979;2:713-4.
18. Kamm MA, Hoyle CH, Burleigh DE et al. *Hereditary internal anal sphincter myopathy causing proctalgia fugax and constipation.* Gastroenterology 1991;100:805-10.
19. Robert R, Labat JJ, Bensignor M, et al. *Bases anatomiques de la chirurgie du nerf pudendal. Conséquences thérapeutiques dans certaines algies périnéales.* Lyon Chir 1993;89:183-7.
20. Lautard M, Fribourg B, Larpent JL, Gorce D. *Cavernous hemangioma of the rectum: an uncommon cause of pelvic pain.* Chirurgie 1997;122:149-52.
21. Thompson WS, Dotterval G, Drossman DA, et al. *Irritable bowel syndrome: guidelines for the diagnosis.* Gastroenterol Int 1989;2:92-5.
22. Longstreth GF. *Irritable bowel syndrome and chronic pelvic pain.* Obstet Gynecol Surv 1994;49:505-7.
23. Roseff SJ, Murphy AA. *Laparoscopy in the diagnosis and therapy of chronic pelvic pain.* Clin Obstet Gynaecol 1990;33:196-204.
24. Farquhar CM, Rogers V, Franks S, et al. *A randomized controlled trial of medroxy-progesterone acetate and psychotherapy for the treatment of pelvic congestion.* Br J Obstet Gynaecol 1989;96:1153-62.

25. Edwards RD, Robertson IR, Mac Lean AB, Hemingway AP. *Case report: pelvic pain syndrome, successful treatment of a case by ovarian vein embolization.* Clin Radiol 1993;47:429-31.
26. Hull TL, Milsom JW, Church J, et al. *Electrogalvanic stimulation for levator syndrome: how effective is it in the long term?* Dis Colon Rectum 1993;36:731-4.
27. Kames LD, Rapkin AJ, Naliboff BD, et al. *Effectiveness of an interdisciplinary pain management program for treatment of chronic pelvic pain.* Pain 1990;41:41-6.



*ADDRESS FOR CORRESPONDENCE*

**DELVAUX M, MD, PhD**

Gastroenterology Unit

CHU Rangueil

31403 Toulouse Cédex 04 France

Fax: +33 561 32 22 29

E-mail: 106521.3337@compuserve.com

# EXTRAGASTROINTESTINAL CHRONIC PAIN
# THE EXAMPLE OF MYOGENIC PAIN

*HC Traue, M Kessler, T Rudisch*

Pain is an unpleasant sensory and emotional experience associated with actual or potential tissue damage or described in terms of such damage[1]. More than 50% of all symptoms leading to medical treatment are pain symptoms and one should note that pain reports leading to medical treatment are always subjective. There is no way to distinguish between pain, with or without tissue damage on the basis of pain reports. It is important to use different definitions for acute and chronic pain. Generally, acute pain is provoked by noxious stimulation of skin, deep somatic structures or visceral organs or abnormal functional changes. Fortunately, most acute pain can be limited by effective therapy or is self-limiting in days or weeks.

Chronic pain is not a distinguished quality or nature of pain, but pain which persists beyond the usual course of an acute disease or a reasonable time for an injury to heal or that is associated with a chronic pathological process[1]. Therefore, chronic pain can be observed within a wide spectrum of medical disorders. In general, there is no sharp definition of chronic pain patients. The classification systems of the International Association for the Study of Pain, the International Headache Society or the Diagnostic and Statistical Manual of the American Psychiatric Association use arbitrary figures between 2 to 6 months of duration which classify a pain disorder as chronic. This time period, is of course, artificial and incorrect, in some cases. For example, the healing process of a simple fracture should result in a pain free state within two weeks. If a therapist waits six months to diagnose a chronic pain problem, the development of a reflex dystrophy is probably overlooked, which should have been treated immediately. Nevertheless, chronic pain is hard to treat, it is challenging for therapists, it is time consuming and expensive.

### What are the differences between acute and chronic pain?

Pain stimulation is processed in the central nervous system with a high priority. This is a quality of acute pain, since acute pain functions as a behavioural self-control system at different levels in order to enhance healing, protect the body from further damage, stimulate social support and prevent future noxious stimulation. In chronic pain, most of the protective mechanisms of acute pain, become part of the suffering inasmuch as these behaviours have lost their biological alarm function and have no healing function, they are unable to protect the patient against further damage and they can not prevent the patient from suffering.

## Essentials of developing a chronic condition

Our knowledge of chronic pain developing mechanisms is still incomplete and much more complex than those of acute pain. From a clinical point of view, it is useful to distinguish three levels of processing.

*Neurophysiological system*

Spinal reflexes induced by pain stimuli increase muscle activity, in certain muscle groups, leading to additional load and decreased mobility. Over time, the patients become fatigued and/or restless. Neuroendocrine responses, for example peripheral increase of serotonin or substance P, sensitize nociceptors. By neuronal plasticity of the neuronal structures within the spinal cord, the spatial processing of the pain stimuli changes. Both result in increased intensity and spatially extended pain experience. Sympathetic hyperactivity, in itself, adds to a subjective increase in pain experience by several pathways. Sympathetic activity is simultaneously part of emotional responses. Since pain acts as a stressor, emotions like anxiety or anger are induced, because the neuronal information of pain stimuli is projected into the limbic system processing the affective quality of pain. The sympathetic arousal increases the intensity of this affective processing of the pain stimuli and adds psychic energy to the subjective suffering.

*Behavioural regulation*

A major function of acute pain is the regulation, control and conditioning of avoidance behaviour in order to protect the body against further damage. In response to pain, the organism develops guarding and protecting motor behaviour[2]. Facial expression of pain for the communication of suffering becomes aversive to the social environment over time, isolating the patient sooner or later. In addition, the inhibition of emotional expressiveness is related to physiological hyperactivity, particularly to muscle hypertension[3].

Part of this process is the vicious circle between pain and anxiety. From earlier experience with acute pain, patients consider their pain as a signal for potential damage. Anxiety as part of their avoidance reaction, is induced. Particularly patients with low back pain, show dramatic avoidance behaviour.

Not only the patients, but also their doctors, in prescribing bed rest and time off. Bed rest and retreat from daily activities is one of the usual, but wrong pieces of advice[4]. In addition, patients avoid social activities including social contact and work. Social isolation is only one negative consequence. Since external and internal cues are processed by a limited capacity attentional system, pain information concurs with other information on the attentional level. Social isolation and physical reductive life style increase the probability of pain information processing.

*Cognitive processing*

Prognosis of future events and the conscious anticipation of quality of events are genuine human abilities. In chronic pain patients, these abilities become maladaptive and dysfunctional. Chronic pain undermines the prognosis of future events like the ability to work, general quality of life, partnership, sexual functioning, leisure time activities and holidays. A major problem is the development of depressive disorders. There is an overwhelming empirical body of evidence that chronic pain induces depressive development. Among the various hypotheses on the relationship between chronic pain and depression, the hypothesis of a cognitive drift into depression is most evident and based on a rich data base[5].

Development of depression and the negative evaluation of the future contribute to the demand for job compensation and premature retirement. Low back pain is the most frequent reason for early retirement[6,7].

## Diagnostic tools for chronic pain

Therapy is based on proper diagnosis. Every therapist involved in chronic pain patients should be familiar with the standards of diagnostic classification systems and specific diagnostic procedures for pain. The classification of the International Association of the Study of Pain (IASP) is a multiaxional system and easy to apply in all fields of medicine. The proper use of international diagnostic schemata help to reduce the Babylonic speech muddle in the diagnosis and classification of pain in general and the myogenic pain disorders in particular (Table 1).

SCHEME AND SOME EXAMPLES OF THE FIVE AXIS FOR CODING PAIN DIAGNOSIS ACCORDING TO MERSKEY & BOGDUK[8]

| Axis | Description | Examples |
|---|---|---|
| I | Regions | Abdominal region<br>Head, face, and mouth<br>and others |
| II | Systems | Musculoskeletal system<br>Gastrointestinal system<br>and others |
| III | Temporal characteristics of pain: pattern of occurrence | Single episode<br>Recurrent regularly<br>and others |
| IV | Patients statement of intensity: time since onset of pain | Mild: more than 6 months<br>Severe: 1 month or less<br>and others |
| V | Aetiology | Neoplasm<br>Dysfunctional<br>and others |

Table 1

*The example of myogenic pain*

The IASP classification is not complete and does not include all conditions and factors relevant to the diagnosis of chronic pain. The classification of pain along the five axis is not sufficient to describe neurophysiological, psychological or social pain mechanisms underlying the pain problem in a specific pain disorder. Among other pain disorders, myogenic pain is one of the most common pain disorders with a high risk of developing chronic condition. According to the IASP classification musculoskeletal pain is of multifactorial origin and various somatic, psychological and social factors as well as their interrelations should be considered for an appropriate interdisciplinary treatment protocol[9,10]. A central problem is the insufficient functional diagnosis which alone can characterize a multifactorial pain event. This holds true for most pain disorders, with or without organic findings. In addition, a Babylonic speech confusion muddles the diagnosis and classification of myogenic pain disorders such as psychogenic rheumatism, fibromyalgia, lumbago, shoulder-arm syndrome, Repetitive Strain Injury (RSI), cervical vertebral syndrome, low-back pain, myofascial pain, tension headache, myalgia, premenstrual tension (PMT), to name just a few. Epidemiological assessment with the IASP classification of chronic pain showed that more than half of all patients suffer from myogenic pain[11].

According to the concept of myogenic pain, general and specific factors may be differentiated. General physiological factors include muscle hyperactivity, localized ischaemic conditions, reduced mean power frequency of the electromyography (EMG) and lowered pain threshold for mechanosensitive nociceptive stimulation. Trigger points result from prolonged muscle hyperactivity and are frequent in myogenic pain. Psychophysiological feedback mechanisms constitute a tension-pain-circle. Anticipation of stress or pain, in particular, can give rise to a muscle reaction which contributes to an accumulation of tension[10,12-14]. Muscular and Autonomic Nervous System (ANS) hyperactivity, in myogenic pain patients, are part of the symptom-specific psychophysiological reactivity to stress. It has been demonstrated in several studies on myogenic pain patients that physical overload, pain expectation and social stress resulted in localized muscle hyperactivity[15]. Muscle activity as a physiological correlate of movements, positions or expressive emotional behaviour is subject to classical and operant learning mechanisms, which result from attention paid to pain expression (positive reinforcement) or withdrawal from uncomfortable tasks (negative reinforcement)[3]. Among specific factors, vertebral instability is the most common for myogenic back pain. Ever since the fifties, numerous studies on back pain patients have described altered EMG samples with abnormally high or low EMG values in the lumbar region and asymmetry. Asymmetry seems first to emerge as a result of pain. Analysis of the connection between EMG values from the back and subjective pain reports dependent on topography, yielded a positive correlation in the upper back region and negative correlations in the lumbar area. This finding can be interpreted as a form of unbalanced muscle activity along the vertebral column in those patients who have not yet reached the chronic phase of back pain. While the pain source may actually be located in the upper back musculature, pain in the lower back area may arise from connective tissue or in ligaments.

A specific factor for tension type headache may be a deficit in the interoceptive perception of physiological hyperactivity. This perception deficit results in intra- and interindividual dysregulation. For example, muscle activity gives a person important information about their emotional state and the amount of excertion used during a task. The deficient interoception can have a disrupting effect on muscle activity when managing a stressful situation, so that, for example, daily stress can be underestimated[14,16].

Dysfunctional chewing behaviour is a specific factor for temporomandibular joint syndrome, another myogenic pain diagnosis. Dysfunctional chewing (raised biting rate and shortened chewing pauses) can give rise to pain due to ischaemia. Organic reasons for an abnormal chewing cycle are considered to be loss of rear teeth and a faulty bite. Oral habits may emerge as learned behaviour in the form of incorrect jaw and tongue positions, pressing lips and cheeks tightly together or as bruxism. When such behaviour forms are practiced intensively over a longer period of time they eventually damage the masticatory organs.

Work-related muscle pain (repetitive strain injury) is caused by fast frequently repeated uniform finger, hand and arm movements accompanied by a large static effort expended over a prolonged period of time[17,18].

In clinical practice, myogenic pain is usually diagnosed by exclusion of organic causes. Although there is a need to demonstrate muscular dysfunction accompanying pain mechanisms when diagnosing myogenic pain, clinicians rarely find appropriate diagnostic procedures. Only diagnostic procedures beyond routine, according to the IASP classification, enables the identification of myogenic pain mechanisms in individuals. Examples of procedures to diagnose myogenic pain mechanisms are: EMG-scanning, psychophysical stress profiling, dynamic evaluation, ambulatory EMG monitoring, muscle fatigue measures, deficits in muscle tension awareness, pain, stress and activity diaries[19].

## Therapy for chronic pain patients

First of all, a general rule: pain patients have no right to get pain free, but they have a right to be treated properly. That means in terms of general treatment recommendations:

- they have the right to have their pain believed
- they have the right to have their pain controlled
- they have the right to be treated with respect
- they have the right to know the truth
- they have the right to get psychological and spiritual support.

The second general rule of pain therapy concerns the partnership between patients and the treatment team. A good partnership makes a complex treatment possible and prevents negative effects of disappointment and unrealizable treatment expectations. Good partnership means in detail:

- avoid authoritarian behaviour (be aware of conflicting empirical data on therapeutic success)
- explain pain processes and develop a joint pain model with the patient
- discuss and propose treatment possibilities (be aware of individuality in treatment responding)
- tell the truth and do not promise more than necessary
- be respectful with the patients wishes (be aware of strong impact on treatment protocol by the patients treatment expectations).

As a third rule, one may conclude from several empirical treatment studies that the treatment of chronic pain patients is no one-man show. The team model with an interdisciplinary treatment protocol is most effective[4].

Medical treatment of chronic pain patients includes pharmacological therapy, behavioural techniques, physical interventions, electrical stimulation, regional analgesia, ablative neurosurgical operations and interdisciplinary pain management. For pharmacological treatment, one should follow the recommendations of the 1990 WHO ladder schemata particularly in the care for cancer patients[20].

For the application of behavioural treatment for chronic pain, three levels of psychological interventions may be considered for different subgroups of patients. The first level is general education about chronic pain, the second level is introduction into pain management, and the third level is psychotherapy. General education is to be given to every chronic patient that enters treatment. Pain management should be provided for those who demonstrate poor coping with pain or who show emotional consequences that indicate failure of coping like catastrophizing cognitions, depression or anxiety. Psychotherapy should be provided for those patients who demonstrate personality disorders or severe emotional dysfunction that either preceded the pain problem or in response to it.

***Pain management*** consists of standardized training programmes for the enhancement of coping with the pain problem that are usually limited to ten sessions. They comprise relaxation and imagination, cognitive restructuring, and techniques to improve the quality of life. Patients who participate may either be self-selected or encouraged to attend as a consequence of an initial screening. Patients with elevated scores in psychological questionnaires that indicate poor coping are the primary target of such an intervention. In patients with functional pain processes, behavioural treatment like relaxation, hypnosis or biofeedback may be effective. This treatment should be provided by psychologists. Patients who have a diagnosis of personality disorder or severe depressive or anxiety disturbance should be referred for psychological treatment either on a psychodynamic or behavioural basis. This treatment should be provided by professional psychotherapists.

*Therapy for myogenic pain*

Several meta-analyses of biobehavioural treatment protocols proved their therapeutic efficiency with myogenic pain. Techniques such as EMG-biofeedback which targets the reduction of muscular activity and promotes sensitivity to muscle tension are successful. At present, a combination of cognitive-behavioural treatment and biofeedback is promising. By means of two-channeled EMG-biofeedback during movement a reduction in muscle tension and a correction in the asymmetry can be trained. Neuromuscular training without biofeedback may be sensible, when a functional vertebral instability has been diagnosed by dorsal-Cybax or through raised EMG activity in the shoulder and neck area in combination with reduced muscle tension in the lumber region in EMG scanning has been established[21]. Specific muscle groups could be trained with such training devices, so that a balanced muscle growth can be stimulated. Pain caused by trauma can act as a stressor through which a pain-tension-pain-cycle develops and is subsequently extensively independent. In such cases, behaviour therapy in pain and stress coping is drawn on in view of success. Along with muscle relaxation, the mediation of imaginative processes is an important part in this programme in the control and prevention of pain.

## *References*

1. Bonica JJ. *Definition and taxonomy of pain.* In: Bonica JJ, editor. The management of pain. Philadelphia: Lea & Febiger; 1990.
2. Frymoyer JW, Cats-Baril W. *Predictors of low back pain disability.* Clin Orthop 1987;221:89-98.
3. Traue HC. *Inihibition and muscle tension in myogenic pain.* In: Pennebaker JW, editor. Emotion, disclosure, and health. Washington, DC: APA; 1995;155-76.
4. Pfingsten M, Hildebrandt J, Leibing E, et al. *Effectiveness of a multimodal treatment program for chronic low-back pain.* Pain 1997;73:77-85.
5. Kessler M, Kronstorfer R, Traue HC. *Depressive symptoms and disability in acute and chronic back pain patients.* Internat J Behav Med 1996;3:91-103.
6. Kessler M, Hrabal V, Traue HC. *Typologie unspezifischer Rückenschmerzen.* Zeitschr Gesundheitspsychol 1996;4:97-112.
7. Kessler M, Hrabal V, Wetzel R, Traue HC. *Schmerzintensität, Stimmung und medizinische Maßnahmen bei prä-chronischen Rückenschmerzpatienten.* Der Schmerz 1997;2:85-90.
8. Merskey H, Bogduk N. *Classification of chronic pain.* Seattle: IASP Press; 1994.
9. Teufel R, Traue HC. *Myogenic factors in low back pain.* In: Bischoff C, Traue HC, Zenz H, editors. Clinical perspectives on headache and low back pain. Toronto:

Hogrefe & Huber Publishers; 1989;64-86.
10. Rudisch T, Traue HC, Kessler M, Petö Z. *A myogen fájdalmak etiológiája.* Lege Artis Medicinae 1998;8:156-63.
11. Raspe H, Kohlmann T. *Rükenschmerzen-eine Epidemie unserer Tage?* Deutsch Ärzteblatt 1993;44:B2165-B2169.
12. Traue HC, Kessler M. *Rückenschmerz: Ätiologie zwischen Psychologie und Medizin.* Zeitschr Psychol Praxis (Psychomed) 1993;5:152-63.
13. Traue HC, Kessler M, Cram JR. *EMG topography and pain distribution in pre-chronic back pain.* Internat J Psychosom 1992;39:18-27.
14. Bischoff C, Müller K-J. *Portable EMG biofeedback: a single-case study with a muscle contraction headache sufferer.* In: Bischoff C, Traue HC, Zenz H, editors. Clinical perspectives on headache and low back pain. Toronto: Hogrefe & Huber Publishers; 1989;201-18.
15. Dickson-Parnell B, Zeichner A. *The premenstrual syndrome: psychophysiologic concomitants of perceived stress and low back pain.* Pain 1988;34:161-9.
16. Traue HC. *Emotion und Gesundheit: Die psychobiologische Regulation durch Hemmungen.* Heidelberg: Spektrum Akademischer Verlag; 1998.
17. Traue HC, Kessler M. *Myogene Schmerzen.* Zeitschr Medizin Psychol 1992;1,1:10-22.
18. Simons D. *Muscular pain syndromes.* In: Fricton JR, Awad EA, editors. Myofascial pain and fibromyalgia. New York: Raven Press; 1990;1-42.
19. Hrabal V, Kessler M, Traue HC. *Rückenschmerz und Alltagsaktivität: Erste Ergebnisse zum Ulmer Schmerztagebuch (UST).* Praxis Klin Verhaltensmed Rehabil 1991;4:290-9.
20. World Health Organization. *Cancer pain relief and palliative care. Report of a WHO Expert Committee.* Geneva; 1990.
21. Kessler M, Traue HC, Cram JR. *EMG muscle scanning in pain patients and controls: a replication and new data.* Am J Pain Management 1993;3:20-8.

## *ADDRESS FOR CORRESPONDENCE*

**TRAUE HC, Prof, Dr**
University of Ulm, Dept. of Medical Psychology
Am Hochsträß 8, 89081 Ulm Germany
Fax: +49 731 5025620
E-mail: harald.traue@medizin.uni-ulm.de

PART **FOUR**

# CHRONIC GASTROINTESTINAL DISORDERS

APPROACH TO THE PATIENT WITH CHRONIC GASTROINTESTINAL DISORDERS

# Clinical approach to management of gastro-oesophageal reflux disease in adults

*J-P Galmiche, HR Galmiche*

Gastro-Oesophageal Reflux Disease (GORD) is a very common disorder caused by retrograde flow of gastric contents through an incompetent gastro-oesophageal junction. It encompasses a wide range of clinical disorders from heartburn without mucosal breaks at endoscopy (i.e., "endoscopy-negative GORD") to severe oesophagitis and complications such as strictures, deep ulcers and metaplasia of the distal oesophageal mucosa (Barrett's oesophagus). As a result of recent progress in pharmacological therapy and laparoscopic antireflux surgery, different options are now available for the treatment of GORD.
This overview article refers to several reviews which have been published in recent years[1,2]. Because of the frequency of GORD and its increasing cost to society, the management of this disease requires consideration of its epidemiology and natural history. As most patients are not treated by specialists but by general practitioners, it is sometimes difficult to apply data from therapeutic trials conducted in tertiary centres to the conditions of a primary care setting.

## Epidemiology and natural history of GORD

The prevalence of heartburn, the most typical symptom together with regurgitation, is extremely high, affecting roughly 10 to 20% of adults at least weekly[3-5]. However, moderate to severe symptoms are present in only 1 to 4% of cases. Interestingly, epidemiological studies have shown that heartburn and regurgitation are significantly associated with such different symptoms or clinical presentations as dysphagia, globus sensation, chest pain of non-cardiac origin, respiratory disorders and dyspepsia, a condition frequently overlapping the GORD spectrum[4,5].
From a clinical standpoint, it seems relevant to distinguish those subjects (the bottom of the iceberg) in whom heartburn or regurgitation occurs

intermittently but who do not seek medical help and/or use self-medication (mainly with antacids) from those who need medical management. For instance, in a study in Finland[3], 10.3% of responders to a questionnaire mailed to a random sample of 2,500 people aged ≥20 years in the general population reported daily heartburn and/or regurgitation. However, only 5.5% had sought medical advice for symptoms during the previous year.

The prevalence of oesophagitis is far lower than heartburn, probably affecting about 2% of the general population and no more than half of those referred to an endoscopy unit because of symptoms suggestive of GORD[6]. In all recent therapeutic studies with a primary care enrollment[7,8] it has been consistently determined that most patients with macroscopic changes at endoscopy ("mucosal breaks") have mild-to-moderate lesions (non-circumferential lesions). On the contrary, severe oesophagitis or complications such as strictures or deep ulcers are very rare, especially in young subjects[9].

The natural history of GORD shows great variations[10-12]. In most patients seen by gastroenterologists or surgeons, GORD appears as a chronic disease which relapses shortly after discontinuation of treatment, therefore requiring maintenance drug therapy (or surgery) to prevent relapses. One reason for performing an endoscopy relatively early in the course of the disease (at least once in a lifetime) is that the severity of lesions seen at initial endoscopy is predictive of therapeutic response and the risk of recurrence after cessation of treatment[13]. However, in the primary care setting, the disease usually develops in a less severe manner, consisting of intermittent attacks, and most patients are endoscopy-negative or have mild oesophagitis. In this group of patients, there is little (if any) evidence that oesophagitis worsens with time. In most of these cases, lesions never develop or, if already present at first assessment, wax and wane without further worsening[11]. For instance, in a recently published study[12], only 2 patients out of 101 with oesophagitis followed up for more than 10 years developed an oesophageal stricture, and only one Barrett's oesophagus. Similarly, during a 6.5-year follow-up of 582 patients discharged from U.S. Veterans Administration hospitals with a diagnosis of oesophagitis, only 2.6% developed a stenosis, and an additional 2.2% an ulcer of the oesophagus[14]. The marked age-dependency of strictures and oesophageal ulcer suggested that these complications may take a long time to develop. Finally, most patients with complications are ≥ 60 years of age.

## What are the primary aims of treatment in GORD?

Until the 1990s, most therapeutic trials of drug therapy concentrated on endoscopic lesions, and the healing of oesophagitis was considered to be the primary end-point by which treatment efficacy should be evaluated. In fact, the relation between symptoms and the presence or grade of oesophagitis in an individual patient is very poor. For example, GORD can remain completely asymptomatic in Barrett's oesophagus[15], or dysphagia can frequently reveal peptic stricture in a patient without any previous history of heartburn or regurgitation. On the contrary, in the large group of "endoscopy-negative" patients, symptoms can severely impact quality of life and thus justify a more active management than previously admitted. Moreover, a relapse of symptoms frequently occurs after discontinuation of treatment, even in the absence of oesophagitis. Therefore, the classical criteria for judgement of therapeutic efficacy in GORD have been revisited during the last decade, and there is now wide consensus that symptom relief and long-term control of the disease are actually the primary aims of therapy for most patients. The inclusion of quality of life assessments in therapeutic trials is recommended[16] for evaluation of both drug therapy and antireflux surgery. However, in patients with moderate to severe oesophagitis and/or complications, healing also remains an important therapeutic goal.

## Medical therapy

*Lifestyle and dietary recommendations* - together with antacids - have been the mainstay of GORD treatment for decades. Physiological studies using oesophageal pH monitoring have suggested that measures such as raising the head of the bed or elimination of fatty foods may be of benefit because they are able to reduce mucosal acid exposure[17,18]. In fact, their therapeutic efficacy has not really been established by well-controlled trials. Similarly, the role of obesity in GORD, as well as the benefit of weight loss, has not been demonstrated. The same holds true for cessation of smoking or discontinuance of drugs such as bronchodilators in asthmatic subjects. In practice, it seems reasonable to retain recommendations such as raising the head of the bed and avoiding recumbency within 3 hours after dinner, especially for patients with regurgitation and/or nocturnal symptoms. Similarly, when specific foods or drugs are poorly tolerated, the clinician should consider the situation case by case. However, a too systematic application of lifestyle and dietary recommendations may affect quality of life adversely in many patients without providing any evident benefit.

## Antacids and alginate/antacids

This class of drugs is very useful for self-medication. Though several placebo-controlled trials have failed to establish their efficacy for heartburn, other studies, as well as epidemiological data, suggest that they are likely to be effective in alleviating symptoms[19]. The combination of antacids with alginate (which floats like a raft on gastric contents) seems more effective than antacid alone. In a large open trial of alginates/antacids taken on-demand, most patients with mild oesophagitis remained in clinical remission throughout the 6-month study period[20]. However, antacids and alginates/antacids are not effective enough to heal moderate/severe oesophagitis and prevent further relapses.

## $H_2$-receptor antagonists

Many placebo-controlled trials have demonstrated that $H_2$-blockers are effective in short-term treatment of GORD (for review see 21). They relieve heartburn more effectively than placebo, even when administered at low dosages (e.g., ranitidine 75 mg or cimetidine 200 mg[22]. Moreover, in patients with reflux oesophagitis, healing is significantly more frequent after 6 to 12 weeks of treatment with cimetidine, ranitidine, famotidine or nizatidine than after placebo. However, $H_2$-blockers are not effective enough in patients with moderate or severe oesophagitis, for whom the average gain in terms of healing does not exceed 25 or 10% respectively. Furthermore, maintenance therapy with standard doses of $H_2$-blockers (e.g., 150 mg ranitidine b.i.d.) does not consistently prevent further relapses. The main reasons for this limited efficacy of $H_2$-blockers in GORD are tolerance and insufficient inhibition of acid secretion in the postprandial period. In this respect, increasing doses (e.g., 1.6 g ranitidine per day) and greater dosing frequency (i.e., a q.i.d. regimen instead of twice daily) can improve efficacy, though at the risk of reducing compliance and at higher cost. Yet, $H_2$-blockers, because of their excellent safety profile despite limited efficacy, are still useful drugs in the primary care setting. Their role as OTC (over-the-counter) medications has been exploited in several countries where they, at least partly, replace antacids for self-medication. Special formulations (e.g., famotidine wafer or cimetidine effervescent tablets) may be especially appropriate for this specific indication.

## Cisapride

Although some cholinergic (e.g., bethanechol) and anti-dopaminergic drugs (e.g., metoclopramide and domperidone) are effective in GORD, their marginal benefit is offset by frequent side effects. These compounds have been abandoned as anti-reflux drugs since the development of cisapride, a drug that enhances oesophageal peristaltic waves, increases lower oesophageal sphincter (LOS) basal tone and accelerates gastric emptying. However, it does not affect LOS transient relaxations, which represent the basic underlying motor mechanism of most reflux episodes.

In the short term, cisapride (10 mg q.i.d. or 20 mg b.i.d.) is more effective than placebo and approximately as effective as $H_2$-blockers for symptom relief and healing of oesophagitis. Cisapride 10 mg b.i.d. (or 20 mg at bedtime) also provides effective prophylaxis of oesophagitis relapse[23,24]. However, this benefit is mainly limited to patients with mild oesophagitis. Combined therapy with an $H_2$-blocker is more effective than monotherapy with either compound, but the combination is more expensive and less convenient than a proton pump inhibitor (PPI) given alone[25]. Therefore, combined therapy has very few indications and is not a first-choice treatment in GORD.

Cisapride is usually well-tolerated, the most frequent side effects being mild diarrhoea, abdominal pain and headache. However, exceptional but lethal cardiac complications (i.e., torsades de pointes) have recently been noted. This risk may reduce the role of cisapride considerably in the treatment of GORD since safe, effective, well-tolerated drugs are now available. The clinician should also be aware that an association of cisapride with several other drugs such as spiramycin or ketoconazole is strictly prohibited[26].

## Proton pump inhibitors (PPI)

Omeprazole (20 and 40 mg o.d.) was the first PPI extensively evaluated for the treatment of reflux oesophagitis, whereas lansoprazole (30 mg o.d.), pantoprazole (40 mg o.d.) and rabeprazole (20 mg o.d.) have been developed more recently. A meta-analysis of 43 therapeutic trials[27] conducted in moderate/severe oesophagitis has confirmed the clear advantage of PPI over $H_2$-blockers. The proportion of patients successfully treated was nearly double, and the rapidity of healing and symptom relief was approximately twice as fast with PPI than with $H_2$-blockers (Figure 1).

The superiority of PPI is obvious, not only in severe cases or in patients refractory to $H_2$-blockers, but also in mild oesophagitis and endoscopy-negative patients[8,28]. Quality of life is restored to a normal level after 4 to 6 weeks of PPI therapy. Although few studies are available [7], omeprazole (20 mg or 10 mg daily) clearly provides better results than cisapride (10 mg q.i.d.).

Continuous maintenance therapy with PPI is significantly superior to ranitidine (150 mg b.i.d.) and is effective in preventing relapses. For example, our meta-analysis[29] showed that after 6 months of maintenance with 20 or 10 mg omeprazole daily, 80 and 70% of patients, respectively, were still in remission. As relief of heartburn during PPI treatment is highly predictive of healing, there is no need for endoscopic monitoring in asymptomatic patients, unless the initial endoscopy shows severe oesophagitis or premalignant conditions such as

Barrett's oesophagus. In the primary care setting, intermittent on-demand therapy[30] with omeprazole has also provided excellent results for symptom relief and quality of life. In several countries, PPI in low dosages are now available for symptomatic treatment of GORD (e.g., omeprazole 10 mg or lansoprazole 15 mg). In fact, it is important to titrate PPI therapy according to individual needs.

Figure 1

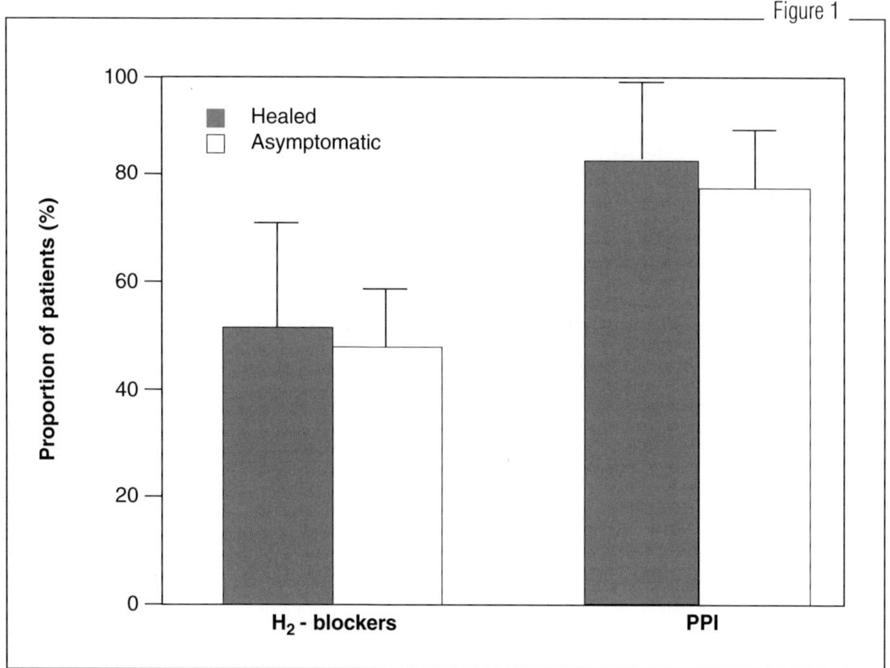


Proportion of patients with healed and asymptomatic oesophagitis after initial therapy with $H_2$-blockers or proton pump inhibitors. Results of a meta-analysis of 43 articles including 7,635 patients (drawn from Chiba N, De Cara CJ, Wilkinson JM, Hunt RH[27]).

Finally, the major issue concerning PPI therapy is not efficacy but safety and economics. Although PPI are extremely well-tolerated drugs, there is some concern about the risks of potent acid suppression in the very long-term. Mild hypergastrinaemia is a direct consequence of acid suppression, which has no clinical relevance. The risk of developing atrophic gastritis during PPI treatment has been reported by Kuipers et al.[31] in patients infected by *Helicobacter pylori (H. pylori)*. However, this result needs to be confirmed in prospective studies. At the present time, the need to eradicate *H. pylori* before embarking on long-term acid suppression with PPI is not supported by sufficient scientific evidence and, therefore, remains controversial.

## Antireflux surgery

The principle of any surgical procedure is to restore an effective anti-reflux barrier. This can be achieved by different types of fundoplication performed through classical open surgery or by laparoscopy. The preferred and probably most efficient anti-reflux procedure is "floppy" Nissen fundoplication, which has been developed to avoid (as far as possible) dysphagia, gas bloat syndrome and inability to burp. With this technique, dividing the short gastric vessels to mobilise the fundus ensures that the wrap will be loose and without tension. Fundic mobilisation is supposed to restore belching ability without compromising antireflux efficacy, but has no advantage regarding flatus or bloating. Toupet fundoplication is a posterior hemifundoplication with the theoretical potential advantage of causing less postoperative gas bloat or dysphagia. Modern advances in equipment and techniques have made it possible to perform the same procedures with minimally invasive laparoscopic techniques.

With open surgery, a high success rate (up to 80%) can be achieved concomitant with almost no mortality and morbidity. Several controlled trials have clearly established that open antireflux fundoplications are more effective than continuous or intermittent therapy, together with lifestyle recommendations and various associations of antacids, $H_2$-blockers, metoclopramide and sucralfate[32]. Recently, a well-designed Scandinavian trial showed that open surgery is at least as effective or even slightly better than continuous omeprazole treatment [33]. However, some deterioration of surgical results may occur with time, usually in association with wrap disruption [34]. Furthermore, open surgery implies an extensive abdominal or even thoracic incision, resulting in patient discomfort, an extended recovery period, notable overall costs and potential risk of incisional hernia.

With laparoscopic fundoplication, a nasogastric tube is unnecessary and a soft diet can be introduced on the first postoperative day. Patients are generally discharged on the first or second postoperative day. Most patients are able to return to work within two weeks, which provides a significant reduction in the overall cost of surgical treatment. However, laparoscopic Nissen fundoplication is a demanding technique, requiring different skills from those generally needed for other procedures such as cholecystectomy or appendectomy. Experience and training in laparoscopic surgery are mandatory[35], and the learning curve is a determinant factor in the risk of postoperative morbidity. In selected centres, postoperative mortality is extremely low (less than 0.5%) and sometimes nil. Complications and/or significant postoperative morbidity[36], especially severe dysphagia, are noted in 2 to 5% of cases. Excellent results are reported in 70 to 90% of cases, but the length of follow-up in most published series does not exceed one or two years. Recurrent reflux is usually due to a breakdown of the repair. A direct comparison of laparoscopic anti-reflux surgery versus long-term PPI therapy is urgently awaited. In these trials, comparisons should include quality of life and economic end-points since this information is needed to define cost-effective strategies for long-term management of GORD. At the present time, mathematical models suggest that laparoscopic surgery may be more cost-effective than continuous omeprazole therapy after 5 to 10 years. However, these estimates are extremely sensitive to drug costs (which may be reduced by the development of generics) and to postoperative morbidity[37].

## Practical approach to GORD management

GORD management should be tailored to the individual patient. It depends not only on the severity of the disease but also on variables such as age, patient preferences and/or concomitant illnesses. Moreover, severity of the disease refers not only to the grade of oesophagitis at endoscopy, but also includes the impact of symptoms on quality of life and responsiveness to drug therapy as well as the individual outcome of the disease as evaluated over a sufficient period of time, usually one or two years.

## Initial therapy (Figure 2)

In patients with mild/moderate heartburn, an initial approach combining lifestyle modifications and alginate/antacids is traditionally recommended and generally sufficient to achieve symptom relief in a large proportion of reflux patients seen in the primary care setting. However, in young adults presenting with no alarm symptoms (such as dysphagia, anaemia or weight loss), the consensus is now to use acid-suppressors empirically (i.e., without any endoscopic assessment).

Figure 2

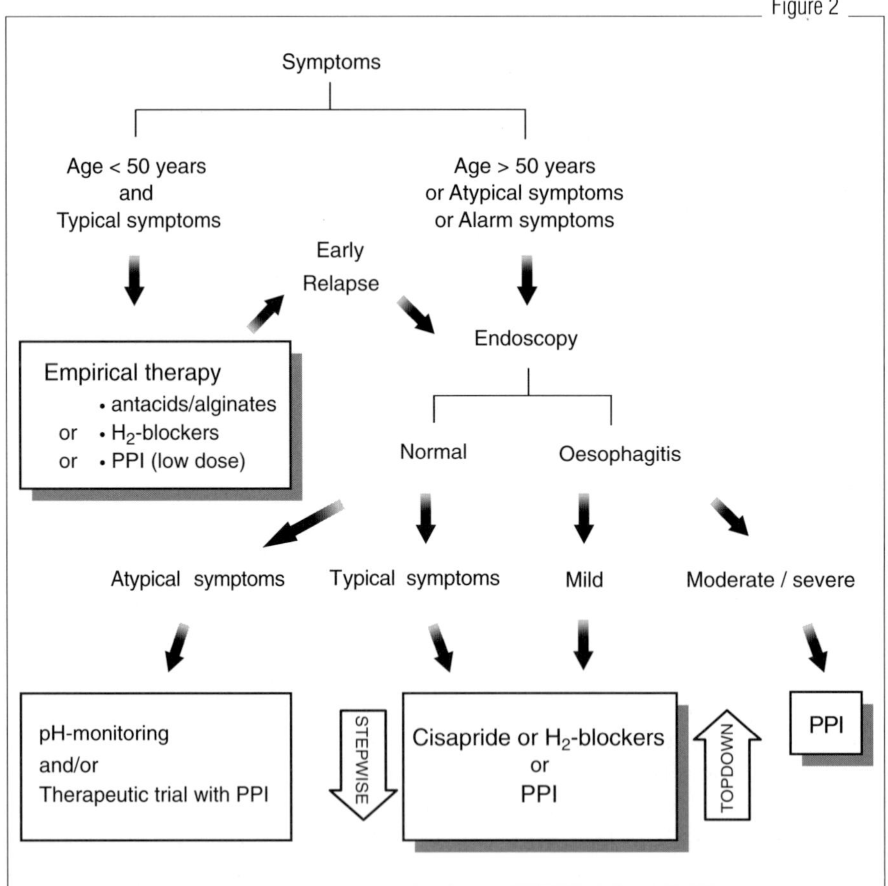


Suggested flowchart for initial management of gastro-oesophageal reflux disease.

Hence, one or two courses of $H_2$-blockers or PPI (e.g., 10 mg omeprazole o.d. for 4 to 6 weeks) can be administered without any risk of missing a life-threatening condition. In contrast, in patients over 50 years of age, or in those with alarm symptoms, it is mandatory to perform endoscopic investigation to exclude malignancy of the upper gastrointestinal tract as well as to assess the degree of oesophageal injury. Two drug strategies are possible in endoscopy-negative patients with typical heartburn or mild oesophagitis: a step-wise approach (with cisapride or $H_2$-blockers prescribed first and PPI administered only in cases of insufficient or no response) or a top-down approach using PPI directly[38,39]. At the present time, there is no definite evidence based on randomised clinical trials in favour of one of these approaches. However, the cost/effectiveness of the top-down strategy usually becomes greater with the severity of the disease.

When endoscopy is normal in a patient with atypical symptoms, it is important first to establish the diagnosis of GORD. Twenty-four-hour pH-monitoring with symptom analysis may be useful, but in clinical practice a "PPI-test" (e.g., omeprazole 20 mg b.i.d. for 2 weeks or 40 mg bid for one week) is more attractive for the patient and probably less expensive. A clear symptomatic response is sensitive (but not very specific) for the diagnosis of GORD[40-42].

In patients with moderate or severe oesophagitis, PPI are now the therapy of choice in GORD. The dosage is increased in the event of insufficient therapeutic response in order to bring acid exposure into the physiological range. Very few compliant patients are truly resistant to PPI, although this eventuality should lead to reconsideration of the diagnosis and further investigations. In such cases, pH-monitoring, both with and without PPI treatment, may be useful in establishing the diagnosis of GORD as well as in assessing the efficacy of the drug regimen[43].

Complications require a specific approach. Strictures are usually successfully managed by endoscopic dilatation in association with PPI, which are more cost-effective than $H_2$-blockers in this specific indication[44,45]. Patients with Barrett's oesophagus are at risk of developing adenocarcinoma, but the indication and modalities of endoscopic and histologic surveillance depend largely on the general status of the patient. Neither surgery nor specific medical therapy reduces the risk of malignancy. Trials combining photochemotherapy and PPI are now in progress, but mainly in patients who have already developed dysplasia[46,47].

## Long-term management

In most cases, symptom relief and healing of oesophagitis are achieved after initial treatment, so that the key issue is long-term control of the disease. Three strategies can then be proposed:

1. intermittent on-demand drug therapy
2. maintenance drug therapy (usually with PPI), or
3. antireflux (open or laparoscopic) surgery

These strategies are not mutually exclusive, e.g., a patient dissatisfied with long-term drug therapy may eventually prefer surgery, even though the former strategy is effective and well-tolerated.
Finally, intermittent on-demand treatment is suitable for patients with mild or moderate symptoms and infrequent relapses, who should be treated in the same way as initially if symptoms recur. Conversely, for patients with severe oesophagitis or whose symptoms recur shortly after treatment has been stopped, maintenance treatment with PPI is highly effective for ensuring excellent remission. However, PPI do not cure the disease, and motor abnormalities remain unchanged even after complete healing of oesophagitis. Therefore, surgery may be preferable to a lifetime of medical therapy [48] in young fit patients with frequent relapses (e.g., more than three per year). Laparoscopic surgery is now the preferred approach for many patients and surgeons, but should be further evaluated and compared with other strategies before the extension of its indications in GORD.

## *REFERENCES*

1. Galmiche JP, Letessier E, Scarpignato C. *Treatment of gastro-oesophageal reflux disease in adults*. Br Med J 1998;316:1720-3.

2. Kahrilas PJ. *Gastroesophageal reflux disease.* JAMA 1996;276:983-8.
3. Isolauri J, Laippala P. *Prevalence of symptoms suggestive of gastro-oesophageal reflux disease in an adult population.* Ann Med 1995;27:67-70.
4. Ruth M, Mänsson I, Sandberg N. *The prevalence of symptoms suggestive of esophageal disorders.* Scand J Gastroenterol 1991;6:73-81.
5. Locke GR, Talley NJ, Fett SL, et al. *Prevalence and clinical spectrum of gastroesophageal reflux: a population-based study in Olmsted County, Minnesota.* Gastroenterology 1997;112:1448-56.
6. Johnsson F, Joelsson B, Gudmundsson K, Greiff L. *Symptoms and endoscopic findings in the diagnosis of gastroesophageal reflux disease.* Scand J Gastroenterol 1987;22:714-8.
7. Galmiche JP, Barthélémy P, Hamelin B. *Treating the symptoms of gastroesophageal reflux disease: a double-blind comparison of omeprazole and cisapride.* Aliment Pharmacol Ther 1997;11:765-73.
8. Carlsson R, Dent J, Watts R, et al. *Gastro-oesophageal reflux disease in primary care: an international study of different treatment strategies with omeprazole.* Eur J Gastroenterol Hepatol 1998;10:119-24.
9. Ben Rejeb M, Bouché O, Zeitoun P. *Study of 47 consecutive patients with peptic esophageal stricture compared with 3880 cases of reflux esophagitis.* Dig Dis Sci 1992;37:733-6.
10. Kuster E, Ros E, Toledo-Pimentel V, et al. *Predictive factors of the long-term outcome in gastro-oesophageal reflux disease: six-year follow-up of 107 patients.* Gut 1994;35:8-14.
11. Schindlbeck NE, Klauser AG, Berghammer G, et al. *Three-year follow-up of patients with gastro-oesophageal reflux disease.* Gut 1992;33:1016-9.
12. McDougall NI, Johnston BT, Kee F, et al. *Natural history of reflux oesophagitis: a 10-year follow-up of its effect on patient symptomatology and quality of life.* Gut 1996;38:481-6.
13. Galmiche JP, Bruley des Varannes S. *Symptoms and disease severity in gastro-oesophageal reflux disease.* Scand J Gastroenterol 1994;29(Suppl 201):62-8.
14. Sonnenberg A, Massey BT, Jacobsen SJ. *Hospital discharges resulting from esophagitis among Medicare beneficiaries.* Dig Dis Sci 1994;39:183-8.
15. Cameron AJ, Zinsmeister AR, Ballard DJ, Carney JA. *Prevalence of columnar-lined (Barrett's) esophagus. Comparison of population-based clinical and autopsy findings.* Gastroenterology 1990;99:918-22.
16. Tebaldi M, Heading RC. *Quality of life assessment in reflux disease.* Eur J Gastroenterol Hepatol 1998;10:451-4.
17. Kitchin LI, Castell DO. *Rationale and efficacy of conservative therapy for gastroesophageal reflux disease.* Arch Intern Med 1991;151:448-54.

18. Galmiche JP. *Gastro-oesophageal reflux: does it matter what you eat?* Gut 1998;40:318-9.
19. Scarpignato C, Galmiche JP. *Antacids and alginates in the treatment of gastroesophageal reflux disease: how do they work and how much are they clinically useful?* In: Scarpignato C, editor. Advances in drug therapy of gastroesophageal reflux disease. Front Gastrointest Res Basel: Karger; 1992;20:153-81.
20. Poynard T, and the French Co-operative Study Group. *Relapse rate of patients after healing of oesophagitis - a prospective study of alginate as self-care treatment for 6 months.* Aliment Pharmacol Ther 1993;7:385-92.
21. Scarpignato C, Galmiche JP. *The role of $H_2$-receptor antagonists in the era of proton pump inhibitors.* In: Lundell L, editor. Guidelines for management of symptomatic gastro-oesophageal reflux disease. London: Science Press Ltd; 1998;55-66.
22. Galmiche JP, Shi G, Simon B, et al. *On-demand treatment of gastro-oesophageal reflux symptoms: a study comparing ranitidine 75 mg with placebo and cimetidine 200 mg.* Aliment Pharmacol Ther 1998;12:909-17.
23. Tytgat GNJ, Janssens J, Reynolds JF, Wienbeck M. *Update on the pathophysiology and management of gastro-oesophageal reflux disease: the role of prokinetic therapy.* Eur J Gastroenterol Hepatol 1996;8:603-11.
24. Blum AL, Adami B, Bouzo MH, et al. *Effect of cisapride on relapse of esophagitis. A multinational placebo-controlled trial in patients healed with an antisecretory drug.* Dig Dis Sci 1993;38:551-60.
25. Vigneri S, Termini R, Leandro G, et al. *A comparison of five maintenance therapies for reflux esophagitis.* N Engl J Med 1995;333:1106-10.
26. Coffin B. *Reflux gastro-oesophagien: quels sont les résultats des traitements médicaux? Les prokinétiques.* Gastroenterol Clin Biol 1999; 23: S90-S96.
27. Chiba N, De Cara CJ, Wilkinson JM, Hunt RH. *Speed of healing and symptom relief in grade II to IV gastroesophageal reflux disease: a meta-analysis.* Gastroenterology 1997;112:1798-1810.
28. Bate CM, Griffin SM, Keeling PWN, et al. *Reflux symptom relief with omeprazole in patients without unequivocal oesophagitis.* Aliment Pharmacol Ther 1996;10:547-55.
29. Carlsson R, Galmiche JP, Dent J, et al. *Prognostic factors influencing relapse of oesophagitis during maintenance therapy with antisecretory drugs: a meta-analysis of long-term omeprazole trials.* Aliment Pharmacol Ther 1997;11:473-82.
30. Bardhan KD, Muller-Lissner S, Bigard MA, et al. *Symptomatic gastroesophageal reflux disease (GERD): intermittent treatment (IT) with omeprazole (OM) and ranitidine (RAN) as a strategy for management.* Gastroenterology 1997;112(Suppl 4):A165.
31. Kuipers EJ, Lundell L, Klinkenberg-Knol EC, et al. *Atrophic gastritis and Helicobacter*

*pylori infection in patients with reflux esophagitis treated with omeprazole or fundoplication.* N Engl J Med 1996;334:1018-22.

32. Spechler SJ. *Comparison of medical and surgical therapy for complicated gastroesophageal reflux disease in veterans.* The Department of Veterans Affairs Gastroesophageal Reflux Disease Study Group. N Engl J Med 1992;326:786-92.
33. Lundell L, Dalenbäck J, Hattlebakk J, et al. *Omeprazole (OME) or antireflux surgery (ARS) in the long term management of gastroesophageal reflux disease (GERD): results of a multicentre, randomised clinical trial.* Gastroenterology 1998;114:A207.
34. Luostarinen M, Isolauri J, Laitinen J, et al. *Fate of Nissen fundoplication after 20 years. A clinical, endoscopical, and functional analysis.* Gut 1993; 34:1015-20.
35. Watson DI, Jamieson GG, Baigrie RJ, et al. *Laparoscopic surgery for gastro-oesophageal reflux: beyond the learning curve.* Br J Surg 1996;83:1284-7.
36. Collet D, Cadière GB. *Conversions and complications of laparoscopic treatment of gastroesophageal reflux disease.* Am J Surg 1995;169:622-6.
37. Heudebert GR, Marks R, Wicox CM, Centor RM. *Choice of long-term strategy for the management of patients with severe esophagitis: a cost utility analysis.* Gastroenterology 1997;112:1078-86.
38. Hillman AL. *Economic analysis of alternative treatments for persistent gastro-oesophageal reflux disease.* Scand J Gastroenterol 1994;29(Suppl 201):98-102.
39. Eggleston A, Wigerinck A, Huijghebaert S, et al. *Cost effectiveness of treatment for gastro-oesophageal reflux disease in clinical practice: a clinical database analysis.* Gut 1998;42:13-6.
40. Schindlbeck NE, Klauser AG, Voderholzer WA, Müller-Lissner SA. *Empiric therapy for gastroesophageal reflux disease.* Arch Intern Med 1995;155:1808-12.
41. Schenk BE, Kuipers EJ, Klinkenberg-Knol EC, et al. *Omeprazole as a diagnostic tool in gastroesophageal reflux disease.* Am J Gastroenterol 1997;92:1997-2000.
42. Johnsson F, Weywadt L, Solhaug JH, et al. *One-week omeprazole treatment in the diagnosis of gastro-oesophageal reflux disease.* Scand J Gastroenterol 1998;33:15-20.
43. Kahrilas PJ, Quigley EMM. *Clinical esophageal pH recording: a technical review for practice guideline development.* Gastroenterology 1996;110:1982-96.
44. Smith PM, Kerr GD, Cockel R, et al. *A comparison of omeprazole and ranitidine in the prevention of recurrence of benign esophageal stricture.* Gastroenterology 1994;107:1312-8.
45. Marks RD, Richter JE, Rizzo J, et al. *Omeprazole versus $H_2$-receptor antagonists in treating patients with peptic stricture and esophagitis.* Gastroenterology 1994;106:907-15.
46. Gossner L, Stolte M, Sroka R, et al. *Photodynamic ablation of high-grade dysplasia and*

*early cancer in Barrett's esophagus by means of 5-aminolevulinic acid.* Gastroenterology 1998;114:448-55.

47. Overholt BF, Panjehpour M. *Photodynamic therapy for Barrett's esophagus: clinical update.* Am J Gastroenterol 1996;91:1719-23.
48. Anvari M, Allen C, Borm A. *Laparoscopic Nissen fundoplication is a satisfactory alternative to long-term omeprazole therapy.* Br J Surg 1995;82:938-42.

## *ADDRESS FOR CORRESPONDENCE*

**GALMICHE J-P, MD**
CHU Hotel Dieu
Department of Hepatology and Gastroenterology
Nantes 44035 France
Fax: +33 2 40 08 31 68
E-mail: galmiche@easynet.fr

# Helicobacter pylori, gastritis and functional dyspepsia

*R Corinaldesi, G Barbara, V Stanghellini*

Functional dyspepsia is highly variable in its clinical presentation and certainly multifactorial in its underlying causes. Since many of the symptoms included in the definition of dyspepsia intuitively suggest different pathogenetic mechanisms, the existence of distinct dyspepsia subgroups has been postulated.

Three working teams have proposed definitions of dyspepsia subgroups with the endorsement of international experts in the field[1-3], and other similar (although not identical) definitions have been proposed[4]. Unlike other published subgroup definitions, previous Rome Criteria proposed not to include the reflux-like subgroup in the context of dyspepsia[3]. Indeed, heartburn and regurgitation are extra-abdominal symptoms and, if severe enough to influence the usual activities, they have been proven of diagnostic value for gastro-oesophageal reflux disease (GORD)[5].

Although clinical features and response to treatment of the milder forms of these symptoms have, as yet, received little attention, their underlying pathogenetic mechanisms are likely better characterized than other dyspeptic symptoms and there is no apparent scientific advantage in considering them as part of dyspepsia.

Two main hypothetical subgroups were identified in all the reports: "ulcer-like" and "dysmotility-like" dyspepsia. The former being characterized by several aspects of pain, the latter by distinct symptoms other than pain and suggest impaired gastroduodenal motility. Two working team reports introduced numeric limitations by requiring the concomitant presence of at least two[2] or three[3] specific symptoms to be included in a subgroup, thus introducing the concept of "cluster of symptoms".

Finally, all reports suggested the existence of the possible presentation of symptoms different from those characterized in specific subgroups. All these definitions of dyspepsia subgroups were totally arbitrary and were proposed to direct research toward selections of dyspeptic patients and analysis of their symptoms.

## Testing the validity of *"a priori"* definitions of dyspepsia subgroups

Overlapping between groups ranges between 15%[6] and 83%[7] and, on average, it is quite substantial thus challenging the validity of the subgroup hypothesis. Interestingly, some of these studies adopted definitions of subgroups that are slightly or considerably modified with respect to those originally proposed, and this may have influenced their findings. For instance, in several studies[7-10], only patients complaining of pain (centered) in the upper abdomen were included (and classified into different subgroups) and this may have favoured overlapping. Talley et al.[11], by quantitating the severity of symptoms, failed to detect any difference between dyspeptic subgroups. Mansi et al.[12] reported a significantly higher prevalence of negative endoscopy in patients with dysmotility-like dyspepsia, as opposed to those with ulcer-like and reflux-like dyspepsia in over two thousand dyspeptic patients.

Klauser et al.[13] subdivided 220 patients with negative upper GI endoscopy into subgroups according to a substantially modified version of the classification proposed by Colin-Jones et al.[1]. They identified only three subgroups: reflux-like, dysmotility-like, and unspecified. Surprisingly, the dysmotility-like group was characterized by features such as abdominal distension, diffuse pain, food intolerance that were not included in the original definition by Colin-Jones et al. An extended work-up was carried out in half the patients including oesophageal manometry and pH-metry, lactose tolerance test and scintigraphic evaluation of oesophageal, gastric and biliary transits. An abnormal finding was detected in approximately half of the investigated patients, but none of the symptoms cluster reliably predicted the underlying pathogenetic abnormality.

Some studies evaluated whether predefined symptom subgroups may by characterized by differences in Helicobacter pylori (H. pylori) infection and its clinical manifestations. Histological H. pylori status, gastric acid secretion, gastrin levels, cutaneous electrogastrography and gastric emptying were evaluated[14] in 144 Japanese patients with functional dyspepsia who were subdivided according to Colin-Jones et al. All the parameters were similar between the subgroups with the exception of gastric emptying, which was more frequently delayed in patients with dysmotility-like and reflux-like dyspepsia. The criteria proposed by Drossman et al.[2] were modified by Trespi et al.[15] to evaluate the symptomatic response to medical therapy in 70 Italian H. pylori positive patients with functional dyspepsia. Ulcer-like patients differed from reflux-like patients in their higher score of antritis activity, and from dysmotility-like patients in achieving a significant regression of dyspeptic score, three and six months after treatment.

## Associations between dyspeptic symptoms and H. pylori infection

The main pathophysiologic abnormalities potentially associated with dyspeptic symptom perception are gastric acid hypersecretion, H. pylori infection, gastrointestinal dysmotility, and visceral hypersensitivity. Interpretation of the studies carried out to investigate abnormalities of these functions and specific dyspeptic symptoms or subgroups of symptoms is difficult since they suffer from the same problems as other studies in the field. A cultural bias of investigators seems particularly relevant in this area. In fact, most of the studies investigating gastric acid secretion and H. pylori status were carried out on patients complaining mainly of pain/ulcer-like dyspepsia and, conversely, patients with dysmotility-like dyspepsia have been more frequently included in studies investigating gastric emptying or other digestive motility functions.

The role of H. pylori in determining functional dyspepsia is, as yet, controversial, leave alone its association with specific dyspepsia subgroups. No specific symptom profile has been identified that could help to distinguish H. pylori positive from H. pylori negative patients.

In the majority of published studies no associated symptom was identified. Kemmer et al.[16] identified five factors with a predictive value of H. pylori infection in functional dyspepsia (pain relief after food intake, body weight, past history of peptic ulcer and absence of fat intolerance and of diarrhoea).

The value of this study is questionable since patients with a history of peptic ulcer were erroneously included in the functional dyspepsia group, and also because of the low sensitivity of the symptoms which makes it of negligible clinical utility[17]. Acute infection was found to be associated with symptoms of gastritis or upper GI pain[18]. If confirmed, these data, taken together, would suggest that an acute infection is associated with ulcer-like symptoms, but that this association would persist only sporadically in the long-term. It is likely that the relationship (if any) between H. pylori and dyspeptic symptoms and/or the identification of a subset of patients in whom such an association exists will be identified only by monitoring the effects of H. pylori eradication and of the subsequent changes in mucosal inflammation. The available studies are flawed by important limitations and therefore, difficult to interpret[9]. Even the most recent studies with a prolonged follow-up period often failed to analyze individual symptoms and produced conflicting results[6,15,19-24]. Only a few studies have analyzed outcomes in different subgroups of patients separately. Trespi et al. reported a more consistent improvement in symptoms in patients with ulcer-like dyspepsia, as compared to other subgroups[15]. A recent preliminary report also seems to point in this direction[23], although conflicting results have been published.

Well designed and conducted studies are needed to evaluate whether eradication of the bacterium and/or improvement of gastritis are associated with an improvement in dyspeptic symptoms and, if so, which symptoms in which patients.

A significant correlation has been described between the degree of gastric mucosal inflammation and some symptoms including epigastric pain, burping-belching and nausea[24]. Mucosal inflammation affects both afferent and efferent enteric neurons, thus potentially influencing visceral perception[25]. H. pylori infection has been shown to be associated with increased concentrations of neuropeptides such as somatostatin, substance P, and Calcitonin Gene Related Peptide in the gastric mucosa, particularly of patients with ulcer-like dyspepsia[26].

### Relationship between H. pylori infection and other objective findings in functional dyspepsia

Several studies have evaluated the relationship between putative pathogenetic factors of functional dyspepsia, in an attempt to further explore the nature of symptoms. The majority of these studies focused on the relationship between H. pylori status and gut dysmotility or hypersensitivity, while a few others explored the relationship between visceral hypersensitivity, on the one hand, and gut dysmotility or psychological disturbances, on the other.

*H. pylori/gut dysmotility*

Testoni et al., in manometric studies, recorded fasting and postprandial motility of the gastric antrum and proximal small bowel in 25 patients with functional dyspepsia[27]. All the patients had gastritis but, surprisingly, up to 40% were found to be H. pylori negative. H. pylori infected patients had decreased fasting and postprandial antral motility, as compared to both healthy controls and H. pylori negative patients. Pieramico et al.[28] showed a lower antral contractile activity in dyspeptic patients and failed to detect significant differences between H. pylori positive and negative patients, but reported a return to normal of interdigestive motility after eradication.

The majority of published studies failed to detect any difference between the two groups. However, some studies showed a higher prevalence of motility disturbances in uninfected patients[29-31]. Indeed, these two putative mechanisms of dyspepsia do not seem to interact since H. pylori eradication does not influence gastric emptying dysmotility[32-33]. If these observations will be confirmed, one would argue that H. pylori infection and gut dysmotility characterize two subgroups of patients with functional dyspepsia[30]. The different relationship of H. pylori with manometric and scintigraphic measurements of gastric motility is difficult to interpret.

*Hypersensitivity/H. pylori/luminal contents/dysmotlity*

The gut wall contains three kinds of neural receptors: chemoreceptors, in the mucosa, which respond to chemical stimuli, mechanoreceptors, in the smooth muscle layer, which respond to stretch or compression; nociceptors, the most numerous receptors, which are commonly silent, but can be "recruited" by any stimulus strong enough to induce pain. H. pylori infection can not be implicated as a consistent feature of the hypersensitivity to gastric[34] distension which characterize functional dyspepsia.

## Conclusions

The role of H. pylori infection in the pathogenesis of functional dyspepsia is far from being established. If the infectious gastritis is involved in determining the syndrome, it is certainly limited to a subset of patients. Indeed, current evidence does not support the existence of different subgroups in patients with functional dyspepsia, nor categorically disproves it.

Although not proven, the existence of dyspepsia subgroups is "de facto" already influencing doctors' attitudes. "A priori" definitions based on presence/absence of symptoms, or of clusters of symptoms are useless and future studies should not adopt this approach. Instruments to measure individual symptoms, their respective severity and possibly also their influence on the quality of life must be developed and validated in the specific settings where they will be applied. If subgroups exist they may be very different from one another in terms of homogeneity, prevalence, natural history. H. pylori infection is very unlikely to identify a homogenous subgroup.

H. pylori positive patients with functional dyspepsia present a wide variety of symptom presentations, and, compared to the H. pylori negative patients, wider ranges of gastric acid secretion, gastrin levels[35], and antral motility index scores[25].

Also patients presenting with pain as their main complaint are unlikely to represent a homogenous group, since any peripheral stimulus intense enough to recruit the otherwise silent nociceptors will end up inducing pain. Conversely, idiopathic nausea is likely to identify a distinct subgroup of patients, although further research is needed to clarify its features. Some recent data suggest that also female gender, body weight, relevant postprandial fullness/vomiting, and overlapping irritable bowel syndrome may identify a distinct subset of patients[36], but again more data are needed.

Finally, patients complaining of dyspeptic symptoms and presenting psychological disturbances are less likely to have other underlying pathophysiological abnormalities.

This is probably an important aspect to be further explored in future studies.

## *References*


1. Colin-Jones DG, Bloom B, Bodemar G, et al. *Management of dyspepsia: report of a working party.* Lancet 1988; l: 576-9.
2. Drossman DA, Thompson WG, Talley NJ, et al. *Identification of subgroups of functional gastrointestinal disorders.* Gastroenterol Int 1990; 3:159-72.
3. Talley NJ, Colin-Jones D, Koch KL, et al. *Functional dyspepsia: a classification with guidelines for diagnosis and management.* Gastroenterol Int 1991;4:145-60.
4. Heading RC. *Definitions of dyspepsia.* Scand J Gastroenterol 1991; 26 (Suppl.182): l-6.
5. Klauser AG, Schindlebeck NE, Muller-Lissner SA. *Symptoms in gastro-oesophageal reflux disease.* Lancet 1990; 335:205-8.
6. Sheu B, Lin C, Lin X, et al. *Long-term outcome of triple therapy in Helicobacter pylori related non-ulcer dyspepsia: a prospective controlled assessment.* Am J Gastroenterol 1996; 91:441-7.
7. Holtmann G, Goebell H, Talley NJ. *Dyspepsia in consulters and non-consulters: prevalence, health care seeking behaviour and risk factors.* Eur J Gastroenterol Hepatol 1994; 6: 917-24.
8. Talley NJ, Zinsmeister AR, Schleck CD, Melton III LJ. *Dyspepsia and dyspepsia subgroups: a population based study.* Gastroenterology 1992;102:1259-68.
9. Talley NJ. *A critique of therapeutic trials in Helicobacter pylori-positive functional dyspepsia.* Gastroenterology 1994;106:1174-83.
10. Agreus L, Svardsudd K, Nyrèn O, Tibblin G. *Irritable bowel syndrome and dyspepsia in the general population: overlap and lack of stability over time.* Gastroenterology 1995; 109:671-80.
11. Talley NJ, Weaver AL, Tesmer DL, Zinsmeister AR. *Lack of discriminant value of dyspepsia subgroups in patients referred for upper endoscopy.* Gastroenterology 1993;105: 1378-86.
12. Mansi C, Savarino V, Mela GS, et al. *Are clinical patterns of dyspepsia a valid guideline for appropriate use of endoscopy? A report on 2253 dyspeptic patients.* Am J Gastroenterol 1993;88:1011-5.
13. Klauser AG, Voderholzer WA, Knesewitsch PA, et al. *What is behind dyspepsia?* Dig Dis Sci 1993;38:147-54.
14. Takayasu H, Harasawa S, Miwa T, Yamada Y. *Investigation of gastric function and prevalence of Helicobacter pylori in non-ulcer dyspepsia.* Nippon Shokakibyo Gakkai Zasshi (Jap J Gastroenterol) 1993;90:743.

15. Trespi E, Broglia F, Villani L, et al. *Distinct profiles of gastritis in dyspepsia subgroups. Their different clinical responses to gastrin healing after Helicobacter pylori eradication.* Scand J Gastroenterol 1994;29:884-8.
16. Kemmer TP, Dorninguez-Munoz JL, Klingel H, et al. *The association between non-ulcer dyspepsia and Helicobacter pylori infection.* Europ J Gastroenterol Hepatol 1994;6:571-7.
17. Talley NJ. *A relationship between Helicobacter pylori and non-ulcer dyspepsia: is there enough data to know?* Eur J Gastroenterol Hepatol 1994;6:567-70.
18. Parsonnett J, Blaser MJ, Perez-Perez GI, et al. *Symptoms and risk factors of Helicobacter pylori infection in a cohort of epidemiologists.* Gastroenterology 1992;102:41-6.
19. Elta GH, Scheiman JM, Barnett JL, et al. *Long-term follow up of Helicobacter pylori treatment in non ulcer dyspepsia patients.* Am J Gastroenterol 1995;90:1089-93.
20. McCarthy C, Patchett S, Collins RM, et al. *Long-term prospective study of Helicobacter pylori in nonulcer dyspepsia.* Dig Dis Sci 1995;40:114-9.
21. Veldhuyzen van Zanten SJ, Malatjalian D, Tanton R, et al. *The effect of eradication of Helicobacter pylori on symptoms of non-ulcer dyspepsia: a randomized double-blind placebo controlled trial.* EHPSG 1995.
22. Greenberg PD, Cello JP. *Prospective, double-blind treatment of Helicobacter pylori in patients with non-ulcer dyspepsia.* Gastroenterology 1996;110:A-123.
23. Buda A, Bortolon M, Saladin S, et al. *Usefulness of symptomatological pattern in predicting the outcome of dyspeptic patients after HP eradication: a prospective six months study.* Gut 1996;39 (Suppl 3) A147.
24. Czinn SJ, Bertram TA, Murray PD, Yang P. *Relationship between gastric inflammation response and symptoms in patients infected with Helicobacter pylori.* Scand J Gastroenterol 1991;26 (Suppl 181)33-7.
25. Mearin F, Cucala M, Azpiroz F, Malagelada JR. *The origin of symptoms on the brain-gut axis in functional dyspepsia.* Gastroenterology 1991;101:999-1006.
26. Kaneko H, Mitsuma T, Uchida K, et al. *Immunoreactive-somatostatin, substance P, and calcitonin gene-related peptide concentrations of the human gastric mucosa in patients with nonulcer dyspepsia and peptic ulcer disease.* Am J Gastroenterol 1993;88:898-904.
27. Testoni PA, Bagnolo F, Masci E, et al. *Different interdigestive antroduodenal motility patterns in chronic antral gastritis with and without Helicobacter pylori infection.* Dig Dis Sci 1993;38:2255-61.
28. Pieramico O, Distchuneit H, Malfertheiner P. *Gastrointestinal motility in patients with non-ulcer dyspepsia: a role for Helicobacter pylori infection?* Am J Gastroenterol 1993;88: 364-8.
29. Barnett JL, Behler EM, Appelman UD, Elta GH. *Campylobacter pylori is not associated with gastroparesis.* Dig Dis Sci 1989; 34: 1677-80.

30. Tucci A, Corinaldesi R, Stanghellini V, et al. *Helicobacter pylori infection and gastric function in patients with chronic idiopathic dyspepsia.* Gastroenterology 1992;103:768-74.
31. Scott AM, Kellow JE, Shuter B, et al. *Intragastric distribution and gastric emptying of solids and liquids in functional dyspepsia. Lack of influence of symptom subgroups and H. pylori-associated gastritis.* Dig Dis Sci 1993;38:2247-54.
32. Peitz U, Blaudszun S, Aygen S, et al. *No significant change of delayed gastric emptying in functionally dyspeptic (FD) patients after cure of Helicobacter pylori (HP).* Gastroenterology 1996;110:A732.
33. Parente F, Maconi G, Imbesi V, et al. *H. pylori (HP) eradication does not modify gastric emptying of solids but reduces gastrin and pepsinogen I release in patients with non-ulcer dyspepsia.* Gastroenterology 1997;112:A251.
34. Mearin F, de Ribot X, Balboa A, et al. *Does Helicobacter pylori infection increase gastric sensitivity in functional dyspepsia?* Gut 1995;37:47-51.
35. El-Omar E, Penman I, Ardill JE, McColl KEL. *A substantial proportion of non-ulcer dyspepsia patients have the same abnormality of acid secretion as duodenal ulcer patients.* Gut 1995;36:534-8.
36. Tosetti C, Stanghellini V, Paternicò A, et al. *An appropriate symptom questionnaire allows to identify separate subgroups among patients with functional dyspepsia.* Gastroenterology 1996;110:A771.

*Address for correspondence*

**CORINALDESI R, MD**
Dipartimento Medicina Interna e
Gastroenterologia
Università di Bologna
Policlinico S. Orsola - Malpighi
Via Massarenti 9
40138 Bologna Italia
Fax: +39 051 345864

# FUNCTIONAL DYSPEPSIA
## CLINICAL MANAGEMENT

*M Lazzaroni, G Bianchi Porro*

### Definition

Nomenclature in this area has been subject to considerable debate and confusion. The actual definition of functional dyspepsia is based on the Rome criteria[1], that is:

1. chronic or recurrent abdominal pain or discomfort in the upper abdomen for a duration of more than 1 month, with symptoms present >25% of the time
2. no clinical, biochemical, endoscopic or ultrasonographic evidence of any known organic disease likely to explain the symptoms.

For clinical purposes, functional dyspepsia has been classified on clinical grounds, and while this may be of use in individual patients, the categories are difficult to define and separate clearly for research purposes, and moreover, there is a significant overlap between the groups.

Three clinical groups have been proposed: ulcer-like dyspepsia, dysmotility-like dyspepsia and non-specific dyspepsia.

Gastro-Oesophageal Reflux Disease (GORD) can be regarded as a separate condition from functional dyspepsia, but, in pratice, there may be a large overlap, because 24-hr pH monitoring is not usually performed on most patients.

***Ulcer-like dyspepsia*** is characterized by predominant epigastric pain or discomfort which may worsen with hunger and may often be relieved by food or antacids. As with ulcer disease, symptoms may relapse and remit spontaneously over months.

***Dysmotility-like dyspepsia*** has clinical features suggestive of disturbed upper gastrointestinal motility, most notably nausea or vomiting, bloating. belching, early satiety, upper abdominal discomfort often aggravated by food, anorexia.

***Non-specific dyspepsia*** refers to symptoms not suggestive of any subgroup.

## Aetiology

Many aetiological factors have been implicated in the dyspepsia subgroups: altered acid secretion, dysmotility, altered symptoms threshold, psychological factors, diet and social factors, enterogastric reflux, Helicobacter pylori (H. pylori) infection.
The role of acid secretion is unclear. A hypersecretory status has been excluded on the basis of basal and peak acid output measurement[2]; however, the best evidence of an acid role is provided by the 20% average advantage of $H_2$ receptor antagonists as compared to placebo in the control of symptoms in the ulcer-like dyspepsia subgroup[3].
Other factors considered to be aetiologically important in the pathogenesis of functional dyspepsia are:

1. abnormal gastric emptying
2. altered symptoms threshold (possibly associated with psychosocial or mechanosensory factors or both)
3. H. pylori, the role of which, as a primary factor or cofactor is however, unclear.

*Gastric motor abnormalities*
Both experimental and clinical studies have suggested a possible role of gastric motor abnormalities in patients suffering from dysmotility-like dyspepsia. Antral hypomotility, impaired gastric emptying of solids or abnormal gastric distribution of a solid meal were observed in some 40 to 50% of these patients[4,5].
Furthermore, the treatment designed to correct the impaired motor function has also proved of some use in symptom improvement in these patients[6,7]
The underlying mechanism for the impaired motor function is unknown. Efferent vagal dysfunction and impaired gastric emptying were recently confirmed, together with increased responsiveness of central serotoninergic 1A receptors[8,9]. These abnormalities, however, were not universal, and further studies are needed to relate these to other malfunctions in dyspeptic patients.

*Altered gastric sensation and compliance*
Data on fasting gastric compliance as measured by gastric barostat are

conflicting. Some authors claim that proximal stomach accommodation may be abnormal in dyspeptic patients[10]; others, on the contrary, showed that, when compared to normal healthy subjects, patients with dysmotility-like dyspepsia have similar fasting gastric compliance but lower thresholds for pain induction and bloating by balloon distention[11,12].

*H. pylori*

The role of H. pylori in chronic functional dyspepsia is still controversial. A number of elements can be cited to account for this discrepancy:

1. the aetiology of non-ulcer dyspepsia is multifactorial and mainly unknown
2. dyspepsia is a symptom complex and, if H. pylori causes symptoms, it may produce different symptoms in different people
3. current definitions of dyspepsia include a variety of symptoms that probably reflect a number of underlying pathophysiological processes
4. both dyspeptic symptoms and H. pylori infection are very common conditions, in particular H. pylori gastritis is common in asymptomatic subjects, thus making it hard to interpret the results of prevalence studies on H. pylori in non-ulcer dyspepsia.

However, the possible aetiologic role of H. pylori in functional dyspepsia has been sought in epidemiological, pathophysiological and eradication studies.

The validity of the epidemiological relationship between H. pylori infection and non-ulcer dyspepsia is challenged by the high prevalence of dyspeptic symptoms and H. pylori infection in the community. Since it is now clear that the prevalence of H. pylori is related to age, socio-economic status and geographic origin[13], most of the studies are open to criticism due to the absence of an appropriate control group as well as the type of population studied (blood donors) and the different definitions used. Another short-coming of these studies in non-patients is the uncertainty as to whether the reported dyspepsia is functional or organic.

However, although some Authors found no difference in the prevalence of H. pylori infection in dyspeptic patients and controls[14,15], a recent meta-analysis of the available data by Armstrong[16] shows that the prevalence of H. pylori is greater in patients with dyspepsia than in controls with a rate difference of 23% (95% CI (confidence interval) 13-32%) and an odds ratio of 2.3% (95% CI 1.9-2.7%)[15].

The analysis of symptoms and symptom patterns in patients with H. pylori infection has also yielded conflicting results. Some Authors have found an association between H. pylori infection and ulcer-like symptoms, others between H. pylori infection and reflux-like symptoms or dysmotility-like symptoms, but most of them failed to detect any typical clinical picture in H. pylori positive dyspeptic patients[17-19].

Whether the CagA status of the infecting organism is associated with more severe or a distinct pattern of dyspeptic symptoms with specific pathophysiologic alterations is also a matter of debate.

Recent observations have suggested that CagA positive and negative H. pylori strains are simultaneously present in the stomach of most patients with functional dyspepsia[20]; furthermore the CagA positive status is not accompanied by disturbances of acid secretion or gastric emptying or by differences in the type and severity of symptoms[21].

The pathophysiological mechanism linking H. pylori infection and non-ulcer dyspepsia is poorly understood. However, findings suggest that chronic gastroduodenal inflammation due to H. pylori, abnormal gastroduodenal motility and psychological disturbances may modify the perception system of the brain, resulting in increased awareness of stimuli from the gut.

### *Psychosocial factors*

There is no unique personality profile identifiable in patients with functional dyspepsia; these patients have more anxiety, neuroticism and depression than healthy subjects[22]. How might these psychological issues impact on the biological expressions of the syndrome? Psychological factors may account for a substantial amount of the variance in vagal activity (reduced), antral motility (depressed) and somatostatin levels (lowered) in mucosal biopsies from the antrum of the human stomach[8].

## Treatment

### *Diet*

Patients frequently attribute their symptoms to dietary indiscretion, or

specific foods, but evidence for such a relationship is poor. Equally, doctors often suggest that smoking or alcohol may be the cause of their patient's symptoms, but no such relationship has been shown. Studies looking at the prevalence of drinking tea, coffee, alcohol, and smoking in dyspeptic patients have failed to identify a relationship, and alcohol and tobacco usage do not correlate with histological gastritis.
No specific dietary advice can, therefore, be recommended for dyspepsia, although patients should stop smoking and reduce alcohol intake, if indicated, on general health grounds.

### *Symptomatic treatment*

#### *Ulcer-like dyspepsia*

***Antacids*** Most dyspeptic patients will self-medicate with antacids before consulting a doctor, but there is no evidence to suggest that antacid therapy is better than placebo[23]. However, there is a place for short-term empirical antacid therapy in low-risk patients in primary care, and it has been suggested that such a treatment strategy reduces endoscopy requests without any significant associated risk[24].
***Antisecretory drugs*** While it is not clear how the reduction in acid secretion improves symptoms in ulcer-like dyspepsia, $H_2$-receptor antagonists (cimetidine 800-1200 mg, ranitidine 300 mg, famotidine 40 mg, nizatidine 300 mg, roxatidine 150 mg daily), have been shown to produce a significant improvement in such patients, with a therapeutic gain of 20% when compared with antacids or placebo[23,25].
Despite the fact that proton pump inhibitors (PPIs) are widely prescribed for dyspepsia, their efficacy in functional dyspepsia not associated to gastro-oesophageal reflux has not been proven.
It has been proposed that a symptomatic response to PPIs could be a useful diagnostic test for GORD[26], but is unknown whether such a test could distinguish between ulcer-like dyspepsia and GORD with adequate sensitivity.
A major role of PPIs in functional dyspepsia is actually limited to H. pylori eradication therapy.
***Cytoprotective drugs*** The role of sucralfate (1 g before each meal and at bedtime or 2 g twice daily, for 4 weeks) is not well defined. Few studies have been published so far. Sucralfate was significantly more effective than placebo or ranitidine in inducing improvement of endoscopic and

histological gastritis, but was similar to placebo and significantly less effective than ranitidine at relieving epigastric pain[27].

### *Dysmotility-like dyspepsia*

***Prokinetic drugs*** Prokinetic drugs available up to now in clinical practice include antidopaminergic compounds (metoclopramide and domperidone) and cisapride.

Metoclopramide has been extensively evaluated in various conditions including gastroparesis secondary to diabetic dysautonomia or vagotomy; unfortunately, few studies deal specifically with functional dyspepsia. It is important to underline the fact that with effective doses (30 - 40 mg daily) adverse events are frequent (up to 10% in young adults and women)[28].

Domperidone has nearly the same pharmacodynamic action as metoclopramide on oesophageal and gastric motility. However, the drug does not cross the blood-brain barrier and seldom causes untoward extrapyramidal effects. A meta-analysis of several controlled studies[3] concluded that this well-tolerated agent (at doses of 40-60 mg daily) was effective in functional dyspepsia with an overall therapeutic gain as compared to placebo of 56%.

Cisapride releases acetylcholine and acts both as an agonist (5-$HT_4$) and an antagonist (5-$HT_3$) of serotonin. Cisapride strengthens the basal tone of the lower oesophageal sphincter (LES) and the amplitude of the oesophageal body contractions, and accelerates gastric emptying without affecting gastric acid secretions.

This agent (at a dose of 10 mg tid or qid) has been found to be better than placebo in patients with both dysmotility and ulcer-like dyspepsia[28], and one large study has suggested that it is more effective than ranitidine in symptom control, although this has not been reproduced[25].

### *H. pylori eradication*

Several controlled studies have investigated the effect of H. pylori eradication on dyspeptic symptoms. However, these results are also contradictory. This can be blamed on short follow-up time, the multiplicity of symptom scores used and other methodological problems (such as selection of patients with or without irritable bowel syndrome, lack of double-blind condition, absence of placebo-controlled conditions). Of the recent long-term (6-12 months) (Table 1) follow-up studies few failed to show any improvement in dyspeptic symptoms after H. pylori eradication[29-34].

SYMPTOMATIC RESPONSE IN DYSPEPTIC PATIENTS AFTER H. PYLORI ERADICATION

| Study, year ref | % Erad. | 8 weeks | 24 weeks | 48 weeks |
|---|---|---|---|---|
| Oddsson et al. 1992[35] | 37 | ↑ | ↑ | |
| Trespi et al. 1994[40] | 97 | ↑ | ↑ | |
| Veldhuyzen van Zanten et al. 1995[34] | 96 | = | = | |
| Lazzaroni et al. 1996[36] | 64 | = | ↑ | |
| Sabbatini et al. 1994[33] | ND | = | | = |
| Elta et al. 1995[29] | 64 | = | | = |
| McCarthy et al. 1996[37] | 49 | = | | ↑ |
| Greenberg et al. 1996[32] | 40-77 | = | = | = |
| Scheu et al. 1996[38] | 75 | ↑ | ↑ | ↑ |
| McColl et al. 1998[39] | 87 | | | ↑ |
| Talley et al. 1998[31] | 85 | | | = |

↑ improved = unchanged **ND** not determined

Table 1

Other Authors, including ourselves, suggest the cure of H. pylori infection improves the course of dyspepsia irrespective of the symptom pattern[35-39] and others found that the improvement was evident only in patients with ulcer-like symptoms[40,41] (Table 2).

DYSPEPSIA SUBGROUPS. IMPROVEMENT OF SYMPTOMS AFTER ERADICATION OF H. PYLORI. POOLED DATA FROM LONG-TERM CLINICAL FOLLOW-UP

| Study, year ref | Follow-up (wks) | DLD | ULD |
|---|---|---|---|
| Trespi et al. 1994[40] | 24 | = | >> |
| Veldhuyzen van Zanten et al. 1995[34] | 24 | = | = |
| Lazzaroni et al. 1996[36] | 24 | >> | >> |
| Sabbatini et al. 1994[33] | 48 | = | = |
| Elta et al. 1995[20] | 48 | = | = |
| McCarthy et al. 1995[37] | 48 | > | >> |
| Greenberg et al. 1996[32] | 48 | = | = |
| Scheu et al. 1996[38] | 48 | ND | >> |

**DLD** dysmotility-like dyspepsia **ULD** ulcer-like dyspepsia
= no difference **>** improved, but not significantly **>>** significantly improved
**ND** not determined

Table 2

In view of these positive results, even if H. pylori eradication is not recommended, it is difficult to deny this treatment to a patient with severe functional dyspepsia and H. pylori infection.

## Clinical management

Dyspepsia is a common problem, and it seems neither necessary nor practical to subject every dyspeptic patient to investigation. However, the major fear associated with any strategy that delays or avoids upper gastrointestinal endoscopy is that organic illness, gastric cancer, in particular, may be missed. Therefore, the practical management of dyspeptic patients is not easy.

Some important problems are a matter of debate concerning the patient to treat (all patients or selected patients?), the therapeutic strategy (scope and treat or treat and scope only if necessary?) and the diagnosis and treatment of H. pylori infection (test and treat strategy or test and scope strategy?).

Attempts to diagnose dyspepsia by history and examination alone are generally unsatisfactory. Only patients with some demographic characteristics (aged over forty-five years, heavy smokers or drinkers, regular non-steroidal anti-inflammatory drug users, and with a strong family history of peptic ulcer or gastric cancer) or with sinister symptoms (anaemia, weight loss, dysphagia, persistent severe vomiting or upper gastrointestinal blood loss which can indicate an organic disease), should be given priority and scoped, whenever possible.

However, the majority of dyspeptic patients do not complain of alarm symptoms and dividing patients into "ulcer-like" or "dysmotility-like" subgroups does not correspond reliably with endoscopic findings and is, therefore, of little use.

The British Society of Gastroenterology, has recently avoided identifying dyspepsia subgroups in its new guidelines on the management of dyspepsia[42].

Provided that alarm symptoms have been excluded, it has been suggested[43] that all patients with H. pylori unrelated functional dyspepsia, should first be treated empirically with antacids, $H_2$-blockers, and only the non-responding or relapsing patients should be referred for endoscopy. It was felt that this strategy would reduce costs with minimal impact on missed diagnoses. However, two well designed studies[44,45] have shown that prompt endoscopy with treatment based on the results was preferable to blind empirical treatment, although it was initially more expensive. They also found a noticeable decrease in drug consumption, visits to doctors and sick leave in the year after the endoscopy compared with the year before. Patients were more satisfied with their management, although the symptomatic outcome was similar with both strategies.

As far as H. pylori is concerned, it has been suggested that the test and treat strategy (without endoscopic control) in dyspeptic patients without alarm signs:

1. will probably improve symptoms in some patients
2. may prevent development of ulcer disease and its complications
3. may reduce spending on antisecretory drugs and the requirement of endoscopy controls, therefore saving money and, lastly
4. may remove a risk factor of gastric cancer.

However some considerations may hamper the practical use of such a strategy:

1. up to now the diagnosis of infection with $^{13}$C-urea breath test has not been easily available and office based blood tests may record false positive results in a percentage of patients varying from 31 to 53%[46]
2. serious diseases such a adenocarcinoma and lymphoma or oesophagitis without typical symptoms may be misdiagnosed
3. the clinical benefit in the short- and long-term follow-up after H.pylori eradication in dyspeptic patients is unclear
4. widespread use of eradication therapy may give rise to resistant strains of bacterium.

In effect, results from decision analysis and from a controlled clinical study have shown that "surprisingly, the choice of optimal management strategy was a "toss-up". Only a modest saving may result from practice guidelines that recommend empirical therapy in the management of patients with dyspepsia"[47].

## Conclusions

Several questions related to the pathophysiology and clinical management of functional dyspepsia remain unanswered. Some patients have unequivocal evidence of impaired gastric emptying, but that is not always the cause of their symptoms. Although decreased perception thresholds to unphysiologic distension with a balloon have been observed in fasting patients, it is unclear whether this holds true in the postcibal state. Finally, whether H. pylori and how psychosocial factors are associated with pathophysiologic changes in motorial or sensory function require further elucidation. Meanwhile, pressure of restricted reimbursement will require development and comparison of practical management guidelines. The algorithms proposed by the Maastricht Consensus Conference[48] (Figure 1) and other authors[46] may offer a valid aid for the management of dypeptic patients in general practice, but need to be formally tested in well designed community trials that compare different management strategies, the respective outcome and cost utility.

Figure 1

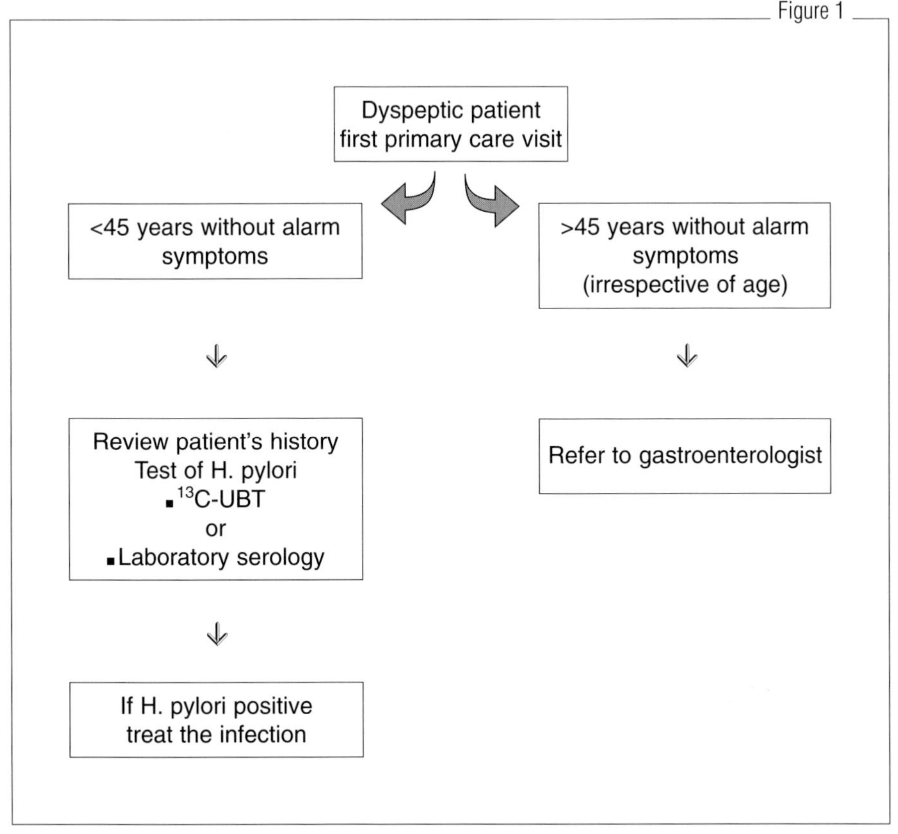


Suggested practical guidelines for the treatment of patients with functional dyspepsia.
Reproduced from Bytzer P, Hansen JM, Schaffalitzky de Muckadell OB[44].

## *REFERENCES*

1. Talley NJ, Colin-Jones D, Koch KL, et al. *Functional dyspepsia: a classification with guidelines for diagnosis and management.* Gastroenterol Int 1991;4:145-60.
2. Collen MJ, Loenbenberg MJ. *Basal gastric acid secretion in non ulcer dyspepsia with or without duodenitis.* Dig Dis Sci 1989;34:246-50.
3. Dobrilla G, Comberlato M, Steele A, Vallaperta P. *Drug treatment of functional dyspepsia. A meta-analysis of randomized clinical trials.* J Clin Gastroenterol 1989;11:169-77.
4. Camilleri M, Malagelada JR, Kao PC, Zinsmeister AR. *Gastric and autonomic responses to stress in functional dyspepsia.* Dig Dis Sci 1991;36:1249-54.
5. Greydanus MP, Vassallo M, Camilleri M, et al. *Neurohormonal factors in functional dyspepsia: insights on pathophysiological mechanisms.* Gastroenterology 1991;100:1311-8.
6. Halter F, Miazza B, Brignoli R. *Cisapride or cimetidine in the treatment of functional dyspepsia.* Scand J Gastroenterol 1994;29:618-23.
7. Corinaldesi R, Stanghellini V, Raiti C, et al. *Effect of chronic administration of cisapride on gastric emptying of a solid meal and on dyspeptic symptoms in patients with idiopathic gastroparesis.* Gut 1987;28:300-5.
8. Haug TT, Svebak S, Hausken T, et al. *Low vagal activity as mediating mechanism for the relationship between personality factors and gastric symptoms in functional dyspepsia.* Psychosom Med 1994;56:181-6.
9. Chua A, Keating J, Hamilton D, et al. *Central serotonin receptors and delayed gastric emptying in non-ulcer dyspepsia.* Br Med J 1992;305:280-2.
10. Troncon LEA, Bennet RJM, Ahluwalia NK, Thompson DG. *Abnormal intragastric distribution of food during gastric emptying in functional dyspepsia patients.* Gut 1994;35:327-32.
11. Mertz H, Fullerton S, Naliboff B, Mayer EA. *Symptoms and visceral perception in severe functional and organic dyspepsia.* Gut 1998;42:814-22.
12. Coffin B, Azpiroz F, Guarner F, Malagelada JR. *Selective gastric hypersensitivity and reflex hyporeactivity in functional dyspepsia.* Gastroenterology 1994;107:1345-51.
13. Marshall BJ. *Helicobacter pylori.* Am J Gastroenterol 1994;89(Suppl):s116-s128.
14. Collins JSA, Hamilton PW, Watt PCH, et al. *Superficial gastritis and Campylobacter pylori in dyspeptic patients - a quantitative study using computer-linking image analysis.* J Pathol 1989;158:303-10.
15. Wilhalmsen I, Tangen Huang T, Sipponen P, Berstad A. *Helicobacter pylori in*

*functional dyspepsia and normal controls.* Scand J Gastroenterol 1994;29:522-7.

16. Armstrong D. *Helicobacter pylori infection and dyspepsia.* Scand J Gastroenterol 1996;31(Suppl 215):38-47.
17. Tucci A, Corinaldesi R, Stanghellini V, et al. *Helicobacter pylori infection and gastric function in patients with chronic idiopathic dyspepsia.* Gastroenterology 1992;103;768-74.
18. Bianchi Porro G, Parente F. *Nature of non-ulcer dyspepsia and related conditions.* Clin Gastroenterol 1995;9:549-62.
19. Rokkas T, Pursy C, Uzoechina E, et al. *Campylobacter pylori and non-ulcer dyspepsia.* Am J Gastroenterol 1987;11:49-52.
20. Figura N, Vindigni C, Covacci A, et al. *CagA positive and negative Helicobacter pylori strains are simultaneously present in the stomach of most patients with non-ulcer dyspepsia: relevance to histological damage.* Gut 1998;42:772-8.
21. Parente F, Imbesi V, Maconi G, et al. *Influence of bacterial Cag-A status on gastritis, gastric function indices, and pattern of symptoms in H. pylori-positive dyspeptic patients.* Am J Gastroenterol 1998;83:1-6.
22. Richter JE. *Stress and psychologic and environmental factors in functional dyspepsia.* Scand J Gastroenterol 1991;182:40-6.
23. Gotthard R, Bodemar G, Brodin U, Jonsson KA. *Treatment with cimetidine, antacids or placebo in patients with dyspepsia of unknown origin.* Scand J Gastroenterol 1988;23:7-18.
24. Goodson JD, Richter JM, Lane RS, et al. *Empiric antacids and reassurance for acute dyspepsia.* J Gen Int Med 1986;1:90-3.
25. Carvalhinos A, Fidalgo P, Freire A, Matos L. *Cisapride compared with ranitidine in the treatment of functional dyspepsia.* Eur J Gastroenterol Hepatol 1995;7:411-7.
26. Schindlbeck NE, Klauser AG, Voderholzer WA, Muller-Lissner SA. *Empiric therapy for gastro-oesophageal reflux disease.* Arch Int Med 1995;155:1808-12.
27. Guslandi M. *Comparison of sucralfate and ranitidine in the treatment of chronic non erosive gastritis. A randomized multicentre trial.* Am J Med 1989;86:45-8.
28. Galmiche JP, Vallot T. *Therapeutic strategy.* In: Galmiche JP, Jian R, Mignon M, Ruszniewski P, editors. Non-ulcer dyspepsia. London: John Libbey. 1991;247-64.
29. Elta G, Scheiman J, Barnett J, et al. *Long term follow-up of Helicobacter pylori treatment in non ulcer dyspepsia patients.* Am J Gastroenterol 1995;90:1089-93.
30. Marshall BJ, Valenzuela JE, McCallum RW, et al. *Bismuth subsalicylate suppression of Helicobacter pylori in nonulcer dyspepsia: a double-blind placebo-controlled trial.* Dig Dis Sci 1993;38:1674-80.
31. Talley NJ, Janssen J, Lauritsen K, et al. *Long term follow-up of patients with non-ulcer*

*dyspepsia after Helicobacter pylori eradication. A randomised double-blind placebo controlled trial.* DDW, May 17-20, 1998, A-503.

32. Greenberg PD, Cello JP. *Prospective double blind treatment of Helicobacter pylori in patients with non-ulcer dyspepsia.* Gastroenterology 1996;110:A123.
33. Sabbatini F, Castiglione F, Piai G, et al. *The long term outcome of dyspeptic patients after Helicobacter pylori eradication.* Gastroenterology 1994;104:A182.
34. Veldhuyzen van Zanten S, Malatjalian D, Tanton R, et al. *The effect of eradication of Helicobacter pylori on symptoms of non ulcer dyspepsia: a randomised double blind placebo controlled study.* Gastroenterology 1995;108:A250.
35. Oddsson E, Gudjonsson H, Theodors A, et al. *DeNol+Metronidazole in the treatment of H. pylori positive patients with non ulcer dyspepsia: symptomatic response and eradication rate.* Scand J Gastroenterol 1992;27(Suppl 190):42A.
36. Lazzaroni M, Bargiggia S, Sangaletti O, et al. *Eradication of Helicobacter pylori and long-term outcome of functional dyspepsia. A clinical endoscopic study.* Dig Dis Sci 1996;41:1589-94.
37. McCarthy C, Patchett S, Collins RM, et al. *Long term prospective study of Helicobacter pylori in non ulcer dyspepsia.* Dig Dis Sci 1995;40:114-9.
38. Sheu B, Lin C, Lin X, et al. *Long term outcome of triple therapy in Helicobacter pylori-related non ulcer dyspepsia: a prospective controlled assessment.* Am J Gastroenterol 1996;91:441-7.
39. McColl KEL, Murray LS, El-Omar E, et al. *U.K. MRC trial of H. pylori eradication therapy for non-ulcer dyspepsia.* Gut 1998,42(Suppl 1):T10.
40. Trespi E, Broglia F, Villani O, et al. *Distinct profiles of gastritis in dyspepsia subgroups. Their clinical response to gastritis healing after Helicobacter pylori eradication.* Scand J Gastroenterol 1994;29:884-8.
41. Hovelius B, Andersson SI, Hagander B, et al. *Dyspepsia in general practice: history and symptoms in relation to Helicobacter pylori serum antibodies.* Scand J Gastroenterol 1994;29:506-10.
42. British Society of Gastroenterology. *Dyspepsia management guidelines.* London, BSG;1996.
43. Health and Public Policy Committee, American College of Physicians: *Endoscopy in the evaluation of dyspepsia.* Ann Intern Med 1985;102:266-9.
44. Bytzer P, Hansen JM, Schaffalitzky de Muckadell OB. *Empirical H2-blocker therapy or prompt endoscopy in management of dyspepsia.* Lancet 1994;343:811-6.
45. Hungin AP, Thomas PR, Bramble MG, et al. *What happens to patients following open access gastroscopy? An outcome study from general practice.* Br J Clin Pract 1994;44:519-21.

46. Agreus L, Talley N. *Challenges in managing dyspepsia in general practice.* Br Med J 1997;315:1284-7.
47. Silverstein MD, Petterson T, Talley N. *Initial endoscopy or empirical therapy with or without testing for Helicobacter pylori for dyspepsia: a decision analysis.* Gastroenterlogy 1996;110:72-83
48. Current European Concepts in the management of Helicobacter pylori infection. The Maastricht Consensus Conference. Gut 1997;41:8-13.

*Address for correspondence*

**LAZZARONI M, MD**

Divisione di Gastroenterologia e Endoscopia digestiva
Polo Universitario
Ospedale "L. Sacco"
Via G.B. Grassi 74
20157 Milano Italia
Fax: +39 02 35799232

# CHRONIC INTESTINAL PSEUDO-OBSTRUCTION

*M Camilleri*

## Objectives

- ✓ To review the normal motor functions of the human small intestine and colon.
- ✓ To introduce recent advances in understanding the genetic basis for dysmotility.
- ✓ To review the clinical manifestations and use of transit and manometric evaluations to diagnose chronic intestinal pseudo-obstruction.
- ✓ To understand the rationale for current approaches to management (nutritional support, pharmacotherapy, and judicious use of surgery) in pseudo-obstruction.
- ✓ To review colonic dysmotility in slow transit constipation (chronic colonic pseudo-obstruction).

## Normal small intestinal and colonic motility

Gastrointestinal motor function is controlled by the extrinsic supply from the brain and spinal cord, the complex plexi within the wall of the intestine, called the enteric brain, and the effects of locally released transmitters, such as amines and peptides, that alter the excitability of the smooth muscle of the intestine (Figure 1). The enteric nervous system includes the interstitial cells of Cajal, which will be discussed below. Small intestinal motility cycles as part of the interdigestive motor complex during fasting. Postprandially, the small bowel produces irregular contractions that mix the digesta with enzymes to facilitate digestion and absorption (Figure 2). The terminal ileum produces high amplitude or giant propagated contractions that sweep into the colon[1]. The rate of transit of solids and liquids through the entire small bowel is approximately equal; the ileum itself may transfer solids slower than liquids[2]; ileocolonic transfers occur as bolus movements[3] and the ileum thus serves as a temporary reservoir to allow salvage of nutrients before being transferred to the colon where bacterial metabolism would deprive the human of the benefit of these nutrients.

Figure 1

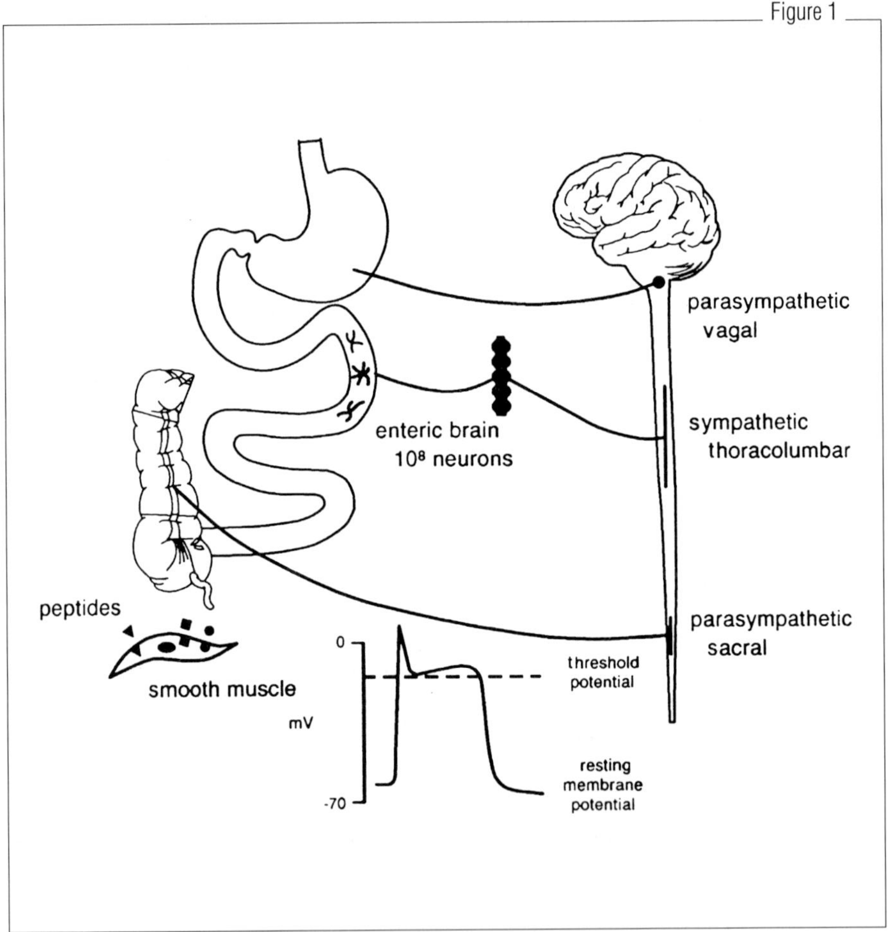


Neuromuscular control of gut motility: extrinsic, enteric and myogenic.
Reproduced with permission from Camilleri M, Phillips SF[71].

The colon has three functional units: a proximal reservoir consisting of the ascending and transverse regions; a conduit (descending colon[4]) and a volitional reservoir (rectum and sigmoid).

In slow transit constipation, emptying of the proximal reservoir is typically prolonged.

In outlet obstruction to defecation, the sigmoid cannot be emptied, and this may secondarily prolong overall colonic transit.

Four types of colonic contractile events are recognized:

1. stationary or segmenting contractions
2. propagated contractions
3. high amplitude propagated contractions (or giant migrating contractions) which occur on average 5 times per day and are sometimes associated with defecation
4. tonic contraction of the colon.

   All forms of contractile activity are increased after ingestion of a meal of >500 kcal[5].

Figure 2

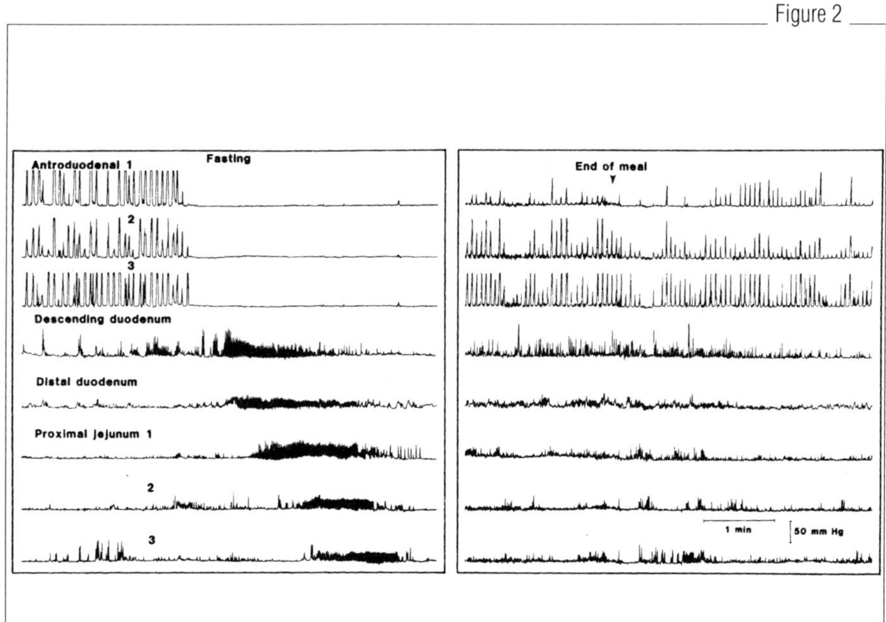


Normal gastric and small intestinal motility during fasting and postprandially. Note the interdigestive complex (left panel) and the sustained but irregular response to the meal (postprandially).

Reproduced with permission from Malagelada J-R, Camilleri M, Stanghellini V[72].

The role of colonic tone in propulsion of content is unclear; it is hypothesized that increased colonic tone may facilitate lumen occlusion by phasic contractions.

## Normal defecation

The process of normal defecation[6] requires:
- the presence of stool within colon and/or rectum
- the ability to raise intra-abdominal pressure, such as by Valsalva maneuver
- contractions of the colon to aborally propel residue
- straightening of the rectoanal angle by relaxation of the puborectalis muscle
- relaxation of the external anal sphincter.

These functions are shown schematically in Figure 3.

Figure 3

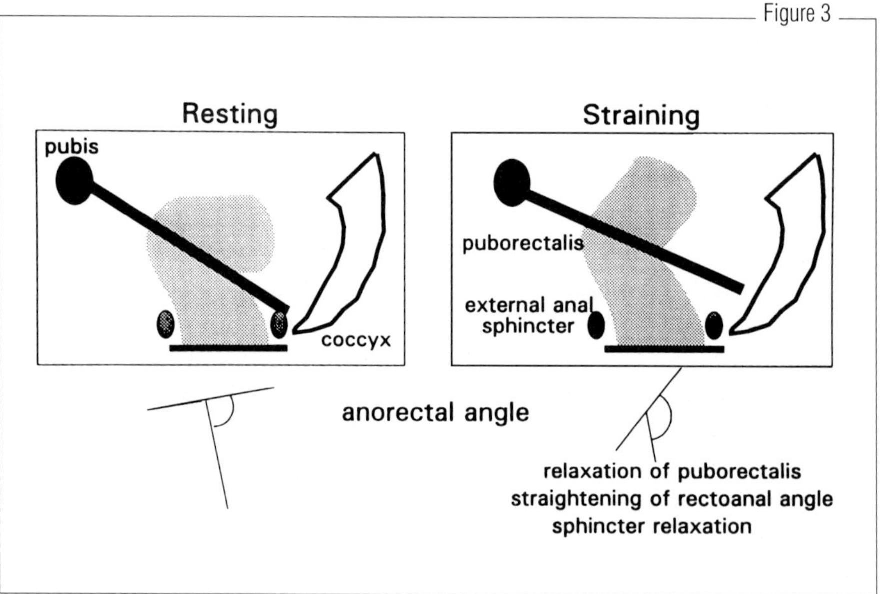


Normal evacuation of the rectum entails relaxation of the puborectalis, straightening of the rectoanal angle and sphincter relaxation.

Reproduced with permission from Camilleri M, Thompson WG, Fleshman JW, Pemberton JH[73].

## Genetic basis for dysmotility? Interstitial cells of Cajal: the new genetics and chronic dysmotility

In recent years, there has been an increasing body of literature supporting a role for the interstitial cells of Cajal as pacemakers of the gut[7]. In diseases associated with dysmotility, such as infantile pyloric stenosis, Hirschsprung's disease, and chronic intestinal pseudo-obstruction, marked decreases in the number of interstitial cells were documented. Genetic mutations in three main loci have been studied.

The proto-oncogene, C-kit, encodes for a receptor, tyrosine kinase, which has extracellular, transmembrane and cytoplasmic domains. The extracellular domain is a receptor for steel factor.

Mutants for the latter component of the C-kit protein (that is steel factor) resulted in mice with abnormal development of interstitial cells of Cajal and absence of small intestinal rhythmicity (spontaneous slow waves[8]). Mutation of dominant-white spotting (w) locus in mice also results in inhibition of the tyrosine kinase activity and disturbances of gastric and small bowel motility[9,10]. Abnormalities in the C-kit receptor in myenteric plexus neurons have been reported in Hirschsprung's disease[11-13].

A major gene causing Hirschsprung's disease was recently mapped in chromosome 10q11.2. Its physical location is restricted to a 250-Kb region containing the RET (rearranged during transfection) proto-oncogene. Point mutations in the RET proto-oncogene were identified in patients with Hirschsprung's disease[14], including mutations in the tyrosine kinase domain[15]. In mice, RET deficiency is associated with Hirschsprung's disease and renal agenesis[16]; in humans, mutations in RET result in Hirschsprung's disease and multiple endocrine neoplasia type IIA[17]. Examples of the RET gene loci mutated in Hirschsprung's disease or mouse models and related genetic disorders are shown in Figure 4.

Recent studies on embryological development of the enteric nervous system suggest that neural crest cells' migration to the bowel is markedly impaired by C-RET deficiency[18]. Mutations in endothelin-B receptor gene and endothelin-3 gene have also been recognized as susceptible genes for Hirschsprung's disease[19].

Figure 4

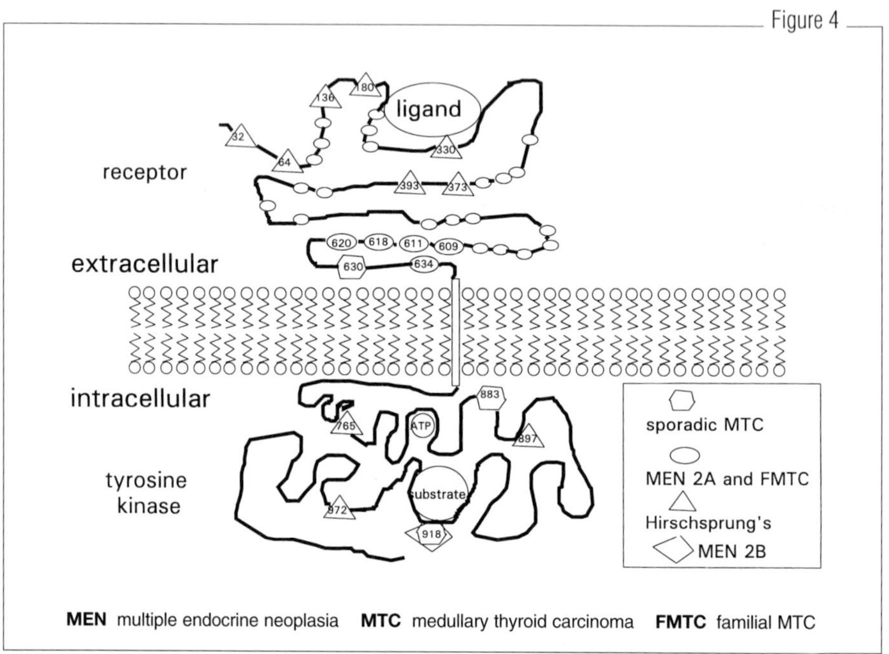


RET proto-oncogene domains and mutations associated with disease.
Reproduced with permission from: Donis-Keller H[74].

## Chronic intestinal pseudo-obstruction or dysmotility

Chronic intestinal pseudo-obstruction is a syndrome that suggests obstruction in the absence of an anatomic lesion that obstructs flow of intestinal content[20].

In pseudo-obstruction, segments of affected bowel appear dilated on radiography. A similar motor disorder of small bowel or colon unassociated with dilatation is referred to as chronic intestinal dysmotility (Table 1).

Although the causes of chronic intestinal pseudo-obstruction and dysmotility are many, they can be summarized under three broad headings: disturbances of the enteric nervous system, extrinsic nervous system, and smooth muscle[21]. These disorders are rarely familial and more often secondary to an underlying disorder affecting neuromuscular function (Table 2).

GI MOTILITY DISORDERS AND DILATATION: EXAMPLES

| Region | With dilatation | Without dilatation |
|---|---|---|
| Esophagus | Achalasia with mega-esophagus | Achalasia |
| Stomach | Acute gastric dilatation | Gastroparesis |
| Small bowel | Pseudo-obstruction | Chronic intestinal dysmotility |
| Colon | Megacolon/pseudo-obstruction | Slow transit constipation/colonic inertia |

Table 1

VARIATIONS OF PSEUDO-OBSTRUCTION

- Familial or sporadic
- Tempo: Acute, recurrent, chronic
- Idiopathic or secondary
- Region: Small bowel ± others; colon ± others
- Pathophysiologic/etiologic types: Neuropathic (e.g., amyloidosis, diabetes, paraneoplastic); myopathic (e.g., scleroderma); combination (e.g., scleroderma, amyloidosis)

Table 2

## Histopathology of the neuromuscular apparatus in chronic pseudo-obstruction syndromes

By using Masson's trichrome stain to identify fibrosis and silver stains of longitudinal sections of the myenteric plexus, several morphological abnormalities have been described in small bowel and colonic pseudo-obstruction syndromes[12,22-28].

In summary, the main findings have been:

- changes in the proportion of argyrophilic neurons
- plasma cell or lymphocytic infiltrations of the myenteric plexus
- neuronal intranuclear inclusions
- fall out of smooth muscle cells and replacement fibrosis; however, the pathologic findings of progressive systemic sclerosis and idiopathic hollow visceral myopathy show considerable overlap
- loss of interstitial cells of Cajal, the likely pacemakers of the intestine
- Lewy bodies in myenteric neurons of patients with Parkinsonism and achalasia.

Generally, these studies require resection of dilated segments or a full-thickness biopsy of the intestines.
The introduction of laparoscopic surgery has facilitated procurement of tissue, but there are still no critical assessments of the risk-benefit ratio of obtaining small bowel full-thickness biopsies. Specifically, it is unclear whether knowledge obtained from the biopsy significantly alters patient management and whether this outweighs the risk of prolonged postoperative ileus, perforation, adhesions and similar complications of the resection.

## Clinical symptoms of chronic intestinal pseudo-obstruction

The clinical symptoms of chronic intestinal pseudo-obstruction are those that suggest upper gut stasis (e.g., nausea, vomiting, easy satiety, anorexia), weight loss, abdominal distention and alteration in bowel movements[20]. An antecedent viral infection may suggest an associated infectious cause; this has been best documented with Epstein-Barr virus infection. These symptoms occur in the absence of mechanical obstruction of the gastrointestinal tract.
Systems review may identify disturbances of neuromuscular function or collagen vascular disease that may be associated with gastrointestinal manifestations[21,29]. The main physical findings are abdominal distention, a succussion splash, and evidence of the underlying collagen vascular or neuromuscular disease. A careful family history should be obtained in all

patients; the presence of general neuromuscular disorder and a positive family history suggest mitochondrial myopathy, amyloidosis or, rarely, porphyria.

## Investigation of patients with suspected chronic intestinal pseudo-obstruction

*Step 1: Radiology and nutritional status*

While radiology is essential to exclude mechanical obstruction or an alternative diagnosis such as Crohn's disease, X-rays rarely provide an etiologic diagnosis. An exception is systemic sclerosis affecting the small intestine, which is characterized by dilated segments, edema and abnormal texture and motility of the valvulae conniventes. More typically, radiology demonstrates air-fluid levels or distended loops of small bowel and, rarely, dilatation in the urinary tract.

While investigating patients, care is taken to assess the nutritional effects of the motility disorder and exclude mechanical obstruction of the intestine or a neoplastic process such as a small cell cancer of the lung. When clinically indicated, patients should also be screened for endocrinopathies, myositis, mitochondrial myopathies with thyroid hormone, cortisol, muscle enzymes and lactate and pyruvate levels.

*Step 2: Confirm dysmotility*

The next step is to confirm the presence of a motility disorder, usually with a gastric and small bowel transit test[30-34]. Scintigraphy is now the method of choice (Figure 5), and novel approaches have been devised to simplify the evaluation of gastric and small bowel transit (Figure 6), as well as reduce costs incurred in documenting the presence of disturbance of transit. Scintigraphy can also evaluate transit through the colon which may also be affected by the pseudo-obstructive process (see below). In patients with abnormal transit in whom there is a known underlying disease, no further investigation is usually necessary, and treatment is indicated (see below).

*Step 3: Specialized tests: manometry and beyond*

If there is no known underlying disease, a manometric study of the stomach and small intestine can be useful[35]. First, it may exclude mechanical obstruction of the intestine, which is sometimes missed on barium follow-through examination, and which typically shows simultaneous, prolonged contractions at the level of the small intestine[36,37]. Second, manometry provides a reasonably accurate method to differentiate a myopathic process, which is typically associated with low amplitude contractions, from a neuropathic process in which the amplitude of contractions is typically normal, but the organization of the contractile response is abnormal (Figure 7).

A neuropathic process may result from a disorder of the enteric or extrinsic nervous system.

Figure 5

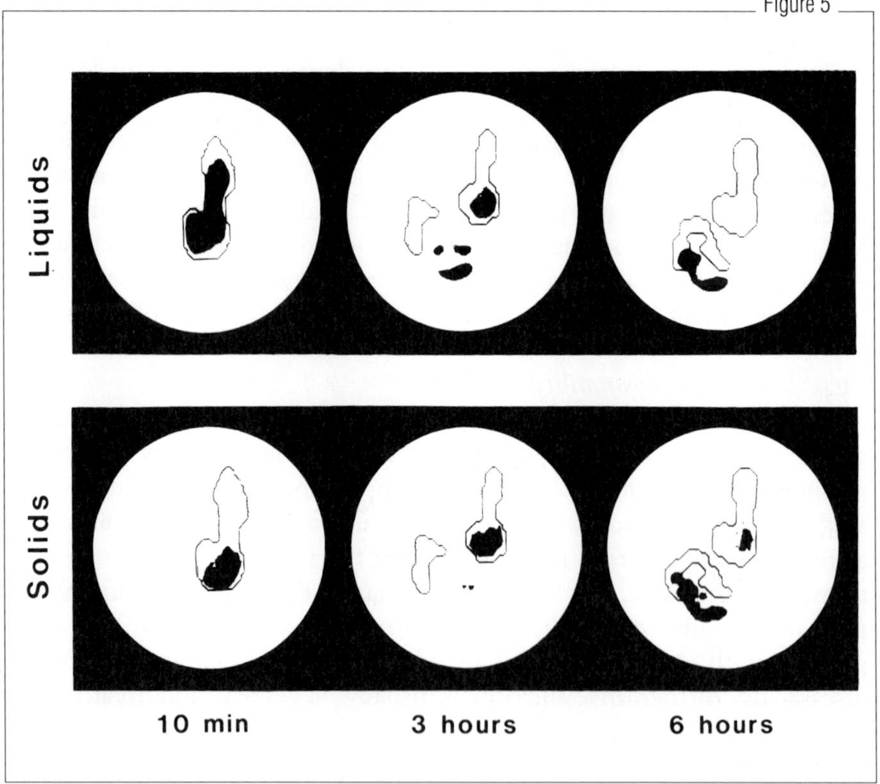


Scintigraphic assessment of chronic intestinal pseudo-obstruction showing the delayed emptying of liquids and solids from the stomach.

Reproduced with permission from Camilleri M, Brown ML, Malagelada J-R[75].

Figure 6

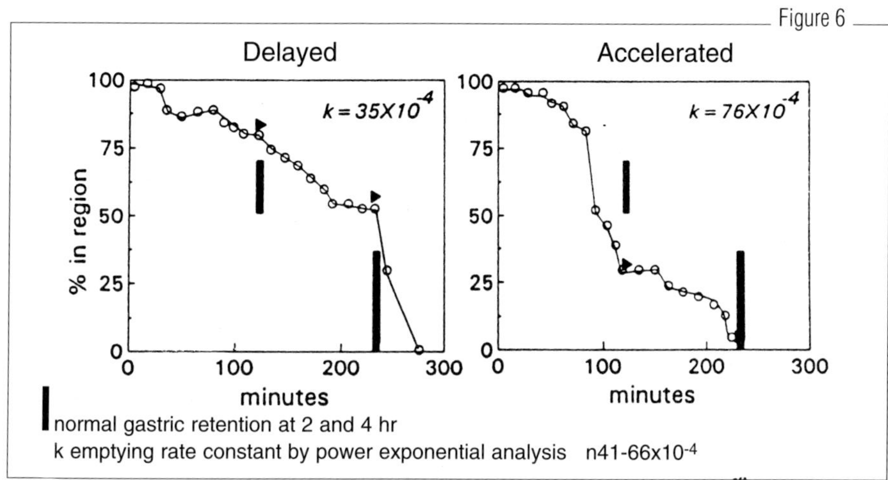


Example of application of simple tests to evaluate delayed and accelerated gastric emptying. Note that, with a well established normal range, it is possible to accurately identify abnormal emptying relative to k, the expression of the instantaneous slope of the gastric emptying curve by power exponential analysis.

Reproduced with permission from Thomforde GM, Camilleri M, Phillips SF, Forstrom LA[76].

Figure 7

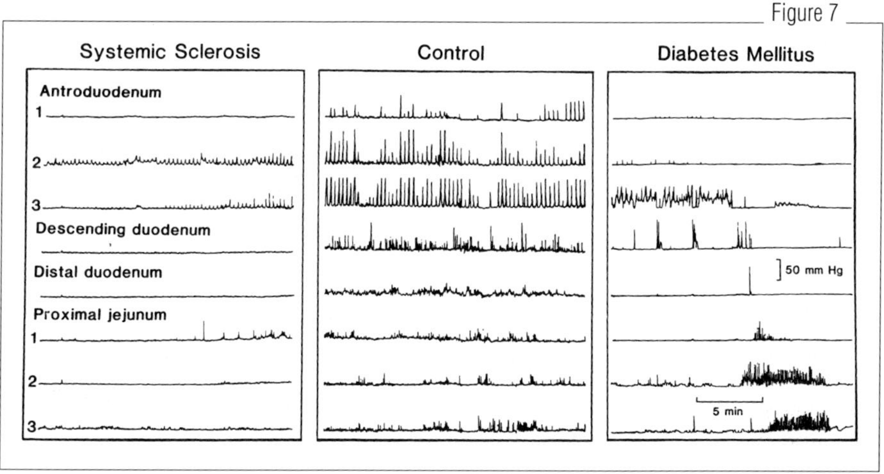


Postprandial tracings from the upper gut in patients with a myopathy (systemic sclerosis) characterized by low amplitude contractions, or a neuropathy (diabetes mellitus) characterized by normal amplitude but disorganized contractions. Note the reduced antral contractile frequency and the persistence of MMC-like activity postprandially.

Reproduced with permission from Camilleri M[77].

## Use of autonomic tests in evaluating neuropathic dysmotilities

Autonomic tests are useful to identify the cause of diseases affecting extrinsic neural control when there is no known underlying neurologic disorder. Several common neurologic disorders may affect gastrointestinal motility, either by altering the parasympathetic or sympathetic supply to the gut[21]. Such diseases include brainstem tumors or strokes, diabetes, spinal cord injury, multiple sclerosis, Parkinson's disease, and autonomic system degenerations[38]. Hence, a careful evaluation of the patient during the office visit is important, with particular emphasis on a past history of such a neurologic disorder or diabetes, concomitant use of medications (including the $\alpha_2$-adrenergic agonist, clonidine, anticholinergic antidepressants, and calcium channel blockers) and a family history of siblings or first degree relatives with similar clinical presentations.

COMMONLY PERFORMED AUTONOMIC TESTS

| Test | Principle | Nerves assessed |
|---|---|---|
| Sweat test | Heat stimulates thermo-regulatory center | Central sympathetic adrenergic and peripheral sympathetic cholinergic |
| BP lying, standing | Postural BP control by adrenergic nerves | Sympathetic adrenergic |
| RR interval with deep breathing | Vagal reflex bradycardia | Cardiac vagus |
| Plasma PP after modified sham feeding | Sham feeding stimulates vagal center and efferents | Efferent vagus to abdomen |

**BP** Blood pressure **PP** pancreatic polypeptide

Table 3

A battery of autonomic tests is available to evaluate the sympathetic adrenergic, sympathetic cholinergic, and vagal innervation of the viscera[21]. The principles explaining the tests most commonly performed are summarized in Table 3.

On the basis of these autonomic tests, it is possible to differentiate a preganglionic or central lesion from a peripheral neuropathy associated with autonomic dysfunction. In patients in whom a central lesion is suspected, brain and spinal cord magnetic resonance imaging is essential. A peripheral dysautonomia requires further screening for a toxic, metabolic or paraneoplastic process (e.g., lead poisoning, porphyria, lung cancer, respectively).

## Paraneoplastic immune-mediated pseudo-obstruction

In recent years, several patients have been described with small cell lung cancers or, rarely, carcinoid tumors in association with a paraneoplastic gastrointestinal motility disorder that is characterized by inflammation of the myenteric plexus (Figure 8).

Lennon et al. at Mayo Clinic[39] developed an immunofluorescence-based test to detect the presence of an antineuronal nuclear (or anti-Hu) antibody which is typically associated with small cell lung cancer. Among those patients with neurologic manifestations, 12% have gastrointestinal disturbances such as achalasia, gastroparesis, or chronic intestinal pseudo-obstruction (unpublished observation, Lennon 1995). This antibody is thought to be directed toward an epitope that is shared between the neuronal elements within the enteric nervous system and the underlying malignancy. Some patients with achalasia and scleroderma or no underlying disease associated with pseudo-obstruction have a similar circulating antibody directed to myenteric neurons[40-42]. The specificity of the assay in the reference laboratory is, therefore, an important factor that guides the subsequent diagnostic search.

Full-thickness intestinal biopsy is rarely needed in clinical practice, but it may reveal abnormal neuronal elements on silver staining[43]; laparoscopy is performed if mechanical obstruction is suspected or a venting/feeding tube is needed.

Figure 8

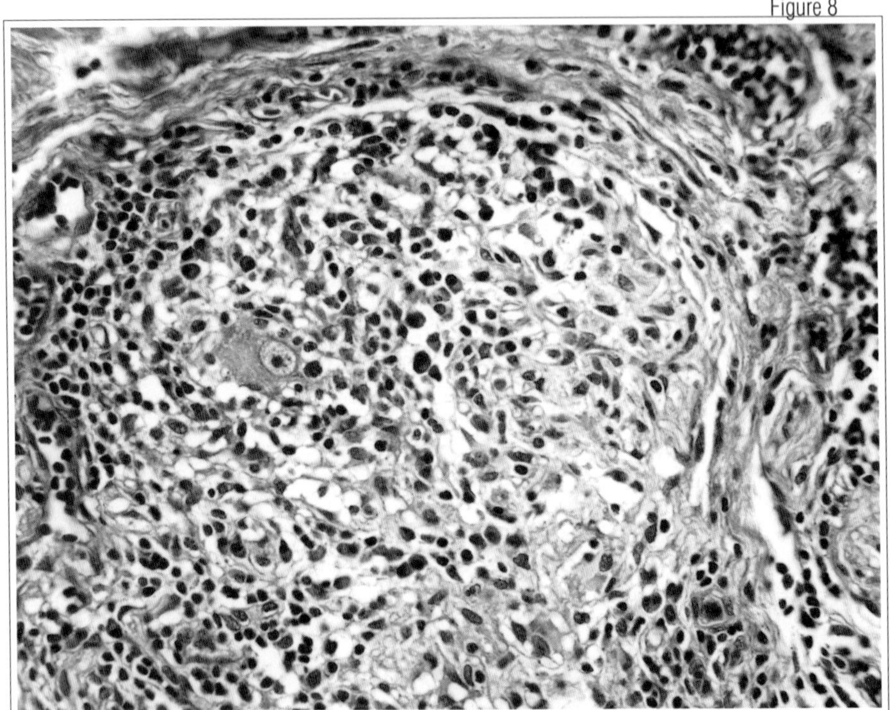

High power (x 400 magnification) photomicrograph showing inflammatory cells infiltrating the myenteric plexus of the stomach in a patient with paraneoplastic gastroparesis associated with positive ANNA serological test.
Reproduced with permission from Lennon VA, Sas DF, Buska J, Scheithauer B et al.[39]

## Bacterial overgrowth

This may complicate pseudo-obstruction and result in steatorrhea or weight loss. Culture of small bowel aspirates are more accurate than breath tests[44] in patients with myopathic forms of pseudo-obstruction.

## Principles of management of chronic intestinal pseudo-obstruction

The principles of management have been based predominantly on clinical experience, although recent reports from medium- and long-term trials have clarified the role of prokinetic medications[45].

*Step 1: Restore hydration and nutrition*

Nutritional support provides oral or enteral nutrition, typically for neuropathic disorders, and parenteral nutrition for patients with severe dysmotilities, typically myopathic pseudo-obstruction. In patients in whom there is evidence of small bowel bacterial overgrowth, as suggested by steatorrhea, vitamin $B_{12}$ malabsorption or folate excess and confirmed by culturing aspirates from the small intestine[44], it is useful to use antibiotics for 7 to 10 days every month. We typically use ciprofloxacin (500 mg, b.i.d.), doxycycline (100 mg, b.i.d.), and metronidazole (250 mg, t.i.d.) to suppress bacterial overgrowth.

*Step 2: Stimulate organized motility*

Recent clinical trials suggest that intravenous erythromycin (3 mg/kg every 8 hours) is effective during acute exacerbations and oral cisapride (up to 20 mg, q.i.d.) as maintenance therapy. During acute exacerbation, with the patient typically in hospital and on intravenous fluids, intravenous erythromycin lactobionate at a dose of 3 mg/kg every 8 hours should be started and continued for at least 5 to 7 days. During this period, the patient should not be dosed with oral cisapride since there is a potential risk of drug interaction leading to significant arrhythmias (torsades de pointes). An alternative to erythromycin is intravenous metoclopramide at dosages that are tolerated (usually 10 mg, 4 times per day), ensuring that the patient does not have a previous history of extrapyramidal reactions to these agents. Metoclopramide has the added advantage of being an antiemetic; it should be used with caution in patients with anxiety, depression or sleeping disorders.

As maintenance therapy, oral cisapride at a dose of up to 20 mg, 4 times per day is probably the treatment of choice. There is evidence among those who initially respond to cisapride that it is effective in controlling symptoms over a period of up to one year[23], and that a 20 mg dose is preferable[46] to the 10 mg dose with which tolerance was seen after a few months of therapy. Use of these prokinetic approaches is associated with maintenance of body weight and an ability to keep patients out of hospital and off parenteral nutrition[47]. Octreotide stimulates migrating motor complex-like activity in scleroderma and reduced symptoms in an open trial[48].

*Step 3: Symptom relief*

It is appropriate to combine a prokinetic with an antiemetic medication, such as a trifluoperazine compound (e.g., prochlorperazine 5-12.5 mg suppositories every 12 hours). There is some theoretical evidence that patients with scleroderma might benefit from subcutaneous octreotide, 50 mg at bedtime[48]. Octreotide should probably not be used in pseudo-obstruction patients if there is clinical evidence of bacterial overgrowth because it has been demonstrated to slow small bowel transit time in healthy individuals[49]. Symptomatic improvement with octreotide may reflect its effects in reducing visceral afferent function rather than its effects on transit through the intestine.

## Role of the surgeon in management of chronic intestinal pseudo-obstruction

Surgery is indicated for the resection of localized disease, although this is performed with great caution since there are several examples of "recurrence" following initial surgery. Bypass of dilated segments has been suggested for megaduodenum, but, in our experience, it tends to be quite ineffective with persistent symptoms. The surgeon's role is, therefore, predominantly in resection of the colon for chronic colonic pseudo-obstruction associated with constipation or for providing access to the stomach or small bowel for venting (decompression to relieve symptoms) and feeding[50]. Recently, we have used laparoscopy to place venting/feeding tubes since it also facilitates exclusion of mechanical obstruction and provides a full-thickness biopsy of the intestinal wall for histologic and electrophysiological examination. Although there are reports of subtotal enterectomy for pseudo-obstruction in the literature, these have been performed predominantly for relief of severe pain associated with markedly distended loops of intestine[51]. The patient is obviously committed to total parenteral nutrition for life after that operation.

At the present time, pacing of the intestine, electrical stimulation of the stomach or intestine, and transplantation are considered experimental. In particular, transplantation for patients with motility disorders has been performed very infrequently, and the risk-benefit ratio is unclear. From the application of small intestinal transplantation for patients with short gut syndrome, it appears that graft rejection, graft vs host disease, and immunosuppression-related lymphoproliferative disorders are more common than after other organ transplants.

## Chronic colonic pseudo-obstruction

The main manifestation of chronic colonic pseudo-obstruction is constipation. Constipation describes a reduced frequency of bowel movements (≤2/week) or the need for excessive straining to pass bowel movements. There is much confusion in the literature because of the lack of standard definitions of constipation syndromes[52,53]. In clinical practice, we identify the following subgroups:

- ***Slow transit constipation (synonyms: chronic colonic pseudo-obstruction, colonic inertia)*** constipation associated with delayed mean colonic transit time (≥72 hr) or retention of >25% of markers in the colon after 5 days. This condition is associated with delayed transit through the proximal colon[54]. We refer to inertia when there is the failure of colonic motility to respond to physiological or pharmacological stimulation in vivo[55-58].
- ***Outlet obstruction to defecation*** describes syndromes associated with excessive straining, need for anal disimpaction, failure to evacuate enemas. Four common conditions associated with outlet obstruction to defecation[6] are: puborectalis spasm (pelvic floor dyssynergia), anismus, excessive perineal descent, and anatomical rectal defects such as rectal intussusception or rectocele. The latter are best identified by defecation proctography.
- ***Normal transit constipation or functional constipation*** describes the symptom of constipation in the absence of prolonged transit or evidence of abnormal defecation such as excessive straining.

The localized dysmotility of Hirschsprung's disease results in a spastic segment associated with proximal dilatation. This is to be contrasted with the generalized or localized megacolon syndromes, which are unassociated with a localized spastic segment. The literature often includes Hirschsprung's, localized or generalized megacolon in the category of colonic pseudo-obstructions.

Abnormal colonic motility in syndromes associated with constipation is most effectively assessed by transit tests[33,59,60] and simple tests of the defecation process such as the balloon expulsion test, anorectal manometry, and defecation proctography[6].
Motor patterns described in various constipation disorders[61-64] are summarized in Table 4. Chronic colonic pseudo-obstruction may result from extrinsic denervation (e.g., multiple sclerosis, spinal cord injury[65]) or an intrinsic neuropathy of the colonic myenteric plexus. Koch et al.[66] showed that inhibitory intrinsic innervation was decreased in patients with severe colonic pseudo-obstruction who underwent subtotal colectomy. Others have observed reduced substance P, CGRP and other peptide deficiencies[67-70]. The role of neuropeptide loss in colonic pseudo-obstruction requires formal, systematic evaluation.

MOTOR PATTERNS IN CONSTIPATION

| | HAPC | Propagated contractions | Tone | MI DC | MI SC |
|---|---|---|---|---|---|
| Slow transit constipation | ↓ | ↓ | ↓orN | ↓ | ↓ |
| Outlet obstruct. to defecat. | N | ? | ↓orN | ↓ | ↓ |
| Injury to spinal cord | ? | ? | ↓ | ↓ | ↓ |
| Injury to cauda equina | ? | ? | ↓ | N | N |
| Megacolon | ? | ↓ | ↓ | N | N |

**MI** Motility index **DC** Descending colon **SC** Sigmoid colon
**HAPC** High amplitude propagating contraction
↓ decrease ↑ increase
**N** normal **?** unknown

Table 4

## Treatment of chronic colonic pseudo-obstruction

Slow transit constipation is treated with fiber, osmotic laxatives and stimuli (e.g., bisacodyl, anthraquinones) and rarely requires subtotal colectomy with ileorectostomy.

## *References*


1. Quigley EM, Phillips SF, Dent J. *Distinctive patterns of interdigestive motility at the canine ileocolonic junction.* Gastroenterology 1984;87:836-44.
2. Kerlin P, Phillips S. *Differential transit of liquids and solid residue through the human ileum.* Am J Physiol 1983;245:G38-G43.
3. Camilleri M, Colemont LJ, Phillips SF, et al. *Human gastric emptying and colonic filling of solids characterized by a new method.* Am J Physiol 1989;257:G284-290.
4. Proano M, Camilleri M, Phillips SF, et al. *Transit of solids through the human colon: regional quantification in the unprepared bowel.* Am J Physiol 1990;258:G856-862.
5. Ford MJ, Camilleri M, Wiste JA, Hanson RB. *Differences in colonic tone and phasic responses to a meal in the transverse and sigmoid human colon.* Gut 1995;37:264-9.
6. Pezim ME, Pemberton JH, Levin KE, et al. *Parameters of anorectal and colonic motility in health and in severe constipation.* Dis Colon Rectum 1993;36:484-91.
7. Sanders KM. *A case for interstitial cells of Cajal as pacemakers and mediators of neurotransmission in the gastrointestinal tract.* Gastroenterology 1996;111:492-515.
8. Ward SM, Burns AJ, Torihashi S, et al. *Impaired development of interstitial cells and intestinal electrical rhythmicity in steel mutants.* Am J Physiol 1995;269:C1577-1585.
9. Isozaki K, Hirota S, Nakama A, et al. *Disturbed intestinal movement, bile reflux to the stomach, and deficiency of c-kit-expressing cells in Ws/Ws mutant rats.* Gastroenterology 1995;109:456-64.
10. der-Silaphet T, Malysz J, Hagel S, et al. *Interstitial cells of Cajal direct normal propulsive contractile activity in the mouse small intestine.* Gastroenterology 1998;114:724-36.
11. Yamataka A, Kato Y, Tibboel D, et al. *A lack of intestinal pacemaker (c-kit) in aganglionic bowel of patients with Hirschsprung's disease.* J Pediatr Surg 1995;30:441-4.
12. Vanderwinden JM, Rumessen JJ, Liu H, et al. *Interstitial cells of Cajal in human colon and in Hirschsprung's disease.* Gastroenterology 1996;111:901-10.
13. Yamataka A, Ohshiro K, Kobayashi H, et al. *Intestinal pacemaker c-kit+ cells and synapses in allied Hirschsprung's disorders.* J Pediatr Surg 1997;32:1069-74.
14. Edery P, Lyonnet S, Mulligan LM, et al. *Mutations of the RET proto-oncogene in Hirschsprung's disease.* Nature 1994;367:378-80.
15. Romeo G, Ronchetto P, Luo Y, et al. *Point mutations affecting the tyrosine kinase domain of the RET proto-oncogene in Hirschsprung's disease.* Nature 1994;367:377-8.
16. Schuchardt A, D'Agati V, Larsson-Blomberg L, et al. *RET-deficient mice: an animal model for Hirschsprung's disease and renal agenesis.* J Intern Med 1995;238:327-32.
17. Borst MJ, VanCamp JM, Peacock ML, Decker RA. *Mutational analysis of multiple endocrine neoplasia type 2A associated with Hirschsprung's disease.* Surgery 1995;117:386-91.

18. Rothman TP, Chen J, Howard MJ, et al. *Increased expression of laminin-1 and collagen (IV) subunits in the aganglionic bowel of ls/ls, but not c-ret-/- mice.* Develop Biol 1996;178:498-513.
19. Robertson K, Mason I, Hall S. *Hirschsprung's disease: genetic mutations in mice and men.* Gut 1997;41:436-41.
20. Stanghellini V, Camilleri M, Malagelada J-R. *Chronic idiopathic intestinal pseudo-obstruction: clinical and intestinal manometric findings.* Gut 1987;28:5-12.
21. Camilleri M. *Disorders of gastrointestinal motility in neurologic diseases.* Mayo Clin Proc 1990;65:825-46.
22. Schuffler MD, Beegle RG. *Progressive systemic sclerosis of the gastrointestinal tract and hereditary hollow visceral myopathy: two distinguishable disorders of intestinal smooth muscle.* Gastroenterology 1979;77:664-71.
23. Krishnamurthy S, Schuffler MD, Belic L, Schweid AI. *An inflammatory axonopathy of the myenteric plexus producing a rapidly progressive intestinal pseudoobstruction.* Gastroenterology 1986;90:754-8.
24. McDonald GB, Schuffler MD, Kadin ME, Tytgat GN. *Intestinal pseudo-obstruction caused by diffuse lymphoid infiltration of the small intestine.* Gastroenterology 1985;89:882-9.
25. Krishnamurthy S, Schuffler MD, Rohrmann CA, Pope CE II. *Severe idiopathic constipation is associated with a distinctive abnormality of the colonic myenteric plexus.* Gastroenterology 1985;88:26-34.
26. Krishnamurthy S, Kelly MM, Rohrmann CA, Schuffler MD. *Jejunal diverticulosis. A heterogenous disorder caused by a variety of abnormalities of smooth muscle or myenteric plexus.* Gastroenterology 1983;85:538-47.
27. Schuffler MD, Lowe MC, Bill AH. *Studies of idiopathic pseudo-obstruction. I. Hereditary hollow visceral myopathy: clinical and pathological studies.* Gastroenterology 1977;73:327-38.
28. Qualman SJ, Haupt HM, Yang P, et al. *Esophageal Lewy bodies associated with ganglion cell loss in achalosia: similarity to Parkinson's disease.* Gastroenterology 1984; 87:848-56.
29. Colemont LJ, Camilleri M. *Chronic intestinal pseudoobstruction: diagnosis and treatment.* Mayo Clin Proc 1989;64:60-70.
30. Camilleri M, Brown ML, Malagelada J-R. *Impaired transit of chyme in chronic intestinal pseudo-obstruction: correction by cisapride.* Gastroenterology 1986;91:619-26.
31. Greydanus MP, Camilleri M, Colemont LJ, et al. *Ileocolonic transfer of solid chyme in small intestinal neuropathies and myopathies.* Gastroenterology 1990;99:158-64.
32. Camilleri M, Zinsmeister AR, Greydanus MP, et al. *Towards a less costly but accurate test of gastric emptying and small bowel transit.* Dig Dis Sci 1991;36:609-615.
33. Camilleri M, Zinsmeister AR. *Towards a relatively inexpensive, noninvasive, accurate test*

*for colonic motility disorders.* Gastroenterology 1992;103:36-42.

34. von der Ohe MR, Camilleri M. *Measurement of small bowel and colonic transit: indications and methods.* Mayo Clin Proc 1992;67:1169-79.
35. Camilleri M. *Study of human gastroduodenojejunal motility: applied physiology in clinical practice.* Dig Dis Sci 1993;38:785-94.
36. Camilleri M. *Jejunal manometry in distal subacute mechanical obstruction: significance of prolonged simultaneous contraction.* Gut 1989;30:468-75.
37. Frank JW, Sarr MG, Camilleri M. *Use of gastroduodenal manometry to differentiate mechanical and functional intestinal obstruction: an analysis of clinical outcome.* Am J Gastroenterol 1994;89:339-44.
38. Vassallo M, Camilleri M, Caron BL, Low PA. *Gastrointestinal motor dysfunction in acquired selective cholinergic dysautonomia associated with infectious mononucleosis.* Gastroenterology 1991;100:252-8.
39. Lennon VA, Sas DF, Buska J, et al. *Enteric neuronal autoantibodies in pseudoobstruction with small-cell lung carcinoma.* Gastroenterology 1991;100:137-42.
40. Howe S, Eaker EY, Sallustio JE, et al. *Antimyenteric neuronal antibodies in scleroderma.* J Clin Invest 1994;94:761-70.
41. Verne GN, Sallustio JE, Eaker EY. *Anti-myenteric neuronal antibodies in patients with achalasia. A prospective study.* Dig Dis Sci 1997;42:307-13.
42. Smith VV, Gregson N, Foggensteiner L, et al. *Acquired intestinal aganglionosis and circulating autoantibodies without neoplasia or other neural involvement.* Gastroenterology 1997;112:1366-71.
43. Krishnamurthy S, Schuffler MD. *Pathology of neuromuscular disorders of the small intestine and colon.* Gastroenterology 1987;93:610-39.
44. Valdovinos MA, Camilleri M, Thomforde GM, Frie C. *Reduced accuracy of* $^{13}$*C-D-xylose breath test for detecting bacterial overgrowth in gastrointestinal motility disorders.* Scand J Gastroenterol 1993;28:963-8.
45. Camilleri M. *Appraisal of medium- and long-term treatment of gastroparesis and chronic intestinal dysmotility.* Am J Gastroenterol 1994;89:1769-74.
46. Camilleri M, Balm RK, Zinsmeister AR. *Determinants of response to a prokinetic agent in neuropathic chronic intestinal motility disorder.* Gastroenterology 1994;106:916.
47. Abell TL, Camilleri M, DiMagno EP, et al. *Long-term efficacy of oral cisapride in symptomatic upper gut dysmotility.* Dig Dis Sci 1991;36:616-20.
48. Soudah HC, Hasler WL, Owyang C. *Effect of octreotide on intestinal motility and bacterial overgrowth in scleroderma.* N Engl J Med 1991;325:1461-67.
49. von der Ohe MR, Camilleri M, Thomforde GM, Klee GG. *Differential regional effects of octreotide on human gastrointestinal motor function.* Gut 1995;36:743-8.
50. Murr MM, Sarr MG, Camilleri M. *The surgeon's role in the treatment of chronic*

*intestinal pseudo-obstruction*. Am J Gastroenterol 1995;90:2147-51.

51. Mughal MM, Irving MH. *Treatment of end stage chronic intestinal pseudo-obstruction by subtotal enterectomy and home parenteral nutrition*. Gut 1988;29:1613-7.
52. Surrenti E, Rath DM, Pemberton JH, Camilleri M. *Audit of constipation in a tertiary-referral gastroenterology practice*. Am J Gastroenterol 1995;90:1471-5.
53. Camilleri M, Thompson WG, Fleshman JW, Pemberton JH. *Clinical management of intractable constipation*. Ann Intern Med 1994;121:520-8.
54. Stivland T, Camilleri M, Vassallo M, et al. *Scintigraphic measurement of regional gut transit in idiopathic constipation*. Gastroenterology 1991;101:107-15.
55. Preston DM, Lennard-Jones JE. *Pelvic motility and response to intraluminal bisacodyl in slow-transit constipation*. Dig Dis Sci 1985;30:289-94.
56. Bassotti G, Imbimbo BP, Betti C, et al. *Impaired colonic motor response to eating in patients with slow transit constipation*. Am J Gastroenterol 1992;87:504-8.
57. Bassotti G, Morelli A, Whitehead WE. *Abnormal rectosigmoid myoelectric response to eating in patients with severe idiopathic constipation (slow transit type)*. Dis Colon Rectum 1992;35:753-6.
58. Bassotti G, Chiarioni G, Imbimbo BP, et al. *Impaired colonic motor response to cholinergic stimulation in patients with severe chronic idiopathic (slow transit type) constipation*. Dig Dis Sci 1993;38:1040-5.
59. Arhan P, Devroede G, Jehannin B, et al. *Segmental colonic transit time*. Dis Colon Rectum 1981;24:625-9.
60. Metcalf AM, Phillips SF, Zinsmeister AR, et al. *Simplified assessment of segmental colonic transit*. Gastroenterology 1987;92:40-7.
61. O'Brien MD, Camilleri M, von der Ohe MR, et al. *Motility and tone of the left colon in constipation: a role in clinical practice?* Am J Gastroenterol 1996;91:2532-8.
62. Choi M-G, Camilleri M, O'Brien MD, et al. *A pilot study of motility and tone of the left colon in diarrhea due to functional disorders and dysautonomia*. Am J Gastroenterol 1997;92:297-302.
63. Bruninga K, Camilleri M. *Colonic motility and tone after spinal cord and cauda equina injury*. Am J Gastroenterol 1997;92:891-4.
64. von der Ohe MR, Camilleri M, Carryer PW. *A patient with localized megacolon and intractable constipation: evidence for impairment of colonic muscle tone*. Am J Gastroenterol 1994;89:1867-70.
65. Johanson JF, Sonnenberg A, Koch TR, McCarty DJ. *Association of constipation with neurologic diseases*. Dig Dis Sci 1992;37:179-86.
66. Koch TR, Carney JA, Go L, Go VLW. *Idiopathic chronic constipation is associated with decreased colonic vasoactive intestinal peptide*. Gastroenterology 1988;94:300-10.
67. Dolk A, Broden G, Holmstrom B, et al. *Slow transit chronic constipation (Arbuthnot*

*Lane's disease). An immunohistochemical study of neuropeptide-containing nerves in resected specimens from the large bowel.* Intl J Colorectal Dis 1990;5:181-7.

68. Tzavella K, Riepl RL, Klauser AG, et al. *Decreased substance P levels in rectal biopsies from patients with slow transit constipation.* Eur J Gastroenterol Hepatol 1996;8:1207-11.
69. Hutson JM, Chow CW, Hurley MR, et al. *Deficiency of substance P-immunoreactive nerve fibres in children with intractable constipation: a form of intestinal neuronal dysplasia.* J Paediatr Child Health 1997;33:187-9.
70. Goldin E, Karmeli F, Selinger Z, Rachmilewitz D. *Colonic substance P levels are increased in ulcerative colitis and decreased in chronic severe constipation.* Dig Dis Sci 1989;34:754-7.
71. Camilleri M, Philips SF. *Disorders of small intestinal motility.* In Ouyang A, editor. Gastroenterol Clin N Am. Philadelphia: WB Saunders; 1989, Vol. 18;405-24.
72. Malagelada J-R, Camilleri M, Stanghellini V. *Manometric Diagnosis of Gastrointestinal Motility Disorders.* New York: Thieme Medical Publischers, Inc.; 1986.
73. Camilleri M, Thompson WG, Fleshman JW, Pemberton JH. *Clinical management of intractable constipation.* Ann Intern Med 1994;121:520-8.
74 Donis-Keller. *The RET proto-oncogene and cancer.* J Intern Med 1995;238:319-25.
75. Camilleri M, Brown ML, Malagelada J-R. *Relationship between impaired gastric empying and abnormal gastrointestinal motility.* Gastroenterology 1986;91:94-9.
76. Thomforde GM, Camilleri M, Philips SF, Forstrom LA. *Evaluation of an inexpensive screening scientigraphic test of gastric emptying.* J Nucl Med 1995;36:93-6.
77. Camilleri M. *Medical treatment of chronic intestinal pseudo-obstruction.* Practical Gastroenterol 1991;15:10-22.

*Address for correspondence*

**CAMILLERI M, MD**
Mayo Clinic, Gastroenterology Research Unit
Rochester, 55905 Minnesota USA
Fax: +1 507 255 6318
E-mail: camilleri. michael@mayo.edu

# Chronic diarrhoea

*R Caprilli, G Latella, A Viscido*

Chronic diarrhoea has been defined as the presence of two or more loose stools per day for at least 3-6 weeks[1,2]. However, this definition does not take into consideration either the severity or the kind of diarrhoea observed in clinical practice. Furthermore, it does not consider other features of diarrhoeal illness beyond stool frequency including abdominal pain or cramps, bloating, urgency, tenesmus, discomfort, perianal pain. All these features, however, should be taken into account both for the diagnostic orientation and for the evaluation of treatment effectiveness. It is important to underline that diarrhoea is not a disease but it is a clinical sign. Reduction in the number of stool movements is not the only goal of treatment.

Most patients want a definitive cause of the diarrhoea to be found. A number of conditions may be responsible for chronic diarrhoea, the most common being Irritable Bowel Syndrome (IBS), Inflammatory Bowel Disease (IBD) and laxative abuse. Laxative abuse with resulting factitious diarrhoea is found in about 4% of new patients visiting gastroenterologists for evaluation of chronic diarrhoea and about 15-20% of those evaluated by tertiary referral centres. Patients with laxative-related diarrhoea have severe psychological abnormalities; they always deny laxative ingestion[2]. In the elderly, recurrent diarrhoea is frequently associated with diverticula of the colon. Chronic diarrhoea is a very common and specific sign of all malabsorption syndromes. It is also frequent after gastrointestinal surgery. Less frequently, it is due to infection (bacterial, parasitic, fungal) or endocrine diseases. Chronic diarrhoea in hosts positive for the Human Immunodeficiency Virus (HIV), with or without the Acquired Immunodeficiency Syndrome (AIDS), is due to an identifiable infectious agent in 75-85% of the cases[2].

Whatever the cause, diarrhoea is characterized by an increase in stool water. Normally, the daily loss of stool in Western diet populations is about 150 ml per day, 60-85% being accounted for by water. Thus, diarrhoea can also be defined by a daily stool weight of more than 200 g. However, daily stool weight does not allow us to distinguish between the functional and organic origin of diarrhoea.

In clinical practice, it is important to identify some factors which may

predict the organic or functional cause of chronic diarrhoea. Some criteria suggesting an organic disorder include: short duration of the diarrhoea (less than 3 months), predominantly nocturnal diarrhoea, continual rather than intermittent diarrhoea, diarrhoea not responsive to fasting, weight loss of more than 5 kg, a high Erythrocyte Sedimentation Rate (ESR), low haemoglobin and albumin levels, and an average daily faecal weight of more than 400 g. The specificity for an organic disorder is more than 90% when at least 3 of these criteria are present, although the sensitivity is poor[3-6].
Some features can orientate us towards the site involved by the disease. The passage of a large volume of stools associated with periumbelical pain usually indicates a small bowel disease, whereas the passage of frequent but small volume of stools, especially with blood, associated with low abdominal pain, tenesmus and urgency, may indicate a colorectal disease. Furthermore, the presence of fever may indicate mucosal inflammation, either of infectious or non infectious origin.
Evaluation of several clinical signs and some faecal characteristics may allow us to distinguish different categories of diarrhoea: secretory, osmotic and inflammatory (Tables 1, 2).

CLINICAL SIGNS IN CHRONIC DIARRHOEA

| Clinical signs | Secretory | Osmotic | Inflammatory |
|---|---|---|---|
| Stools | watery | watery | bloody |
| Urgency | - | - | + |
| Dehydration | ++ | - | + |
| Anaemia | - | - | + |
| Base - acid | acidosis | normal | alkalosis |
| Fasting test | - | + | - |

Table 1

Stool features in chronic diarrhoea

| Stools | Secretory | Osmotic | Inflammatory |
|---|---|---|---|
| Weight (g/day) | >1000 | 500 -1000 | <500 |
| Osmolality | n | n/+ | n |
| Osmotic gap | - | + | n |
| Na, Cl | + | - | + |
| K, $HCO_3$ | + | - | - |
| SCFA | ? | + | - |
| Lactate | - | + | + |
| pH | high | low | low |

**SCFA** short chain fatty acid **n** normal

Table 2

Secretory diarrhoea is characterized by watery stools, dehydration, metabolic acidosis, high faecal volume, reduction of the faecal osmotic gap, increase in faecal concentration of Na, Cl, K, $HCO_3$ and high faecal pH.

Osmotic diarrhoea presents with watery stools, normal acid-base balance, a positive response to the fasting test, high stool weight, high faecal osmolality and osmotic gap, reduction in faecal concentrations of Na, Cl, K, $HCO_3$, increase in faecal concentration of Short Chain Fatty Acids (SCFA) and lactic acid with a low faecal pH.

Inflammatory diarrhoea is characterized by bloody faeces, urgency, dehydration, anaemia, metabolic alkalosis, moderate increase in faecal volume, increase in faecal concentrations of Na, Cl, reduction in faecal concentrations of K and $HCO_3$, increase in concentration of lactic acid and a low faecal pH.

In a step-wise diagnostic approach, after the initial clinical examination and a laboratory evaluation, the presence of blood in the faeces may provide correct orientation in the choice of instrumental examinations (Figure 1).

Figure 1

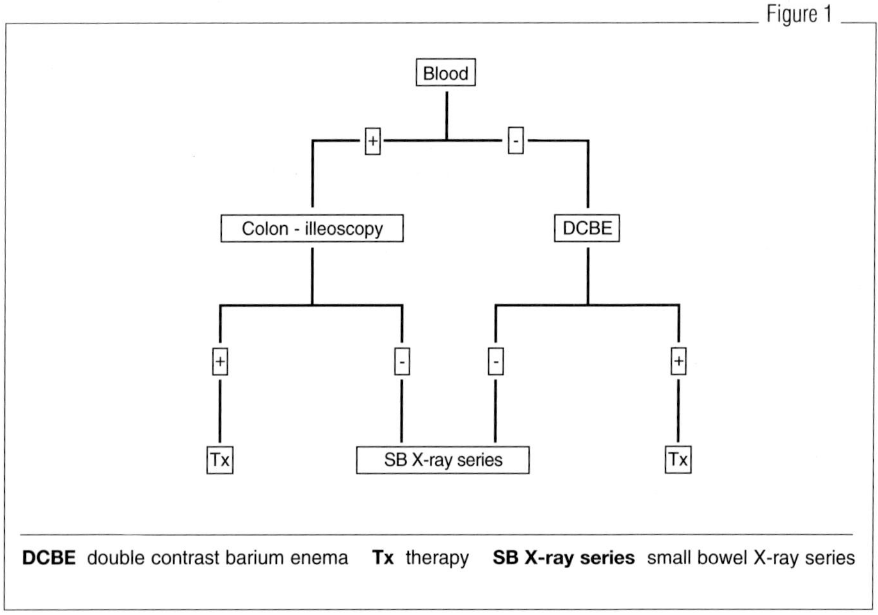


Flow charts for diagnostic procedures in chronic diarrhoea.

In the presence of bloody diarrhoea, colonoscopy should be performed as first line procedure and if negative, small bowel X-ray series should be performed. On the other hand, in the absence of blood in the stools, double contrast barium enema is more useful on account of the greater accuracy for diverticula of the colon compared to colonoscopy; if negative, small bowel X-ray series should be performed. If endoscopic, histologic and radiologic examinations are negative, more specific laboratory and instrumental investigations (CT, NMR, scintigraphy) should be taken into account before classifying the diarrhoea as functional.

In the clinical approach to chronic diarrhoea, besides the clinical signs and their underlying diseases, patient's subjective perception and function should also be taken into consideration. In fact, from the patient's point of view, chronic diarrhoea represents a condition which causes prolonged and, at times, even permanent disability. This also occurs in those patients in whom diarrhoea is found to be of functional origin. Besides the most traditional evaluation of disease status including symptoms, signs, laboratory data and underlying disease, the health status should also be evaluated. This takes into account, in addition to disease activity, also the illness experience and social and economic performance of the patient. For this purpose, in the last few years, the Health Related Quality of Life (HR-QoL) assessment has become of major importance in the evaluation of disease. The HR-QoL describes the physical, emotional and social impact of disease from the patient's point of view. Available HR-QoL instruments include a global assessment, as well as generic and specific disease instruments[7-9]. The potential applications of the HR-QoL assessment include identification of the problems and needs of individuals or groups of patients, assessment of standards of health care, enhancement of knowledge concerning the clinical course of the disease and evaluation of treatment efficacy in clinical trials[10]. Finally, HR-QoL assessment is critical for cost effectiveness and cost/utility analysis[11].

HR-QoL, to our knowledge, has not been evaluated in chronic diarrhoea, but only in some specific conditions such as IBD, both Ulcerative Colitis (UC) and Crohn's Disease (CD) and IBS[12-15]. HR-QoL is impaired, in both conditions, compared to normal subjects. Patients with IBS show a similar impairment in HR-QoL to that in patients with UC. Patients with CD have a more impaired HR-QoL than those with UC.

Health status in IBD depends on specific disease features (symptoms, severity, site, duration, age at onset) and its management (need for surgery, drug efficacy and toxicity), but also upon features not related to the disease, such as gender, cultural factors and "environment".

Psychological factors affect the health status much more in IBS than in IBD. Due to these influences psychotherapeutic approaches provide new forms of treatment which are really effective in a considerable proportion of patients with IBS, especially those with the more severe forms[13,16,17]. In fact, due to the link between the enteric nervous system and the mind through the brain-gut connection, psychologic treatments can improve symptoms, not only by influencing the patient's perception, but also by determining a return to normal of the presumed altered stimuli that are transmitted from the mind to the bowel wall determining the disorder[18].

Finally, it is important to bear in mind that management of chronic diarrhoea represents an important socio-economic problem both for the patient and the community. IBD and IBS, which are the major causes of chronic diarrhoea, have a marked socio-economic impact in Italy.

The incidence of IBD in Italy is 8 new cases per 100,000 people per year, with presumably 70,000 persons affected[19]. Management of IBD costs overall 240 billion Lit, with a mean cost per patient of 3.5 million, the annual breakdown of costs being 20 billion for diagnosis, 149 for hospital charges, 65 for drug treatment and 4.5 for surgery[20].

The prevalence of IBS is 10-20% in Western countries with 20-50% of appointments in a gastroenterology outpatient centre due to IBS. Furthermore, patients with IBS often undergo surgery without specific indications. In Italy, the overall costs for IBS are 1,000 billion Lit per year: 105 billion for clinical visits, 406 for instrumental investigations, 112 for hospital charges, 300 for drug treatment and 92 for consumption of fibres[20]. The medical charges for IBS to the USA white population have been estimated to exceed 8 billion dollars yearly[21].

In conclusion, the principal aims in the management of chronic diarrhoea, are two-fold, namely, to improve the HR-QoL and to reduce the health costs of these patients. Medical management plays a pivotal role in attaining these two aims which can be better achieved in a gastroenterology department.

## *REFERENCES*

1. Fine KD. *Diarrhea.* In: Feldman M, Scharschmidt BF, Sleisenger MH, editors. Gastrointestinal and liver disease. Philadelphia: WB Saunders; 1998; 128-52.
2. Donowitz M, Kokke FT, Saidi R. *Current concepts: evaluation of patients with chronic diarrhea.* N Engl J Med 1995;332:725-9.

3. Read NW, Krejs GJ, Read MG et al. *Chronic diarrhea of unknown origin.* Gastroenterology 1980;78:264-71.
4. Geraedts AAM, Esseveld MR, Tytgat GNJ. *The value of non-invasive examinations of patients with chronic diarrhea.* Scand J Gastroenterol 1988;154(Suppl):46-56.
5. Bytzer P, Stokholm M, Andersen I et al. *Aetiology, medical history, and fecal weight in adult patients referred for diarrhea: prospective survey.* Scand J Gastroenterol 1990;25:572-8.
6. Bertomeu A, Ros E, Barragan V et al. *Chronic diarrhea with normal stool and colonic examination: organic or functional?* J Clin Gastroenterol 1991;13:531-6.
7. Garrett JW, Drossman DA. *Health status in inflammatory bowel disease: biological and behavioural considerations.* Gastroenterology 1990;99:90-6.
8. Drossman DA. *The role of psychosocial factors in gastrointestinal illness.* Scand J Gastroenterol 1996;221(Suppl):1-4.
9. Irvine EJ. *Measuring quality of life: a review.* Scand J Gastroenterol 1996;221(Suppl):5-7.
10. Fitzpatrick R, Fletcher A, Gore S. *Quality of life measures in health care. I: applications and issues in assessment.* Br Med J 1992;305:1074-7.
11. Jonsson B. *Quality of life and health economics: where is the link?* Scand J Gastroenterol 1996;221(Suppl):33-6.
12. Drossman DA, Leserman J, Mitchell CM et al. *Health status and health care use in persons with inflammatory bowel disease. A national sample.* Dig Dis Sci 1991;36:1746-55.
13. Irvine EJ. *Quality of life in inflammatory bowel disease and other chronic diseases.* Scand J Gastroenterol 1996; 221(Suppl):26-8.
14. McLeod RS, Baxter NN. *Quality of life of patients with inflammatory bowel disease after surgery.* World J Surg 1998;22:375-81.
15. Patrick DL, Drossman DA, Frederick IO et al. *Quality of life in persons with irritable bowel syndrome. Development and validation of a new measure.* Dig Dis Sci 1998;43:400-11.
16. Drossman DA, McKee DC, Sandler RS et al. *Psychosocial factors in the irritable bowel syndrome. A multivariate study of patients and nonpatients with irritable bowel syndrome.* Gastroenterology 1988;95:701-8.
17. Heymann-Monnikes I, Amold R, Florin I, Monnikes H. *Evaluation of a multi-component behavioral treatment for the irritable bowel syndrome.* Gastroenterology 1998;114:A764.
18. Camilleri M, Ford MJ. *Review article: colonic sensorimotor physiology in health, and its alteration in constipation and diarrhoeal disorders.* Aliment Pharmacol Ther 1998;12:287-302.

19. Tragnone A, Corrao G, Miglio F et al. *Incidence of inflammatory bowel disease in Italy: a nationwide population based study.* Int J Epidemiol 1996;25:1044-52.
20. Caprilli R, Taddei G, Viscido A, Assisi D. *Le malattie del colon: criteri di gestione.* In: Attanasio E, Delle Fave G, editors. Criteri farmacoeconomici e terapia delle malattie digestive (CIMAD). Genova: Forum Service Ed; 1995. p. 19-24.
21. Talley NJ, Gabriel SE, Harmsen WS et al. *Medical costs in community subjects with irritable bowel syndrome.* Gastroenterology 1995;109:1736-41.

*ADDRESS FOR CORRESPONDENCE*

**CAPRILLI R, MD**
I Cattedra di Gastroenterologia, Dipartimento di Scienze Cliniche
Università di Roma "La Sapienza"
Policlinico Umberto I
Viale del Policlinico, 155
00161 Roma Italia
Fax: +39 06 4463737
E-mail: caprilli@aconet.it

# Clinical approach to management of Crohn's disease

*L Biancone, P Doldo, F Pallone*

Crohn's Disease (CD) is a chronic inflammatory bowel disease of unknown etiology[1,2].

The intestinal lesions may involve any segment of the gastrointestinal tract, with a typical transmural and patchy distribution[3,4]. The more frequently involved segments include the terminal ileum and the colon. CD is an heterogeneous condition in both clinical and anatomical terms. This is related to the different site, extent and type of gross lesions. The intestinal lesions may show a more prevalent fibrostenotic, inflammatory or fistulizing feature, leading to different disease behaviour[5]. The various combinations of the different anatomical characteristics (site, extent, type) account for the wide spectrum of symptoms and course of the disease in different patients. The more common symptoms related to CD are abdominal pain, chronic remittent diarrhoea with or without macroscopic blood, abdominal mass and weight loss. Periodical anorexia, low grade fever and extraintestinal manifestations[6] may also occur. The disease course is chronic remittent and is characterised by the high tendency to recur after surgical resection of the entire segment involved[1,2,7]. Despite these common features of the CD course, different symptoms and local or systemic complications may occur during the natural history of the disease, being related to the involved segment and to the characteristics of the lesions. Local complications include intestinal obstruction, perforation, abdominal abscesses, perianal disease, fistulae either internal (entero-enteric, entero-vesical, entero-vaginal) or external (entero-cutaneous). Possible extra-intestinal complications may involve the joints (arthritis, ankylosing spondylitis, sacroileitis, "finger clubbing"), the skin (erithema nodosum, pyoderma gangrenosum), the eyes (uveitis, episcleritis) and the biliary tract (sclerosing cholangitis, cholangiocarcinoma). None of the reported symptoms and no haematochemical parameters are diagnostic for Crohn's Disease.

## Clinical management

The multiple clinical and anatomopathological features of CD require a patient-specific treatment with continuous monitoring, assessment and optimization during the natural history of the disease[8,9]. An appropriate clinical management of CD is the result of several variables which need to be known before choosing the patients' treatment. Among these:

- ✓ the characteristics of the disease
- ✓ the characteristics of the host
- ✓ the specific purpose of treatment in each patient at that time
- ✓ therapeutic options in our hands.
- ✓ the resulting drugs

***Characteristics of the disease*** which influence patient management include the site, extent and type of gross lesions, the disease course and duration as well as the possible presence of complications or previous surgery (Figure 1). CD subtypes implies relevant therapeutic implications[5,8,9]. The fibrostenotic subtype is characterized by a greater need for surgery mainly related to recurrent obstructions and by temporary improvement induced by bowel rest and anti-inflammatory drugs. The inflammatory subtype is associated with a marked responsiveness to anti-inflammatory drugs, which is significantly affected by the disease extent, and with a high tendency to recurrent relapses related to incomplete remission. Finally, fistulizing/perforating CD is significantly associated with severe complications, with early post-operative recurrence and with a marked responsiveness to immunosuppressive drugs and bowel rest.

***Characteristics of the host*** which affect patient management include age, sex, lifestyle, risk factors (including smoke, use of contraceptives), psycho-social background, ability to cope, defence mechanisms and family history of inflammatory bowel disease[10-13] (Figure 2). In patients below 20 at diagnosis, CD is significantly associated with a greater need for surgery, upper GI involvement, responsiveness to immunosuppressive drugs and familial IBD. Moreover, paediatric active CD is highly responsive to bowel rest. Smoking habits and the use of contraceptives are associated to a more severe course of the disease, representing the first one a significant risk factor for an earlier post-operative recurrence[13].

CHARACTERISTICS OF THE DISEASE AFFECTING THE CLINICAL APPROACH TO MANAGEMENT OF CROHN'S DISEASE

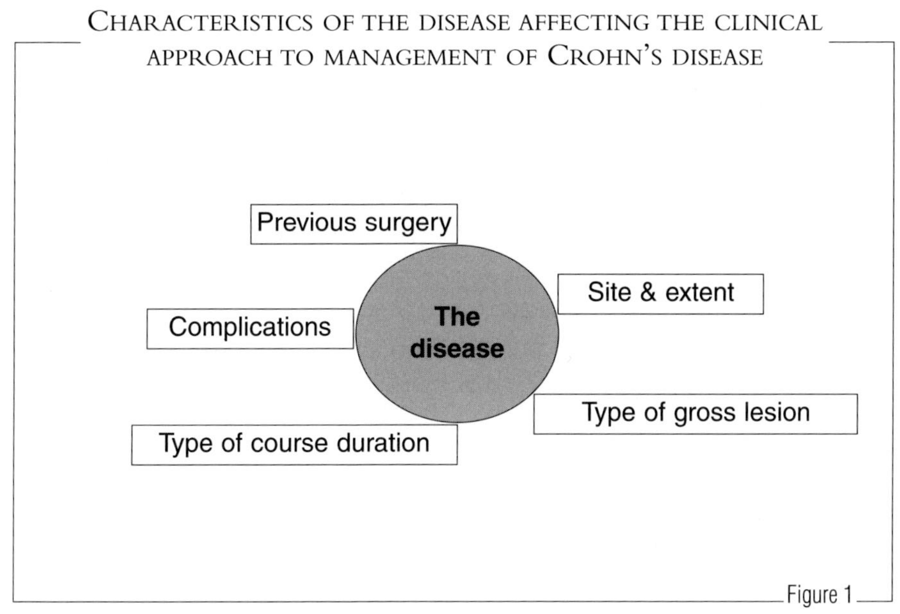


Figure 1

CHARACTERISTICS OF THE HOST AFFECTING THE APPROACH TO MANAGEMENT OF CROHN'S DISEASE

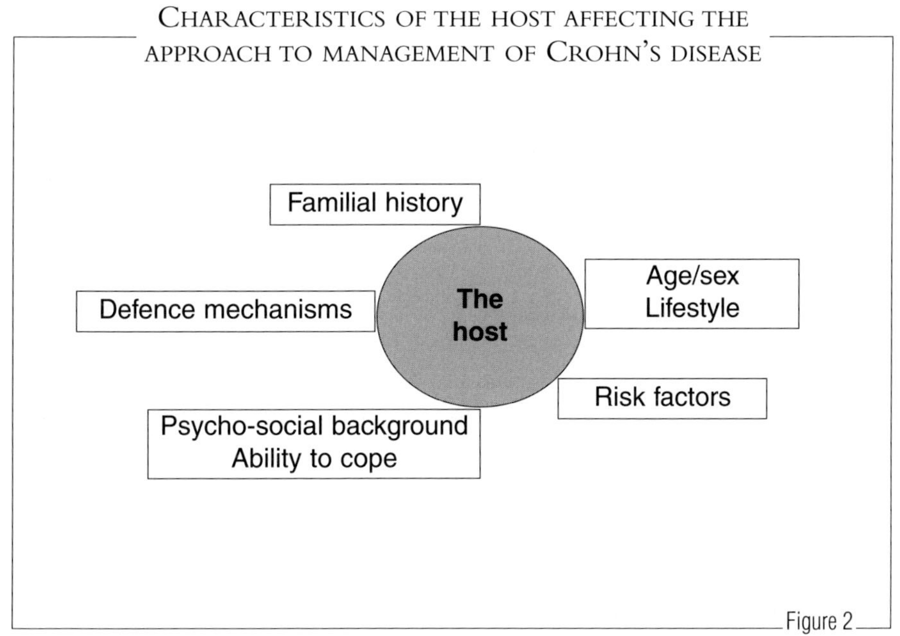


Figure 2

A familial history of IBD also represents a risk factor for earlier onset and a more severe course of CD[10,11,14].

Although the reported characteristics of the host represent predictive markers of the disease course, the efficacy of drug treatments in CD shows marked inter- and intra-individual variation. These observations taken together, stress the need of repeated optimizations of CD management in each patient in each step of the natural history of the disease (Figure 3). Among the factors leading to discrepant results in terms of drug responsiveness there is also the difficult assessment of CD activity[15].

NATURAL HISTORY OF CROHN'S DISEASE

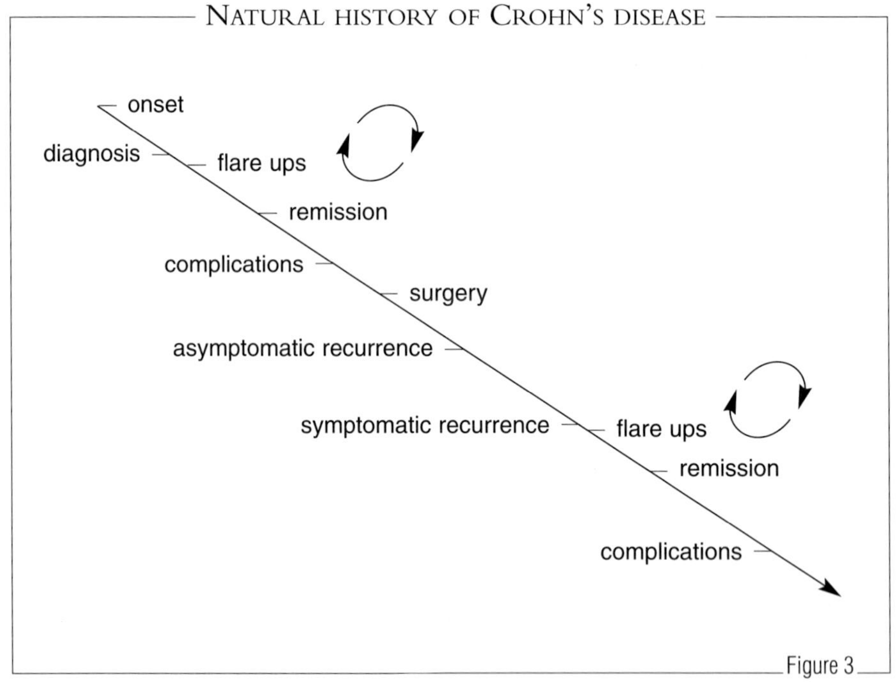


Figure 3

A careful consideration of past history is also an important factor affecting the clinical approach[16].

The specific purposes of treatment, in each patient, at any particular time, play an important role in estabilishing the appropriate management of CD, once information regarding the characteristics of the disease and of the host have been collected (Figure 4). Aims of treatment include inducing symptom relief or improving the quality of life of the patient, treating/preventing complications (Table 1), relapse, post-operative recurrence, maintaining remission or rather reaching individual goals.

INDIVIDUAL GOALS TO BE REACHED IN CROHN'S DISEASE MANAGEMENT

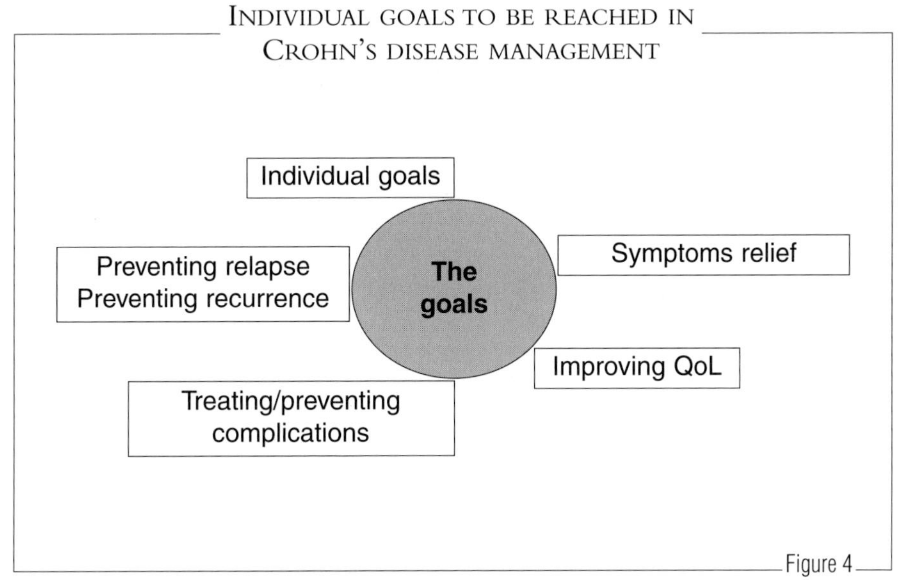


Figure 4

COMPLICATIONS OF CROHN'S DISEASE ACCORDING TO DISEASE SITE (%)

| | ileum | ileum+colon | colon |
|---|---|---|---|
| **Obstruction** | **34** | **44** | **17** |
| **Fistulas** | | | |
| Anal, perirectal | **22** | **50** | **51** |
| Internal, cutaneous | **18** | **34** | **13** |
| **Systemic manifestations** | **27** | **28** | **47** |

Table 1

Among these, steroid-sparing, fistula healing, controlling extraintestinal manifestations, restoring normal growth, managing osteopenia, relief of individual symptoms (e.g. diarrhoea) or managing unrelated disorders.
Among the extraintestinal manifestations, ankylosing spondylitis and arthritis frequently occur in CD, being associated with colonic disease and HLA-B27 genotype.
Osteopenia is also a frequent complication in CD, since not only is it related to malabsorbtion and corticosteroid use, but may also be observed at the onset of the disease.

## Choice of the drugs

Drug treatment of CD may be used for managing flare-up, maintenance of remission, management of complications or prevention of post-operative recurrences.
The appropriate treatment also depends on the characteristics of the suitable drugs, including their mode of action, active moiety, delivery system, modes of administration, optimal doses and side effects (Figure 5).

CHARACTERISTICS OF THE DRUGS AFFECTING THE CLINICAL MANAGEMENT OF CROHN'S DISEASE

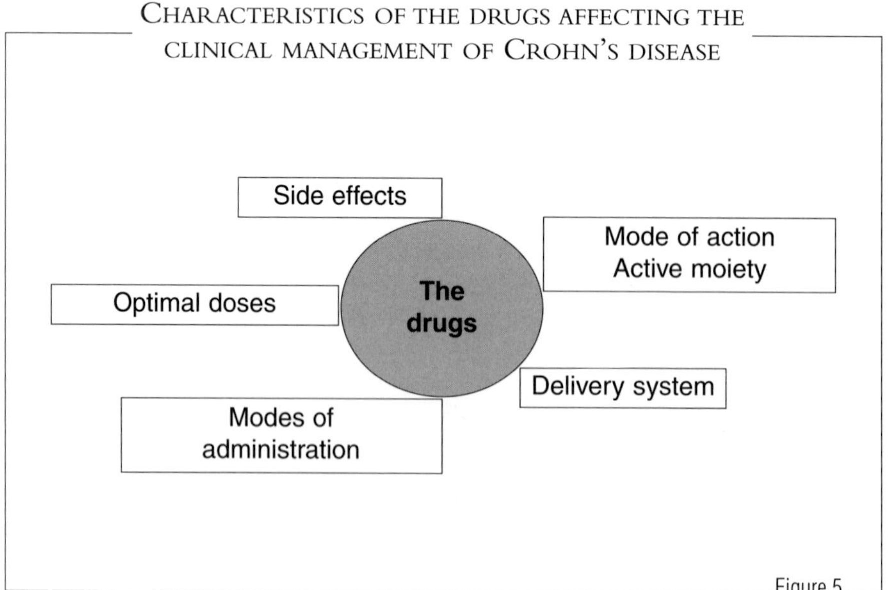


Figure 5

Among the drugs effective in CD we may identify:
a. "conventional drugs", including oral and topical salicylates, corticosteroids, immunosuppressive agents (e.g., azathioprine, 6-mercaptopurine, cyclosporine, methotrexate) and antibacterial drugs;
b. "new drugs", including new steroids, anti-cytokines/cytokines, newer biologics compounds and probiotics.

## *Conventional drugs*

### *Induction of remission*

***Corticosteroids*** As shown in Table 2, among the conventional drugs, corticosteroids represent the most effective drugs for treatment of active CD with any location. 6-Methylprednisolone (i.v. or i.m.) and prednisolone (by mouth)(1 mg/kg/day) treatment are associated with a 65%-85% remission rate at 4 weeks much higher than that observed with high doses sulphasalazine (3-5 g/day) or 5-aminosalicylic acid (5-ASA)(4 g/day) compounds[8,9,17,18].

EFFICACY OF CONVENTIONAL DRUGS IN CROHN'S DISEASE

| | % Response rate | | |
|---|---|---|---|
| | 5-ASA | Steroids | AZA/6MP |
| Inducing remission | ? | 65-85 | 35 |
| Remission maintenance | 55 | 40 | 65 |
| Managing complications | -- | ? | 50-65** |
| Preventing recurrence* | 48 | 30 | ? |

* endoscopic recurrence ** fistulae healing

Table 2

Bowel rest (parenteral nutrition or enteral feeding) and antibiotic treatment (ciprofloxacin 500 mg x 2/day and metronidazole 250 mg x 3/day) may enhance the efficacy of corticosteroids.

***Immunosuppressive drugs/agents*** Azathioprine (AZA) and its metabolite 6-mercaptopurine (6MP) are purine analogues competitively inhibiting purine ribonucleotide production and cell proliferation[19]. 6-Mercaptopurine is metabolized to thioinosinic acid, the active compound. The mechanisms whereby these immunosuppressive drugs are effective in CD have not been fully elucidated. Both drugs modulate the cell-mediated immune response, inhibiting the activity of cytotoxic T-cells and natural killer cells. Azathioprine (2-2.5 mg/kg/day) and 6-mercaptopurine (1-1.5 mg/kg/day) show a lower percent of response rate in inducing remission than steroids (1 mg/kg/day)(30-40% vs 65%-85%) when considering the whole group of active CD[20-24]. However, they are highly effective in managing complications of the disease. In particular, in chronic, unremitting steroid-dependent active CD, azathioprine and 6-mercatopurine are highly effective in achieving individual goals, with a 73% control of refractory individual symptoms, 76% steroid "sparing" effect and a 63% rate of fistula closure. These percentages for both groups are significantly higher than placebo[20-24].
Methotrexate is an immunosuppressive drug interfering with DNA synthesis and cellular replication. Its mechanism of action in CD is not yet fully elucidated, although it has been shown to modulate IL-1 activity[25]. Methotrexate has been shown to induce remission in 39% of patients versus 19% on placebo at 16 weeks ($p=0.002$), with a steroid-sparing effect and a lower mean CDAI score than control group[26]. However, further studies are needed.
Cyclosporine A is an inhibitor of the T-cell mediated perpetuation of the pro-inflammatory cascade. This drug blocks the IL-1-mediated action of macrophages on helper T-cells, thus inhibiting the release/action of other pro-inflammatory cytokines[27]. Results regarding the efficacy of cyclosporine in CD are conflicting[28-31]. Brynskov et al. reported the efficacy of this drug (5-7 mg/kg/day) at 3 months in steroid-refractory-active disease[28], although the remission appeared not long lasting. Malabsorption of the drug in 27% of patients requires careful control of serum levels[27]. A cyclosporin preparation with a higher absorption has recently become available. A controlled study showed no efficacy of oral

cyclosporine in active disease[28], while an uncontrolled study reported its efficacy in fistulous steroid-refractory disease[29].
Tacrolimus (FK506) is a T-cell immunosuppresive drug similar to cyclosporine. Preliminary studies reported its efficacy in fistolous active CD[32].
Taken together, present knowledge indicates that azathioprine and 6-mercaptopurine represent the most effective immunosuppressive drugs showing a proven efficacy in terms of "steroid-sparing" effect and of achieving individual goals (e.g. fistula closure) in active CD.

***Antibiotics*** Although no specific aetiologic agent has been detected in CD, several antibacterial drugs showed efficacy in reducing intestinal inflammation, extraintestinal manifestations as well as symptoms related to bacterial overgrowth[33,17].
Metronidazole is an imidazole with an antimicrobial spectrum including gut anaerobes[34]. Metronidazole (1 g/day) shows efficacy in perianal CD[34]. Controlled studies versus placebo and prednisone also showed its efficacy in ileo-colonic as well as in colonic active CD[35-37]. The more frequent dose-related side effects (10-20% of cases) include metallic taste, gastrointestinal intolerance and neurotoxicity. The long-term use of metronidazole can lead to peripheral neuropathy in 50-80% of cases[33-37].
Ciprofloxacin is a derivative of the quinolones showing a significant bactericidal activity against enteric pathogens with no significant effects on anaerobic flora[38]. Long-term therapy with ciprofloxacin and metronidazole has shown efficacy in perianal CD[39]. Combined treatment with metronidazole (250 mg x 4/day) and ciprofloxacin (500 mg x 2/day) for 12 weeks has shown efficacy comparable to that of methylprednisolone (0.7-1 mg/kg/day) in inducing CD remission (CDAI <150)(% remission in antibiotic- vs steroid-treated group: 45.5% vs 63%; p=n.s.)[40,41]. Although further studies are needed, these data suggest that this combined antibiotic therapy is efficacious in CD.

*Maintenance of remission*
Conventional corticosteroids show no efficacy in maintaining CD remission at 0.25–0.7 mg/kg/day[18]. Azathioprine and 6-mercaptopurine have shown efficacy in terms of a "steroid-sparing effect" in steroid-dependent patients[42,43]. A controlled trial showed that parenteral methotrexate 25 mg i.m. or s.c. weekly is effective in discontinuing or tapering prednisone in steroid-dependent patients[26], while cyclosporine

showed no efficacy[44]. The optimal use and duration of conventional immunosuppressive drug treatments in maintaining remission of CD needs to be determined in long-term studies. Sulfasalazine showed no efficacy as a maintenance drug in CD[17,18]. Conversely, several studies demonstrated that mesalamine (2.4 g/day) is effective in maintaining CD remission[45-49]. This drug regimen, therefore, represents the treatment of choice in this group of patients, also in relation to the long-term safety of the drug.

*Prevention of post-operative recurrence*

As the aetiology of CD is unknown, no drugs have shown proven efficacy in preventing CD recurrence after resection of the whole entire involved segment. Mesalamine (2.4 g/day) showed a certain efficacy in delaying the post-operative endoscopic and clinical recurrence after resection for ileal CD[50-52].

However, recent controlled studies showed conflicting results requiring further trials and evaluation of the role of an appropriate drug absorption and dosage for optimal efficacy.

Azathioprine treatment (2.5 mg/day) recently showed a significant efficacy in preventing post-operative CD recurrence, as also in inducing healing of the early recurrent lesions[53].

## *Alternative approaches*

*Induction of remission*

Reasons for alternative approaches to conventional treatment of active CD, represented by steroids, include: refractory disease, steroid-dependence, drug side-effects and local or systemic complications. In steroid-dependent/refractory chronic active CD alternative drugs include:

1. Luminal/topical drugs, including high dose mesalazine, the new corticosteroid budesonide, antibacterial drugs (see above), probiotics
2. Immunomodulatory drugs such as cytokines/anti-cytokines monoclonal antibodies (Interleukin-10, IL-10; anti-tumor necrosis factor-α, TNF-α; ICAM-1 antisense; anti-IL-12; IL-11). The efficacy of this last group of drugs is still under investigation.

High dose sulfasalazine (3-6 g/day) or mesalamine (3.2-4.8 g/day) are more effective than placebo, but less than conventional steroids, as they induce clinical remission in about one-half of patients with active CD[17,18,54-56] respectively with colonic or ileal involvement.
Budesonide in capsules is a relatively new steroid inducing a low systemic bioavailability (10-15%) after oral intake, due to its first-pass metabolism in the liver[57].
Budesonide per os (9 mg/day) has shown an efficacy comparable to conventional steroids (prednisone 1 mg/kg per os) in inducing clinical remission (CDAI <150) in active small bowel CD. This efficacy was associated with a significantly lower induction of steroid-related side effects[57-59]. Budesonide, therefore, represents a useful alternative drug treatment for mild/moderate active small bowel Crohn's Disease, particularly in young steroid-dependent, chronic active patients.

***Cytokines/anticytokines treatment*** Increasing "in vitro" evidence showing quantitative alterations of the intestinal mucosal immune response[19,60-63] has led to the development of new drugs capable of specifically targeting the host immune response. Among these, chimeric monoclonal antibody anti-TNF-$\alpha$[66]. Recent studies demonstrated that anti-TNF-$\alpha$ monoclonal antibody treatment shows a greater efficacy than placebo in inducing remission in patients with active CD. This efficacy was observed in almost two/thirds of the patients, being most effective in those with fistulizing disease[70]. The remission induced by anti-TNF-$\alpha$ MoAb is associated with endoscopic healing of the lesions associated with histological remission[71].
One of the problems arising from the use of this drug is the difficult identification, before treatment, of the subgroup of responsive patients, particularly in relation to the possible incidence of severe side effects associated with the use of this drug. Multicentre trails are currently investigating the safety, tolerability and optimal use of this highly promising new drug in CD.

*Maintenance of remission*
Therefore, the standard treatment in this subgroup of patients is represented by mesalamine per os (2.4 mg/day)[45-49]. The possible efficacy of higher mesalamine dosage (>3.2 g/day) is currently under

investigation. Azathioprine and 6-mercaptopurine represent alternative drugs for chronic active, steroid-dependent or steroid-refractory CD[20,21,72-74]. Ciprofloxacin and metronidazole (1 g/day) associated with mesalazine are effective in maintaining clinical remission in patients with ileo-colonic or colonic CD with or without perianal involvement[33-41]. Fish oil has been reported, in one study, to be effective in preventing clinical relapse in CD[75]. However, no other studies have confirmed this observation. Anti-TNF regiments for relapse prevention are currently under investigation.

***Prevention of post-operative recurrence*** Clinical trials are currently investigating the possible efficacy of higher mesalamine regimens (2.4 vs 3.6 g/day) in delaying/preventing the post-operative recurrence of ileal CD. Results from a recent study also demonstrated, for the first time, the efficacy of metronidazole in preventing CD recurrence[76]. More recently, azathioprine[53] has also shown efficacy in this regard.
However, no current data demonstrate the certain effectiveness of any drug in preventing the post-operative recurrence of CD.

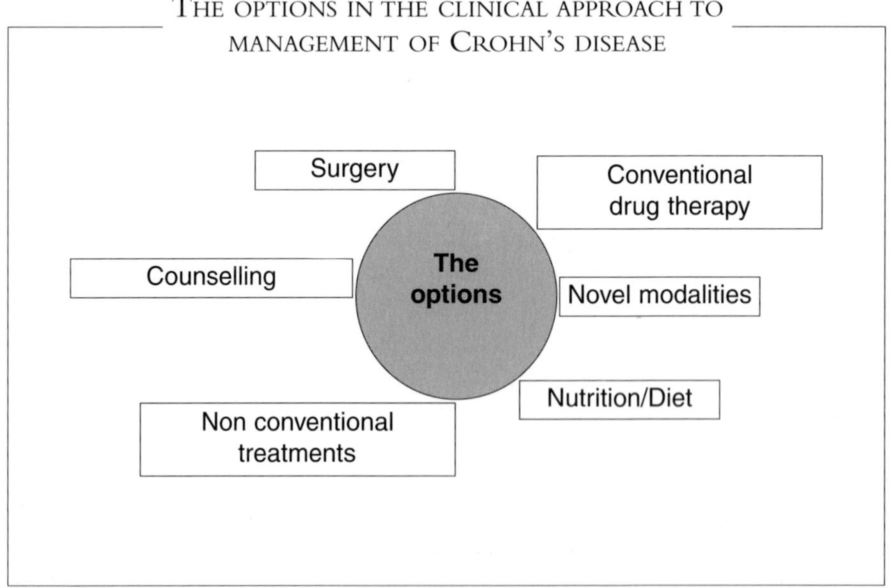

## Options

Mild/moderate active CD indicates patients tolerating oral feeding with no toxicity, dehydratation, abdominal tenderness, painful mass, local or systemic complications[9]. In CD involving the ileum, the ileum-colon or the colon only, treatment is represented by high dose oral amino salicylates (SASP or 5-ASA)[7,8,21,22,78] with the possible addition of metronidazole and/or ciprofloxacin in cases of colonic involvement. In contrast, CD involving the ileum-colon or the upper gastrointestinal tract is highly responsive to immunomodulatory drugs.

When considering moderate/severe active CD as patients not responsive to the therapy reported above, with relevant symptoms but no complications, current treatment modalities include: prednisone or methylprednisolone (1 mg/kg) until symptom resolution and weight gain (7-28 days), antibiotics (metronidazole 1 g/day). Elemental diets and bowel rest may represent an alternative to steroids mainly in paediatric CD. Chronic active CD regardless of the location is highly responsive to immunosuppressive drugs[77-80].

Finally, patients with severe CD presenting persistent symptoms despite steroids, complications and/or systemic symptoms, require hospitalization. In these patients, in the presence of local complications as suggested also by imaging techniques, surgery may be required. In contrast, patients with uncomplicated disease may be treated with parenteral prednisone antibiotics and/or bowel rest.

## References

1. Sartor RB. *Current concepts of the etiology and pathogenesis of Crohn's disease and ulcerative colitis.* Gastroenterol Clin North Am 1995;24:475-507.
2. Targan SR, Murphy LK. *Clarifying the causes of Crohn's.* Nature Medicine 1995; 1:1241-3.
3. Crohn BB, Ginzburg L, Oppenheimer GD. *Regional enteritis: a pathobiological and clinical entity.* JAMA 1932;99:1323-5.

4. Morson BC, Dawson IMP, Day DW, et al. *Inflammatory disorders of the small intestine.* In: Morson BC, Dawson IMP, editors. Gastrointestinal Pathology, 3rd ed. Chicago: Blackwell; 1990.
5. Sachar DB, Andrews HA, Farmer RG, et al. *Proposed classification of patient subgroups in Crohn's disease. Working Team Report.* Gastroenterol Int 1992;3:141-54.
6. Greenstein AJ, Janowitz HD, Sachar DB. *The extraintestinal manifestations of Crohn's disease and ulcerative colitis: a study of 700 patients.* Medicine 1976;55:401-7.
7. Rutgeerts P, Geboes K, Vantrappen G, et al. *Natural history of recurrent Crohn's disease at the ileocolonic anastomosis after curative surgery.* Gut 1984;25:665-72.
8. Elton E, Hanauer SB. *Review article: the medical management of Crohn's disease.* Aliment Pharmacol Ther 1996;10:1-22.
9. Hanauer SB, Meyers S. *Management of Crohn's disease in adults.* Am J Gastroenterol 1997;92:559-66.
10. Cottone M. *Stress and physical activity: are they risk factors for inflammatory bowel disease?* Ital J Gastroenterol Hepatol 1998;30:252-3.
11. Cottone M, Rosselli M, Orlando O, et al. *Smoking habits and recurrence in Crohn's disease.* Gastroenterology 1994;106:643-8.
12. Bayless TM, Tokayer AZ, Polito LM, et al. *Crohn's disease: concordance for site and clinical type in affected family members – potential hereditary influences.* Gastroenterology 1996;111:573-9.
13. Peeters M, Nevens H, Baert F, et al. *Familial aggregation in Crohn's disease: increased age-adjusted risk and concordance in clinical characteristics.* Gastroenterology 1996;111:597-603.
14. Polito JM II, Rees RC, Childs B, et al. *Preliminary evidence of a genetic anticipation in Crohn's disease.* Lancet 1996;347:798-800.
15. Best WR, Becktel LM, Singleton JW, Kern F. *Development of a Crohn's Disease Activity Index.* Gastroenterology 1976;70:439-44.
16. Pallone F, Boirivant M, Stazi MA, et al. *An analysis of clinical course of postoperative recurrence in Crohn's disease of distal ileum.* Dig Dis Sci 1992;37:215-9.
17. Malkow H, Ewe K, Brandes JW. *European Cooperative Crohn's Disease Study (ECCDS): results of drug treatment.* Gastroenterology 1984;86:249-66.
18. Summers RW, Switz DM, Sessions JT. *National Cooperative Crohn's Disease Study: results of drug treatment.* Gastroenterology 1979;77:847-69
19. Lugering N, Kucharzik T, Stoll R, Domschke W. *Current concepts of the role of monocytes/macrophages in inflammatory bowel disease. Balance of pro-inflammatory and immunosuppressive mediators.* Am J Gastroenterol 1998;30:338-44.

20. Ewe K, Press AG, Singe CC. *Azathioprine combined with prednisolone or monotherapy with prednisolone in active Crohn's disease.* Gastroenterology 1993;105:367-72.
21. Hawthorne AB, Hawkey CJ. *Immunosuppressive drugs in inflammatory bowel disease: a review of their mechanism of efficacy and place in therapy.* Drugs 1989;38:267-88.
22. Present DH, Korelitz BJ, Wisch N, et al. *Treatment of Crohn's disease with 6-mercaptopurine. A long-term double blind study.* N Engl J Med 1980;302:981-7.
23. Colonna T, Korelitz BJ. *The role of leukopenia in the 6-mercaptopurine-induced remission of refractory Crohn's disease.* Am J Gastroenterol 1994;89:362-6.
24. Present DH. *6-Mercaptopurin and other immunosuppressive agents in the treatment of Crohn's disease and ulcerative colitis.* Gastroenterol Clin North Am 1989;18:57-71.
25. Miller LC, Cohen SE, Orencole SG. *Interleukin-1 is structurally related to dihydrofolate reductase: effects of methotrexate on IL-1.* Lymphokine Res 1988;7:272.
26. Feagan BG, Rochon J, Fedorak RN. *Methotrexate for treatment of Crohn's disease.* N Engl J Med 1995;332:292-7.
27. Bendtzen K, Petersen J. *Effects of cyclosporin A (CyA) and methylprenisolone (MP) on the immune response. T-cell activating factor 1 (Il-1) abrogates CyA- but not MP-induced suppression of antigen-induced lymphokine production.* Immunol Lett 1982;5:79-82.
28. Brynskov V, Freund L, Rasmussen SN. *A placebo-controlled, double-blind, randomized trial of cyclosporine therapy in active Crohn's disease.* N Engl J Med 1989;321:845-50.
29. Brynskov J, Freund L, Campanini MC, Kampmann JP. *Cyclosporine pharmacokinetics after intravenous and oral administration in patients with Crohn's disease.* Scand J Gastroenterol 1992;27:961-7.
30. Jewell DP, Lennard-Jones JE. *Oral cyclosporine for chronic active Crohn's disease: a multicenter controlled trial. The Cyclosporine Study Group of Great Britain and Ireland.* Eur J Gastroenterol 1994;6:499-505.
31. Hanauer SB, Smith MB. *Rapid closure of Crohn's disease fistulas with continuous intravenous cyclosporin A.* Am J Gastroenterol 1993;88:646-9.
32. Reynolds JC, Treills DR, Abu-Elmagd K, Fung J. *The rationale for FK506 in inflammatory bowel disease.* Can J Gastroenterol 1993;7:208-10.
33. Peppercorn MA. *Is there a role for antibiotics as primary therapy in Crohn's ileitis?* J Clin Gastroenterol 1993;17:235-7.
34. Brandt LJ, Bernstein LH, Boley SJ, Frank MS. *Metronidazole therapy of perineal Crohn's disease: a follow up study.* Gastroenterology 1982;983:383-7.
35. Ursing B, Kamme C. *Metronidazole for Crohn's disease.* Lancet 1975;1:755-7.
36. Ursing B, Lam T, Barany F. *A comparative study of metronidazole and sulfasalazine for active Crohn's disease. The Cooperative Crohn's disease Study in Sweden. II Result.* Gastroenterology 1982;83:550-62.

37. Sutherland L, Singleton J, Sessions J. *Double-blind placebo-controlled trial of metronidazole in Crohn's disease.* Gut 1991;32:1071-5.
38. Norel CE. *Effect of new quinolones on the human gastrointestinal microflora.* Rev Infect Dis 1988;10:5193-6.
39. Solomon MJ, LcLeod RS, O'Connor BI, et al. *Combination ciprofloxacin and metronidazole in severe perianal Crohn's disease.* Can J Gastroenterol 1993;7:571-3.
40. Prantera C, Kihgna A, Zammoni F, et al. *Metronidazole plus ciprofloxacin in the treatment of active refractory Crohn's disease: results of an open study.* J Clin Gastroenterol 1994;19:79-88.
41. Prantera C, Zannoni F, Scribano ML, et al. *An antibiotic regimen for the treatment of active Crohn's disease: randomized, controlled clinical trial of metronidazole plus ciprofloxacin.* Am J Gastroenterol 1996;91:328-32.
42. Pearson DC, May GR, Fick GH. *Azathioprine and 6-mercaptopurine in Crohn's disease: a meta-analysis.* Ann Int Med 1995;122:132-42.
43. Meyers S, Sachar DB. *Medical therapy of Crohn's disease.* In: Kirsner JB, Shorter RG, editors. Inflammatory Bowel Disease. 4th ed. Baltimore: Williams & Wilkins; 1995;695-714.
44. Feagan BG, McDonald JW, Rochon J. *Low-dose cyclosporine for the treatment of Crohn's disease. The Canadian Crohn's Relapse Prevention Trial Investigators.* N Engl J Med 1994;330:1846-51.
45. Sachar DB. *Maintenance therapy in ulcerative colitis and Crohn's disease.* J Clin Gastroenterol 1995;20:117-22.
46. Steinhart HA, Hemphill D, Greenberg R. *Sulphasalazine and mesalazine for maintenance therapy of Crohn's disease. A meta-analysis.* Am J Gastroenterol 1994;89:211-24.
47. Messori A, Brignola C, Trallori G. *Effectiveness of 5-aminosalicylic acid for maintaining remission in patients with Crohn's disease: a meta-analysis.* Am J Gastroenterol 1994; 89:692-8.
48. Gendre JP, Mary JY, Florent C. *Oral mesalamine (Pentasa) as maintenance treatment in Crohn's disease: a multicenter placebo-controlled study. The Group d'Etudes Therapeutiques des Affections Inflammatoires Digestives (GETAID).* Gastroenterology 1993;104:435-9.
49. Modigliani R, Colombel JF, Dupas L. *Mesalamine in Crohn's disease with steroid-induced remission: effect on steroid withdrawal and remission maintenance.* Gastroenterology 1996; 110:688-93.
50. Caprilli R, Andreoli A, Capurso L, et al. *5-ASA in the prevention of Crohn's disease*

*post-operative recurrence. An interim report of the Italian Study Group of the Colon (GISC).* Aliment Pharmacol Ther 1994;8:35-43.

51. Brignola C, Cottone M, Pera A, et al. *Mesalamine in the prevention of endoscopic recurrence after intestinal resection for Crohn's disease. Italian Cooperative Study Group.* Gastroenterology 1995;108:345-49.
52. Mclead RS, Wolff BG, Steinhart AM. *Prophylactic mesalanine treatment decreases post-operative recurrence of Crohn's disease.* Gastroenterology 1995;109:404-13.
53. D'Haens G, Geboes K, Ponette E, et al. *Healing of severe recurrent ileitis with azathioprine therapy in patients with Crohn's disease.* Gastroenterology 1997;112:1475-81.
54. Singleton JW, Hanauer SB, Gitnick GI, et al. *Mesalamine capsules for the treatment of active Crohn's disease: results of a 16-week trial.* Gastroenterology 1993;104:1293-301.
55. Salomon P, Kombluth A, Aisemberg J, et al. *How effective are recurrent drugs for Crohn's disease? A meta-analysis.* J Clin Gastroenterol 1992;14:211-15.
56. Prantera C, Cottone M, Pallone F. *Mesalamine in the treatment of mild to moderate active Crohn's ileitis: results of a randomized, multicenter trial.* Gastroenterology 1999; 116(3):521-6.
57. Dahlberg E, Thalen A, Brattsand R. *Correlation between chemical structure, receptor binding and biological activity in some novel, highly active 16α-acetyl-substituted glucocorticoids.* Mol Pharmacol 1984;25:70-8.
58. Greenberg GR, Feagan BG, Martin F and the Canadian Inflammatory Bowel Disease Study Group. *Oral budesonide for active Crohn's disease.* N Engl J Med 1994;331:836-41.
59. Lofberg R. *Critical review: new steroids for inflammatory bowel disease.* Inflamm Bowel Dis (CCFA Journal) 1995;1:135-41.
60. Fiocchi C. *Inflammatory Bowel Disease: etiology and pathogenesis.* Gastroenterology 1998;115:182-205.
61. Sartor RB. *Cytokines in inflammatory bowel disease.* Gastroenterology 1994;106:533-9.
62. Pallone F, Fais S, Squarcia O, et al. *Activation of peripheral blood and intestinal lymphocytes in Crohn's disease:* in vivo *states of activation and* in vitro *response to stimulation as defined by the expression of early activation antigens.* Gut 1987; 28:745-53.
63. Monteleone G, Biancone L, Marasco R, et al. *Interleukin 12 is expressed and actively released by Crohn's disease intestinal lamina propria mononuclear cells.* Gastroenterology 1997;112:1169-78.
64. Breese EJ, Michie CA, Nicholls SW, et al. *Tumor necrosis factor-α-producing cells in the intestinal mucosa of children with inflammatory bowel disease.* Gastroenterology 1994;106:1455-66.

65. Braegger CP, Nicholls S, Murch SH, et al. *Tumor necrosis factor alpha in stool as a marker of intestinal inflammation.* Lancet 1992;339:89-91.
66. Scallon BJ, Nicholls S, Murch SH, et al. *Chimeric anti-TNF-α and activated immune effector functions.* Cytokine 1995;7:251-9.
67. VanDullemen HMN, VanDeventer SJH, Hommes DW, et al. *Treatment of Crohn's disease with anti-tumor necrosis factor chimeric monoclonal antibody (cA2)* Gastroenterology 1995;109:129-35.
68. Targan SR, Hanauer SB, van Deventer SJH, et al. *A short-term study of chimeric monoclonal antibody (cA2) to tumor necrosis factor α for Crohn's disease.* N Engl J Med 1997;337:1029-35.
69. Baert FJ, D'Haens GR, Peeters M, et al. *Tumor necrosis factor α antibody (Infliximab) therapy profoundly down-regulates the inflammation in Crohn's ileocolitis.* Gastroenterology 1999;116:22-8.
70. Present DH, Rutgeerts MD, Targan S, et al. *Infliximab for the treatment of fistulas in patients with Crohn's disease.* N Engl J Med 1999;340:1398-405.
71. D'Haens G, Van Deventer S, Van Hogezand P. *Endoscopical and histological healing with infliximab anti-tumor necrosis factor antibody in Crohn's disease: a European Multicenter Trial.* Gastroenterology 1999;116(5):1029-34.
72. O'Donoghue DP, Dawson AM, Powell-Tuck J, et al. *Double-blind withdrawal of azathioprine as maintenance treatment of Crohn's disease.* Lancet 1978;2:955-7.
73. Hanauer SB, Meyer S, Sachar DB. *The pharmacology of anti-inflammatory drugs in inflammatory bowel disease.* In: Kirsner JB, Shorter RG, editors. Inflammatory Bowel Disease. 4th ed. Baltimore: Williams & Wilkins; 1995;643-63.
74. Present DH, Meltzer SJ, Krumholz MP, et al. *6-Mercaptopurine in the management of inflammatory bowel disease: short- and long-term toxicity.* Ann Intern Med 1989; 111:8641-9.
75. Belluzzi A, Brignola G, Campieri M, et al. *Effect of enteric-coated fish oil perpetuation in relapses of Crohn's disease.* N Engl J Med 1996;334:1557-60.
76. Rutgeerts O, Hiele M, Geboes K, et al. *Controlled trial of metronidazole treatment for prevention of Crohn's recurrence after ileal resection.* Gastroenterology 1995;108:1617-21.
77. Gorard DA, Hunt JB, Payne-James JJ, et al. *Initial response and subsequent course of Crohn's disease treated with elemental diet or prednisolone.* Gut 1993;34:1198-202.
78. Raouf AF, Hildrey V, Daniel J, et al. *Enteral feeding as sole treatment for Crohn's disease: controlled trial of whole protein versus amino acid based feed and a case study of dietary challenge.* Gut 1991;32:702-7.
79. Griffiths AM, Ohlsson A, Sherman PM, et al. *Meta-analysis of enteral nutrition as a*

*primary treatment of active Crohn's disease.* Gastroenterology 1995;108:1056-67.

80. Lochs H, Steinhart HJ, Kalus-Wentz B, et al. *Comparison of enteral nutrition and drug treatment in active Crohn's disease: results of the European Cooperative Crohn's Disease Study.* IV. Gastroenterology 1991;101:881-8.

*ADDRESS FOR CORRESPONDENCE*

**PALLONE F, MD**
Dipartimento di Medicina Interna
Università di Roma "Tor Vergata"
Via di Tor Vergata 135
00133 Roma Italia
Fax: +39 06 72596934
E-mail: pallone@med.uniroma2.it

# Clinical approach to irritable bowel syndrome
## A six-point management strategy

*WG Thompson*

The Irritable Bowel Syndrome (IBS) affects up to 20% of adults worldwide[1,2]. Most people with the syndrome do not see doctors for it, and most of those that do are managed in primary care. The IBS is more common in women, and women are more likely than men to report their symptoms to doctors. While the IBS is benign, it is chronic and recurrent, and consumes a substantial portion of the health care budget.

The reasons for consulting a General Practitioner (GP) include stress and worry about serious disease. The GP (at least in the UK) refers only a minority of his or her patients (20%) to specialists and the stated reasons include an uncertain diagnosis and an unsatisfied patient[3-5].

Referred patients are less likely to admit to stress, a feature that others have noted to describe those patients who respond poorly to treatment. The cause of IBS is unknown, and no drug or psychological treatment is shown to cure the disease, nor to have a benefit beyond placebo. Therefore, the clinical approach to IBS must be based upon a careful interview, empathy, what is known about the symptoms and their epidemiology, and common sense. The following is a 6-point management strategy (Table 1).

**A six-point management plan for IBS**

- ✓ A positive diagnosis
- ✓ Consideration of the patient's agenda
- ✓ Dietary advice and fibre
- ✓ Strategic use of drugs
- ✓ A graded therapeutic response
- ✓ Continuing care

Table 1

## *A positive diagnosis*

A careful history should disclose the clinical features of the IBS such as those described by the Manning and Rome Criteria (Tables 2 and 3).

### THE MANNING CRITERIA

**Chronic or recurrent abdominal pain for at least 6 months and two or more of:**

1. Abdominal pain relieved with defaecation
2. Abdominal pain associated with more frequent stools
3. Abdominal pain associated with looser stools
4. Abdominal distension
5. Feeling of incomplete evacuation after defaecation
6. Mucus in the stools

Table 2

Reproduced from Manning AP, Thompson WG, Heaton KW, et al.[6]

### ROME II DIAGNOSTIC CRITERIA

**At least 12 weeks, which need not to be consecutive, in the preceding 12 months of abdominal discomfort or pain that has two of three features:**

a. relieved with defaecation; and/or
b. onset associated with a change in the frequency of stool; and/or
c. onset associated with a change in form (appearance) of stool

**Supportive symptoms of IBS:**

a. abnormal stool frequency
b. abnormal stool form (lumpy/hard or loose/watery stool)
c. abnormal stool passage (straining, urgency, or feeling of incomplete evacuation)
d. passage of mucus
e. bloating, or feeling of abdominal distension

Table 3

Reproduced from Thompson WG, Longstreth GF, Drossman DA, et al.[7]

The diagnosis can be safely made if there are no alarm symptoms or physical findings. Alarm symptoms include: intestinal bleeding, fever, weight loss, and anaemia. In a young person, tests are usually unnecessary, but a colon examination is wise in people over 50 years of age or those with risk factors for colon cancer. A small bowel X-ray or ultrasound (US) of the intestines may be done if there is suspicion of Inflammatory Bowel Disease (IBD), as in the case of patients with a family history. In endemic areas it makes sense to search for giardia, although stool examination is notoriously unreliable. A firm diagnosis is especially important in primary care. Uncertainty of diagnosis is a frequent cause for referral to a gastroenterologist. Patients with persistent diarrhoea are more likely to be referred, since there are many specific causes for diarrhoea. Armed with a firm diagnosis, the doctor is in a position to explain the symptoms, and reassure the patient that there is no serious disease. The patient should know that having IBS creates no greater risk of serious disease developing in the future. Reassurance is the cornerstone of treatment, but the patient must also realize that the symptoms are often chronic, or may recur frequently during a lifetime.

*The patient's agenda*

One should then discover why the patient is consulting the doctor. In primary care, the stress and fear of cancer are likely, and the primary care doctor should be at pains to deal with these. A young person with IBS symptoms may not take them seriously until he or she loses a loved-one to colon cancer. Here the objective is clear; reassure the patient that IBS symptoms do not mean cancer. This usually requires a colon examination.

Psychosocial issues, depression, and panic should not be overlooked, since the gut symptoms are unlikely to improve until these are effectively treated. Research also shows that people with IBS often consult their doctor following a stressful life event such as a divorce, loss of employment or death in the family. Such phenomena should be a subject of a sympathetic discussion with the patient.

The specialist may be consulted because the general practitioner is uncertain of the diagnosis. It is, therefore, essential that he or she convince the patient (and the referring doctor) that the diagnosis is IBS. Any required tests should be done promptly, and not repeated unless there is a significant change in the symptoms that suggest new organic disease. Repeated testing undermines confidence in the diagnosis. Most difficult are those unhappy, referred patients who tend not to recognize any relationship of stress to their IBS symptoms. These may have difficulty coping with the symptoms, and are more likely to be referred to specialists. Many of these suffer from a history of abuse, depression or loss. The IBS is unlikely to be better tolerated until the often unspoken, but troublesome patient's agenda is addressed.

*Dietary advice and fibre*

Dietary fibre helps many patients in primary care provided it is in sufficient amount prescribed. It helps constipation, and is a safe, cheap way of eliciting the placebo response. It is most effective for constipation, and patients should be instructed to look for bulkier, more easily passed stools as end-points indicative of an effective dose of fibre. Specialists tend to see "bran failures." A practical approach is to advise patients to start with one tablespoonful of bran with breakfast and add more at lunch and supper until the maximum effect is achieved. He or she should take it good days and bad to try to even out the defaecation response to bulkier stools. Since it takes a few days to achieve a new steady state, changes in dose should be made weekly. If bran is poorly tolerated, a commercial bulking agent such as psyllium may be substituted.

The patient should be advised to minimize gut irritants such as caffeine and alcohol. Artificial sweeteners such as sorbitol, fructose and mannitol have a laxative effect. They are found in "sugar-free" gums, soft drinks and some preservatives. In non-Caucasians, lactose intolerance is likely, but even these can tolerate a modest amount of milk. The risk of lactose intolerance is exaggerated, and one must be careful not to unnecessarily deprive people, especially women, of an important source of calcium.

It goes without saying, that many drugs affect bowel habit and these should be inquired about. Irregular eating habits promote similarly irregular bowel habits, and should be corrected, if practical. Many IBS patients try alternate medicine. Most such treatment is harmless but the doctor should beware of dangerous diets that may seriously impair nutrition, or herbal medicines that contain drugs such as senna in herbal teas.

*Strategic use of drugs*

The large number of drugs promoted for IBS, the national differences in drug approval, and the lack of satisfactory clinical trials bespeak the absence of cure. If an 'approved' drug is used, it should be for a short period and carefully monitored. Once the placebo effect wears off, symptoms will usually resume.

Nevertheless, certain drugs targeted against a specific symptom may be used if it interferes with work or social life. For example, loperamide may be taken strategically for episodes of urgent diarrhoea, or for important occasions which the patient fears may be interrupted by an irresistible urge to attend the toilet. When the pain becomes chronic, and interrupts daily functioning, low dose antidepressant therapy may help. Theoretically, a pre-prandial anticholinergic drug may suppress an overactive, post-prandial gastro-colonic response. We have already discussed the usefulness of dietary fibre in constipation.

None of the existing IBS drugs has a viable rationale. The old idea that IBS symptoms were due to gut spasm has been discredited. A new idea is that the gut is "hypersensitive". This derives largely from studies that indicate that many IBS patients are aware of, and experience rectal pain at lower intrarectal pressures than controls. Moreover, this hypersensitivity may be due to higher nervous centres that control the enteric nervous system. This intriguing notion has led to the development of serotonin agonists and antagonists that are believed to act on these higher centres. Some of these are in advanced stages of clinical development.

*Graded therapeutic response*

It is important to tailor therapy to the patient's needs. In addition to attending to the "hidden agenda", the physician should determine how much the IBS is interfering with a patient's life.

"Mild" patients are usually satisfied by a firm diagnosis, reassurance and some dietary advice.

"Moderately severe" patients usually return and may require more reassurance. Counselling and discussion of psychosocial factors may be necessary. If one symptom, such as diarrhoea seems to be restricting the patient's life, a drug that targets that symptom may help.

The "severely affected or disabled" patient with IBS is often referred to a specialist. Such patients require much time, counselling and reassurance. Some may benefit from psychoactive drugs or the intervention of psychologists, psychiatrists or a pain clinic. Depending upon the resources of the community, special psychological treatment may be tried. These include cognitive behavioural therapy, hypnotherapy, and special relaxation treatments. Naturally, these treatments have not been proven effective by clinical trial, but they are not harmful. They at least provide the close attention that some troubled patients need.

*Continuing care*

Troubled, unsatisfied patients need assurance that help is nearby - a service best provided by a primary care doctor, backed up as needed by a specialist. Such patients are prone to alternative medicines and diets, some of which are harmful. Doctor shopping and multiple referrals should be discouraged, since they usually lead to repeated and unwarranted tests and greater uncertainty about the diagnosis in the patient's mind. The objective here is not cure, but psychosocial support, development of coping skills and normal pursuit of work and play.

## General comments

The future may bring new insights into the nature of IBS, but a cure is not imminent. We simply know too little about the enteric nervous system and gut physiology. We may hope that by serendipity a cause will appear such as Helicobacter pylori did for peptic ulcer. It seems more likely that the IBS will continue for some time to confound investigators and trouble many people. The psychosocial difficulties often associated with the syndrome as it presents to specialists will always be with us. We must consider both the physical and the psychological forces at work to interfere with our patients' functioning and enjoyment of life.

## Summary

Any strategy for managing IBS patients will have to take into account the very great number of people with the condition, most of whom do not consult doctors for it, the hidden agenda of those that do, the lack of a known cause, the consequent absence of cure, and the very great cost of the disorder. This paper proposes a management strategy based on a firm diagnosis, consideration of the patient's agenda, the use of dietary advice, the strategic use of drugs only in resistant cases, a graded therapeutic response and continuing care. Rather than specific treatment, it is the success of the doctor-patient interaction that is most important in the end.

## *References*


1. Thompson WG. *Gut Reactions*. New York: Plenum;1989.
2. Drossman DA, Richter J, Talley NJ, et al. *Functional gastrointestinal disorders*. Boston: Little, Brown;1994.
3. Drossman DA, Thompson WG. *Irritable bowel syndrome: a graduated, multicomponent treatment approach.* Ann Int Med 1992;116:1009-16.
4. Thompson WG. *The irritable bowel syndrome: pathogenesis and management.* Lancet 1993;341:1569-72.
5. Thompson WG, Heaton KW, Smyth GT, Smyth C. *Irritable bowel syndrome in general practice: Prevalence, management and referral.* Gut 1999;45(in press).
6. Manning AP, Thompson WG, Heaton KW et al. *Towards positive diagnosis of the irritable bowel.* Br Med J 1978;2:653-4.
7. Thompson WG, Longstreth GF, Drossman DA, et al. *Functional bowel disorders and functional pain*. Gut 1999;45(Suppl II):II43-II47.


## *Address for correspondence*


**THOMPSON WG, MD, FRCPC**

7 Nesbitt St

Nepean, Ontario K2H 8C4 Canada

Fax: +1 7613 828 7300

E-mail: wgthompson@compuserve.com

# FUNCTIONAL BOWEL DISORDERS IN INFLAMMATORY BOWEL DISEASE

*EJ Irvine*

The Functional Bowel Disorders (FBD) are a group of disorders in which the symptoms are referable to the mid or lower gastrointestinal tract. The symptoms include abdominal pain, bloating or distension and various symptoms of disordered defecation[1]. Irritable Bowel Syndrome (IBS) is the most common FBD, and the others include functional abdominal bloating, functional constipation and functional diarrhea. The FBD, functional abdominal pain and functional anorectal disorders (incontinence, anorectal pain, pelvic floor and sphincter disorders) may be associated with altered gut sensory or motor function with no apparent alteration in the gross, endoscopic or microscopic appearance of the gut[1,2]. In contrast, the Inflammatory Bowel Diseases (IBD), Crohn's disease, ulcerative colitis and indeterminate colitis are chronic inflammatory diseases of the gastrointestinal tract with well defined macroscopic and endoscopic features and the presence of microscopic chronic inflammation[3-5].

Most experienced gastroenterologists have encountered patients with a new diagnosis of IBD who have carried a previous diagnosis of IBS or alternatively have patients with IBD but with limited or no disease activity in the face of substantial symptoms. As many of the symptoms of the functional gut disorders and IBD overlap, this raises two important questions:

1. Is one diagnosis a risk factor for developing the other?
2. Are there other factors which predispose subjects to one or both conditions?

To date, there is no conclusive evidence to answer these questions. However, there is a growing body of evidence to support substantial common pathways in the development of the FBD and IBD. Below, two cases are presented to illustrate some of the features which are discussed later in this report.

*Case A*

Mr. RH, a 32 year old smoker, has been unable to work as a crane operator for 8 years. He was diagnosed to have small bowel Crohn's disease 12 years ago and has had a terminal ileal resection, anastomotic revision and two stricturoplasties of the neoterminal ileum. He claims no response to cholestyramine, 5-ASA, metronidazole, or steroids for symptoms of increased stool frequency and abdominal pain. He developed nausea on 6-mercaptopurine. He has been narcotic dependent in the past, is unable to reduce smoking, and two ileo-colonoscopies 9 months apart revealed healing of small bowel aphthous and linear ulcers following treatment with azathioprine 150 mg/day. A small bowel X-ray is normal. He continues to complain of abdominal pain and loose stools after eating which has prompted several visits to the emergency department. During these visits, he has had a benign abdomen and normal blood work. Fluoxetine has been attempted with no benefit.

*Case B*

Mrs. PH, a 35 year old hospital clerk, presented 5 years ago with a one year history of loose stools and abdominal pain. Imaging and biopsies of the small and large bowel were normal and she responded to trimebutine 200 mg three times daily. Two years later, with increasing pain, looser stools and weight loss, a repeat work-up revealed aggressive stricturing Crohn's disease of the terminal ileum.

## Epidemiology of FBD and IBD

The incidence of IBD is highly variable with the highest incidence in Scandinavia and the United Kingdom for ulcerative colitis at approximately 141/$10^6$ population, and lower rates for Crohn's disease of 62/$10^6$ for females and 41/$10^6$ for males[6]. The U.S. Householder Survey reported that up to 69% of individuals surveyed had symptoms suggestive of at least one FBD with 44.5% having a FBD and 26% a functional anorectal disorder[7]. However, incidence rates for FBD are not well documented[8]. A recent study suggested that the cumulative onset of abdominal pain over a 3 year period was 19.6%, while that for disturbed defecation was 6.1%[9]. Thus, it appears that the incidence of FBD is approximately two orders of magnitude greater than the incidence of IBD. Both IBD and IBS are commonly diagnosed between the ages of 15 and 40. Other FBD and functional abdominal pain also occur commonly in young subjects while functional anorectal disorders are more frequent in an older age group[2]. All, except functional diarrhea, have a female predominance, although this is much more frequent for the FBD than for IBD[7]. As well, there appears to be substantial geographic variability in the incidence and prevalence rates for FBD and IBD[1,6]. This may be due to etiologic factors, to accessibility to health care, to demographic or cultural factors.

## Clinical features

Both FBD and IBD have considerable heterogeneity in their phenotypic presentation. For example, the extent of ulcerative colitis will determine whether patients have constipation, as in proctitis or looser stools with more extensive colitis. Patients with Crohn's colitis may have diarrhea and rectal bleeding, like ulcerative colitis or obstructive symptoms (pain, bloating, nausea, vomiting) or appendicitis-like symptoms. Rectal bleeding generally occurs during episodes of active ulcerative or Crohn's colitis as do night time diarrhea, urgency, tenesmus and incontinence[3,10,11]. Many of these problems are common to both FBD and IBD. Isgar et al. showed that abdominal pain, pain relieved by bowel movements, incomplete evacuation, distension, diarrhea and nausea occurred significantly more frequently in patients with inactive ulcerative colitis than in healthy controls, while frequent or looser stools and constipation were not significantly different between the two groups[12]. Extraintestinal symptoms also occur in both groups, and in IBD series, a consistent figure of approximately 40% of patients has been observed with musculoskeletal, skin, liver or eye inflammation[3]. Maxton et al.[13] noted 36% to 88% of IBS patients had extraintestinal symptoms of disturbed micturition, headaches, backpain and lethargy, almost twice that of IBD patients ($p<0.05$). However, the frequency of extraintestinal symptoms may relate more to the degree of psychological disturbance.

## Risk factors

While the etiologies for FBD and IBD are not well delineated, there are clear similarities in known risk factors for these entities. Based on twin studies, association and linkage studies, there is evidence for familial clustering, congruence of disease type and pattern and the presence of specific genes which increase or decrease the risk of IBD[6,14]. Familial clustering has been suggested in IBS but no genetic association has yet been demonstrated. Environmental risk factors appear to play a role in both FBD and IBD and, in the latter, interactions between genetic and environmental factors appear to be strong. Perinatal infection, bacterial or viral infections, early life influences and thrombogenic factors (smoking and oral contraceptives) may also play a role, in particular as promoters, in the development of Crohn's disease[14]. FBD (especially IBS) have also been shown to follow infectious enteritis and may be more common in patients who are particularly anxious or stressed beforehand[15].

## Natural history

Episodic disease exacerbation and periods of prolonged remission are common in IBD[3]. IBD patients who have entered remission and are followed for a year on placebo will experience a relapse rate of approximately 60%[16]. Multiple factors including previous duration of remission, drug or surgery induction, extent of disease, clinical features, biological activity and use of tobacco all affect the duration of remission. Factors such as enteric or respiratory infection, use of non-steroidal anti-inflammatory drugs may provoke an exacerbation. Stress also appears to play a role in producing disease exacerbations.

Factors predicting the natural history of FBD are less well worked out. Nevertheless, certain dietary components may worsen symptoms (such as fiber increasing pain, bloating, diarrhea), medications, alcohol, caffeine, tobacco, chronic stress, and psychological factors[17]. Allergic reactions have been proposed in subgroups of patients with IBD or FBD as playing a causative role in symptoms[18].

## Pathophysiology

There are well-defined changes in the function of the gut epithelium, immune cells, neuromuscular function and in interactions between the central, autonomic and enteric nervous systems which control these functions in both IBD and FBD[19].

Both basal and meal-stimulated colonic motility as well as sensory perception are altered in IBD[20] and are similar to changes found in patients with IBS[21]. Some patients with functional constipation appear to have delayed intestinal transit, while those with diarrhea have rapid gut transit[22,23]. Studies in animal models of inflammation suggest an increased muscle contractility in the small bowel and a decreased muscle contractility in the large bowel which appears to be T-lymphocyte dependent. As well, changes in neurotransmitter profiles occur following inflammation which correlate well with changes in cytokine profiles[20]. These residual changes may explain the colonic hyper-responsiveness or reactivation of inflammation noted in the rat following imposed stress[24].

Heightened perception due to altered afferent nerve function throughout the gut could explain the predominance of pain in some of the FBD and in IBD and may also explain the increased gut responses to stimuli such as food, bile acids, physical and psychological stress[1,25, 26]. Studies of psychosocial function suggest that there is an increased history of psychological disturbance, particularly depression and anxiety, as well as physical and sexual abuse in subjects seeking healthcare for FBD[27]. The perception of symptoms of similar severity appears to be greater in patients with IBS than with IBD[28]. However, a few small studies in IBD suggest that there is an increased perception of symptom severity which correlates with daily stress and an increased functional disability in the presence of psychiatric disorders[28,29].

## Therapy

A discussion of the therapy of IBD and FBD is beyond the scope of this presentation. Nevertheless, in IBD patients, in the absence of obvious endoscopic inflammation, or increased biological markers of disease activity, or other obvious causes of specific symptoms, evidence of psychoneurosis and acute or chronic stress should be sought and treated accordingly. If neither active inflammation or psychopathology is found, patients should be treated symptomatically depending upon the specific symptom profile as for a functional bowel disorder.

In patient A, the use of either anti-depressants, in low dose for pain modulation or relaxation or cognitive behavioral therapy, could be considered together with antidiarrheal agents [27]. In patient B, surgical therapy followed by aggressive anti-inflammatory therapy should be considered. Both patients should be strongly encouraged to stop smoking.

## Summary

Inflammatory bowel disease and functional bowel disorders have considerable overlap in demographic features, symptoms, the phenotypic heterogeneity, multifactorial etiology and pathophysiology (Table 1).

| SIMILARITIES IN IBD AND FBD |
| --- |
| Chronicity |
| Episodic exacerbation |
| Heterogeneous presentation |
| Symptoms |
| Risk factors |
| Altered gut function |
| Altered psychosocial function |
| Supportive therapies |

Table 1

Alterations in gut sensory and motor function have been documented as have perturbations in psychological and social status in both groups of conditions. The functional bowel disorders encompass the irritable bowel sydrome, functional abdominal bloating, functional constipation and functional diarrhea. Functional bowel disorders, functional abdominal pain syndrome and functional anorectal disorders seem to occur in patients with Crohn's disease, ulcerative colitis or indeterminate colitis. For example, irritable bowel syndrome symptoms occur in up to 33% of ulcerative colitis patients in clinical remission, almost five times the rate in healthy controls. Theories of the etiology and risk factors associated with inflammatory bowel disease and functional bowel disorders are surprisingly similar. These include familial clustering, dietary, drug, infection, behavioral factors and chronic stress as triggers of disease. Alterations in epithelial, neuromuscular, immune and psychosocial function occur in both functional bowel disorders and inflammatory bowel disease. Many patients with inflammatory bowel disease carry a prior diagnosis of functional bowel disorders. Others with inflammatory bowel disease have functional bowel disorders symptoms that are more severe than objective evidence of inflammation supports. These observations suggest that inflammatory bowel disease or other inflammatory conditions may predispose subjects to functional bowel disorders. Management of functional bowel disorders-type symptoms in the absence of active disease is often symptom driven, similar to the treatment of functional bowel disorders.

## *References*

1. Thompson WG, Creed F, Drossman DA, et al. *Functional bowel disorders and functional abdominal pain*. Gastroenterol Int 1992;5:75-91.
2. Whitehead WE. *Functional disorders of the anus and rectum*. In: Drossman DA, Richter JE, Talley NJ, Thompson WG, Corazziari E, Whitehead WE, editors. The Functional Gastrointestintal Disorders. Boston: Little Brown and Company; 1994;217-63.
3. Vermeire S, Peeters M, Rutgeerts P. *The primary diagnosis of inflammatory bowel disease.* In: Campieri M, Bianchi-Porro G, Fiocchi C, Schölmerich J, editors. *Clinical challenges in inflammatory bowel disease: diagnosis, prognosis and treatment.* Dordrecht: Kluwer Academic Publishers; 1998;31-5.

4. Coremans G, Rutgeerts P, Geboes K, et al. *The value of ileoscopy with biopsy in the diagnosis of intestinal Crohn's disease.* Gastrointest Endosc 1984;30:167-72.
5. Pera A, Bellando P, Caldera D, et al. *Colonoscopy in IBD-diagnostic accuracy and proposal of an endoscopic score.* Gastroenterology 1987;92:181-5.
6. Logan RFA. *Inflammatory bowel disease incidence: up, down or unchanged?* Gut 1998;42:309-11.
7. Drossman DA, Li Z, Andreuzzi E, et al. US *Householder survey of functional gastrointestinal disorders. Prevalence, sociodemography and health impact.* Dig Dis Sci 1991;9:1569-80.
8. Locke GR. *The epidemiology of functional gastrointestinal disorders in North America.* Gastroenterol Clin N Am 1996;25:1-19.
9. Talley NJ, Weaver AH, Zinmeister AR, Melton LJ III. *Onset and disappearance of gastrointestinal symptoms and functional gastrointestinal disorders.* Am J Epidemiol 1992;136:165-77.
10. Farmer RG, Hawk WA, Turnbull RB. *Long-term follow-up of patients with Crohn's disease.* Gastroenterology 1985;88:1818-25.
11. Langholz E, Munkholm P, Davidsen M, et al. *Changes in extent of ulcerative colitis. A study on the course and the prognostic factors.* Scand J Gastroenterol 1996;31:260-6.
12. Isgar B, Harman M, Kaye MD, Whorwell PJ. *Symptoms of irritable bowel syndrome in ulcerative colitis in remission.* Gut 1983;24:190-2.
13. Maxton DG, Morris J, Whorwell PJ. *More accurate diagnosis of irritable bowel syndrome by the use of non-colonic symptomatology.* Gut 1991;32:784-6.
14. Russel MGVM, Stockbrugger RW. *Epidemiology of inflammatory bowel disease: an update.* Scand J Gastroenterol 1996;31:417-27.
15. Gwee KA, Graham JC, McKendrick MW, et al. *Psychometric scores and persistence of irritable bowel after infectious diarrhea.* Lancet 1996;347:150-3.
16. Modigliani R. *Definition of patient groups: remission.* In: Campieri M, Bianchi-Porro G, Fiocchi C, Schölmerich J, editors. *Clinical challenges in inflammatory bowel disease: diagnosis, prognosis and treatment.* Dordrecht: Kluwer Academic Publishers; 1998;85-91.
17. Borum ML. *Gastrointestinal diseases in women.* Med Clin N Am 1998;82:21-50.
18. Bischoff SC, Herrmann A, Manns MP. *Prevalence of adverse reactions to food in patients with gastrointestinal disease.* Allergy 1996;51;811-8.
19. Berin MC, Perdue MH. *Effect of psychoneural factors on intestinal epithelial function.* Can J Gastroenterol 1997;11:353-7.
20. Collins SM. *Is the irritable gut an inflamed gut?* Scand J Gastroenterol 1992;27 (Suppl 192):102-5.
21. McKee DP, Quigley EMM. *Intestinal motility in irritable bowel syndrome: is IBS a*

*motility disorder?* Part I. Definition of IBS and colonic motility. Dig Dis Sci 1993;38:1761-72.

22. Vassallo M, Camilleri M, Phillips SF, et al. *Transit through the proximal colon influences stool weight in the irritable bowel syndrome.* Gastroenterology 1992;102:102-8.
23. Stivland T, Camilleri M, Vassallo M, et al. *Scintigraphic measurement of regional gut transit in idiopathic constipation.* Gastroenterology 1991;101:107-15.
24. Collins SM, McHugh K, Jacobson K, et al. *Previous inflammation alters the response of the rat colon to stress.* Gastroenterology 1996;111:1509-15.
25. Mertz H, Naliboff B, Munakata J, et al. *Altered rectal perception is a biological marker of patients with irritable bowel syndrome.* Gastroenterology 1995;109:40-52.
26. Galati JS, McKee DP, Quigley EMM. *Response to intraluminal gas in irritable bowel syndrome. Motility versus perception.* Dig Dis Sci 1995;40:1381-7.
27. Drossman DA, Creed FH, Fava GA, et al. *Psychosocial aspects of the functional gastrointestinal disorders.* Gastroenterol Int 1995;8:47-90.
28. Walker EA, Gelfand MD, Creed F, Katon WJ. *The relationship of current psychiatric disorder to functional disability and distress in patients with inflammatory bowel disease.* Gen Hosp Psychiatry 1996;18:220-9.
29. Garrett VD, Brantley PJ, Jones GN, McKnight GT. *The relation between daily stress and Crohn's disease.* J Behav Med 1991;14:87-96.

*Address for correspondence:*

**IRVINE EJ, MD, FRCP(C), MSc**
4w8-HSC, McMaster University
1200 Main St. West
Hamilton, Ontario L8N3Z5 Canada
Fax: +1 905 521 4957
E-mail: irvinej@fhs.csu.mcmaster.ca

# Approach to the patient with chronic functional constipation

*E Corazziari, D Badiali*

*Definition of functional constipation*

Functional constipation is regarded as a long-standing symptomatic manifestation of abnormal defaecation expressed by either a reduced frequency of bowel movements and/or an altered act of evacuation.

Accordingly the above symptomatic aspects are the essential elements of the Rome diagnostic criteria for functional constipation: two or more of

- ✓ straining at defaecation
- ✓ lumpy and/or hard stools
- ✓ sensation of incomplete evacuation, and/or
- ✓ two or fewer bowel movements in a week[1].

In clinical practice, most of the patients with manifestations of abnormal defaecation complain also, and oftentimes mainly, of abdominal symptoms and/or other constipation-related conditions.

In the Italian Cooperative study on Chronic Constipation[2], the most relevant symptoms referred by patients who self-reported constipation were: abdominal pain and/or distension, flatulence, and headache.

Thus chronic constipation presents clinically as a syndrome the core of which is represented by two or more of the Rome diagnostic criteria accompanied by none, one, or more, other symptom(s).

*Prevalence*

Prevalence of functional constipation varies with the different definitions used and in the different populations investigated.

Prevalence of functional constipation, on the basis of undefined, self-reported, complaints of the disturbance is about 20% of the general population[3,4].

The condition increases with age[5,6] and is more frequent in adult females than adult males[7].

Using the Rome diagnostic criteria that take into consideration reduced bowel frequency and/or impaired defaecation, the mean prevalence of functional constipation was 3.0% in a US national householder survey, varying from 2.4% in adult males to 4.8% in adult females[8].
In an Italian nationwide survey[9] constipation, defined on reduced bowel frequency and on paediatric diagnosis, showed a prevalence of about 10% of children.

*Health status*
Functional constipation may affect health status to variable degrees.
Abdominal, and even more gynaecological, surgery is more frequently performed in constipated than in normal subjects.
Constipated patients have an increased prevalence of chronic illnesses and an increased use of non-laxative medications. Only 22.9% of chronic constipated patients have ever seen a doctor and most of them have sought medical advice for non-gastrointestinal symptoms[8].
Despite the low request for medical health care for constipation, about 13% of these patients may feel too sick to perform working activities and the days missed from work or school for constipation averages 22 per year[8].
Furthermore, 30% of chronic constipated patients are habitual consumers of laxatives that increase bowel frequency but do not improve general well-being, abdominal or extra-abdominal symptoms and may induce from negligible to serious side-effects[6].
Score evaluation for Quality of life (QoL) is lower in patients with functional constipation than in healthy controls.
QoL may differ markedly from patient to patient. QoL appears to be inversely related to the severity of bowel dysfunction, such as the feeling of incomplete evacuation and tenesmus, and to the severity of constipation-related symptoms such as abdominal pain, nausea, vomiting. It would also appear that an objective delay in gastrointestinal transit plays an important role in reducing QoL[10] but this observation has not been confirmed[11].

*Co-morbid conditions*
The high rate of familial cases suggests that functional constipation may

be a genetic disorder, but environmental factors, such as parental behaviour and lifestyle, appear to play a substantial role in causing and maintaining the disorder[2,12,13]. A low ratio between the number of family members and house rooms which limits privacy and toilet availability is associated with a reduced bowel frequency in children[9].
Patients with constipation frequently have psychological disturbances[5,14] and there is evidence that symptoms of depression may be considered as an independent risk factor for constipation[3]. Eating behaviour disorders may also be associated with chronic constipation.
Conflicting data have been reported concerning the relationship between psychological disorders and the different types of constipation. Wald et al[15] indicated that only patients with normal gastrointestinal transit, as opposed to patients with prolonged transit, show psychological disturbances.

## Diagnostic approach

*First visit*
A circumstantial and detailed clinical interview together with a rectoanal examination are of great importance for the physician to reach at least six goals when a patient complaining of constipation first comes for medical advise.

1. To establish a trusting doctor-patient relationship
2. To determine the onset and the subsequent development of the clinical condition
3. To find out why the patient decided to seek medical advice, if in the presence of a long-standing clinical condition
4. To evaluate the many cofactors: psychological, environmental, dietary, behavioural, comorbid, which usually contribute, alone or in combination, to the clinical condition.
5. To look for the presence of faecal impaction or other rectoanal disorders.
6. To find out whether the patient's complaints match the operational definition of constipation and deserve further diagnostic investigations.

*Diagnostic investigations*

Diagnostic investigations are indicated because the presence of symptoms complying with the definition of constipation do not offer any clue as to the aetiology, pathophysiologic mechanism(s) or severity of the disorder.

Metabolic assessment and morphological investigation of the large bowel are initially performed to evaluate possible organic causes of constipation.

In those patients who have been taking laxatives, detailed assessment of their use and of the possible occurrence of side-effects should be made. The chronic use of laxatives and enemas is a complex issue that often interferes with the diagnosis and treatment of constipation and with the patient-doctor relationship itself. The continuous use of laxatives and/or enemas does not enable the patient to provide indications concerning spontaneous bowel habits, as to stool consistency, and straining pattern. The doctor thus remains uncertain whether the patient is constipated but could anyway manage his/her disorder with less, or even without, laxatives or whether he/she is not at all constipated and thus the lack of urge to defaecate, which follows the laxative-induced bowel emptying, is the only affliction of the patient. A diary in which the patient is instructed to report bowel frequency, stool consistency, straining pattern, as well as other relevant symptoms while off laxatives/enemas would be useful to evaluate the patient's spontaneous complaints[16]. Some, especially elderly, patients, however, may object to staying off laxatives or may offer opposition to other types of treatment and this behaviour may even give rise to a patient-doctor conflict.

Although the excessive use of laxatives may cause relevant side effects, there are no hard data to support the widespread belief that laxatives per se are detrimental and should be avoided at all costs. This widespread and deep-rooted belief may affect both the patient's and the doctor's behaviour.

Some patients may feel guilty for having used laxatives/enemas and look for alternative treatments that might not be as successful or can be frustrated by doctors prescribing other types of laxatives. It is also possible that, for the same belief, the doctor may oppose the use of laxatives that the patient has been using profitably and without side-effects. The above-mentioned behaviours may lead to a conflictual relationship between the patient and his/her physician. A practical and constructive approach is for the doctor to offer suggestions and indications on the use, if any, of laxatives /enemas, taking into account the patient's cultural attitude on bowel emptying and habits on the use of laxatives.

Functional tests of the colon, rectum and anus may be helpful to assess the pathophysiologic mechanism(s) of chronic constipation. Assessment of the segmental large bowel transit time is of value to identify whether and in which part of the large bowel there is faecal retention[17]. According to results of this investigation, patients can be classified into four subtypes:

1. with normal transit
2. with slow colonic transit
3. with slow rectal transit
4. with slow rectal and colonic transit.

Anorectal manometry, defaecography, and electromyography of the anal and pelvic floor muscles[18,19] may be indicated in those patients with normal transit or slow rectal transit in whom a defaecatory dysfunction may be found. Manometry of the colon is indicated in those patients with slow colonic transit who do not respond to dietary and laxative treatment (severe constipation).

## Therapeutic approach

### *General measures*

Treatment of functional constipation is based, in all cases, on a good patient-doctor relationship as well as patient's education. It is necessary to carefully study the patient's history to check dietary and/or behavioural habits possibly responsible for constipation. Fibre intake correlates with faecal output and transit through the large bowel. A low intake of fibre should be modified either by increasing the amount of vegetables to reach at least 15-18 g of dietary fibres and/or by adding fibre integrators (bran, psyllium, etc.) with adequate intake of water (1500 ml/day). Bulking agents accelerate large bowel transit, and increase frequency of bowel movements. It is likely that intraluminal distention secondary to bulking agents, speeds up the large bowel transit by eliciting propulsive and/or inhibiting segmenting contractions. Bulking agents are generally recommended as a first therapeutic step in chronic constipation but not all patients benefit from them. Patients with slow rectal transit may not be responsive to bulking agents[20] and furthermore, patient's compliance to bulking agents may be reduced due either to palatability and/or bloating.

Some subjects may ignore or defer the call to evacuate because of lack of time and/or suitable toilet facilities. In this condition, it may be useful to retrain bowel habits by attempting to empty the bowel in a favourable setting, possibly in a mentally and physically relaxed state, and after a meal in order to take advantage of the gastro-colonic response.

Some patients believe it is necessary to evacuate daily or more than once/day. Others, with normal bowel habits, believe that symptoms such as abdominal bloating and/or pain, nausea, headache will improve with more frequent evacuations. These subjects may interpret their symptoms as due to inadequate bowel emptying and use laxatives chronically, with no improvement in abdominal symptoms that, on the contrary, may even be made worse by laxatives. These patients should be informed about normal bowel frequency and the origin of their symptoms that are not caused by constipation.

Some patients report a distressing need to evacuate repeatedly for any minimal amount of faeces retained in the rectum. This type of problem is usually associated with an obsessive-compulsive behaviour and is interpreted by the patients as constipation. In these patients and in those complaining mainly of pain and/or bloating, low dose trycyclic antidepressants may be helpful[5,21].

In those patients in the habit of continuously using laxatives, it is advisable to assess bowel movements and to perform functional tests during a laxative-free period.

### *Normal transit and normal anorectal function*

Patients with normal intestinal transit and normal anorectal function may only need reassurance, education about bowel physiology and symptom interpretation and, if necessary, dietary advice with fibre supplementation.

*Slow colonic transit* (Figure 1)
With bran treatment (30 g/die) transit time and frequency of bowel movements may return to normal in patients with slow colonic transit constipation[20].

Figure 1

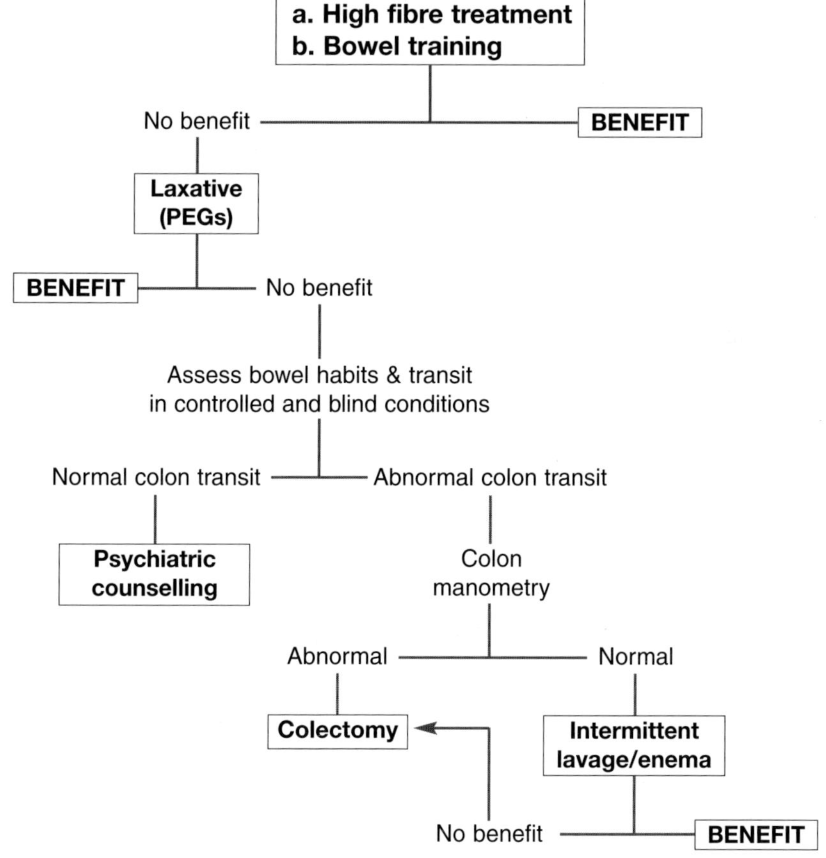


**PEGs** Polyethylene glycol solution.

Possible diagnostic-therapeutic algorithm in constipated patients with slow colon transit.

A subgroup of patients with slow transit through the colon may be unresponsive to bulking agents, and, in these subjects, a trial with oral laxatives should be attempted.

Those patients who still complain of the impossibility to empty the bowel despite laxatives should have their bowel frequency and intestinal transit assessed after blind administration of radiopaque markers. This blind evaluation may require hospital admission in order to control ingestion of disguised markers and bowel emptying as well as to perform radiographic assessment, with the patient being unaware of the test[22]. In these conditions, if markers are not evacuated spontaneously, bowel emptying and marker transit should be assessed after oral administration of one litre, or more, of isosmotic polyethylene glycol solution (PEGs).

In those patients refractory to any conservative, even aggressive, approach, surgical treatment with colectomy and ileo-rectum anastomosis, should be taken into consideration. These are often young women with a depressive syndrome, and absence of colonic motor activity; before surgery, it is necessary to assess whether motor abnormalities affect the stomach and/or the small bowel and whether a condition of marked psychopathology is also present[23].

The Malone antegrade colonic enema through a non-refluxing appendicular stoma may offer a valid alternative to colectomy[24]. However, the Malone procedure is associated with a high failure rate when used in neurologic constipated adults[25]; it may not be successful in patients with obstructed defaecation and severe constipation.

*Rectal faecal impaction and megarectum*

Slow transit through the rectum can lead to faecal impaction and megarectum. In this condition, which is frequent both in children and the elderly, rectal impaction must first be removed using either oral administration of PEGs[26-28] or iso- or hyper-osmotic enemas (2000 ml/die until satisfactory emptying of the large bowel has been achieved)[29]; effects may be enhanced by prior administration of mineral oil per rectum.

Treatment is then based on scheduled bowel evacuations, bowel habit retraining with regular use of laxatives and/or anorectal biofeedback[30].

In children and non-cooperative patients, large daily doses of oral laxatives can be used.

*Anorectal dysfunction* (Figure 2)

In normal conditions, evacuation is the result of the synergism between the contraction of abdominal muscles and appropriate inhibition of the pelvic floor triggered by the arrival of adequate amounts of faeces in the rectum that elicit the urge to defaecate. Hard and pellety stools, impairment of rectal sensation and/or lack of relaxation or paradoxical contraction of the external anal sphincter and puborectalis during straining (pelvic floor dyssynergia) can impede evacuation[31].

Figure 2

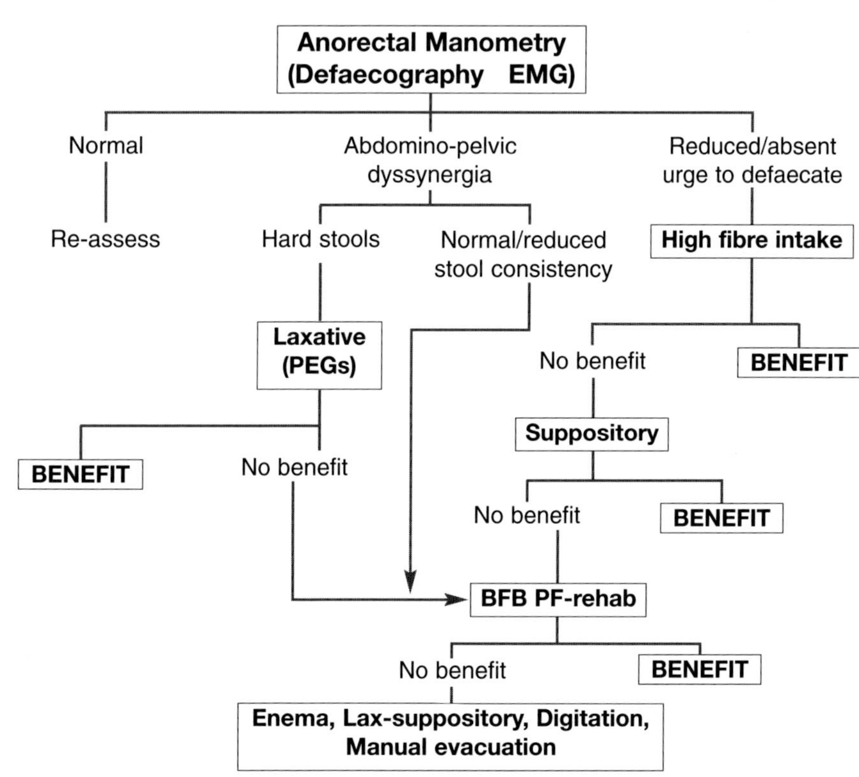


**EMG** Electromyography **PEGs** Polyethylene glycol solution **BFB** Biofeedback **PF-rehab** Pelvic Floor rehabilitation.

Possible diagnostic-therapeutic algorithm in constipated patients with either slow rectal transit or normal transit.

Treatment of these anorectal dysfunctions is based on biofeedback and bowel habit training once stools have been brought to within normal consistency[32].

When perception of the stimulus to defaecate is reduced, prescription of a high residue diet, integrated with additional fibre supplements, may be required to increase stool volume so that efficient rectal distension may more rapidly reach the threshold of rectal perception triggering defaecation. Bowel habit training consists in attempting to open the bowels after a meal, either spontaneously or using a defaecatory stimulus; it is aimed to induce defaecation, at regular time intervals and to avoid rectal impaction.

If patients are unresponsive to fibre supplementation a glycerine suppository can be added in order to train the bowel by inducing defaecation at regular time intervals.

If stools are still hard and pellety, it may be useful to give a low daily dosage of isosmotic PEGs to reduce faecal consistency[33].

In patients with low rectal sensitivity and in those with proven abdomino-pelvic dyssynergia, biofeedback and other rehabilitative measures should be attempted in order to improve rectal sensitivity and synergism between the abdominal wall contraction and pelvic floor relaxation.

*Psychological disturbances*

When symptoms of constipation are believed to be caused by, or associated with, psychosocial conditions, the patient may require psychological counselling.

The presence of a psychological disorder should be suspected when patients deny bowel emptying, when complaints are not proportional to the objective finding of the functional tests, when abdominal pain or bloating or defaecatory disturbances are continuous, unrelated to bowel emptying and do not improve irrespectively of treatment.

Psychological support is also needed in those patients with eating behaviour disorders.

*Drug treatment*

Although the long-term treatment of chronic constipation with oral or rectal laxatives is generally discouraged, there are conditions for which their continued use is necessary:

1. patients who need to avoid straining (cardiac disease etc)
2. patients not responding to other conservative treatments and for whom surgery is not possible
3. patients with cognitive or physical impairment which interferes with self-toileting.

Both stimulant and osmotic laxatives facilitate evacuation by softening stool consistency and/or speeding bowel transit. Laxatives must be chosen bearing in mind possible side-effects, patient compliance and long-term efficacy. Prescription is aimed at obtaining adequate voiding of the bowel, preventing colo-rectal impaction, without causing diarrhoea and other side-effects, which are rarely reported[34]. Of the available stimulant laxatives, it may be recommended to use the non absorbable type in order to lessen the risk of side-effects. Stimulant and/or hyperosmotic laxatives should be administered 2-3 times/week; however, their effect may wear off in the long-term treatment. Non-purging daily dose (125-500 ml) of isoosmotic PEG electrolyte balanced solutions can profitably be used for long-term treatment since the therapeutic efficacy is maintained with few side-effects[34].
Prokinetic drugs such as cisapride that increase motor activity of the colon, may be useful in children[36] and in patients with constipation-predominant irritable bowel syndrome[37,38]. More recently $5HT_4$-agonists[39-42] (Tegaserod, Prucalopride) and CCK-antagonists[43] have been reported to improve bowel habits as well other symptoms in constipated patients.

## *References*

1. Thompson WG, Longstreth GF, Drossman DA, et al. *Functional bowel disorders and functional pain.* Gut 1999;45(Suppl II):II43-II47.
2. Corazziari E, Bausano G, Torsoli A et al. *Italian cooperative study on chronic constipation.* In: Wienbeck M, editor. Motility of digestive tract. New York: Raven Press; 1982;523-5.

3. Everhart JE, Go VLW, Johannes RS, et al. *A longitudinal survey of self-reported bowel habits in the United States.* Dig Dis Sci 1989;34:1153-62.
4. Thompson WG, Heaton KW. *Functional bowel disorders in apparently healthy people.* Gastroenterology 1980;79:283-8.
5. Whitehead WE, Drinkwater D, Cheskin LJ, et al. *Constipation in the elderly living at home. Definition, prevalence and relationship to life style and health status* J Am Geriatr. Soc 1989;37:423-9.
6. Corazziari E, Materia E, Bausano G, et al. *Laxative consumption in chronic nonorganic constipation.* J Clin Gastroenterol 1987,9:427-30.
7. Martelli H, Devroede G, Arhan P, Duguay C. *Mechanisms of idiopathic constipation: outlet obstruction.* Gastroenterology 1978;75:623-31.
8. Drossman DA, Li Z, Andruzzi E, et al. *U.S. householder survey of functional gastrointestinal disorders. Prevalence, sociodemography, and health impact.* Dig Dis Sci 1993; 38:1569-80.
9. Corazziari E, Staiano E, Greco L and SIGEP. *Italian national survey on bowel frequency and anorectal disorders in children.* Gastroenterology 1994;106:A481.
10. Glia A, Lindberg G. *Quality of life in patients with different types of functional constipation.* Scand J Gastroenterol 1997;32:1083-9.
11. Pace F, Molteni G, Bollani S, et al. *Psychological state, life events and quality of life in patients with inflammatory bowel disease or irritable bowel syndrome.* NeUroGastroenterologia; 1998; 4 (Suppl):88.
12. Bellman MM. *Studies on encopresis.* Acta Paed Scand 1996; 56(Suppl 170):1-151.
13. Federici A, Mangia M, Bausano G. *Indagine di prevalenza sulla stipsi e il dolore addominale ricorrente nei bambini in età scolare.* NeUroGastroenterologia 1999,4:132-8.
14. Whitehead WE, Chaussade S, Corazziari E, Kumar D. *Report of an international workshop on management of constipation.* Gastroenterol Int 1991;4:99-113.
15. Wald A, Hinds JP, Caruana B. *Psychological and physiological characteristics of patients with severe idiopathic constipation.* Gastroenterology 1983;97:932-7.
16. Wald A, Whitehead WE. *AGA technical review on anorectal testing techniques.* Gastroenterology 1999;116:735-60.
17. Corazziari E, Dani S, Pozzessere C, et al. *Colonic segmental transit time in non-organic constipation.* Rend Gastroenterol 1975;7:67-9.
18. Wald A, Caruana BJ, Freimainis MG, et al. *Contributions of evacuation proctography and anorectal manometry to evaluation of adults with constipation and defecatory difficult.* Dig Dis Sci 1990;35:481-7.
19. Jorge JMN, Wexner SD, Ger GC, et al. *Cinedefecography and electromyography in the diagnosis of non-relaxing puborectalis syndrome.* Dis Colon Rectum 1993;36:668-76.

20. Badiali D, Corazziari E, Habib FI, et al. *The effect of wheat bran in the treatment of chronic non-organic constipation. A double-blind controlled trial.* Dig Dis Sci 1995;40:349-56.
21. Cadau G, Pallotta N, Badiali D, Corazziari E. *L'impiego degli antidepressivi triciclici a basso dosaggio nel trattamento dei disturbi funzionali del tratto gastrointestinale superiore e inferiore.* NeUroGastroenterologia 1998,4:16-20.
22. Costa E, Biondi M, Badiali D, et al. *Caso Clinico. Stipsi cronica: reale, fittizia o simulata? Diagnosi con misurazione in cieco dei tempi di transito.* NeUroGastroenterologia 1997, 3:114-7.
23. Wexner SD, Daniel N, Jagelman DG. *Colectomy for constipation: physiologic investigation is the key to success.* Dis Colon Rectum 1991;34:851-6.
24. Krogh K, Laurberg S. *Malone antegrade continence enema for faecal incontinence and constipation in adults.* Br J Surg 1998;85:974-7.
25. Gerharz EW, Vik V, Webb G, et al. *The value of MACE (Malone antegrade colonic enema) procedure in adult patients.* J Am Coll Surg 1997;185:544-7.
26. Puxty JA, Fox RA. *Golytely: a new approach to fecal impaction in old age.* Age Ageing 1986,15:182-4.
27. Tolia V, Lin CH, Elitsur Y. *A prospective randomized study with mineral oil and lavage solution for treatment of fecal impaction in children.* Aliment Pharmacol Ther 1993,7:523-9.
28. Ferguson A, Culbert H, Gillet H, Barras N. *New PEG/electrolyte solution for the treatment of constipation and fecal impaction.* Ital J Gastroenterol Hepatol 1999; (in press).
29. Cucchiara S, Coremans G, Staiano A, et al. *Gastrointestinal transit time and anorectal manometry in children with fecal soiling.* J Pediatr Gastroenterol Nutr 1984;3:545-50.
30. Loening-Baucke V. *Constipation in children.* In: MA Kamm and JJ Lennard-Jones editors, Constipation. Petersfield (UK) and Bristol (USA), Wrightson Biomedical Publishing LTD; 1994;361-8
31. Kuijpers HC, Bleienberg G, De Moiree H. *The spastic pelvic floor syndrome. Large bowel outlet obstruction caused by pelvic floor dysfunction: a radiologic study.* Int J Colorectal Dis 1986;1:44-8.
32. Rao SSC, Kimberly DW, Retta EP. *Effects of biofeedback therapy on anorectal function in obstructive defecation.* Dig Dis Sci 1997;42:2197-205.
33. Corazziari E, Badiali E, Habib FI, et al. *Small volume isosmotic PEG electrolyte balanced solution in the treatment of chronic non-organic constipation.* Dig Dis Sci 1996; 41:1636-42.
34. Müller-Lissner SA. *Adverse effects of laxatives: fact and fiction.* Pharmacology 1993;47 (Suppl 1):138-45.

35. Corazziari E, Badiali D, Bazzocchi G, et al. *Long-term efficacy, safety and tolerability of low daily doses of isosmotic PEG electrolyte solution (PMF-100) in the treatment of functional chronic constipation.* Gastroenterology 1999;116:A976.
36. Staiano A, Cucchiara S, Andreotti MR, et al. *Effect of cisapride on chronic idiopathic constipation in children.* Dig Dis Sci 1991;36:733-6.
37. Müller-Lissner SA and the Bavarian Constipation Study Group. *Treatment of chronic constipation with cisapride and placebo.* Gut 1987;28:1033-8.
38. Van Outryve M, Milo R, Toussaint J, Van Eeghem P. *"Prokinetic" treatment of constipation-predominant irritable bowel syndrome: a placebo-controlled study of cisapride.* J Clin Gastroenterol 1991; 3:49- 57.
39. Langaker KJ, Morris D, Pruitt R. et al. *The partial 5-HT4 agonist (HTF 919) improves symptoms in constipation-predominant Irritable Bowel Syndrome (C-IBS).* Digestion 1998;59:S3.
40. Lefkowitz MP, Rüegg P, Shi Y, Dunger-Baldauf C. *Relief of overall GI symptoms and abdominal pain and discomfort as outcome measure in clinical trials of irritable bowel syndrome with HTF 919.* Gastroenterology 1999;116:A1027.
41. Miner PB Jr, Nichols T, Silvers DR, et al. *The efficacy and safety of Prucalopride in patients with chronic constipation.* Gastroenterology 1999;116:A1043.
42 Felt-Bersma RJF, Bouchoucha M, Wurzer H, et al. *Effects of a new enterokinetic drug, Pricalopride, on symptoms of patients with chronic constipation: a double-blind, placebo - controlled, multicenter study in Europe.* Gastroenterology 1999;116:A992.
43. D'Amato M, Whorwell PJ, Thompson DG, et al. *The CCK-A receptor-antagonist dexloxiglumide in the treatment of IBS.* Gastroenterology 1999; 116:A981.


*ADDRESS FOR CORRESPONDENCE*


**CORAZZIARI E, MD**

Dipartimento di Scienze Cliniche
Clinica Medica II
Policlinico Umberto I
00161 Roma Italia
Fax: +39 06 49382437
E-mail: anemgi@mclink.it

# Dyschezia and tenesmus

*SSC Rao*

The term "dyschezia" was first proposed in 1909 by Sir Arthur Hurst in his book, "Constipation and Allied Intestinal Disorders." He used the term dyschezia to describe the "inability to defecate completely." But there are many other definitions. The Dorland's medical dictionary defines dyschezia as "difficult, painful evacuation of feces from the rectum." The gastroenterology textbook by Bockus 1944, defined dyschezia as "constipation due to chronic neglect of a desire to defecate". An international working team defined dyschezia as "difficult defecation occurring on at least 25% of bowel movements over a period of at least 3 months"[1]. In my view, a more appropriate definition for dyschezia is "a chronic inability to evacuate or difficulty with defecation."

In reality, "dyschezia" is an artificial, confusing and poorly understood term. Most patients never use it and most physicians either use this inappropriately or are unclear as to what it really means. Consequently, at a recent international experts meeting in Rome[2], it has been proposed that this term should be abandoned in favor of simpler and more definitive descriptions of altered bowel function (see below/under Clinical presentation). In contrast, tenesmus describes "painful, and often, ineffectual effort to defecate." These and many other bowel symptoms are commonly lumped by patients and physicians under the umbrella term "constipation". Therefore, in a given patient, it is the responsibility of the physician to determine the exact nature of bowel dysfunction. The overriding issue is can we distinguish patients with anorectal or pelvic floor disorders from those with generalized colonic dysfunction purely on the basis of the aforementioned symptoms. In clinical practice, we find that it is often difficult to make this distinction.

## Epidemiology

In the general population, the prevalence of symptoms associated with defecatory dysfunction varies between 10 to 20%[3,4] with a two-to three-fold higher prevalence in the elderly[4]. In a large study, it was reported that symptoms suggestive of dyschezia were present in 13.8% of the population[4]. But only 13% sought medical help. In contrast, the prevalence of Irritable Bowel Syndrome (IBS) was 11.5% and 46% of these patients visited a physician[3]. What are the reasons for this discrepancy?

- Patient behavior: it is possible that patients with defecatory dysfunction do not belong to the "health care seeking" category or they believe either from self-experience or those of friends and relatives that physicians do not have good remedies for their problem
- Illness behavior: this refers to the nature of illness itself, i.e., the lack of life threatening or alarm symptoms such as weight loss, protracted pain or bleeding; and
- Physician's behavior: this refers to a lack of adequate training and awareness among physicians about recent developments in the pathophysiology and treatment of defecation disorders and, to some extent, either a lack of interest or a lack of empathy for these problems.

Whatever the reason, the fact remains that a majority of these patients suffer silently.

## Clinical presentation

Patients with defecation problems present with a variety of symptoms (Table 1).

**BOWEL SYMPTOMS**

- ✓ Tenesmus
- ✓ Feeling of incomplete evacuation
- ✓ Excessive straining (prolonged time in rest-room)
- ✓ Hard stools
- ✓ Digital disimpaction/vaginal splinting
- ✓ Proctalgia fugax/levator ani syndrome
- ✓ Lump-like sensation or perianal heaviness
- ✓ Dyschezia

Table 1

Often, most do not volunteer their symptoms but require prodding. Not uncommonly, they misrepresent their symptoms. For example, digital disimpaction of stool or vaginal splinting to facilitate defecation are symptoms that patients do not readily describe. But, by establishing a trustworthy relationship, it is often possible to unearth the nature of bowel disturbance. It is essential to determine the precise symptom or constellation of symptoms, because only then can a physician approach the investigations or treatment of this problem more rationally.

## Pathophysiology

Three important factors may play a role (Figure 1).
In a given patient one or more factors may play a role and there could be a significant overlap.

Figure 1

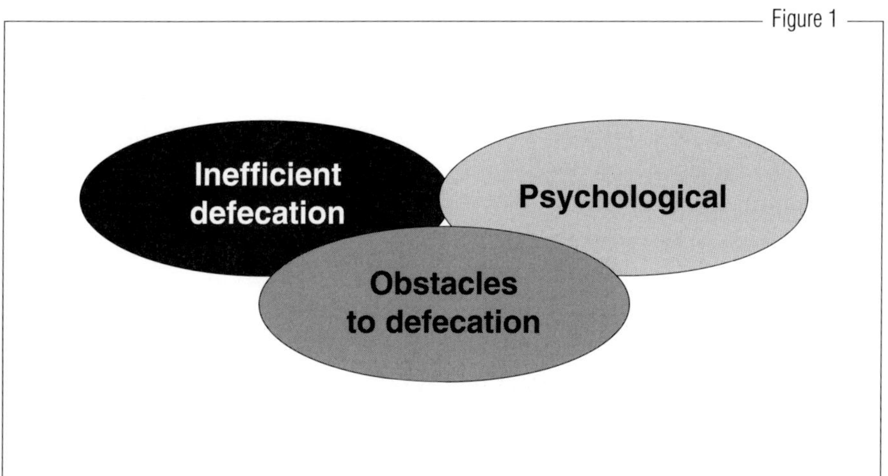


Pathophysiology of dyschezia and tenesmus.

*Inefficient defecation*

Habitual disregard to nature's call can induce a vicious cycle of stool retention, purgation and, eventually, severe constipation. That one can postpone defecation was elegantly demonstrated in a study where normal volunteers were enticed to withhold defecation for as long as possible[5]. During the study period, the stool frequency decreased, and the mean colon transit time increased significantly. Because defecation is a private act, many subjects, particularly kids often tend to avoid defecation in public places such as schools, churches or work places. A strong volitional effort to postpone defecation can lead to fecal stasis. Subsequently, the bulkier and harder stool may not only be difficult to expel but also can overwhelm the rectal and anal capacity to evacuate thus, setting the stage for a chronic defecation disorder.

The "early morning rush"- perhaps a curse of modern civilization - can also play an important role. Recent studies of prolonged colonic motility have shown that waking is associated with a 3-5 fold increase in colonic motor activity[6-8]. In other words, the colon is optimally primed to empty stools in the morning. If the morning hour is preoccupied with other necessities of life, and the individual does not capitalize on nature's call, over time such neglect can lead to significant difficulty with defecation. Dietary factors may also play a role. Infrequent meals, inadequate meals or meals with low fiber content may each cause problems with defecation. Because ingestion of meals stimulates colonic motor activity[9-11], by skipping meals one can deprive the colon of a natural stimulant. Finally, it is well known that 25-30 g/of fiber a day is important to produce stools that are soft and bulky and, therefore, dietary fiber deficiency can lead to dyschezia.

*Obstacles to defecation*

This problem may arise from a variety of structural or functional abnormalities. Common structural abnormalities include the presence of rectocele, hypertensive anal sphincter, hemorrhoids, anal fissure, anorectal growth, mucosal intussusception, rectal prolapse or proctitis. Such conditions are readily diagnosed by most physicians and are appropriately treated. The functional problems are, however, less well recognized and are poorly managed.

Functional abnormalities that cause difficulty with defecation include: dyssynergic defecation (obstructive defecation, pelvic floor dyssynergia, anismus)[12-15], excessive perineal descent, and mucosal intussusception. The volitional act of defecation involves a coordinated effort which consists of intraabdominal and intrarectal pushing forces along with relaxation of the puborectalis and the anal sphincter muscle[16]. Patients with dyssynergic defecation exhibit impaired rectal pushing force, paradoxical anal contraction or inadequate anal relaxation[13,16]. In other words they exhibit poor coordination of the rectoanal muscles that, in turn, leads to incomplete evacuation of stools and fecal stasis.

Solitary rectal ulcer syndrome is a hybrid because, in this condition, there may be structural, functional and self-induced habitual dysfunction of the anorectum. Many of these patients have rectal mucosal intussusception and have a history of prolonged and excessive straining with defecation[17]. Additionally, they may report tenesmus and a history of digital disimpaction of stool[17]. Manometrically, many of these patients exhibit a pattern of obstructive defecation[18,19].

*Psychological*

Patients with defecation disorders have several psychological abnormalities[20-23]. This includes problems such as obsessive compulsive disorder-where the patient believes that having a bowel movement every day or sometimes several times a day is the norm. Consequently, a deviation from this process compels the individual to use laxatives, enemas, suppositories or any other means to induce an unphysiological pattern of bowel movement. These vain attempts eventually fail.

There are others who have a phobia for stool impaction or a delusion about normal bowel habit. Many, particularly children, learn quickly to exploit minor disturbances in defecation as a means of seeking attention[21,22]. This can be driven by psychosocial issues such as interparental, or parental-child conflicts or sibling rivalry. It has also been shown that parental disattachment during childhood can lead to bowel dysfunction in adult life[23]. Patients with bulimia or anorexia nervosa and others with physical or sexual abuse may also develop profound defecatory problems[24].

## Diagnostic evaluation

After a careful history and detailed physical examination, it is essential to perform a systematic evaluation in order to define the underlying pathophysiology. Historical evaluation should be supplemented by symptom and stool diaries for one or two weeks, because a patient's recall of bowel habit is poor[25]. At the bedside, digital examination of the rectum can be very helpful. With the finger in the rectum, the physician must ask the patient to bear down. Normally, this physiological act should produce three changes; an increase in intraabdominal pressure, perineal descent and relaxation of the external anal sphincter[14]. If these changes are present, it would be unlikely that a patient has significant functional obstructive defecation.

On the other hand, absence of these changes would suggest a clinical diagnosis of pelvic floor dysfunction.

Before embarking on physiological testing, it is essential to exclude structural and mucosal abnormalities of the anorectum by performing a proctosigmoidoscopy or flexible sigmoidoscopy. Subsequently, evaluation with anorectal manometry, simulated defecation test, pudendal nerve terminal latency or defecography may prove to be extremely useful in a majority of patients[18,26]. When performing manometry, it is useful to ask the patient to bear down as if to defecate, preferably in the sitting position on a commode. The normal response should consist of a rise in rectal pressure associated with a coordinated relaxation of the external anal sphincter (Figure 2).

Figure 2

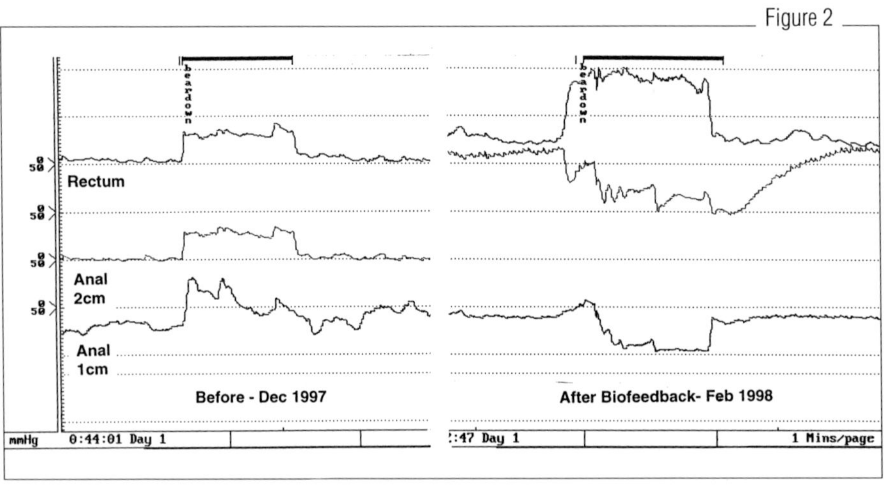


Manometric changes in the rectum and anal canal during simulated defecation in a patient with dyschezia, before and after treatment with biofeedback therapy. Before: "obstructive pattern" of defecation. After: coordinated normal pattern of defecation.

This coordinated movement can be quantified by a simple measure such as the defecation index[13,27]. The normal defecation index is greater than 1.5[13,27]. Defecography may provide new or additional corroborative evidence[28]. For example, it may reveal the inability to activate the pelvic floor and external anal sphincter during defecation, the presence of significant mucosal intussusception, the occurrence of rectal prolapse and the presence of rectocele or enterocele that could interfere with defecation[28,29]. Because no single physiological parameter can reliably diagnose dyssenergic defecation, the presence of at least two or more of the following criteria has been suggested[13,27]:

1. an obstructive pattern of defecation, defined as a paradoxical increase of anal sphincter pressure (Figure 2) or less than 20% relaxation of the resting anal sphincter pressure during straining, as if to have a bowel movement, particularly after inflating a balloon in the rectum with 60 ml air
2. inability to expel a 50 ml water filled balloon within 5 minutes,
3. inability to expel, or greater than 50% retention, of barium during defecography.

## Management of functional defecation disorders

The treatment of functional defecation disorders depends on the underlying pathophysiology.

### *Inefficient defecation*

Patients who ignore nature's call or are preoccupied with the "early morning rush" should be educated about normal colonic function and the need for changing their lifestyle and habits to regulate this important aspect of their body function. Patients with poor posture and inadequate pushing forces can be helped by postural techniques and diaphragmatic breathing exercises[27,30]. Because meal stimulates colonic motor activity[9,10], and recently caffeinated coffee has been shown to stimulate colonic motility[31], it is worth emphasizing the need for consuming an adequate breakfast along with a caffeinated drink, first thing in the morning. Avoiding medications that dessicate stool or impair colonic peristalsis is also important and is often overlooked[32,33].

During habit retraining, it is useful to provide laxatives as an adjunct measure. Saline or osmotic laxatives such as milk of magnesia are preferable over stimulant laxatives[32,33].

*Obstacles to defecation*

If a patient has obstructive defecation or dyssynergic defecation, the best method of treatment is to perform neuromuscular conditioning using biofeedback techniques[13,27,30,31,34-36] There are several methods of performing biofeedback therapy and most centers have reported symptomatic improvement in 60-80% of patients[34,35]. The key element of this training program is to improve rectoanal coordination[13]. Additionally, in those individuals with impaired rectal sensation, sensory conditioning may be performed[13,27,37].

***Maneuvers to improve recto-anal coordination.*** The goal here is to produce a coordinated movement that consists of a rise in abdominal pressure synchronized with relaxation of anal sphincters (Figure 2). This can be performed by placing either an EMG device[35,36] or a manometry catheter[27] into the anorectum, preferably with the patient seated on a commode in front of a monitor[37]. By titrating the degree of abdominal and anal effort to achieve a coordinated movement, the subject instantly learns to improve their defecatory dysfunction. Additionally, it is possible to correct their posture and breathing techniques[37]. If using an EMG device, the goal is to achieve a reduction in the amplitude of the waveforms that depict anal sphincter activity. If using a manometry probe, the goal is to achieve an increase in the intrarectal pressure and simultaneously a decrease in anal resting pressure[27,37]. By distending a balloon in the rectum, and providing a sensation of rectal fullness, it is also possible to enhance the awareness for stooling and facilitate the maneuvers for simulated defecation[27,37].

***Sensory conditioning.*** The goal here is to improve the thresholds for rectal perception by intermittently and repeatedly inflating a balloon in the rectum, and by using progressively smaller volumes of distention. Through a process of trial and error, the patient learns to recognize smaller volumes of inflation, and thereby newer sensory thresholds are established[27,37].

The number of retraining sessions should be customized for each patient and based on the patient's performance and learning ability[27,37]. On average, three to five, one - hour training sessions are required. Patients who splint their vagina or disimpact their stools may also benefit with neuromuscular conditioning[27,30,36].
In the vast majority of patients, rectoceles are unlikely to be a significant source of symptoms. Not surprisingly, surgery is unhelpful[38]. In patients with solitary rectal ulcer syndrome, excessive straining over many years can lead to mucosal intussusception and consequently functional obstruction of the anorectum. Therefore, neuromuscular conditioning can be effective in improving bowel dysfunction, by educating the patient to avoid excessive straining and to coordinate the pelvic floor muscles[18,19]. Painful straining during defecation (tenesmus) can be a consequence of frequently passing small, hard pellet-like stools. These patients may benefit with a high fiber diet, stool softeners, and bulking of stool[32,33] together with education regarding the rectal and anal forces that are involved with defecation.

*Psychological dysfunction*
These patients are best managed in consultation with a psychologist or a psychiatrist. Their inability to defecate is often a somatic manifestation of an underlying psychosocial dysfunction which should be unmasked and appropriately treated[32]. Sexual or physical abuse can have profound effects on pelvic floor function. Many of these patients also present with pelvic pain[40]. The psychological trauma from abuse is deep seated and most patients do not readily admit to this problem. Unless these issues are appropriately dealt with, the physical ailment may prove refractory to treatment. Hence, they are best managed in consultation with a pelvic pain specialist and/or a psychologist[40]. Because many anti-psychotic drugs can adversely affect gut motor and sensory function, they should be used judiciously and their use should be monitored to prevent any worsening of the bowel problem.

## Conclusions

In summary, dyschezia and tenesmus are common symptoms that contribute to chronic bowel dysfunction. Often, they are due to a combination of structural or functional problems of the pelvic floor. Identifying the underlying pathophysiological mechanism(s) such as inefficient defecation, obstacles to defecation or psychosocial dysfunction, usually with the help of detailed history and manometric or radiographic evaluation should facilitate more optimal treatment for these patients. Neuromuscular conditioning and biofeedback therapy can be effective in the management of a majority of these patients[34]. This and other approaches may revolutionize the treatment of these disorders.

## *REFERENCES*


1. Whitehead WE, Devroede G, Habib F et al. *Functional disorders of the anus and rectum.* In: Drossman DA, editor. The Functional Gastrointestinal Disorders. Boston: Little Brown & Company; 1994;217-63.
2. Whitehead WE, Wald A, Diamant N et al. *Functional disorders of the anus and rectum.* Gut 1999 (in press).
3. Drossman DA, Li Z, Andruzzi E et al. *US Householder survey of functional gastrointestinal disorders. Prevalence, sociodemography and health impact.* Dig Dis Sci 1993; 38:1569-80.
4. Talley NJ, O'Keefe EA, Zinsmeister R, Melton LJ III. *Prevalence of gastrointestinal symptoms in the elderly. A population based study.* Gastroenterology 1992;102:895-901.
5. Klauser AG, Voderholzer WA, Heinrich CA, Schindlbeck NE. *Behavior modification of colonic function. Can constipation be learned?* Dig Dis Sci 1990;35:1271-5.
6. Rao SSC, Chamberlain M, Hatfield R et al. *Ambulatory 24 hour colonic motility in health and in patients with constipation.* Gastroenterology 1997;112:A809.
7. Narducci F, Bassotti G, Gaburri M, Morelli A. *Twenty-four hour manometric recordings of colonic motor activity in healthy man.* Gut 1987;28:17-25.
8. Bassotti G, Gaburri, M. *Manometric investigation of high amplitude propagated contractile activity of the human colon.* Am J Physiol 1988; 255:G660-G664.
9. Rao SSC, Hatfield R, Chamberlain M, Stumbo P. *Is the gastrocolonic response influenced by fat or carbohydrate content of a meal?* Gastroenterology 1996;110:A742.
10. Snape WJ, Matarazzo SA, Cohen S. *Effect of eating and gastrointestinal hormones on human colonic myoelectrical and motor activity.* Gastroenterology 1978;75:373-8.

11. Bazzocchi G, Ellis J, Villanueva-Myer J et al. *Postprandial colonic transit and motor activity in chronic constipation.* Gastroenterology 1990; 98:686-93.
12. Preston DM, Lennard-Jones JE. *Anismus in chronic constipation.* Dig Dis Sci 1985;30:413-8.
13. Rao SSC, Happel J. *Obstructive Defecation (O.D.): A failure of recto-anal coordination.* Am J Gastroenterol 1998;93:1042-50.
14. Rao SSC: *Functional colonic and anorectal disorders.* Postgrad Medicine 1995;98:115-25.
15. Wald A. *Colonic and anorectal motility testing in clinical practice.* Am J Gastroenterol 1994;89:2109-15.
16. Rao SSC, Hatfield R, Leistikow J. *Does the rectum generate a pushing force during defecation?* Gastroenterology, 1998;114:G3368.
17. Lam TCF, Lubowski DZ, King DW. *Solitary rectal ulcer syndrome.* Bailliere's Clinical Gastroenterol 1992;6:129-43.
18. Rao SSC, and Patel RS. *How Useful are Manometric Tests of Anorectal Function in the Management of Defecation Disorders.* Am J Gastroenterol 1997; 92:469-75.
19. Vaizey CJ, Roy AJ, Kamm MA. *Biofeedback is an effective treatment for solitary rectal ulcer syndrome.* Gastroenterology 1997;112:A841.
20. Wald A, Hinds JP, Caruanna BJ. *Psychological and physiological characteristics of patients with severe idiopathic constipation.* Gastroenterology 1989;81:879-83.
21. Wald A, Chandra R, Chiponis D, Gabel S. *Anorectal function and continence mechanisms in childhood encopresis.* J Pediatr Gastroenterol Nutr 1986;5:346-351.
22. Hoag JM, Norriss NG, Himeno ET, Jacobs J. *The encopretic child and his family.* J Am Acad Child Psychiatry 1971;10:242-56.
23. Hobbis JCA, Turpin G, Read NW. *Examination of the role of psychosocial factors in the pathogenesis of functional bowel disorders.* Gastroenterology 1995;108:A614.
24. Drossman DA, Leserman J, Nachman G et al. *Sexual and physical abuse in women with functional or organic gastrointestinal disorders.* Ann Intern Med 1990;13:828-33.
25. Ashraf W, Park F, Quigley EMM, Lof J. *An examination of the reliability of reported stool frequency in the diagnosis of idiopathic constipation.* Am J Gastroenterol 1996;91:26-32.
26. Wexner SD, Jorge JMN. *Colorectal physiological tests. Use or abuse of technology?* Eur J Surg 1994;160:167-74.
27. Rao SSC, Welcher KD, Pelsang RE. *Effects of biofeedback therapy on anorectal function in obstructive defecation.* Dig Dis Sci 1997;42:2197-205.
28. Rao SSC, Sun WM. *Current techniques of assessing defecation dynamics.* Dig Dis 1997;15 (Suppl. 1):64-77.

29. Mahieu P. *Defecography. I. Description of a new procedure and results in normal patients.* Gastrointest Radiol 1984:9:247-51.
30. Koutsomanis D, Lennard-Jones JE, Roy AJ, Kamm MA. *Controlled randomized trial of visual biofeedback versus muscle training without a visual display for intractable constipation.* Gut 1995;37:95-9.
31. Rao SSC, Stumbo P, Zimmerman B, Welcher K. *Is coffee a colonic stimulant?* Eur J Gastroenterol Hepatology 1998;10:1113-8.
32. Wald A. *Approach to the patient with constipation.* In: Yamada T, Alpers DH, Owyang C, Powell D, Silverstein F, editors. Textbook of Gastroenterology. Philadelphia: J.B. Lippincott Co.; 1991;779-96.
33. Rao SSC. *Clinical approach to constipation.* In: Gastrointestinal Motility - a multimedia guide. Janssen Pharmaceutica and Research Foundation and Advanced Medical Ventures. Ltd. Pasadena, Ca;1999;79-89.
34. Rao SSC, Enck P, Loening-Baucke V. *Biofeedback therapy for defecation disorders.* Dig Dis 1997; 15:78-92.
35. Bleijenberg G, Kuijpers HC. *Treatment of spastic pelvic floor syndrome with biofeedback.* Dis Colon Rectum 1987;30:108-11.
36. Kawimbe BM, Papachrysostomou M, Binnie NR et al. *Outlet obstruction constipation (anismus) managed by biofeedback.* Gut 1991;32:1175-79.
37. Rao SSC. *The technical aspects of biofeedback therapy for defecation disorders.* The Gastroenterologist 1998;6:96-103.
38. Enck P. *Biofeedback training in disordered defecation: A critical review.* Dig Dis Sci 1993;38:1953-60.
39. Mollen RMHG, vanLaarhoven CJHM, Kuijpers JHC. *Pathogenesis and management of rectoceles.* Seminars in Colon & Rectal Surgery 1996;7:192-6.
40. Rapkin AJ. *Gynecological pain in the clinic: Is there a link with the basic research.* In: Gebhart GF, editor. Visceral Pain. IASP Press; Seattle: 1995;5:469-88.

### *ADDRESS FOR CORRESPONDENCE*

**RAO SSC, MD, PhD, FRCP**
University of Iowa Hospital
College of Medicine Department of Internal Medicine 4612, JCP
200 Hawkins Dr, Iowa City, Iowa 52242 USA
Fax: +1 319 353 6399

# Approach to the patient with faecal incontinence

*F Musial, P Enck*

## Faecal incontinence

The term "Faecal Incontinence" describes a complex of symptoms associated with the uncontrollable loss of smaller or larger volumes of stool. It can occur as faecal soiling or staining of the underwear, but also as the complete inability to voluntarily control the evacuation of the rectum. In our society, incontinence is also a disorder with a strong impact on the patient's personal life, causing shame and insecurity. Therefore, epidemiological data may contain a detection bias leading to the underestimation of the true prevalence of faecal incontinence[1]. According to the few existing studies in the US, UK and Germany, the prevalence of adult-type faecal incontinence ranges between 1% and 6% in the general population. Furthermore, since faecal incontinence is a symptom rather than a diagnosis, it may occur as a consequence of a variety of diseases (Table 1)[2].

These disorders do not have to be associated with urinary or faecal incontinence, however, they may increase the potential risk to develop the symptom if there are other predisposing factors.

The prevalence of faecal and urinary incontinence in elderly people and women is higher, suggesting that age-related alterations of the pelvic floor muscles, the different anatomy in women as well as birth traumas are possible risk factors[3]. In psychiatric and geriatric institutions and in nursing homes, up to 50% of the inhabitants may suffer from faecal incontinence[3,4]. As the variety of disorders which may be associated with incontinence suggests, no single pathomechanism for faecal incontinence exists[5]. The preservation of continence is based upon the correct interplay of muscular (internal and external anal sphincters, puborectal muscle) and sensory (pudendal nerve) functions and their appropriate coordination. Not all of these functions are under central nervous system (CNS) control: only the striated external anal sphincter muscle can be influenced voluntarily. However, any of these functions may be impaired in faecal incontinence. The dysfunctions can be neurological, muscular, inflammatory, traumatic or iatrogenic (Table 2).

## PREVALENCE OF FAECAL INCONTINENCE IN DIFFERENT DISEASES

| Background | Disease/disorder | Prevalence of faecal incontinence |
|---|---|---|
| Gastroenterology | Crohn's disease/ulcerative colitis | 28 - 51% |
| | Diarrhoea | 14 - 20% |
| | Irritable bowel syndrome | 19 - 21% |
| Endocrinology | Diabetes | 7 - 12% |
| Gynaecology | Episiotomy | 16% |
| | Perineal tear | 0.04 - 0.2% |
| Surgery | Excision of anal fistulas | ≤ 10% |
| | Haemorrhoidectomy | ≤ 10% |
| | Rectal prolapse | 20% |
| Neurology | Multiple sclerosis | 50% |

Table 1

Adapted from Enck P, Schäfer R[2].

## POSSIBLE DYSFUNCTIONS ASSOCIATED WITH SYMPTOMS OF FAECAL INCONTINENCE

| Characterisation of faecal incontinence | Suspected dysfunction |
|---|---|
| Urge incontinence | Impaired motor control<br>Muscle defect |
| Involuntary loss of stool during the day | Autonomic neuropathy<br>Cerebral dysfunctions<br>Rectal prolapse |
| Involuntary loss of stool at night<br>Soiling | Autonomic neuropathy (e.g., diabetes)<br>Rectocele<br>Mucosal prolapse<br>Scars in the anal canal |
| Inadequate differentiation of stools and gas | Sensory incontinence (prolapse, scars) |
| Involuntary loss of wind | Lowered tone of the internal anal sphincter |
| Stress incontinence | Impaired innervation (pudendal nerve, spinal, central) |

Table 2

Adapted from Enck P, Schäfer R[2].

Moreover, since anal resting and voluntary anal squeeze pressure are decreased with age and lower in women compared to men[3,6,7], age and gender play an important role in the predisposition to faecal incontinence. Thus, the first step in handling faecal incontinence is the treatment of the underlying disorder. Only if this is not possible or effective, symptomatic treatment may become a goal.

## Diagnostic instruments

### *Anamnesis*

Since faecal incontinence is a socially impairing disorder which often leads to feelings of shame and which may even cause psychological disturbances, most patients feel significantly reduced in their quality of life. Major problems are experienced in professional life and sexuality[8,9]. Anamnesis, therefore, needs to be performed carefully, with empathy and patience in a quiet and neutral atmosphere, and without time stress. The effort is worthwhile since a carefully performed anamnesis can be one of the most powerful diagnostic instruments. We use a semi-standardized interview together with a bowel and eating habits diary, which should be kept for at least one week before the doctor's appointment and for longer periods during treatment[10]. The diaries also leave space to document relevant additional information (medication, sport etc.).

Especially the use of diaries has been helpful. Figure 1 shows a diagram of a one-month diary of a patient with unclear diarrhoea. It turned out that she used a laxative daily without being aware of the fact. After withdrawing the laxative, stool constistency returned to normal and the incontinence disappeared.

The anamnesis should be performed according to the criteria suggested by Engel in 1983[11] and include a careful analysis of the medical history, the characteristics of the problem, and the preceding and contingent factors. Emphasis should not only be placed on the medical history, but also on the psychosocial context, in which the incontinence event occurs. This is especially important in order to evaluate, whether the incontinence event fulfils a social function such as, for example, secondary reinforcement to illness behaviour. This is likely not the most common situation of an incontinent patient, but may play a role in some cases.

Figure 1

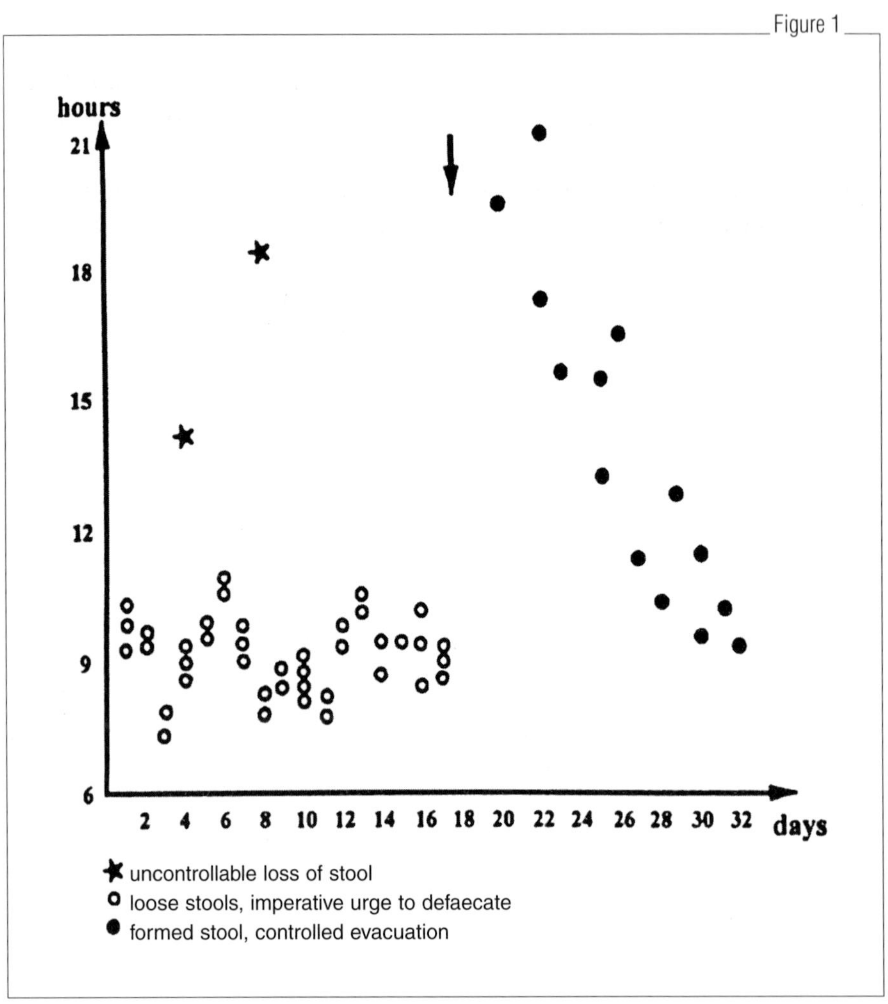


One-month bowel habits diary. Patient used a laxative daily without being aware of it. Arrow marks point where laxative was withdrawn. Loose stools and incontinence improved thereafter.

The most important part of the anamnesis will certainly focus on the medical history and the characteristics of the incontinence event. Medical history should focus on bowel habits trying to identify the type of incontinence, its severity and frequency. Nonetheless, dietary habits may play an important role, especially if incontinence is associated with loose stools or diarrhoea. Possible trauma or surgery of the anorectum, the gynaecologic history with special emphasis on child birth, episiotomies and perianal tears are also important predisposing factors[12]. More than 30% of vaginal first births lead to defects of the anal sphincters, and episiotomies result in faecal incontinence in up to 15% of cases. Haemorrhoidectomies and anal fistula excisions may, like anal traumas, impair sensory discrimination in the anal canal[2, 13].

## Medical examination and diagnostic procedures

Rectoscopy, proctoscopy or even colonoscopy should be the first diagnostic procedures to be carried out. It is important to exclude neoplastic and inflammatory diseases before any additional diagnostic approach is taken. Additional functional testing of the anorectum should include anorectal manometry and defaecography, but may be extended to endoanal ultrasound, and neurophysiological examinations[5,7,14-19].
Important manometric parameters in faecal incontinence are lowered anal resting and squeeze pressures. Other factors of importance are sphincter relaxation after balloon distention and perception of rectal distention stimuli[14]. Defaecography is a dynamic radiological examination with a barium enema. Pictures taken under resting conditions are compared to the dynamic changes during the defaecation process. This procedure allows evaluation of perineal descent and possible changes in anorectal morphology (rectocele, prolapse)[15]. Anal ultrasound is performed with an intra-anal probe and allows evaluation of pelvic floor anatomy, since muscle layers of the internal and external anal sphincter and adjacent structures can easiliy be inspected[16-18]. Electromyographic examination helps to identify nerve dysfunctions and muscle defects of the external sphincter muscle[19]. Table 3 summarizes the suggested diagnostic procedures and their functional relevance (according to[20]).
The major aim of this rather sophisticated diagnostic approach is the exact description of the problem in order to design the most appropriate biofeedback training programme. The evaluation of the diagnostic results may follow the scheme (Figure 2) we use in our outpatient clinic[21]. A patient who shows a decrease in anal resting and squeeze

pressure, unchanged rectal compliance and perception, will most likely benefit from a training programme intended to improve *anal sphincter strength*.

FUNCTIONAL TESTING OF FAECAL INCONTINENCE

| Factors of relevance in faecal incontinence | Manometry | | | | Defaeco-graphy | Ultra-sound | EMG |
|---|---|---|---|---|---|---|---|
| | Anal resting pressure | Anal squeeze pressure | Rectal perception | Rectal compliance | | | |
| ***Anal sphincters*** | | | | | | | |
| Internal | + | | | | | + | |
| External | | + | | | | + | + |
| M. puborectalis | | | | | + | | + |
| ***Rectums*** | | | | | | | |
| Perception | | | + | | | | |
| Compliance | | | | + | | | |
| Reservoir function | | | + | + | + | | |
| Megarectum | | | + | | + | | |
| ***Pelvic floor*** | | | | | | | |
| Perineal descent | | | | | + | | |
| Anorectal angle | | | | | + | | |
| ***Neural*** | | | | | | | |
| Pudendal nerve | | + | | | | | + |

Table 3

Adapted from Wienbeck M, Barnert J[20].

A patient who has appropriate anal resting and squeeze pressures, unchanged rectal compliance, but cannot perceive distending stimuli in the rectum, may benefit from a *sensory discrimination training programme*, directed towards the improvement of rectal sensation. If a patient shows only moderately or no impairment of rectal sensation and good sphincter function, but cannot initiate an appropriate external sphincter contraction as soon as stool arrives in the rectum, a training programme will have to focus on the *coordination of rectal perception and sphincter contraction*.

Patients with gross morphological abnormalities or relevant changes of rectal compliance (e.g., overflow incontinence due to faecal impactation) will most likely not benefit from a biofeedback programme and should first be treated for the underlying disorder or the functional-anatomical deficit. In patients with overflow incontinence, the incontinence may disappear after treatment of constipation. In patients who have undergone surgery, incontinence may be improved but still persistent. These patients may now have a much greater benefit from a biofeedback training programme than before surgical intervention.

Figure 2

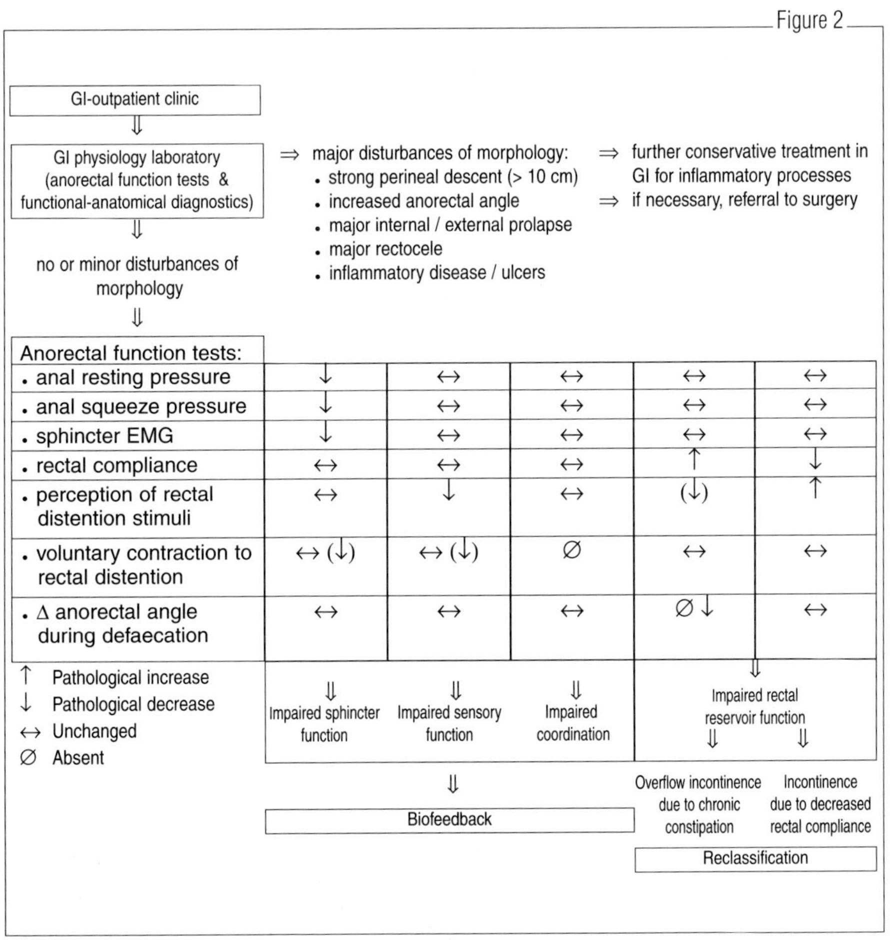


Diagnostic scheme for classification and selection of patients for anorectal biofeedback. Adapted from Musial F, Kalveram KTh, Enck P[21].

## Biofeedback therapy for faecal incontinence

### *What is "biofeedback"?*

The term "biofeedback" describes a therapeutic instrument, which is derived from the "Theory of learning". Its theoretical basis is "learning through reinforcement" in the tradition of Pavlov and Skinner[22]. If a behaviour is followed by reward or punishment, the chance that it is being emitted increases or decreases. This type of learning is also called instrumental learning, type II learning, trial and error learning or operant conditioning. Possible feedbacks are reward or punishment but also knowledge of results[23].

While Skinner and others restricted operant conditioning to observable behaviour, Miller[24] was the first to show that even functions of the autonomic nervous system can be influenced by operant conditioning. In laboratory rats, he used feedback signals from various autonomic systems, like, for example, heart rate or gastrointestinal motility together with CNS stimulation as reinforcement[25]. He was able to show, that the animals were influencing specifically the particular body function that was reinforced, either heart rate or gastrointestinal motility. Thus, he was able to demonstrate, that the learned control over this particular function was specifically directed towards it, and not a generalised effect of the autonomic nervous system[24]. After Miller had proposed this "visceral learning paradigm", it became evident that this technique carried the potential of a variety of applications both in psychology and medicine. Biofeedback is a treatment approach directly derived from Miller's visceral learning paradigm: A body function, which cannot be perceived by the subject under normal conditions is measured by a technical device and shown to the subject. The reinforcer in humans is usually the "knowledge of results", but additional verbal or other positive reinforcement may be helpful under some circumstances.

However, biofeedback is not always the treatment of choice. Before applying a biofeedback programme, possible "rewarding properties of the symptoms"[23] have to be excluded. This means, that if a symptom produces a strong rewarding gain, biofeedback will not be useful. This is the reason why besides the medical history and the current determinants of the symptom, the psychosocial background of the patient has to be an intergral part of the anamnesis. Miller defined four conditions under which biofeedback training is likely to be successful[23]:

1. the medically desirable direction of change is clear
2. when this response is learnable
3. when the desirable learning has been prevented by poor or wrong perception of natural feedback
4. when moment-to-moment measurement can provide prompt artificial feedback that is better than the patient's perception of the natural feedback.

If a successful biofeedback application is available, it is the method of choice, if no low risk, highly effective and less costly medical treatment is available. All these conditions are fulfilled for the three possible types of anorectal biofeedback for faecal incontinence, which is sensory feedback of distention stimuli in the rectum, muscular feedback, which is the feedback of sphincter function, and coordination, which is a combination of both.

*Studies on biofeedback for faecal incontinence*

Kohlenberg was the first investigator able to show improvement of faecal incontinence through biofeedback training[26]. Since then, many studies have evaluated the possible benefits. In 1996, Enck et al.[12] reviewed 15 data-based studies reported in peer-reviewed international journals (see Table 4) which were derived from 11 clinical centres around the world, all of them being either gastroenterological or surgical units or institutions closely associated with them[27-41]. The review focused on biofeedback application in adults with faecal incontinence. Of the 15 studies published, 14 reported a success rate greater than 50%, with efficacy criteria ranging between 75 to 90% improvement in the frequency of incontinence. The overall success (% improved patients) was approximately 70%, supporting the view that even if there are only a few studies incorporating control groups, the effects cannot be attributed to a placebo response alone. In most studies,patients have been followed for up to 2 years after training, but systematic long-term follow-up data have been reported only in one study for 24 patients after 30 months[41]. The authors found an increase in incontinence scores compared to the 6 months' follow-up evaluation and conclude that re-initiation of training may be appropriate for some patients. However, a

5-year follow-up reported by Enck et al.[42] showed that the symptom improvement was maintained even after such a long time.

BIOFEEDBACK STUDIES IN FAECAL INCONTINENCE

| Author, year ref | N. | Age | Range | Sex M:F | Sessions | Control group | Effect (%) |
|---|---|---|---|---|---|---|---|
| Engel et al. 1974[27] | 7 | 40.7 | 6-54 | 5:2 | 1-4 | No | 57 |
| Cerulli et al. 1979[28] | 50 | 46.0 | 5-97 | 36:12 | 1 | No | 72 |
| Goldenberg et al. 1980[29] | 12 | ? | 12-78 | 6:6 | >1 | No | 83 |
| Wald et al. 1981[30] | 17 | 46.9 | 10-79 | 11:6 | 1+1 | Good/poor | 71 |
| Wald et al. 1984[31] | 11 | 52.2 | 25-75 | 8:3 | ? | Manometry only | 73 |
| Latimer et al. 1984[32] | 8 | 30.1 | 8-72 | 4:4 | 8(2/wk) | ABACADA * or ACABADA * | 88 |
| Whitehead et al. 1985[33] | 18 | 72.7 | 65-92 | 15:3 | 8(2/wk) | Behaviour treatment | 77 |
| Buser et al. 1986[34] | 13 | 53.6 | 13-66 | 7:6 | 1-3 | No | 92 |
| MacLeod et al. 1987[35] | 113 | 56.0 | 25-88 | 67:46 | Mean 3.3 | No | 63 |
| Riboli et al. 1988[36] | 21 | 61.0 | 14-84 | 15:6 | 12(2/wk) | Good/poor | 86 |
| Enck et al. 1988[37] | 19 | 47.3 | 10-80 | 10:9 | 5-10 | Manometry only | 63 |
| Loening-Baucke et al. 1990[38] | 8 | 63.0 | 35-78 | 8:0 | 3 | Conventional treatment | 50 |
| Miner et al. 1990[39] | 25 | 54.6 | 17-76 | 17:8 | 3 | 2-arm cross-over | 76 |
| Keck et al. 1994[40] | 15 | 39.0 | 29-65 | 13:2 | Mean 3.0 | No | 73 |
| Guillemot et al. 1995[41] | 24 | 60.7 | 39-78 | 19:5 | ? | Conventional treatment | 68 |

* **A** diary **B** exercise training **C** sensory discrimination training **D** biofeedback training

Table 4

Adapted from Enck P, Schäfer R[12].

## Performance of a biofeedback training session

*Equipment and general preparations*

Biofeedback can be performed with any conventional manometry system. However, some studies suggest, that transcutaneous sphincter electromyography (EMG) is more effective than pressure recordings for sphincter biofeedback[43]. The system used in our hospital (Pelvicheck system, Medicheck GmbH, Essen, Germany) is shown in Figure 3.

Figure 3

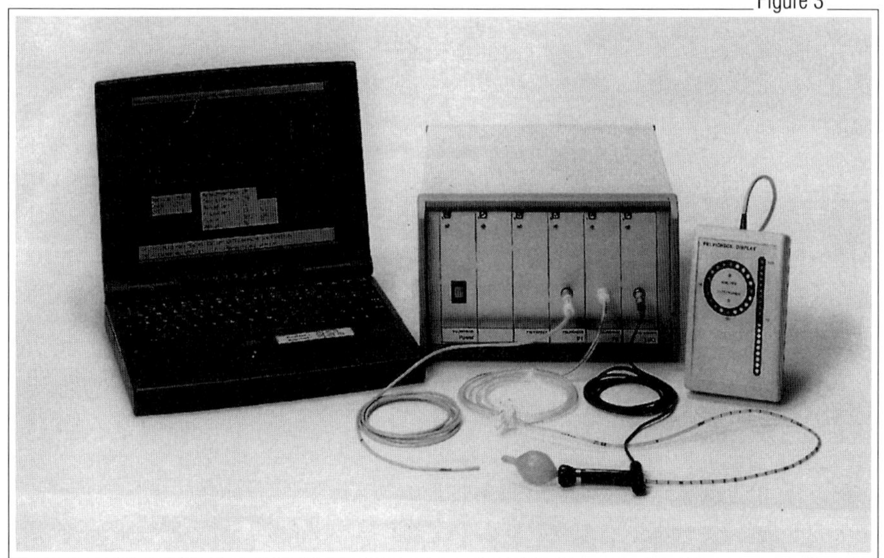

Computer-aided manometry and biofeedback system (Pelvicheck System, Medicheck Co., Essen, Germany).

This unit combines manometry recordings with transcutaneous sphincter EMG. Furthermore, a balloon channel for rectal balloon distention is provided and can be added to the transcutaneous EMG. This setting is essential for coordination training.

The stationary biofeedback system can be combined with an ambulatory version for sphincter biofeedback shown at the very right side of the picture (Figure 3). Both systems use a ring of light as feedback signal. The sensitivity of the EMG channel can be adjusted and the

EMG sensor can be equipped with a rectal balloon probe, if the stationary system is utilized (Figure 4). This is a major benefit of the stationary system, since the rectal balloon probe can be used to control abdominal pressure during sphincter biofeedback and is essential for coordination training.

Figure 4

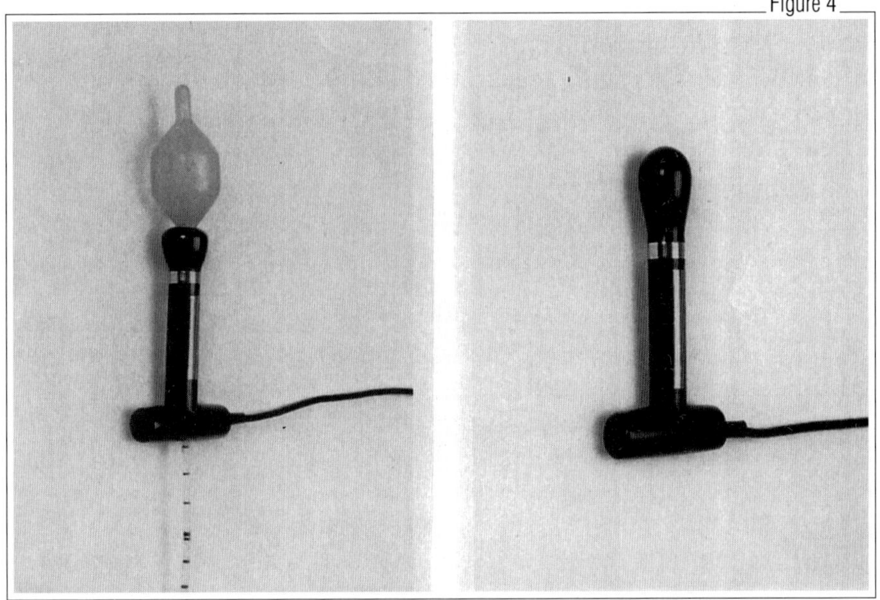

Anal sphincter EMG probe with rectal balloon (Medicheck Co., Essen, Germany).

After the patient has been classified into one of the subcategories "impaired sphincter function", "impaired sensory function" or "impaired coordination" according to Figure 2, the appropriate programme should be selected. If the category is not easily identified and the patient suffers from more than one dysfunction, we recommend to start with sensory discrimination training first and to continue with coordination training[39].

The training sessions are performed in the left lateral position after spontaneous evacuation of the rectum; if that is not possible, a saline based enema can be used. After introducing the probe, a ten-minute resting period for anal sensation to adapt to the probe should be kept.

We recommend training sessions at least twice a week, with a single session not exceeding a duration of 45 minutes. Diaries are kept during the programme and brought to the sessions and evaluated by the therapist. A preset criterion is used to define when a training is successful. Thus, the diaries are the most important information for treatment evaluation. Most groups use a criterion between 75% and 90% decrease of incontinence events[44]. If the criterion is not reached after ten training sessions and no significant improvement in incontinence is seen, alternative treatment strategies should be considered.

*Sphincter biofeedback*

Biofeedback of the external anal sphincter contraction strength is the easiest of the training programmes. The patient should be able to observe the computer screen or the display of the ambulatory system. At the very beginning of the first training session and before introducing the probe, we explain and demonstrate the procedure to the patient, who can be encouraged to self-handle the sensor in order to experience the connection between stimulus and signal. After placing the probe, the patient is instructed to squeeze the sphincters, so that the open ring of lights shown on the display is closed.

A major benefit of the stationary biofeedback system is the combination of balloon and EMG probe. With the rectal probe in place, the patient can learn to differentiate between contractions of the pelvic floor and the abdominal muscles. It is important that the patient learns to squeeze the anal sphincters selectively, without using the abdominal or gluteal muscles. Thus, the instruction is to increase the signal of the EMG channel without producing a signal on the balloon channel. At the beginning of the training session the technique is shaped by trial and error. As soon as the response to the instruction to squeeze is reliable, two different types of exercises are performed. First the patient is asked to squeeze with maximum strength for a short period of time (5 sec). This task is repeated ten times with feedback control. After a five-minute resting period, the patient is asked to keep approximately 50% of the maximum squeeze pressure for at least one minute. This task is repeated five times. After a five-minute rest, both tasks, including the rest periods, are repeated once.

*Sensory discrimination training*

As in every training programme, the procedure should be explained to the patients at the very beginning of the session, and the distention of the balloon should be demonstrated before placement. For sensory discrimination training, no visual feedback is necessary. The first stimuli delivered should be well above the predetermined sensory perception threshold. The patient is then asked to give a prompt response to the stimulus. Any feedback before the patient's response must be avoided in order not to provide additional cues for the filling of the balloon. Thus, either the computer screen has to be covered before the patient's response and then uncovered for feedback, or only verbal feedback is used. We agree with others[39,45], that verbal feedback is sufficient for that particular type of task. After the patient has learned to give a prompt response to perceivable rectal distention, the volume is lowered to the sensory threshold and slightly below. After ten trials a 5 min break is recommended. If the patient perceives the new stimulus in about two thirds of all stimulus presentations, a lower stimulus is used and the procedure is repeated.

The greatest threat to a therapeutic success in this training procedure is premature feedback. Unfortunately, even the sound of air moving through the probe or the balloon can give the patient a "feedback signal" concerning a possible stimulus. One technique to overcome this disadvantage is to use a second balloon for sham inflation through the same three-way perfusion port used for the filling of the rectal balloon providing "false feedback". Which balloon is filled is "determined" by chance and unpredictable to the patient. As a consequence, the patient has to rely exclusivedly on his/her rectal perception.

*Coordination training*

The first instructions to the patient are very similar to those described above (sphincter biofeedback), except that the patient has to understand the function and signal of the balloon and the balloon tracing in addition. It is explained to the patient, that as soon as the balloon is filled, the patient has to squeeze as hard as possible and with an immediate onset. It is important to ensure, that the sensory threshold of the patient is appropriate, otherwise it is recommended to start with sensory discrimination training first. The balloon volume for this task should not exceed the patient's sensory threshold. It should be emphasized by the therapist that the squeeze response has to be as prompt as possible to the distention. Maximum squeeze pressure should be held for at least ten seconds. A five-minute break is recommended after ten repetitions.

## Conclusions

Biofeedback applications for the treatment of faecal incontinence have been available for more than 20 years now and have become an established procedure at least over the last decade. Even though the exact mode of action remains unclear and may include both improvement of sphincter function and sensory discrimination[44] even critical reviews admit, that biofeedback training programmes show an average efficacy (e.g. 79.8% in the studies reviewed by Enck, 1994[46]), which is too high to rely completely on a placebo response. Furthermore, there have been two very well controlled studies over the last few years (for review see[12,44,46]) still supporting the effectiveness of biofeedback training in faecal incontinence.

However, biofeedback training will be more successful if it is integrated into a behavioural medicine approach to treatment combining medically oriented diagnostic procedures and treatments with behaviour modification. Patients treated for faecal incontinence will benefit even more, if they are additionally instructed for toilet training and, at least in cases suffering from loose stools, if they receive dietary advice. Behaviourally oriented treatment approaches are not seen as an alternative strategy in treating a disorder, but as an integral part of routine therapy with low costs and little or no side effects.

Acknowledgements

This paper was supported by grant DFG MU 1241/4-1 from the Deutsche Forschungsgemeinschaft.

### *References*

1. Enck P, Gabor S, von Ferber L, et al. *Häufigkeit von Stuhlinkontinenz und Informationsgrad von Hausärzten und Krankenkassen.* Z Gastroenterol 1991;29:538-40.

2. Enck P, Schäfer R. *Stuhlinkontinenz (inkl. Stoma). Verlust der Selbstkontrolle des Stuhlabgangs.* Klinik der Gegenwart 1996;18:1-13.
3. Enck P, Garbor K-S, Walega P. *Epidemiologie der Stuhlinkontinenz.* Kontinenz 1994;3:59-66.
4. Enck P, Bielefeldt K, Rathmann W, et al. *Epidemiology of fecal incontinence in selected patient groups.* Int J Colorect Dis 1991;6:143-6.
5. Bielefeldt K, Enck P, Erckenbrecht JF. *Sensory and motor function in the maintenance of anal continence.* Dis Colon Rectum 1990;33:674-8.
6. Bannister JJ, Abouzekry L, Read NW. *Effect of aging on anorectal function.* Gut 1987;28:353-7.
7. Enck P, Kuhlbusch R, Lübke H, et al. *Age and sex and anorectal manometry in incontinence.* Dis Colon Rectum 1989;32:1026-30.
8. Enck P, Weber P. *Lebensqualität bei Stuhlinkontinenz Erwachsener.* Kontinenz 1992;1:58-61.
9. O'Keefe EA, Talley NJ, Zinsmeister AR, et al. *Bowel disorders impair functional status and quality of life in the elderly: a population-based study.* Gerontol A Biol Sci Med 1995;50:M184-9.
10. Musial F, Enck P. *Patiententagebücher als Instrument zur Diagnosestellung und Therapieverlaufskontrolle bei Defäkationsstörungen.* In: Wilz G, Brähler E, editors. Tagebücher in Therapie und Forschung. Göttingen: Hogrefe Verlag; 1997;253-69.
11. Engel BT. *Fecal incontinence and encopresis: a psychophysiological analysis.* In: Hölzl R, Whitehead WE, editors. Psychophysiology of the gastrointestinal tract. New York: Plenum Press; 1983;301-10.
12. Enck P, Schäfer R. *Biofeedback applications in gastroenterology.* Eur J Gastroenterol Hepatol 1996;8:534-9.
13. Schäfer R, Enck P. *Physiologie und Pathophysiologie der Defäkation.* In: Jost WH, editor. Neurologie des Beckenbodens. Weinheim: Chapman & Hall; 1997;15-39.
14. Enck P, Fischell B. Gantke B, et al. *Klinische Symptome und Manometrie bei Stuhlinkontinenz.* Kontinenz 1992;1:14-8.
15. Bielefeldt K, Enck P, Zamboglou N, et al. *Anorectal manometry and defecography in the diagnosis of fecal incontinence.* J Clin Gastroenterol 1992;13:661-5.
16. Gantke B, Enck P, Schäfer A, et al. *Sonographic, manometric and myographic evaluation of the anal sphincters morphology and function.* Dis Colon Rectum 1994;36:1037-41.
17. Schäfer A, Enck P, Heyer T, et al. *Endosonography of the anal sphincters: incontinent and continent patients and healthy controls.* Z Gastroenterol 1994;32:328-31.
18. Schäfer R, Heyer T, Gantke B, et al. *Anal endosonography and manometry.* Dis Colon Rectum 1997;40:293-7.

19. Schulz A. *Elektromyografie des Beckenbodens.* In: Müller-Lissner SA, Akkermans LMA, editors. Chronische Obstipation und Stuhlinkontinenz. Berlin: Springer; 1989;119-30.
20. Wienbeck M, Barnert J. *Äthiologie und Pathogenese der Inkontinenz.* In: Müller Lissner SA, Akkermans LMA, editors. Chronische Obstipation und Stuhlinkontinenz. Berlin: Springer; 1989;215-34.
21. Musial F, Kalveram KTh, Enck P. *Therapie der analen Inkontinenz im höheren Lebensalter - Wie effektiv ist das Biofeedbacktraining?* Grant DFG MU 1241/4-1 1997.
22. Skinner BF. *Science and human behavior.* New York: MacMillan; 1953.
23. Miller NE. *General perspective: need for evaluation and basic research.* In: Richter-Heinrich E, Miller NE, editors. Biofeedback - Basic problems and clonical applications. Berlin: Deutscher Verlag der Wissenschaften; 1982;13-8.
24. Miller NE. *Learning of visceral and glandular responses.* Science 1969;163:434-5.
25. Miller NE. *Effect of learning on gastrointestinal functions.* Clin Gastroenterol 1977;6:533-46.
26. Kohlenberg JR. *Operant conditioning of human anal sphincter pressure.* J Appl Behav Anal 1973;6:201-8.
27. Engel BT, Nikoomanesh P, Schuster MM. *Operant conditioning of rectosphincteric responses in the treatment of fecal incontinence.* N Engl J Med 1974;290:646-9.
28. Cerulli MA, Nikoomanesh P, Schuster MM. *Progress in biofeedback conditioning for fecal incontinence.* Gastroenterology 1979;76:742-6.
29. Goldenberg DA, Hodges K, Hersh T, Jinich H. *Biofeedback therapy for fecal incontinence.* Am J Gastroenterol 1980;74:342-5.
30. Wald A. *Biofeedback therapy for fecal incontinence.* Ann Int Med 1981;95:146-9.
31. Wald A, Tunuguntla AK. *Anorectal sensorimotor dysfunction in fecal incontinence and diabetes mellitus.* N Engl J Med 1984;310:1282-7.
32. Latimer PR, Campbell D, Kasperski J. *A components analysis of biofeedback in the treatment of fecal incontinence.* Biofeed Selfregul 1984;9:311-24.
33. Whitehead WE, Burgio KL, Engel BT. *Biofeedback treatment of fecal incontinence in geriatric patients.* J Am Geriatr Soc 1985;33:320-4.
34. Buser WD, Miner PB. *Delayed rectal sensation with fecal incontinence.* Gastroenterology 1986;91:1186-91.
35. MacLeod JH. *Management of anal incontinence by biofeedback.* Gastroenterology 1987;93:291-4.
36. Riboli EB, Frascio M, Pitto G, Reboa G. *Biofeedback conditioning for fecal incontinence.* Arch Phys Med Rehabil 1988;69:29-31.
37. Enck P, Kränzle U, Schwiese J, et al. *Biofeedback - Behandlung bei Stuhlinkontinenz.* Dtsch Med Wschr 1988;113:1789-94.

38. Loening-Baucke V. *Efficacy of biofeedback training in improving faecal incontinence and anorectal physiologic function.* Gut 1990;31:1395-402.
39. Miner PB, Donnelly TC, Read NW. *Investigation of mode of action of biofeedback in treatment of fecal incontinence.* Dig Dis Sci 1990;35:1291-8.
40. Keck JO, Staniunas RJ, Coller JA, et al. *Biofeedback training is useful in fecal incontinence but disappointing in constipation.* Dis Colon Rectum 1995;37:1271-6.
41. Guillemot F, Bouche B, Gower-Rousseau C, et al. *Biofeedback for the treatment of fecal incontinence.* Dis Colon Rectum 1995;38:393-7.
42. Enck P, Däublin G, Gantke B, et al. *Long term efficacy of biofeedback therapy for fecal incontinence.* Dis Colon Rectum 1994;37:97-101.
43. Enck P, Schäfer R. *Verhaltensmedizin in der Gastroenterologie: Biofeedback-Behandlung der Stuhlinkontinenz.* In: Enck P, Musial F, editors. Psychologie und Gastroenterologie. Göttingen: Hogrefe; 1996;108-19.
44. Enck P. *Biofeedback training in disordered defecation: a critical review.* Dig Dis Sci 1993;38:1953-60.
45. McCubbin JA, Surwitt RS, Mansbach, CM. *Case study: sensory discrimination training in a case of chronic constipation.* Behavior Therapy 1987;18:273-8.
46. Enck P. *Biofeedback-Behandlung der Stuhlinkontinenz und der Obstipation.* Therapeutische Umschau 1994;51:203-7.

### *ADDRESS FOR CORRESPONDENCE*

**ENCK P, PhD**
Universitätsklinikum Tübingen
Abt. Allg. Chirurgie - Forschungsbereich
Zentrum Medizinische Forschung (ZMF)
Waldhörnlestr. 22
72072 Tübingen Germany
Fax: +49 7071 29 5142
E-mail: paul.enck@uni-tuebingen.de

PART **FIVE**

# CHRONIC GASTROINTESTINAL DISORDERS IN NEUROLOGICAL PATIENTS

APPROACH TO THE PATIENT WITH CHRONIC GASTROINTESTINAL DISORDERS

# ORO-PHARYNGEAL DYSPHAGIA IN NEUROLOGICAL PATIENTS

*FI Habib, S Torrico, M Ruggeri, C Zampaletta*

Many neurogenic and primary muscle disorders are associated with abnormalities of gut motility. Stroke, even when unilateral, is commonly associated with dysphagia[1] Transcranial magnetoelectric stimulation has established that the pharyngeal phase of swallowing tends to receive its innervation principally from one hemisphere[2]. In many neurological disorders, dysphagia is only a part of the clinical picture[3-6] while in others, dysphagia may be the first symptom, and in the Chiari malformation may be the sole or major feature.
Patients with neurological disease or after brain injury may complain of dysphagia. The symptoms and the complications due to neurogenic dysphagia are primarily due to sensorimotor dysfunction of the oral and the pharyngeal phases of swallowing, and problems related to oro-pharyngeal dysphagia are clinically predominant in most cases. Oro-pharyngeal dysphagia is neurogenic in type in 80% of cases while it is due to structural changes in 20%[7].
Neurogenic dysphagia may present in three ways:

1. A patient with known neurological disease may present with obvious symptoms or complications of dysphagia such as nasal regurgitation, chewing difficulty, problems in initiating the actual swallow, drooling, coughing or choking episodes during eating, dehydration, malnutrition, laryngospasm, aspiration pneumonia[8].
2. A patient with known neurological disease may have substantial oropharyngeal dysfunction but report only subtle clinical clues of its presence for three essential reasons:
   a. compensatory processes,
   b. reduction of the laryngeal cough reflex, and
   c. cognitive impairment.

The ***compensation process*** involves voluntary behavioural modifications and involuntary adjustment in oro-pharyngeal performance[9]. Voluntary forms of compensation include modifications in dietary characteristics and eating methods. When the onset of neurogenic dysphagia is gradual, patients may be relatively unaware of their adaptive changes in eating. It is important for the clinician to enquire specifically about the elimination of difficult-to-swallow dietary items or the development of habits such as cutting food into small pieces, chewing more thoroughly, swallowing liquids after a solid bolus, double swallow, throat clearing during meals, head tilting while eating and taking longer to finish a meal. The process of involuntary compensations seems to involve automatic adaptations in oro-pharyngeal performance in order to avoid the adverse functional consequences of a neurological disease.

***Reduction of the laryngeal cough reflex*** may be due to several factors. Some neurological diseases, such as brain stem stroke, can cause loss of laryngeal sensation and/or the motor response to aspirated material as a direct result of the disease process itself. Other patients may exhibit reduction of the laryngeal cough reflex in response to chronic laryngeal stimulation (i.e., chronic aspiration) and the following desensitization of the reflex, related to either damage of local sensory receptors or centrally mediated adaptation. In other patients the underlying motor disorder may compromise motor function of the components of the cough reflex (the larynx and the diaphragm). Endotracheal intubation, tracheostomy, medications[10] can also impair the cough reflex.

Neurological patients with ***cognitive impairment*** may not present with overt dysphagia. Demented or mentally retarded individuals with dysphagia may have limited capacity to understand or communicate their difficulty in swallowing. The clinician must observe the patient while he/she eats, question the caregivers and bear in mind that neurogenic dysphagia may be silent.

3 The third way in which neurogenic dysphagia can present is in a patient with an underlying neurological disease that is unrecognized but produces dysphagia as an initial or primary problem. Clinicians should be able to recognize the symptoms indicative of oro-pharyngeal dysphagia, and then further evaluate these symptoms. Videofluoroscopy (VFS) of swallowing is sensitive in the detection of neurogenic oropharyngeal impairment but relatively non-specific as far as concerns the responsible neurologic disease[11]. If VFS findings suggest neurologic dysfunction but the specific cause is unclear, neurological consultation is the next step.

Occasionally, what appears to be neurogenic dysphagia turns out to have a psychogenic basis[12]. Such patients tend to be young and otherwise physically healthy and their symptoms of oropharyngeal dysphagia may fluctuate dramatically. These individuals are characterized by the absence of dysphonia or any other objective neurologic impairment, and neurologic investigation is negative. Videofluorographic pharyngeal function is normal once initiated, but oral behaviour is often peculiar. Patients with psychogenic dysphagia are reluctant to initiate swallowing and may complain of their inability to do so even as the intactness of their oral ability is revealed by videofluoroscopic observation. On the other hand, the clinician must be very careful in labelling oropharyngeal dysphagia as psychogenic. Although subtle abnormalities may escape detection, every effort should be made to reach a diagnosis. In a study on 23 referred patients labelled as psychogenic dysphagia, Ravich et al. were able to offer a different explanation for symptoms in 15[13].

There are few distinctive features of oro-pharyngeal dysphagia in the various neurological diseases. Clinical and videofluoroscopic features of dysphagia tend to overlap between patients with stroke, Parkinson's disease, head trauma, motor neuron disease, Multiple Sclerosis (MS), postpolio syndrome, myopathy. The poor specificity is related to factors such as extent and severity of the underlying disease, characteristics of disease in individual patients and the premorbid characteristics of that patient swallowing.

Symptoms and findings that are warning signs for the likely presence of impaired swallowing and the risk of aspiration are listed in Table 1. The bedside evaluation should screen patients for the likelihood and severity of a swallowing impairment. Pain during swallowing, sensation of sticking and obstruction during swallowing or visible effort when swallowing are signs of discrete disease. Oral feeding problems are likely in patients whose neurologic disease had led to confusion and dementia. Patients with poor judgment, sensory deficit or poor motor coordination from brain damage may not possess the vigilance and physical ability to handle their food intake safely. Dysarthric speech with slow slurred articulation, nasal air emission, and a hoarse or wet voice demonstrates impairment of muscle groups essential for effective oropharyngeal swallow. Frequent coughing or choking on food reflect impaired pharyngeal swallowing. Strenuous chewing, laboured swallowing, repetitive swallowing of a single bolus, prolongation of the meal times should be taken in serious consideration, particularly if associated with fear of food or weight loss. Drooling is of aesthetic consequence and is related to poor labial continence and poor pharyngeal clearance of secretions by periodic swallowing.

WARNING SIGNS OF SWALLOWING PROBLEMS

Drooling
Inability to keep the bolus in the mouth
Laborious chewing, repetitive swallowing
Nasal regurgitation
Choke or cough when eating or drinking
Increased need to clear throat
Food sticking in the throat
Meal times take much longer than usual
No enjoyment while eating
Hoarse or wet voice
Weight loss
History of recurrent pneumonia

Table 1

The swallowing history and physical examination determine the likely site and mechanism of the problem and guide in the selection of diagnostic tests and therapeutic measures. The clinician uses history taking and physical examination in the attempt to formulate a preliminary diagnosis and to select appropriate tests. The value of the clinician is determined by the skill with which he/she uses historical and physical clues to direct the search for additional evidence[14], these clues often allow the clinician to design appropriate strategies for care and to predict outcome. In other instances, the bedside examination helps the examiner to select appropriate tests and to determine the need for referrals or management by multiple disciplines. The history proceeds

from the definition of the swallowing problem to investigate associated (change in speech and voice, coughing or choking, nasal regurgitation, drooling) and ancillary (weight loss, dehydration, hoarse voice, apnoea, pneumonia) symptoms. The physical examination proceeds from a general assessment of the patient's physical and mental health to an assessment of swallowing structures and functions. Both history taking and physical examination seek to establish the adequacy and safety of oral food intake and to identify remediable causes of abnormal swallowing. Both provide indications for specific diagnostic tests, referrals or therapeutic plans.
Oropharyngeal dysphagia may present with symptoms related mostly to either the oral phase (oral dysphagia) or the pharyngeal phase of swallowing (pharyngeal dysphagia).

## Oral dysphagia

Oral dysphagia typically presents as difficulty in retaining or manipulating a bolus in the oral cavity. There is a prolonged struggling with the bolus, but the involuntary pharyngeal and oesophageal stages of swallowing may proceed normally once the swallow is triggered. Patients may compensate for failure to push the bolus backward with the tongue by using their fingers or lifting their chins. Oral stage dysphagia is part of the impairment of volitional functions and may be characteristic of dementia, pseudobulbar palsy and cerebral palsy with oral motor incoordination, Parkinson's disease, Amyotrophic Lateral Sclerosis (ALS).

## Pharyngeal dysphagia

Pharyngeal dysphagia may present with patient's complaints of coughing or choking on liquids more than on solids. Patients may report that water and other thin liquids like tea, coffee present their greatest problem. However, they may also complain of the sensation of food sticking because of an inability to propel a viscous bolus through the pharynx. When asymmetric impairments are present, patients may try to compensate by tilting or turning their heads, or by pressing against one side of their neck while swallowing. Saliva management is a frequent problem and may be experienced as an accumulation of phlegm in the throat due to pharyngeal stasis. Concomitant problems of impaired phonation or speech may be reported[15]. In severe cases, aspiration will be evident. In the case of neuromuscular disorders the onset and the duration of dysphagia coincide with the paralysis resulting from cerebro-vascular accidents or other manifestations of a disease. The consistency of foods that produce dysphagia provide diagnostic clues. With neuromuscular dysfunction of the pharynx, liquids frequently cause greater problems. Marked fatigue is characteristic of myasthenia gravis. Patients may function normally early in the day or into a meal and later develop dysphagia. In some cases, the temperature of the bolus can exacerbate problems with swallowing. In muscular dystrophy, cooling can lead to myotonia and clonus of the oro-pharyngeal musculature.

## Videofluoroscopic examination

VFS examination of oro-pharyngeal swallowing function has become the gold standard for assessing the integrity of the oral and pharyngeal stages of the swallow. This procedure is not used simply to determine whether a patient is aspirating or even why the patient is aspirating, it helps the clinician to determine if a patient can receive sufficient alimentation by mouth for well-being and recovery and if there are particular compensatory postures or predefined volumes or bolus viscosity that can help the patient to return to oral intake. There are some limitations to this procedure:

1. The patient is exposed to radiation;
2. The dynamic study is not adequate for assessment of structural abnormalities.

Occasionally, VFS reveals a distinctive pattern of abnormality that is helpful in the diagnosis of the underlying neurological disease. Difficulty initiating swallowing is characteristic of upper motor neuron dysfunction due to MS or to extensive bilateral strokes. Patients with Multiple System Atrophy (MSA) may exhibit lingual resting tremor or reduced range of motion of the tongue. Absence of the pharyngeal swallow response indicates brainstem dysfunction. Asymmetric pharyngeal weakness suggests a unilateral lower motor neuron disorder

of the brain stem or cranial nerves. VFS may show oesophageal motor dysfunction in patients affected by ALS[16], MSA[17] and myotonic dystrophy or Steinert's disease[18].
We examined 52 consecutive patients: 26 with ALS, 12 with MSA and 14 with Steinert's disease. All patients were investigated for symptoms of oral and pharyngeal dysphagia (Table 2) and were submitted to VFS to evaluate the presence of oral and pharyngeal motor abnormalities (Table 3).
At VFS, patients with Steinert's disease more frequently showed pharyngeal than oral motor abnormalities. Such abnormalities, particularly pharyngeal hypotonia, pooling in the valleculae and pyriform sinuses, upper airways penetration were not frequently accompanied by symptoms of pharyngeal dysphagia (cough was referred only in 38% of the patients, but in 74% of the cases, upper airways penetration was detected at VFS).

SYMPTOMS OF ORAL AND PHARYNGEAL DYSPHAGIA

| | **MSA (N=12)** | **ALS (N=26)** | **Steinert's disease (N=14)** |
|---|---|---|---|
| Difficulty in pushing bolus backwards with tongue | 1 | 9 | 1 |
| Difficulty in keeping bolus in oral cavity | 3 | 5 | 1 |
| Impaired chewing | 3 | 0 | 1 |
| Drooling | 6 | 8 | 1 |
| Cough during meals | 5 | 19 | 5 |
| Choking | 2 | 3 | 1 |
| Nasal regurgitation | 1 | 1 | 3 |
| Upper airways inflammation | 3 | 1 | 2 |
| Food sticking in throat | 2 | 3 | 2 |
| Food sticking at jugulus | 2 | 2 | 0 |

**MSA** multiple system atrophy **ALS** amiotrophic lateral sclerosis

Table 2

ORO-PHARYNGEAL MOTOR ALTERATION AT VIDEOFLUOROSCOPY

| | MSA | ALS | Steinert's disease |
|---|---|---|---|
| Tongue incoordination | 5 | 13 | 10 |
| Difficulty in transport of bolus backward | 9 | 11 | 4 |
| Abnormal soft palate movement | 0 | 4 | 3 |
| Leakage in pharynx | 7 | 5 | 1 |
| Nasal regurgitation | 2 | 1 | 7 |
| Pharyngeal hypotonia | 3 | 2 | 12 |
| Incomplete and/or delayed epiglottic tilt | 3 | 11 | 7 |
| Upper airways penetration/aspiration | 7 | 9 | 10 |
| Pooling in valleculae and/or pyriform sinuses | 6 | 18 | 10 |
| Crico-pharyngeal incompetence | 4 | 1 | 6 |

Table 3

In patients with MSA, oral motor alterations were frequently detected at VFS. Difficulty in pushing the bolus backward with the tongue, tongue incoordination and oro-pharyngeal leakage was present in 75%, 41% and 58%, respectively. However, only a few patients (25%) referred symptoms of oral dysphagia. These data confirm previous reports in patients with other types of movement disorders such as Parkinson's disease in which there is a discrepancy between symptoms and VFS results[19-21].
Concerning pharyngeal motor abnormalities, upper airways penetration and pooling in the valleculae and pyriform sinuses were present in 58% and 50%, respectively, at VFS, while cough during eating and upper airways inflammation were the main symptoms and were referred in 42% and 25% of patients with Steinert's disease and MSA, respectively.
In patients with ASL, both oral and pharyngeal motor alterations were well represented at VFS. Tongue incoordination and difficulty in pushing the bolus backward with the tongue, were the most important oral motor alterations revealed at VFS (50% and 42%, respectively), while incomplete and/or delayed epiglottic tilt, pooling in the valleculae and pyriform sinuses and upper airways penetration, (42%, 69% and 35%)

were the main representative pharyngeal motor alterations determined. Concerning the symptoms of oral and pharyngeal dysphagia, 80% of the patients referred cough during eating, while difficulty in pushing the bolus backward with the tongue and difficulty in accommodation of the bolus were the main referred symptoms of oral dysphagia.
Swallow therapy is done with the help of VFS; several therapeutic manoeuvres are used to improve the oro-pharyngeal bolus transport and airways safety. A change in bolus size and consistency is helpful in some patients (Table 4), while in others, swallowing with the head in a specific position may help the safe passage of bolus (Table 5).

DIETARY CHANGES TO COMPENSATE SWALLOWING DIFFICULTIES

***Texture*** Easy to swallow foods that hold together, easy to control by the tongue such as: puddings, egg dishes such as soufflés or quiche, softcheese, egg salad, gelatin, casseroles, minced meat with gravy, creamed vegetables, au gratin potatoes.

***Taste*** Flavourful foods can be more easily swallowed than bland food.

***Temperature*** Cold or warm foods are easier to swallow than lukewarm foods.

***Avoid*** foods that are too hard or that fall apart in the mouth or dry sticky foods.

***Avoid*** thin liquids like water, coffee, tea, milk, - thicken them, or

***Try*** milkshakes, eggnog, yoghurt.

Table 4

POSTURAL TECHNIQUES

Chin tuck

Tilt head toward the stronger side

Turn head toward the weaker side

Tilt all the body backward

Table 5

Chin tuck by displacing the larynx under the mandibula reduces the chance of aspiration, while rotating the head toward the weaker side will improve pharyngeal transit and prevent aspiration. Tilting all the body 30° backward may help the patient with oral dysfunction.
Patients with pre-deglutitive, deglutitive and post-deglutitive aspiration may benefit from specific therapeutic manoeuvres (Table 6).

| SWALLOW MANOEUVRES |
|---|
| Mendelsohn manoeuvre |
| Supra-glottic swallow |
| Super-supra-glottic swallow |
| Effort in swallowing |

Table 6

The Mendelsohn manoeuvre may improve pharyngeal emptying in patients with impaired pharyngeal transit and post-deglutitive aspiration. In this manoeuvre, patients are asked to generate a sustained laryngeal elevation during swallowing thus prolonging the upper oesophageal sphincter (UES) traction and opening. Patients with pre-deglutitive and intra-deglutitive penetration may benefit from the supra glottic or the super-supra-glottic swallow. In this manoeuvre, patients swallow once or twice in apnoea and cough immediately after, during expiration, clearing the larynx of the aspirated material.
In some diseases, such as ALS, the rate of progression may be rapid; in others, such as Parkinson's disease, progression is slow. In MS, on the other hand, rate of progression is highly variable from individual to individual and from one point in time to another for one individual. Typical age of onset ranges from young adulthood in MS to the 60's and 70's in Parkinson's disease. The degree of cognitive impairment also varies from one disease to another. Although dysarthria and dysphagia are common in all these diseases, the characteristics of the speech and swallowing disorders vary. These differences in disease features dictate different approaches to management of the swallowing disorder.

## REFERENCES


1. Perkin GD, Murray-Lyon I. *Neurology and the gastrointestinal system.* J Neurol Neurosurg Psychiatry 1998;65:291-300.
2. Aziz Q, Thompson DG. *Brain-gut axis in health and disease.* Gastroenterology 1998;114:559-78.
3. Johnston BT, Li Q, Castell JA, Castell DO. *Swallowing and esophageal function in Parkinson's disease.* Am J Gastroenterol 1995;90:1741-6.
4. Chen MY, Peele VN, Donati D, et al. *Clinical and videofluoroscopic evaluation of swallowing in 41 patients with neurologic disease.* Gastrointest Radiol 1992;17:95-8.
5. Daniels SK, Brailey K, Priestly DH, et al. *Aspiration in patients with acute stroke.* Arch Phys Med Rehabil 1998;79:14-9.
6. Perie S, Eymard B, Laccourreye L, et al. *Dysphagia in oculopharyngeal muscular dystrophy: a series of 22 French cases.* Neuromuscul Disord 1997;(Suppl 1):896-9.
7. Duranceau A, Lafontaine ER, Taillefer R, et al. *Oropharyngeal dysphagia and operations on the upper esophageal sphincter.* Surg Annu 1987;19:317-62.
8. Martin BJW, Corlew MM, Wood H, et al. *The association of swallowing dysfunction and aspiration pneumonia.* Dysphagia 1994;9:1-6.
9. Bucholz DW, Bosma JF, Donner MW. *Adaptation, compensation and decompensation of the pharyngeal swallow.* Gastrointest Radiol 1985;10:235-9.
10. Greenberg DJ. *The incidence of aspiration in patients with tracheostomies.* Anest Analg 1984;63:1142-1149.
11. Nilsson H, Ekgerg O, Sjöberg S, Olsson R. *Pharyngeal constrictor paresis: an indicator of neurologic disease?* Dysphagia 1993;8:239-43.
12. Buchholz D, Barofsky I, Edwin D, et al. *Psychogenic oropharyngeal dysphagia: report of 26 cases.* Dysphagia 1994;9:267-8.
13. Ravich WJ, Wilson RS, Jones B, et al. *Psychogenic dysphagia and globus: reevaluation of 23 patients.* Dysphagia 1989;4:35-8.
14. Castell DO, Donner MD. *Evaluation of dysphagia: a careful history is crucial.* Dysphagia 1987;2:65-71.
15. Bosma JF. *Deglutition: pharyngeal stage.* Physiol Rev 1967;37:275.
16. Habib FI, Ruggeri M, Inghilleri M, et al. *Videofluoroscopic evaluation of the swallowing act in amyotrophic lateral sclerosis.* Gastroenterology 1997;112:741.
17. Zampaletta C, Stocchi F, Ruggeri M, et al. *Multiple system atrophy: videofluoroscopic evaluation of the swallowing act.* Gastroenterology 1997;112:857.

18. Piretta L, Habib FI, Ruggeri M, et al. *Muscular and neuromuscular oesophageal motor alterations in Steinert's myotonic dystrophy.* Gastroenterology 1995;108:669.
19. Logemann J, Blonsky ER, Boshes B. *Lingual control in Parkinson's disease.* Trans Am Neurol Assoc 1973;98:276-8.
20. Bushmann M, Dobmeyer SM, Leeker L, Perlmutter JS. *Swallowing abnormalities and their response to treatment in Parkinson's disease.* Neurology (Minneap) 1989;39:1309-14.
21. Leopold NA, Kagel MC. *Prepharyngeal dysphagia in Parkinson's disease.* Dysphagia 1996;11:14-22.

*ADDRESS FOR CORRESPONDENCE*

**HABIB FI, MD**
Cattedra di Gastroenterologia I
Dipartimento Scienze Cliniche
Università di Roma "La Sapienza"
Policlinico Umberto I
Viale del Policlinico 155
00161 Roma Italia
Fax: +39 06 4463737
E-mail: me1084@mclink.it

# Lower gastrointestinal dysfunctions in neurological patients

*D Badiali, L d'Alba, F Bracci, E Corazziari*

The autonomic nervous system affects motility of the large bowel by means of parasympathetic acetylcholine and sympathetic norepinephrine outflows. The former (vagus, $S_2$-$S_4$) is excitatory to gastrointestinal smooth muscle and the sacral section controls the External Anal Sphincter (EAS); the latter ($T_5$-$L_3$) is inhibitory to large bowel smooth muscle and excitatory to Internal Anal Sphincter (IAS). Moreover, afferent fibres start from the large bowel to activate viscero-visceral reflexes and convey sensation such as pain, intestinal distension, desire to defaecate.

The extrinsic innervation of the lower gastrointestinal tract thus modulates the motor function of the large bowel and controls the ability to withhold, stop, or trigger defaecation, by the integration of the smooth muscle of the large bowel and IAS with the striated muscle of the EAS and pelvic floor.

Different neurological diseases, irrespective of their aetiology, may affect the lower gastrointestinal tract manifesting clinically with identical symptoms: constipation and anal incontinence. Chronic diarrhoea caused by intestinal pseudo-obstructions with bacterial overgrowth, and chronic visceral pain due to peripheral neuropathy or sensory neuron sensitization, can worsen recto-anal dysfunctions.

Frequency and severity of constipation and/or anal incontinence vary in relation to neurological aetiology and the level, and the degree, of the lesions, but these factors may, also variably interact with the presence of gastrointestinal[1] pathology and dysfunctions or neurological pharmacotherapy (e.g., anticholinergics, anticonvulsivants, antidepressive agents) can cause constipation.

## Constipation

Constipation is closely associated[2] with brain dysfunctions and damage as well as with spinal cord alterations (Table 1). This variety of neurological disorders of the central nervous system suggests that an alteration of the neuronal modulation of the colonic and/or recto-anal motility may lead to the development of constipation.

SIGNIFICANT ASSOCIATION BETWEEN CHRONIC CONSTIPATION AND NEUROLOGIC DISEASES

| Neurological Disease | Confidence Interval (99.99% odds ratio) |
|---|---|
| • Senile organic psychotic condition | 1.4 - 1.8 |
| • Other organic psychotic conditions | 1.1 - 3.3 |
| • Mental disorders due to organic brain damage | 1.2 - 1.7 |
| • Unspecified mental retardation | 1.7 - 6.9 |
| • Parkinson's disease | 2.8 - 3.6 |
| • Other movement disorders | 1.6 - 3.4 |
| • Spinal cord diseases | 1.8 - 4.5 |
| • Other paralytic syndromes | 1.8 - 2.9 |
| • Multiple Sclerosis | 2.5 - 6.1 |
| • Disorders of the autonomic nervous system | 1.1 - 3.0 |

Table 1

Modified from Johanson JF, Sonnenberg A, Koch Tr, Mc Carty DJ[2].

Constipation may be secondary to the slow transit of faeces through the colon (right and/or left) and/or inability to trigger and perform properly the act of defaecation on account of dysfunction in ano-rectal sensitivity and/or motor activity.

The volume and consistency of faeces affect and interact significantly with both transit and defaecation; thus reduced faecal volume secondary to low fibre intake slows colonic transit[3,4]; a prolonged retention time in the large bowel is inevitably followed by segmentation and dehydration of the faeces[5] which are then more difficult to displace distally and to evacuate[6]. In addition, the presence of hard stools, the poor rectal filling, due to the concomitant slow colonic transit, or chronic rectal overdistension may interfere negatively with the act of defaecation.

*Megacolon*

Prolonged faecal stasis can cause faecal impaction and lead to megacolon, megarectum, with risk of volvulus and/or presenting with overflow incontinence. Less frequently, an enlarged colon is not caused by chronic faecal retention and overdistension but by marked hypotonia secondary to alterations of the smooth muscle and/or the enteric nervous system of the large bowel. These conditions may be caused by parietal ischaemia secondary to prolonged colonic distension or lesions of the enteric nervous system as it may occur in Parkinson's disease[7], viral infection such as Herpes Zoster[8], or due to casual association with myopathies.

*Slow transit*

Modulation between non-propagated contraction and peristaltic activity of the large bowel is controlled by central nervous system. Also the increase in motor activity triggered by meals, the gastro-colic reflex, is mediated at the level of the spinal cord.

The right colon, like the upper gastrointestinal tract, is supplied by the vagus; lesions of the anterior part of the brain stem[9] and autonomic neuropathy affecting the vagus nerve[10] may induce slow transit at the level of the right side of the colon. This condition may be associated with delayed gastric emptying and other motor dysfunction of the small bowel.

Complete disconnection of the sacral nuclei from the higher centres is associated with slow transit at the level of the left colon and rectum which are under sacral parasympathetic control. A prolonged gastrointestinal transit time, mainly due to the distal large bowel, has been reported both in paraplegia and in Multiple Sclerosis (MS) with lesions located above $D_9$, between $D_9$ and $L_2$, or below $S_2$, independently of the level of the injury[11,12]. In these patients, recording of electrical activity in the colon showed, an increase in the non-propagated contractions, which slow transit, and the abolition of the gastro-colic reflex with reduction/absence of the propagated contractions[13,14]. The pattern of altered motility cannot easily be related to the level of the lesion(s), because they are often incomplete. However, as a general rule, the involvement of the dorsal sympathetic centres abolishes the inhibiting modulation and consequently increases the non propagated motor activity; peristaltic activity is, instead, reduced with the involvement of the sacral nuclei.

Incomplete and less severe lesions or lesions affecting only one hemisphere or discrete nuclei, as occurs in Parkinson's disease[15], multiple sclerosis[12], and cerebrovascular accidents, may variably affect transit through the colon and/or rectum.

*Obstructed defaecation*

In neurological diseases, one or more mechanisms controlling the sequence of an efficient defaecatory act may be altered. The conscious triggering of the defaecatory act can be affected by a cortex damage or by the disconnection of the afferent visceral fibres from the sensory centres. Faecal evacuation can be negatively affected by the impairment of the recto-anal inhibitory reflex as may occur in patients with suprasacral alterations[16-18] and multiple sclerosis[12,19].

Likewise, faecal expulsion can be blocked by lack of inhibition or the paradoxical contraction of the EAS (Figure 1) and puborectalis muscle during straining in suprasacral alterations[20], Parkinson's disease[21] and multiple sclerosis[22-24].

Figure 1

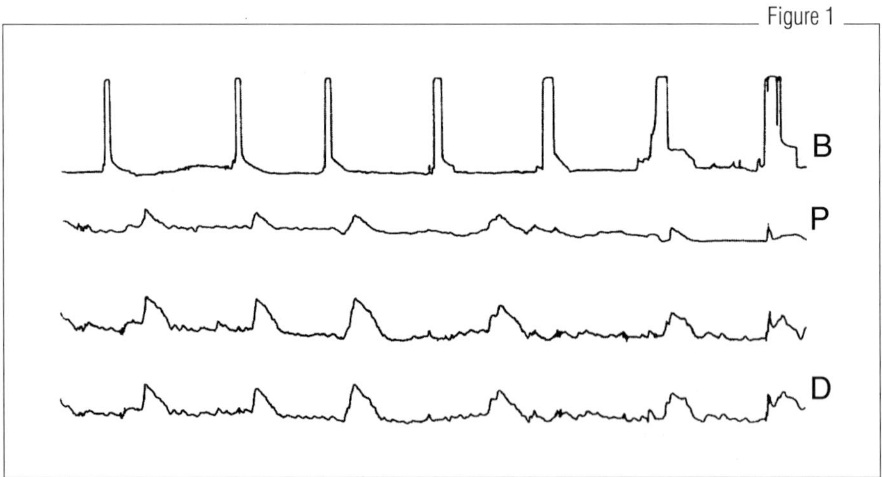


Anorectal manometry in patient with lesion of distal spinal cord; distension of the rectum by means of balloon (B) evokes the hypercontractile response of EAS with increase of pressure both in distal (D) and proximal (P) part of anal canal, which blocks reflex relaxation of internal anal sphincter. Reproduced with permission from Inghilleri M et al. NeUroGastroenterologia 1995,1:12-16.

The lack of inhibition or paradoxical contraction of the EAS and perineal muscles during evacuation in movement disorders, have been interpreted as part of the generalized extrapyramidal motor disorder[21]. Moreover, EAS shows a hypercontractile response during the recto-anal reflex and anal relaxation is blocked. The degree of anal dysfunction fluctuates over time in parallel with the pharmacologically induced "on" and "off" periods[25].

## Anal incontinence

Faecal incontinence was observed in 50% of a group of MS patients[26]; other studies have demonstrated an impairment in the resting and/or squeezing anal pressure, but did not report faecal incontinence, probably because it was prevented by the concomitant presence of constipation.
In normal continence conditions, the arrival of the faecal bolus in the rectum inhibits, via an intramural reflex, the resting tone of the internal anal sphincter. However, this anal relaxation is interrupted by the reflex, and voluntary contraction of the EAS and pelvic muscles. A reflex contraction of the EAS is also observed in response to increases in intra-abdominal pressure (cough) or rectal contractions. The inability to delay evacuation can be caused by an impairment in rectoanal sensitivity, a decrease in resting anal tone, impairment of the conscious and/or reflex contraction of the anal sphincters, or by the reduced rectal compliance, caused by neurological diseases (Table 2).

FAECAL INCONTINENCE AND NEUROLOGIC DISEASES

| Central nervous system | Peripheral nervous system |
|---|---|
| • Dementia | • Cauda equina lesions |
| • Mental retardation | |
| • Stroke | • Polyneuropathies (diabete mellitus, Shy-Drager syndrome, toxic) |
| • Brain tumours | |
| • Spinal cord lesions | |
| • Multiple sclerosis | • Traumatic neuropathy (post-partum, descent pelvic floor) |
| • Tabe dorsalis | |

Table 2

Total loss of sensitivity usually occurs when the rectoanal area is disconnected from the higher centres and the conscious control of continence is decreased or missing[27]. Stroke, MS, myelomeningocele, diabetic neuropathy, which cause different neurological damages from the cortex to the spinal cord and the peripheral nerves, may variably affect rectal sensitivity[28]. In these conditions the failure or delay in perceiving the presence of rectal contents corresponds to failure or delay in activating the conscious contraction of the EAS and pelvic muscles to impair the inhibition of the IAS. Impaired rectoanal sensitivity may also affect the ability to discriminate between faeces and gas allowing the passage of the latter instead of the former.

In addition, denervation of the recto-anal area and the pelvic muscles secondary to damage to the sacral spinal segment and/or its fibres is accompanied by lack of voluntary contraction of the EAS.

Resting anal tone is largely (75-80%) provided by the IAS, the excitatory tone of which is affected by the sympathetic supply. Voluntary or reflex contraction of the EAS, controlled by sacral nuclei and pudendal nerves, hinders intrarectal pressure increases.

Patients with spinal cord injury show a reduced anal resting tone and impairment of EAS contraction. Neurological alterations such as suprasacral lesions may reduce rectal compliance, or cause hypercontractile response of the rectum to distension, all factors challenging anal continence[27].

In movement disorders, there may be a low resting anal pressure and difficulty to maintain squeeze pressure, since the EAS and pelvic muscles display fatigue like other striated muscles[29].

Reduced anal pressures, both resting and squeezing, can be detected in diabetic neuropathy[28] and other damage of the pudendal nerve lesions[30], leading to denervation of the pelvic floor.

In the presence of impaired sensitivity and motor function, anal continence can be easily overcome when faecal impaction of the rectum occurs, or after the use of laxatives which cause liquid faeces and accelerated intestinal transit. These two common situations, associated with constipation, should be sought in any neurological patient with anal incontinence. More than one third of patients with movement disorders use laxatives to treat constipation and complain of faecal incontinence (Figure 2)[31].

Figure 2

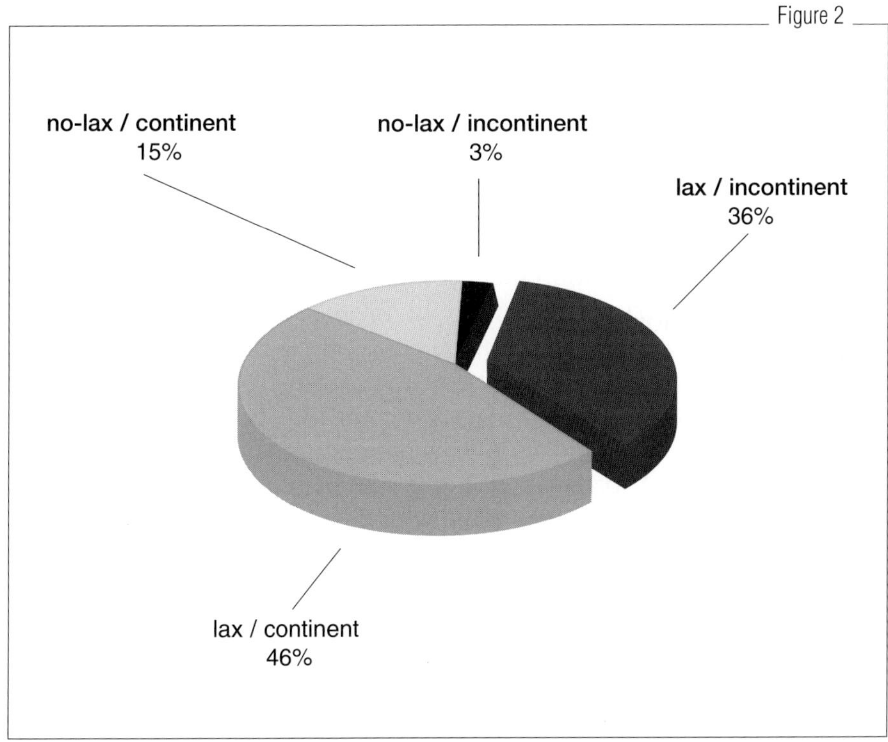


Use of laxatives and faecal incontinence in a personal group of patients with movement disorders. 82% used laxatives of whom 36% (separate slice) reported liquid faeces and faecal incontinence. Of the patients not using laxatives 3% had incontinence, and 15% were continent.

## Management

The management of constipation and anal incontinence is mainly based on therapeutic means aimed at correcting, improving, or compensating for those dysfunctions which are considered responsible for the disturbances and are amenable to treatment. Symptoms reported by patients are of little use to identify the main pathogenetic mechanism because they often bear little relation to the modified function. The type of disease and the level of the lesion should suggest the pathogenetic mechanism, but frequently several concordant factors are found. In Parkinson's disease, 50% of patients complaining of reduced bowel frequency showed anal dyssynergia and conversely 60% of patients complaining of obstructed defecation showed slow transit through the colon[29]. Faecal incontinence can be related to constipation and rectal impaction.

Lower gastrointestinal disturbances caused by neurological diseases are the end result of several different dysfunctions. A rational therapeutic approach to these dysfunctions is necessarily based on knowledge of the underlying lower gastrointestinal tract dysfunctions which should be sought during the diagnostic work-up of the patient. Medical history, rectal examination, measurement of gastrointestinal transit time and anorectal-manometry represent useful means to identify retention of faeces, to evaluate total and segmetal large bowel transit, impairment of motor function and/or sensitivity of the ano-rectum. When indicated defaecography and electromyography should be used to further investigate, respectively, the act of evacuation and the innervation of the EAS. Detection of pathophysiologic mechanisms in the individual patient, is aimed at addressing treatment in a properly integrated time sequence[32]. Schematic guidelines in the management of patients with variable neurological alterations must take into consideration four main conditions: faecal impaction, slow transit constipation, difficult defaecation, and anal incontinence.

Therapeutic efficacy of any treatment should be assessed by weighing benefits in term of patient's autonomy, long term effect and cost-effectiveness.

## Constipation

### *Faecal disimpaction*

In neurologic patients, severe constipation and prolonged retention of faeces may lead to the formation of megacolon. In this condition any therapeutic measures will be of no benefit unless the large bowel has been previously disimpacted. Faecal impaction of the colon and/or rectum can be removed by means of iso- or hyperosmotic enemas (2000 ml/die untill satisfactory emptying of the large bowel); their effect may be enhanced by previous administration of mineral oil either per rectum or orally. Gut irrigation with iso-osmotic PEG electrolyte solutions or large doses of oral laxatives can be used alone or to increase the effect of enemas. Extremely large and hard faecalomas may require digital endoscopic fragmentation or surgical removal.

*Diet*

Colonic transit is directly related to stool weight and dietary fibre intake[3,4]. In patients with idiopathic constipation and slow colonic transit, bran treatment can affect a return to normal of large bowel transit and bowel frequency[33]. In neurologic patients with slow colonic transit an attempt to accelerate transit can be made by means of a high residue diet (15 g/die) and, if necessary, with additional fibre supplements (e.g. bran, psyllium, mucillages) which must be adequately hydrated (1500 ml/die of water). This treatment accelerates colonic transit and improves defaecation in paraplegic and Parkinson's disease patients[34,35]. It is likely that the intraluminal distension secondary to high fibre intake speeds up the large bowel transit by eliciting propulsive and/or by inhibiting segmenting contractions.

Dietary fibre supplements may also be required to increase stool volume and reach the threshold of rectal perception needed to trigger the act of defaecation in patients with reduced rectal sensitivity such as in incomplete cord lesions, and neuropathy (e.g. in diabetics).

*Bowel training*

In impaired evacuation, the aim of treatment is to evoke the defaecatory reflex at regular time intervals, to obtain predictable, effective and painless bowel movements and to avoid rectal impaction and overflow incontinence. In order to take advantage of food-induced hormonal and nervous effects on intestinal motility, patients should attempt to open their bowels after a meal, spontaneously or using a defaecatory stimulus. Whenever rectoanal sensitivity is totally lost, it is necessary to stimulate the defaecation act, if possible, when the faeces are already retained in, or are entering, the rectum. Sometimes, rectal distension may be perceived as a sensation arising from visceral or somatic areas other than the recto-anal region that can be usefully employed to regulate the timing of defaecation.

Exogenous stimuli, such as abdominal massage and percussion, perianal massage, anal digitation, suppositories, should be used to trigger the act of defaecation and it is useful to test them according to a sequential step-by-step programmed schedule[32]. This approach allows us to identify, in each patient, the stimulus that produces the maximal therapeutic benefit with the minimal limitation of patient's autonomy[34].

In patients with less severe Parkinson's disease, the paradoxical contraction of the EAS and the puborectalis muscle is related to the "on-off fluctuations" of the anti-parkinson pharmacological treatment. To facilitate defaecation, Parkinson patients are encouraged to attempt or stimulate defaecation during the "on-period" and, if necessary, after apomorphine administration[25].

*Rehabilitative Treatments*

Biofeedback treatment has been employed with favourable results to enhance rectal sensitivity and to rehabilitate abdomino-pelvic dyssynergia in chronic idiopathic constipation[36,37]. Although the experience of biofeedback treatment refers mainly to conditions other than neurogenic defaecatory disorders, this technique could be attempted to improve rectal sensitivity and recto-ano-pelvic coordination in neurological patients with incomplete lesions.

Many of these neurological conditions also present from slight to total impairment of the abdominal, anal and pelvic muscles which cannot be properly activated during the act of defaecation. Kinesitherapy and/or electrostimulation can be used to increase muscle tone and contractility, as well as to help the patients to improve recruitment of the motor units of the perineal and/or abdominal muscles.

Biofeedback and other rehabilitative measures can be attempted in patients who are cooperative, have residual recto-anal sensitivity and at least partial control of the anal and pelvic muscles.

*Laxatives*

Some of these patients above-mentioned do not behave differently from those with chronic idiopathic constipation and they may benefit from treatment with oral laxatives. The dosage and frequency of laxative prescription is aimed to obtain complete voiding of the rectum and prevent rectal impaction, without causing diarrhoea. Non-purging daily dose of an iso-osmotic PEG electrolyte solutions[38], or of other osmotic laxatives can be profitably used instead of stimulant laxatives to be ingested 2-3 times/week, but, in the long time, have a less predictable and reliable effect.

*Prokinetics*

It has been suggested that cisapride, a benzamide derivative with an indirect cholinomimetic action with no antidopaminergic effect, enhances the amplitude of colonic contractions by increasing acetylcholine release from neurons of the myenteric plexus.

Two case reports[39,40] and a short-term uncontrolled study[41] indicated that cisapride, at a dose of 40 mg/die, could be beneficial in paraplegic patients. On the other hand, two controlled, double-blind clinical trials[42,43] failed to observe any statistical difference between placebo and cisapride treatment in improving large bowel transit and frequency of defaecation. A recent short-term pilot study[44] showed that cisapride (10 mg/die) can accelerate colonic transit and lead to an improvement of defaecatory complaints in patients with Parkinson's disease.

*Surgery*

In patients with megacolon caused by primary changes in the smooth muscle or the enteric nervous system, a colostomy may be an acceptable treatment[45]: it relieves abdominal distension and accompanying symptoms of dyspnoea and anorexia, but it does not necessarily affect abdominal discomfort/pain. When only the colon is affected, surgical treatment may be indicated in slow transit constipation, with and without magacolon, refractory to any conservative approach.

Use of the Malone Antegrade Continence Enema (MACE)[46] has been suggested for colonic washout and emptying. Access to the proximal colon is provided by a non-refluxing continent stoma with the appendix, and the gut is irrigated with saline solution after a phosphate enema (200-400 ml 2-3/week)[47].

*Sacral anterior root electrostimulation*

In paraplegia, posterior root rhyzotomy combined with sacral anterior root electrostimulation is performed to prevent urinary incontinence and vesico-pyelic reflux secondary to reflex bladder contraction. Once implanted for the management of urinary dysfunctions these electrostimulators can be programmed to trigger defaecation. The simultaneous stimulation of the ventral sacral nerve roots $S_2$, $S_3$, and $S_4$ may, in fact, induce rectosigmoid contraction coordinated with anal relaxation[48]. This therapeutic technique is useful in 50% of the patients, who benefit from the acceleration of the large-bowel transit[49] and/or complete unassisted defaecation[48]. This therapeutic approach can be attempted in patients in whom the electrostimulator has already been implanted for the neurological bladder, but the unpredictable and moderately favourable outcome, accompanied by the irreversible sequelae of posterior rhyzotomy, does not support the use of the implant for bowel disorders only. Recently the transcutaneous electrical stimulation of the $S_2$ dermatome has been tested in subjects with spinal cord injuries and, although it induced a change in colonic motility, there was no improvement in bowel function[50].

## Anal incontinence

### *Diet*

Initially, a diet with low fermentable, low liquid and balanced fibre constituents, in addition to the liberal use of pharmaceutical preparations containing chalk, kaolin, or polycarbophyl, can be used to increase consistency and reduce the gaseous and watery contents, as well as the volume, of faeces; a smaller intracolonic bulk reduces the number of peristaltic contractions and thus prolongs large bowel transit which, in turn, enhances dehydration and increases consistency of the stool.

### *Concomitant diarrhoea*

Liquid faeces or frank diarrhoea facilitate anal incontinence and, in many patients with neurological disease, they are the additional cofactors which overwhelm the mechanisms of continence and lead to faecal loss. The management of anal incontinence in diabetic patients may be challenging due to the concomitant presence of diarrhoea refractory to routine therapeutic means. The most frequent causes of refractory diarrhoea in diabetics are autonomic neuropathy (diabetic diarrhoea), bacterial overgrowth, and coeliac disease. Patients with diabetic diarrhoea invariably have evidence of autonomic neuropathy and may benefit from treatment with the alpha-2-adrenergic agonist clonidine, which re-establishes the impaired intestinal net absorption secondary to the loss of adrenergic tone[51]. In the presence of bacterial overgrowth, treatment with antibiotics is indicated.

*Bowel Training*

A toilet training programme is based on the findings obtained by the assessment of the recto-ano-pelvic area.

When voluntary and/or reflex anal contraction is lost, it is advisable to programme timely emptying of the bowel by triggering defaecation at a scheduled time in the appropriate place[32], thus anticipating and avoiding the incontinence loss. The modality of triggering defaecation and the extent of bowel emptying are dependent on the diet, the rectocolonic motility, the degree of vigilance, cooperation, and autonomy, and the assistance available for the patient. So a fully vigilant, cooperative and autonomous patient on a standardized diet and with valid rectocolonic motility can schedule to trigger defaecation from every other day to twice a day with minimal stimuli, such as abdominal percussion, perianal or intrarectal digitation, or glycerin suppository. These stimuli can induce reflex emptying of the rectum and distal part of the colon and thus delay the subsequent arrival of faeces in the rectum for several hours.

In an unconscious, non cooperative, fully dependent patient with sluggish rectocolonic motor activity, it may be necessary to trigger defaecation three or fewer times a week with large-volume cleansing enemas containing, and/or followed by suppository of, stimulant laxatives which can induce total emptying of the large bowel and delay the subsequent arrival of faeces into the rectum for several days.

Also in incontinent patients, it may be useful to follow a step-by-step programmed schedule to identify the minimal intervention which needs obtaining the maximal benefit.

There is evidence, at least in children with spina bifida, that high therapeutic compliance and preserved ano-cutaneous and bulbocavernous reflexes predict favourable response to the bowel training programme[52].

*Drugs*

Opiate derivates and loperamide, which has fewer side effects and is more effective than codeine and dephenoxilate hydrochloride[53,54], can be used to obtain symptomatic control of chronic diarrhoea. It is also reported that loperamide increases anal pressures[54]. In patients with anal incontinence and in whom diarrhoea cannot be controlled by any of the above mentioned means, the use of octreotide can be attempted.

*Rehabilitative treatment*

Cooperative patients with at least partially preserved recto-ano-pelvic sensitivity and contractility[55] may benefit from rehabilitative treatment. It is based essentially on three techniques: kinesitherapy, biofeedback and electrostimulation, which can be used synergically within an integrated therapeutic protocol. In patients with residual function of the pelvic muscles, kinesitherapy can attempt in order to achieve maximal improvement of the impaired movements. The execution and repetition of therapeutic exercises tend to enhance muscle strength on account of the increased trophism as well as the precision and efficiency of movement secondary to the improvement in the neural time recruitment of the participating muscle fibres.

Electrostimulation is used in an attempt to prevent atrophy of denervated muscles with a view to possible reinnervation[56] and/or to reinforce the trophism and strength of innervated muscles. This use of electrostimulation on normally innervated muscles may help the patient to recognize, and reinforce his/her conscious control of the pelvic floor[57]. Recently, it has been demonstrated that the electrostimulation of sacral roots by means of electrodes placed percutaneously can lead to an improvement in faecal incontinence enhancing EAS contraction and reflexes[58].

In the biofeedback technique[59], the relevant stimuli and contractions of the recto-ano-pelvic area are properly amplified and conveyed as visual or audible signals to the patient who recognizes, and attempts to improve, abnormal responses by a process of trial and error. Practising anal contractions in response to decreasing volumes of rectal distensions, initially in the presence, and then in the absence, of the biofeedback signals, is used to progressively lower the threshold of awareness of distension, to enhance rectal sensitivity, and to improve recto-anal synergism.

Biofeedback has been the most widely used technique in the rehabilitation of anal function and although properly randomized double blind clinical trials have yet to be performed, favourable responses have been obtained in the treatment of incontinence in diabetic neuropathy[60] and myelomeningocele[61,62].

*Surgery*

Children and young subjects with spina bifida and poorly controlled incontinence have been treated with the MACE[23]. It cannot be excluded that individual patients may benefit from rational surgical treatment. Anal sphincter reconstruction with the gracilis or the gluteus maximus muscle or implantation of an artificial sphincter may be proposed, but experience of such treatment in neurologic disease is scanty[63].

## Conclusions

Constipation and/or anal incontinence are frequently present in neurologic diseases, decreasing the autonomy and affecting the quality of life of these patients. Different pathophysiologic mechanisms can interact in the same patient according to the level and grade of lesion, and effects of neurological treatment.
Although standardized therapeutic approaches are lacking, it is possible to define management guidelines based on those pathophysiologic alterations which, being amenable to treatment, can be improved with substantial benefit to the patients.

### *References*

1. Camilleri M. *Disorders of gastrointestinal motility in neurological diseases.* Mayo Clin Proc 1990;65:825-46.
2. Johanson JF, Sonnenberg A, Koch TR, McCarty DJ. *Association of constipation with neurologic diseases.* Dig Dis Sci 1992;37:179-86.
3. Burkitt DP, Walker ARP, Painter NJ. *Effect of dietary fibre on stools and transit times and its role in the causation of disease.* Lancet 1972;2:1408-12.
4. Davies GJ, Crowder M, Reid B, Dickerson JWT. *Bowel function measurements of individuals with different eating patterns.* Gut 1986;27:164-9.
5. Devroede G, Soffié M. *Colonic absorption in idiopathic constipation.* Gastroenterology 1973;64:552-61.
6. Aaronson MJ, Freed MM, Burakoff R. *Colonic myoelectric activity in persons with spinal cord injury.* Dig Dis Sci 1985;30:295-300.
7. Kupsky WJ, Grimes MM, Sweeting J et al. *Parkinson's disease and megacolon: concentric hyaline inclusions (Lewy bodies) in enteric ganglion cells.* Neurology 1987;37:1253-5.

8. Debinski HS, Kamm MA, Talbot IC et al. *DNA viruses in the pathogenesis of sporadic idiopathic intestinal pseudo-obstruction*. Gut 1977;41:100-6.
9. Weber J, Denis Ph, Mihout B et al. *Effect of brain-stem lesion on colonic and anorectal motility. Study of three patients.* Dig Dis Sci 1985;30:410-25.
10. Werth B, Meyer-Myss B, Spinas GA et al. *Non-invasive assessment of gastrointestinal motility disorders in diabetic patients with and without cardiovascular signs of autonomic neuropathy.* Gut 1992;33:1199-203.
11. Menardo G, Bausano G, Corazziari E et al. *Large bowel transit in paraplegic patients.* Dis Colon Rectum 1987;30: 924-8.
12. Weber J, Grise P, Roquebert M et al. *Radiopaque marker transit and anorectal manometry in 16 patients with multiple sclerosis and urinary bladder dysfunction.* Dis Colon Rectum 1987;30:95-100.
13. Glick ME, Meshkinpour H, Haldeman S et al. *Colonic dysfunction in multiple sclerosis.* Gastroenterology 1982;83:1002-7.
14. Glick ME, Meshkinpour H, Haldeman S et al. *Colonic dysfunction in patients with thoracic spinal cord injury.* Gastroenterology 1984;86:287-94.
15. Edwards LL, Pfeiffer RF, Quigley EMM et al. *Gastrointestinal symptoms in Parkinson's disease.* Mov Disord 1991;6:151-156.
16. Devroede G, Arhan P, Duguay C et al. *Traumatic constipation.* Gastroenterology 1979;77:1258-67.
17. Beuret-Blanquart F, Weber J, Gouverneur JP et al. *Colonic transit time and anorectal manometric anomalies in 19 patients with complete transection of the spinal cord.* J Auton Nerv Syst 1990;30:199-208.
18. Weber J, Beuret-Blanquart F, Ducrotte P, et al. *External anal sphincter function in spinal patients.* Dis Colon Rectum 1991;34:409-15.
19. Sorensen M, Lorenten M, Peterson J, Christiansen J. *Anorectal dysfunction in patients with urologic disturbance due to multiple sclerosis.* Dis Colon Rectum 1991;34:136-9.
20. Weber J, Delangre T, Hannequin D et al. *Anorecal manometric anomalies in seven patients with frontal lobe brain damage.* Dig Dis Sci 1990;35:225-30.
21. Mathers SA, Kempster PA, Law PJ, et al. *Anal sphincter dysfunction in Parkinson's disease.* Arch Neurol 1989;46:1061-4.
22. Mathers SE, Ingram DA, Swash M. *Electrophysiology of motor pathways for sphincter control in multiple sclerosis.* J Neurol Neurosurg Psychiatry 1990;53:955-60.
23. Gill KP, Chia Y-W, Henry MM, Shorvon PJ. *Defecography in multiple sclerosis patients with severe constipation.* Radiology 1994;191:553-6.
24. Chia Y-W, Gill KP, Jameson JS et al. *Paradoxical puborectalis contraction is a feature of constipation in patients with multiple sclerosis.* J Neurol Neurosurg Psychiatry 1996;60:31-5.

25. Ashraf W, Wszolek ZK, Pfeiffer RF et al. *Anorectal function in fluctuating (on-off) Parkinson's disease: evaluation by combined anorectal manometry and electromyography.* Movem Disord 1995;10:650-7.
26. Chia Y-W, Fowler CJ, Kamm MA et al. *Prevalence of bowel dysfunction in patients with multiple sclerosis and bladder dysfunction.* J Neurol 1995;242:105-8.
27. Sun W-M, MacDonagh, Forster D et al. *Anorectal function in patients with complete spinal transection before and after sacral posterior rhizotomy.* Gastroenterology 1995;108:990-8.
28. Caruana BJ, Wald A, Hinds JP, Eidelman BH. *Anorectal sensory and motor function in neurogenic faecal incontinence.* Gastroenterology 1991;100:465-70.
29. Edwards LL, Quigley EMM, Harned RK et al. *Characterization of swallowing and defecation in Parkinson's disease.* Am J Gastroenterol 1994;89:15-25.
30. Parks AG, Swash M, Urich H. *Sphincter denervation in anorectal incontinence and rectal prolapse.* Gut 1977;18:656-65.
31. D'Alba L, Badiali D, Stocchi F et al. *Faecal incontinence in patients with movement disorders.* Ital J Gastroenterol Hepatol 1997;29: 23A.
32. Corazziari E, Badiali D. *Management of lower gastrointestinal tract dysfunction.* Seminars Neurol 1996;16:289-96.
33. Badiali D, Corazziari E, Habib FI et al. *The effect of wheat bran in the treatment of chronic non-organic constipation. A double-blind controlled trial.* Dig Dis Sci 1995;40:349-56.
34. Badiali D, Bracci F, Castellano V et al. *Sequential treatment of chronic constipation in paraplegic subjects.* Spinal Cord 1997;35:116-20.
35. Ashraf W, Pfeiffer RF, Park F et al. *Constipation in Parkinson's disease: objective assessment and response to psyllium.* Mov Disord 1997;12:946-51.
36. Bleijenberg G, Kuipers JHC. *Treatment of spastic pelvic floor syndrome with biofeedback.* Dis Colon Rectum 1987;30:108-11.
37. Wexner SD, Cheape JD, Jorge JMN et al. *Prospective assessment of biofeedback for the treatment of paradoxical puborectalis contraction.* Dis Colon Rectum 1992;35:145-50.
38. Corazziari E, Badiali E, Habib FI et al. *Small volume isosmotic PEG electrolyte balanced solution in the treatment of chronic non-organic constipation.* Dig Dis Sci 1996;41:1636-42.
39. Binnie NR, Creasey GH, Edmond P, Smith AN. *The action of cisapride on the chronic constipation of paraplegia.* Paraplegia 1988;26:151-8.
40. de Groot GH, de Pagter GF. *Effects of cisapride on constipation due to a neurological lesion.* Paraplegia 1988;26:159-61.
41. Etienne M, Varlinden M, Brassinne A. *Treatment with cisapride of the gastrointestinal and urological sequelae of spinal cord transection: case report.* Paraplegia 1988;26:162-4.

42. Badiali D, Corazziari E, Habib FI et al. *A double-blind controlled trial on the effect of cisapride in the treatment of constipation in paraplegic patients.* J Gastroint Motility 1991;3:263-7.
43. de Both PSM, de Groot GH, Slootman HR. *Effects of cisapride on constipation in paraplegic patients: a placebo-controlled randomized double blind cross-over study.* Eur J Gastroenterol Hepatol 1992;4:1013-7.
44. Jost WH, Schimrigk K. *Cisapride treatment of constipation in Parkinson's disease.* Mov Disord 1993;8:339-43.
45. Stone JM, Wolfe VA, Nino-Murcia M, Parkash I. *Colostomy as treatment for complications of spinal cord injury.* Arch Phys Med Rehabil 1990;71: 514-8.
46. Malone PS, Ransley PG, Kiely EM. *Preliminary report: the antegrade continence enema.* Lancet 1990;336:217-8.
47. Griffith DM, Malone PS. *The Malone antegrade continence enema.* J Pediatr Surg 1995;30:68-71.
48. MacDonagh RP, Sun WM, Smallwood R et al. *Control of defecation in patients with spinal injuries by stimulation of sacral anterior nerve roots.* Br Med J 1990;300:1494-7.
49. Binnie NR, Smith AN, Creasey GH, Edmond P. *Constipation associated with chronic spinal cord injury: the effect of pelvic parasympathetic stimulation by the Brindley stimulator.* Paraplegia 1991;29:463-9.
50. Frost F, Hartwig D, Jaeger R et al. *Electrical stimulation of the sacral dermatomes in spinal cord injury: effect on rectal manometry and bowel emptying.* Arch Phys Med Rehabil 1993;74:696-700.
51. Fedorok RN, Field M, Chang NB. *Treatment of diabetic diarrhea with clonidine.* Ann Int Med 1985;102:197-9.
52. King JC, Currie DM, Wright E. *Bowel training in spina bifida: importance of education, patient compliance, age, and anal reflexes.* Arch Phys Med Rehabil 1994;75:243-7.
53. Palmer KR, Corbett CL, Holdsworth CD. *Double blind cross-over study comparing loperamide, codeine and diphenoxylate in the treatment of chronic diarrhea.* Gastroenterology 1980;70:1271-80.
54. Read M, Read NW, Barber DC. *Effects of loperamide on anal sphincter function in patients complaining of chronic diarrhea and fecal incontinence and urgency.* Dig Dis Sci 1982;27:807-14.
55. Wald A. *Biofeedback for neurogenic faecal incontinence: rectal sensation is a determinant of outcome.* J Pediatr Gastroenterol Nutr 1983;2:302-6.
56. Plas F, Bouchet JY, Chatrenet Y. *Renforcement et entrainement musculaire.* Encyclopedie Med Chir Kinesitherapie 26005 A10-4-9-12.
57. Enok AR. *Muscle strength and his development.* Sport Medicin 1988;6:146-8.

58. Vaozey, Kamm MA, Turner IC et al. *Effects of short term sacral nerve stimulation on anal and rectal function in patients with anal incontinence.* Gut 1999;44:407-12.
59. Cerulli MA, Nikoomanesh P, Schuster MM. *Progress in biofeedback conditioning for faecal incontinence.* Gastroenterology 1979;76:742-6.
60. Wald A, Tunuguntla AK. *Anorectal sensorimotor dysfunction in faecal incontinence and diabetes mellitus. Modification with biofeedback therapy.* N Engl J Med 1984;310:1282-7.
61. Wald A. *Use of biofeedback in treatment of faecal incontinence in patients with myelomeningocele.* Pediatrics 1981;68:45-9.
62. Whitehead WE, Parker E, Basmajian L et al. *Treatment of faecal incontinence in children with spina bifida: comparison of biofeedback and behaviour modification.* Arch Phys Med Rehabil 1986;67:218-24.
63. Christiansen J. *Advances in the surgical management of fecal incontinence.* In: Bailléreʼs Clinical Gastroenterology 1992;6:41-57.

*ADDRESS FOR CORRESPONDENCE*

**BADIALI D, MD**
Dipartimento di Scienze Cliniche
Clinica Medica II
Policlinico Umberto I
00161 Roma Italia
Fax: +39 06 49382437
E-mail: anemgi@mclink.it

PART **SIX**

# THERAPEUTIC ASPECTS OF CHRONIC GASTROINTESTINAL DISORDERS

# PHYSIOPHARMACOLOGY OF RECEPTORS INVOLVED IN GASTROINTESTINAL MOTOR FUNCTION

*M Tonini*

Gastrointestinal receptors play a major role in the regulation of motility and are the predominant targets for drugs[1]. A great variety of receptors involved in gastrointestinal motility are not only located on smooth muscle cells, but they are also present on ganglionic structures and nerve endings of ascending and descending pathways responsible for excitatory and inhibitory reflexes and peristalsis. Within this system, drugs interacting with neurotransmitter, autacoid and hormone receptors may behave as agonists or antagonists and produce direct or indirect excitatory and inhibitory effects on motility[2].

The aim of the present review is to give an outline of receptors that are the target of drugs currently used in the clinical setting, and of investigational agents with therapeutic potential in gastrointestinal motility disorders.

*Cholinoceptors*

It is well known that acetylcholine released from enteric cholinergic nerve terminals evokes a contractile response mediated by muscarinic receptors. In spite of the presence of a preponderant $M_2$ receptor population on smooth muscle cells compared to $M_3$ receptors, only the latter receptor appears to be functionally involved in muscular contraction[3,4]. $M_3$ muscarinic receptors preferentially couple to mobilization of intracellular calcium, by enhancement of phosphoinositide hydrolysis with production of inositol triphosphate ($IP_3$) and diacylglycerol (DAG), whereas activation of $M_2$ receptors inhibits adenylyl cyclase activity[5]. Experimentally, a functional role for the $M_2$ receptor can be demonstrated only after enhancement of cyclic adenosine monophosphate (cAMP) production by appropriate pharmacological treatment (e.g., following administration of a ß-adrenoceptor agonist)[6]. Selective blockade of $M_3$ receptors may be therapeutically useful in the treatment of respiratory, urinary tract and gastrointestinal disorders (i.e., the irritable bowel syndrome: IBS)[7]. The therapeutic potential of selective $M_3$ receptor antagonists such as zamifenacin and darifenacin is under investigation[7-9].

*Tachykinin receptors*

Three tachykinin receptors, namely $NK_1$, $NK_2$ and $NK_3$ receptors, have been identified so far. Endogenous tachykinins (co-stored with acetylcholine on intrinsic sensory, ascending interneurons and ascending motor neurons[10] that preferentially interact with the three sites are substance P (SP) for $NK_1$, neurokinin A (NKA) for $NK_2$ and neurokinin B (NKB) for $NK_3$ receptors. Since NKB is not present in mammalian intestine, the $NK_3$ receptor is probably activated by SP (and other tachykinins) which acts as a full agonist at this site, though with lower potency[11,12]. In general, $NK_1$ and $NK_2$ receptors are distributed on both neuronal and smooth muscle cells (mainly in the latter), whereas $NK_3$ receptors have a prominent neuronal localization[13]. In human isolated intestinal tissues, $NK_2$ receptors are mainly involved in muscular contraction to endogenously released or exogenously applied tachykinins[14,15]. Since $NK_2$ receptors regulate intestinal peristaltic reflex in human isolated tissues[16] and participate in visceral hyperalgesia to rectal distension[17], it is likely that $NK_2$ receptor antagonists might turn out to be drugs of value in the management of the IBS. In fact, $NK_2$ receptor blockade may concomitantly inhibit the function of extrinsic afferent (primary sensory neurons) and intrinsic efferent pathways (cholinergic/tachykinergic motor neurons to the circular muscle), thus leading to the control of visceral perception and intestinal motor activity. Available $NK_2$ receptor antagonists include investigational compounds such as SR 48968A (saredutant) and MEN 11420 (nepadutant)[17,18].

*Adrenoceptors*

The importance of extrinsic adrenergic pathways in the regulation of gastrointestinal motility is well established. In particular, the inhibitory effect of endogenous noradrenaline on intrinsic excitatory pathways is mediated by $\alpha_2$-adrenoceptors[19], while ß-adrenoceptors (both $\beta_1$ and $\beta_2$) are located on the effector cells, where they mediate direct muscular relaxation. Recently, a novel ß-adrenergic receptor (the $\beta_3$-adrenoceptor) has been recognized in the intestine from animals and humans[20,21]. These receptors, like other ß-adrenoceptors, are located postjunctionally where they cause smooth muscle to relax. In this respect, the $\beta_3$-adrenoceptor agonist SR 58611A was found to inhibit colonic motility at doses having only a mild cardiovascular effect. Therefore, selective $\beta_3$-adrenoceptor agonists may represent a new class of putative antispasmodic agents for gastrointestinal disorders associated with cramp-like activity.

*Cholecystokinin receptors*

Cholecystokinin (CCK) at physiological and pharmacological doses causes either direct or a mixture of direct and neurogenic effects, through activation of $CCK_A$ (or $CCK_1$) and $CCK_B$ (or $CCK_2$) receptors[22,23]. Direct myogenic effects are invariably contractile as demonstrated in isolated smooth muscle cells, whereas neurogenic effects are excitatory (as in the small intestine) or inhibitory (as in the lower oesophageal sphincter, stomach and sphincter of Oddi) depending on the type of transmitter released by CCK[24]. At physiological doses, CCK inhibits gastric emptying in man[25], while it stimulates colonic motility only at pharmacological doses[26]. Currently, $CCK_A$ receptor antagonists, such as devazepide, loxiglumide and dexloxiglumide are being evaluated for their ability to reduce transient lower oesophageal sphincter relaxations[27].

*Motilin receptors*

Motilin is a regulatory polypeptide originating in cells scattered in the duodenal epithelium. The distribution of motilin receptors have been recently elucidated[28], and the availability of selective antagonists will allow new insights into the pharmacology of these receptors[29,30]. In humans, the highest receptor density was found in the upper gut[31]. Motilin receptors stimulate motility by a direct action on the musculature, and, indirectly, through activation of cholinergic (such as in the human antrum) and non-cholinergic nerves (such as in the human duodenum)[32]. In the pylorus of the rabbit, motilin receptors are distributed on inhibitory motor neurons, where they cause nitric oxide (NO) and vasoactive intestinal polypeptide (VIP) release, leading to muscular relaxation[33]. A co-ordinated effect on the antrum, pylorus and duodenum might explain the potent gastrokinetic properties exerted by the well-known motilin receptor agonists erythromycin and motilides[34,35]. The latter (e.g., EM-574, GM-611, ABT-229) are motilin-like macrolides without (or with minimal) antibacterial activity compared to erythromycin. To manifest motilin activity, macrolide compounds must have, in their structure, a 14-membered lactone ring with a neutral sugar attached at C3 and an amino sugar at C5 with a glycosidic linkage[35].

*Serotonergic receptors*

In the intestine, serotonin (5-hydroxytryptamine: 5-HT) is contained in enterochromaffin cells and in a subset of descending interneurons[36]. 5-HT markedly affects intestinal motility by activating receptors located on the effector cells, on nerves (excitatory and inhibitory), and on both[37]. Among the best characterized receptors are the 5-$HT_3$ and 5-$HT_4$ receptors. 5-$HT_3$ receptors are ligand-gated cation channels distributed on abdominal vagal afferent fibres (i.e., the site of action of 5-$HT_3$ receptor blockers against emesis induced by cytotoxic drugs) [38] and on intrinsic ascending excitatory and descending inhibitory pathways[37], where they cause the release of excitatory (acetylcholine, tachykinins) and inhibitory (NO, VIP) transmitters[37]. Therefore, it is not surprising that 5-$HT_3$ receptor blockade is associated with constipation both in animals and humans[39,40]. 5-$HT_4$ receptors are G-protein linked receptors, which are located on neural and secretory pathways and on effector cells[41]. Those located on smooth muscle cells cause a relaxant effect by stimulating cAMP production (as in the human colon)[42], whereas prejunctional and presynaptic receptors evoke acetylcholine and tachykinin release from excitatory pathways[1,37,43]. The latter is a well established mechanism through which compounds such as cisapride[1,43] and the novel 5-$HT_4$ receptor agonists R093877 (prucalopride) and SDZ HTF 919 (tegaserod) exert their prokinetic action[44,45]. Prucalopride and tegaserod have been recently found to activate intrinsic sensory neurons in human isolated jejunal specimens, leading to the release of excitatory and inhibitory transmitters[46]. The presence of

5-$HT_4$ receptors on intrinsic inhibitory pathways in the gastrointestinal tract (e.g., guinea-pig stomach) has been reported only occasionally[47].

## REFERENCES


1. Tonini M. *Recent advances in the pharmacology of gastrointestinal prokinetics.* Pharmacol Res 1996;33:217-26.
2. Ruoff H-J, Fladung B, Demol P, Weihrauch TR. *Gastrointestinal receptors and drugs in motility disorders.* Digestion 1991;48:1-17.
3. Eglen RM, Reddy N, Watson N, Challiss RAJ. *Muscarinic receptor subtypes in smooth muscle.* Trends Pharmacol Sci 1994;15:114-9.
4. Eglen RM, Hegde SS, Watson N. *Muscarinic receptor subtypes and smooth muscle function.* Pharmacol Rev 1996;48:531-65.
5. Felder CC. *Muscarinic acetylcholine receptors: signal transduction through multiple effectors.* FASEB J 1995;9:619-25.
6. Thomas EA, Baker SA, Ehlert FJ. *Functional role for the $M_2$ muscarinic receptor in smooth muscle of guinea pig ileum.* Mol Pharmacol 1993;44:102-10.
7. Wallis RM. *Preclinical and clinical pharmacology of selective muscarinic $M_3$ receptor antagonists.* Life Sci 1995;56:861-8.
8. Alabaster VA. *Discovery and development of selective $M_3$ antagonists for clinical use.* Life Sci 1997;60:1053-60.
9. Eglen RM, Watson N. *Selective muscarinic receptor agonists and antagonists.* Pharmacol Toxicol 1996;79:59-68.
10. Costa M, Brookes SJH, Steele PA, et al. *Neurochemical classification of myenteric neurons in the guinea-pig ileum.* Neuroscience 1996;75:949-67.
11. Holzer-Petsche U. *Tachykinin receptors in gastrointestinal motility.* Regul Peptides 1995;57:19-42.
12. Maggi CA. *The mammalian tachykinin receptors.* Gen Pharmacol 1995;26:911-44.
13. Holzer P, Holzer-Petsche U. *Tachykinins in the gut. Part I. Expression, release and motor function.* Pharmacol Ther 1997;73:173-217.
14. Maggi CA, Giuliani S, Patacchini R, et al. *Tachykinin antagonists inhibit nerve-mediated contractions in the circular muscle of the human ileum. Involvement of neurokinin-2 receptors.* Gastroenterology 1992;102:88-96.
15. Patacchini R, Giuliani S, Lazzeri N. *Effects of several bicyclic peptide and cyclic*

*pseudopeptide tachykinin $NK_2$ receptor antagonists in the human isolated ileum and colon.* Neuropeptides 1997;31:71-7.

16. Grider JR. *Identification of neurotransmitters regulating intestinal peristalstic reflex in humans.* Gastroenterology 1989;97:1414-9.
17. Julia V, Morteau O, Buéno L. *Involvement of $NK_1$ and $NK_2$ receptors in viscero-sensitive response to rectal distension in rats.* Gastroenterology 1994;107:94-102.
18. Catalioto RM, Criscuoli M, Cucchi P, et al. *MEN 11420 (Nepadutant), a novel glycosylated bicyclic peptide tachyknin $NK_2$ receptor antagonist.* Br J Pharmacol 1998;123:81-91.
19. Starke K, Göthert M, Kilbinger H. *Modulation of neurotransmitter release by presynaptic autoreceptors.* Physiol Rev 1989;69:864-989.
20. De Ponti F, Cosentino M, Costa A, et al. *Inhibitory effects of SR 58611A on canine colonic motility: evidence for a role of $\beta_3$-adrenoceptors.* Br J Pharmacol 1995;114:1447-53.
21. De Ponti F, Gibelli G, Croci T, et al. *Functional evidence of atypical $\beta_3$-adrenoceptors in the human colon using the $\beta_3$-selective adrenoceptor antagonist, SR 59230A.* Br J Pharmacol 1996;117:1374-6.
22. Wank SA. *Cholecystokinin receptors.* Am J Physiol 1995;269:G628-G646.
23. Silvente-Poirot S, Dufresne M, Vaysse N, Fourmy D. *The peripheral cholecystokinin receptors.* Eur J Biochem 1993;215:513-29.
24. Grider JR, Makhlouf GM. *Regional and cellular heterogeneity of cholecystokinin receptors mediating muscle contraction in the gut.* Gastroenterology 1987;92:175-80.
25. Liddle RA, Morita ET, Conrad CK, Williams JA. *Regulation of gastric emptying in humans by cholecystokinin.* J Clin Invest 1986;77:992-6.
26. Niederau C, Faber S, Karaus M. *Cholecystokinin's role in regulation of colonic motility in health and in irritable bowel syndrome.* Gastroenterology 1992;102:1889-98.
27. Trudgill N, D'Amato M, Riley S. *Loxiglumide inhibits post-prandial oesophageal sphincter relaxations in patients with gastro-oesophageal reflux disease.* Gastroenterology 1997;112:A315.
28. Koutsoviti-Papadopoulou M, Kounenis G, Elezoglou V. *Effect of erythromycin on different parts of the rabbit intestine: comparison with motilin.* Gen Pharmacol 1994;25:93-6.
29. Depoortere I, Macielag MJ, Galdes A, Peeters TL. *Antagonistic properties of [Phe3,Leu13]porcine motilin.* Eur J Pharmacol 1995;286:241-7.
30. Takanashi H, Yogo K, Ozaki K-I, et al. *GM-109: a novel, selective motilin receptor antagonist in the smooth muscle of the rabbit small intestine.* J Pharmacol Exp Ther 1995;273:624-8.

31. Van Assche G, Thijs T, Depoortere I, Peeters TL. *Excitatory effect of motilin on the isolated human colon*. Gastroenterology 1995;108:A703.
32. Boivin M, Pinelo LR, St-Pierre S, Poitras P. *Neural mediation of the motilin motor effect on the human antrum*. Am J Physiol 1997;272:G71-G76.
33. Parkman HP, Pagano AP, Ryan JP. *Erythomycin inhibits rabbit pyloric smooth muscle through neuronal motilin receptors*. Gastroenterology 1996;111:682-90.
34. Peeters TL. *Erythromycin and other macrolides as prokinetic agents*. Gastroenterology 1993;105:1886-99.
35. Itoh Z. *Motilin and clinical application*. Peptides 1997;18:593-608.
36. Meedeniya ACB, Brookes SJH, Hennig GW, Costa M. *The projections of 5 hydroxytryptamine-accumulating neurones in the myenteric plexus of the small intestine of the guinea-pig*. Cell Tissue Res 1998;291:375-84.
37. Tonini M, De Ponti F. *Serotonin modulation of gastrointestinal motility*. In: Gaginella TS, Galligan JJ, editors. Serotonin and gastrointestinal function. Boca Raton (FL): CRC Press; 1995;53-84.
38. Andrews PLR, Rapeport WG, Sanger GJ. *Neuropharmacology of emesis induced by anti-cancer therapy*. Trends Pharmacol Sci 1988;9:334-41.
39. Sanger GJ, Wardle KA. *Constipation evoked by 5-HT$_3$-receptor antagonism: evidence for heterogeneous efficacy among different antagonists in guinea-pigs*. J Pharm Pharmacol 1994;46:666-70.
40. Talley NJ, Phillips SF, Haddad A, et al. *GR 38032F (ondansetron), a selective 5-HT$_3$ receptor antagonist, slows colonic transit in healthy man*. Dig Dis Sci 1990;35:477-80.
41. Hegde SS, Eglen RM. *Peripheral 5-HT$_4$ receptors*. FASEB J 1996;10:1398-407.
42. Tam FSF, Hillier K, Bunce KT. *Characterization of the 5-hydroxytryptamine receptor type involved in inhibition of spontaneous activity of human isolated colonic circular muscle*. Br J Pharmacol 1994;113:143-50.
43. Tonini M, Rizzi CA, Manzo L, Onori L. *Novel enteric 5-HT$_3$ receptors and gastrointestinal prokinetic action*. Pharmacol Res 1991;24:5-14.
44. Bouras EP, Burton DD, McKinzie S, et al. *Dose-related effects of R093877, a benzofurane 5-HT$_4$ agonist, on gastrointestinal and colonic transit in health*. Gastroenterology 1998; 114:A725.
45. Appel S, Kumle A, Meier R. *Clinical pharmacodynamics of SDZ HTF 919, a new 5-HT$_4$ receptor agonist, in a model of slow colonic transit*. Clin Pharmacol Ther 1997;62:546-55.
46. Grider JR, Foxx-Orenstein AE, Jin J-G. *5-hydroxytryptamine4 receptor agonists initiate the peristaltic reflex in human, rat, and guinea pig intestine*. Gastroenterology 1998;115:370-80.

47. Meulemans AL, Briejer MR, Helsen LF, Schuurkes JAJ. *Mechanism involved in the gastric relaxation induced by cisapride*. Neurogastroenterol Motil 1995;7:275.

*ADDRESS FOR CORRESPONDENCE*

**TONINI M, PhD**
Dipartimento di Medicina Interna e Terapia Medica
Sezione di Farmacologia Clinica e Sperimentale
Piazza Botta 10
27100 Pavia Italia
Fax: +39 0382 506419
E-mail: tonini@unipv.it

# NOVEL DRUGS FOR TREATMENT OF FUNCTIONAL GASTROINTESTINAL DISORDERS

*C Scarpignato, I Pelosini*

Functional Dyspepsia (FD) and the Irritable Bowel Syndrome (IBS) are the most frequent functional disorders of the gastrointestinal tract (FGID). Both syndromes comprise a variety of symptoms with no underlying common pathophysiology. Numerous pathogenetic factors may play a role. Motility disorders, disturbances of sensitivity and perception, and psychosocial factors are involved in the pathophysiology of both syndromes[1]. In functional dyspepsia gastric secretion, duodenogastric reflux and the Helicobacter pylori infection are further possible pathogenetic factors[2]. Psychosocial factors in addition to the gut symptoms themselves contribute to the decision of patients to seek medical care[3]. Examination of these not only suggests that the manifestation of symptoms is multifactorial, but also offers clues for management of individuals. There is evidence for both physical and psychological contributions to FGID symptoms and both together may induce illness behavior[1]. In some patients, many factors may be present, in others apparently none, but the more factors involved, the more complex the treatment. Unfortunately, there is no convincing evidence than any therapeutic agent is effective in treating the wide and overlapping symptom complex of FGID. Although, as stated by Parsons & Garner[4], IBS (and other FGID) probably represent too diverse a target for logical research, different classes of new therapeutic agents that may be helpful in their treatment are presently under development. This chapter will summarize the current status of present knowledge on those drugs which have been tested in clinical trials.

## Motor inhibiting drugs

Although it is still unclear to what extent symptoms arising from FGID represent normal perception of abnormal function or abnormal perception of normal function, many believe that they constitute the clinical expression of an underlying motility disorder, affecting either upper and/or lower gut. Indeed, transit and contractile abnormalities have been demonstrated with sophisticated techniques in a subset of patients with FGID[5-7]. As a consequence, drugs affecting gastro-intestinal (GI) motility have been widely employed with the aim of correcting the major FGID manifestations, like, for instance, pain, abdominal discomfort, nausea and vomiting as well as altered bowel function. Besides being often ineffective, available medications have sometimes been associated with unpleasant side effects. Therefore the search for a truly effective and safe drug to control motility disturbances in FGID still continues. There are several classes of drugs which look promising and are currently under evaluation.

Amongst motor inhibiting drugs, gut selective muscarinic antagonists, $NK_2$-antagonists, $\beta_3$-adrenoreceptor agonists and GI selective calcium channel blockers would be able to decrease painful contractile activity in the gut (antispasmodic effect), without significantly affecting other body functions.

*Gut selective muscarinic antagonists*

The excitatory actions (motility and secretion) of acetylcholine on the alimentary tract are well established. Muscarinic receptors are present in smooth muscle from myenteric plexus, longitudinal and circular muscle from the esophagus to the bowel with the stomach and the colon possessing the highest number of $^3$H-QNB binding sites[8]. Muscarinic receptors are heterogeneous and have been classified using pharmacological techniques into $M_1$, $M_2$, $M_3$ and $M_4$ and on genomic cloning into m1, m2, m3, m4 and m5 subtypes[9]. Pharmacologically, $M_1$, $M_2$, $M_3$ and $M_4$ subtypes correlate with m1, m2, m3 and m4 gene products, although a pharmacological correlate of the m5 gene product has not been identified[9].

Available data indicate that most smooth muscles (including human ileum[10] and colon[11]) contract in response to muscarinic $M_3$ receptor activation, even though this receptor forms a small percentage of the total muscarinic receptor population in the tissues studied to date. Gomez et al.[12] have identified muscarinic $M_2$ and $M_3$-receptors in both rat and human colon, although the radioligand binding data suggest that the proportions differed between the two species, with $M_2$-receptors being predominant in the human colon. The difference in these muscarinic $M_2$:$M_3$-receptor proportions between human and rat may reflect genuine species variation or post-mortem changes occurring in human tissue after removal. It is also possible that the proportion of muscarinic $M_2$:$M_3$-receptors is modified by disease. Indeed, human, HT-29 colon carcinoma cells express a homogeneous population of $M_3$ receptors, with no evidence for $M_2$-receptors[13]. Nonetheless, under appropriate experimental conditions, the majority population of muscarinic $M_2$-receptor are functional, principally after depletion of muscarinic $M_3$-receptors. In vitro experiments[14,15] have shown that ileal contraction can be mediated indirectly by $M_2$-receptors (as a result of inhibition of relaxation caused by ß-adrenoceptor stimulation) and directly by $M_3$-receptors. $M_2$-receptors may mediate the dominant parasympathetic control over smooth muscle tone under conditions of highly sympathetic activity or where $M_3$-receptors are dysfunctional. The parasympathetic control of smooth muscle contractility may thus occur directly, via the muscarinic $M_3$-receptor activation and indirectly, via $M_2$-receptor stimulation[16]. In this model (Figure 1), the muscarinic $M_2$-receptor serves to oppose relaxant responses induced by elevation of intracellular cAMP.

Consequently, the regulation of intracellular cAMP levels, as in the myocardium, is reciprocally regulated by the sympathetic and parasympathetic nervous systems. The physiological consequences of this model remain unknown, although one may speculate on its function. Muscle relaxation may occur during the relaxant phase of peristalsis. This phase is presumably dominated by sympathetic drive to the muscle while parasympathetic control is inhibited. Alternatively, when active contraction takes place (during peristalsis), both muscarinic $M_2$ and $M_3$-receptors are activated and the sympathetic system reciprocally inhibited[9].

An important therapeutic indication for muscarinic receptor antagonists is to relax smooth muscle, with the degree of relaxation produced depending upon the level of preexisting cholinergic tone. In general, muscarinic $M_3$-receptors appear to mediate contraction of most types of smooth muscle studied in detail to date. Selective blockade of muscarinic $M_3$-receptors, therefore, should be therapeutically useful in the treatment of painful gastrointestinal disorders, such as IBS[17-19]. The advantage of such compounds lies in the potential for reduced incidence of side effects, including blurred vision, increased heart rate, heat intolerance, sedation and mild confusion[20]. These effects, uncomfortable in the young, may be serious in the elderly, because they are exacerbated with age.

REGULATION OF SMOOTH MUSCLE CONTRACTION BY MUSCARINIC AND ADRENERGIC RECEPTOR ACTIVATION

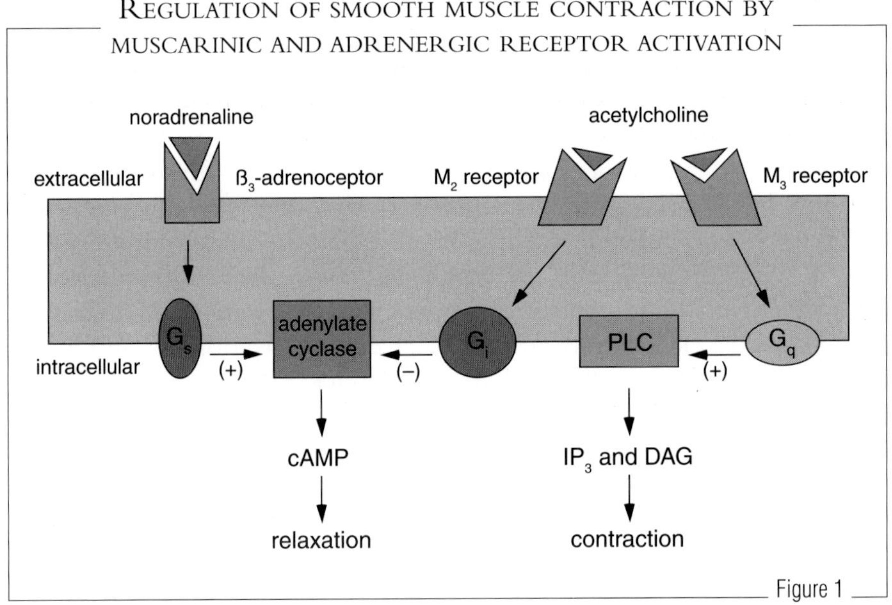


Figure 1

The balance between the relaxant and contractile state of the smooth muscle depends on the prevailing parasympathetic and sympathetic drive. In this model, both muscarinic $M_2$ and $M_3$ receptors modulate the contractile state of the tissue. $M_3$ receptors mediate contraction by coupling to the G protein $G_q$, mobilising inositol (1,4,5)-triphosphate ($IP_3$) and diacylglycerol (DAG) and, consequently, elevating intracellular $Ca^{2+}$ levels. Stimulation of $ß_3$-adrenoceptors causes relaxation by enhancement of adenylate cyclase activity, while activation of $M_2$-receptors, by coupling to $G_i$, inhibits this augmentation.

Reproduced with permission from Eglen RM, Reddy H, Watson N, Challis RAJ[16].

Zamifenacin (UK-76,654) and darifenacin (UK-88,525) are two selective $M_3$ receptor antagonists which are under clinical evaluation for the treatment of IBS. Both compounds inhibit gut motility in the absence of cardiovascular effects and with a certain degree of selectivity over inhibition of salivary secretion[17-19]. In healthy volunteers, zamifenacin was able to inhibit small and large bowel motility and to accelerate gastric emptying over a dose range which was associated with minimal anticholinergic side effects[17]. Resting and postprandial colonic motility was found to be strongly reduced after a single oral dose (40 mg) of zamifenacin in IBS patients[21], thus suggesting that developing selective antimuscarinic agents may be a promising approach in the treatment of pain-predominant IBS. Compared with zamifenacin, darifenacin displays a high affinity (pKi 9.12) and selectivity (9 to 74-fold) for the human cloned muscarinic $M_3$-receptor. Consistent with this profile, the compound potently inhibited $M_3$-receptor mediated responses of smooth muscle preparations (guinea pig ileum, trachea and bladder, $pA_2$ 8.66 to 9.4) with selectivity over responses mediated through the $M_1$ ($pA_2$ 7.9) and $M_2$ receptors ($pA_2$ 7.48)[19]. Interestingly, darifenacin also exhibited functional tissue selectivity for intestinal smooth muscle over the salivary gland. This compound is therefore being developed and clinical studies are presently ongoing.

Although the molecular basis for zamifenacin and darifenacin selectivity is unknown, it seems unlikely that it arises from additional actions since radioligand studies have shown that the compounds do not bind to a wide range of receptors. Since multiple muscarinic receptors, including inhibitory $M_1$-receptors[22,23], control gut function, it is possible that - through selective blockade of excitatory $M_3$-receptors - these drugs reveal the inhibitory actions of acetylcholine acting through $M_1$ receptors. Thus the net functional effect of selective $M_3$-antagonists on gut function may be achieved via blockade of $M_3$-receptors and the revealing of agonist-induced inhibition via $M_1$-receptors.

If one assumes that the model outlined in Figure 1 is physiologically appropriate, responses of smooth muscle to parasympathetic activation should be considered equally in terms of opposing relaxation and augmenting contraction. Participation of both muscarinic $M_2$ and $M_3$-receptors in the maintenance of muscle tone implies that current development of selective muscarinic $M_3$-receptor antagonists is at least arguable. Indeed, studies in isolated tissue, admittedly of animal origin, show that reducing the muscarinic $M_3$-receptor function predisposes the tissue to contraction via the muscarinic may assume a greater importance, because in atopic sensitised rabbit trachea, the muscarinic $M_2$-receptor density and coupling are enhanced[24]. The paucity of information in this area clearly reflects the lack of data reported using human tissue from normal and diseased states.

*$\beta_3$-adrenoceptor agonists*

Since Bayliss and Starling's early studies[25] showing inhibition of intestinal motility after splanchnic nerve stimulation, a large body of literature [for review see[26,27]] has accumulated suggesting the involvement of adrenergic pathways in the physiological control of intestinal motility and secretion. While $\alpha_1$-adrenoceptors are located postsynaptically on smooth muscle cells and, to a lesser extent, on intrinsic neurons, $\alpha_2$-adrenoceptors are present both pre- and postsynaptically, with presynaptic auto- and hetero-receptors playing an important role in the modulation of neurotransmitter release. Postjunctional ß-adrenoceptors (initially characterised as $\beta_1$-adrenoceptors) are found mainly on smooth muscle cells where they mediate muscle relaxation.

Early studies using a variety of synthetic ß-adrenoceptor antagonists suggested the existence of atypical ß-adrenoceptor-mediated responses that were clearly distinct from the traditional effects mediated by the $\beta_1$ and $\beta_2$-adrenoceptors. This atypical ß-adrenoceptor, which was initially proposed to exist in the adipose tissues and later in the digestive tract of rodents, was referred to as $\beta_3$-adrenoceptor. Acceptance of the functionally based concept of a $\beta_3$-adrenoceptor was boosted on structural grounds by molecular biology studies. Sequence analysis indicated the existence in humans and rodents of genes coding for a third subtype of ß-receptor that, when expressed in transfected heterologous cells, had a pharmacological profile distinct from the previously established subtypes[28].

Finally, aryloxypropanolaminotetralins have been synthesised as the first selective antagonists of $\beta_3$-adrenoceptors, thus providing unambiguous conclusive evidence of their distinctive functional features. Several in vitro and in vivo studies have now confirmed the presence of inhibitory $\beta_3$-adrenoceptors in small and large bowel of different animal species[27,29], including man[30]. Expression of these receptors in human tissues is now well documented, since the mRNA of $\beta_3$-adrenoceptors has been detected in adipose tissues and GI tract (stomach, small intestine, colon and gallbladder) of adults[31,32] and children[31].

The therapeutic potential in gastroenterology of the newer compounds targetable on the $\beta_3$-adrenoceptor is suggested by their potent intestinal action in vivo in animal models without any of the cardiovascular or

other unwanted effects of conventional beta -adrenoceptor agonists and antagonists, and by the clinically confirmed importance of ß -adrenergic control of motor function throughout the alimentary canal[26]. Theoretically, the use of a ß-adrenoceptor agonist as an antispasmodic drug might even have an advantage over antimuscarinic agents, since the former compounds directly relax smooth muscle while the latter can only counteract an excessive cholinergic tone. Although several $ß_3$-agonists have been synthesised[33] only phenylethanolaminotetralines (PEAT) proved to be gut-selective compounds[34]. Amongst these derivatives, SR 58611A[35], is now available for human studies and phase II clinical trials are ongoing. Interestingly enough, Delvaux et al.[36] observed an increase in rectal sensory thresholds, without a significant modification of the rectal compliance, after oral administration of the drug (40 mg) in healthy volunteers. SR 58611A was well tolerated and no effect on hearth rate could be detected[36].
However, despite the attractive theoretical advantages of $ß_3$-agonists, an open question concerns the incidence of species-related differences in $ß_3$-adrenoceptors[29], and - as a consequence - the effectiveness of these compounds as antispasmodics in human beings.

*$NK_2$-receptor antagonists*
The tachykinins (TKs) are a family of small peptides whose common structural feature is the C-terminal aminoacid sequence Phe-X-Gly-LeuMet$NH_2$, where X is an aromatic (Phe or Tyr) or hydrophobic (Val or Ile) residue. Three peptides of this family, substance P, neurokinin A (NKA) and neurokinin B (NKB) have an established role as neurotransmitters in mammals[37].
The use of selective agonists in both functional and binding studies has provided unequivocal evidence for the existence of three types of tachykinin receptors: $NK_1$ (Substance P-preferring), $NK_2$ (NKA-preferring) and $NK_3$ (NKB-preferring); there is also preliminary evidence for the existence of further subtypes. These results have been confirmed by the development of selective antagonists and by the identification and cloning of three distinct cDNA sequences[38,39]. All three receptors belong to the superfamily of G protein coupled receptors and are linked to the phosphoinositide transmembrane-signalling pathway[38].

TKs enhance motor activity in virtually all regions and layers of the mammalian gut[40]. In many instances, this action depends not only on a direct activation of the muscle, but also on stimulation of enteric motor neurons that excite the muscle by release of acetylcholine (ACh)[37]. Although ridden by species differences, the distribution of motility-controlling tachykinin receptors is such that, typically, $NK_2$-receptors are located on smooth muscle cells and $NK_3$-receptors on enteric neurons, while $NK_1$-receptors reside on both muscle and nerve[40]. Besides their prominent excitatory action, TKs also exert inhibitory influences on motor activity by stimulating either inhibitory neural pathways or interrupting excitatory relays[40]. There is abundant evidence that endogenous SP and NKA participate in the neural stimulation of motility in synergism with ACh, with which they are co-released from enteric neurons[37]. This synergistic action, which seems to be particularly relevant for the enteric control of peristaltic motor activity, needs to be borne in mind when the implications of TKs in GI motor regulation are analysed and considered as a potential target for therapeutic intervention.

Functional studies with isolated gut segment and autoradiographic receptor mapping indicate that both $NK_1$ and $NK_2$-receptors are expressed in human small intestine. Binding sites for SP occur on the longitudinal muscle, myenteric plexus, circular muscle and muscularis mucosae, while binding sites for NKA are present on the muscle but absent from the plexus[41]. The longitudinal muscle of the ileum is contracted by NKA, SP and $NK_2$-receptor selective agonists, whereas $NK_1$-agonists are virtually inactive[42]. This observation and the much higher potency of NKA compared with that of SP show that it is exclusively $NK_2$-receptors that determine the excitatory action of TKs on the longitudinal muscle. The situation in the circular muscle is not much different, although the existence of functional receptors has been demonstrated[43]. These motor responses apparently are brought about by a direct action on the muscle, since they are not affected by atropine. $NK_3$-receptors seem to be absent from the human small intestine because $NK_3$-agonists fail to stimulate motor activity[43] and specific binding sites for NKB are not demonstrable[41]. The longitudinal and circular muscle layers of the human isolated colon are very sensitive to NKA and $NK_2$-agonists, while SP, $NK_1$ and $NK_3$-agonists are comparatively weak in causing a contraction[44-46]. It appears therefore that TKs contract the human colon too predominantly via stimulation of $NK_2$-receptors. However, the muscle layers of the human colon exhibit also specific binding for SP, which is thought to reflect $NK_1$-receptors[43,47]. Additional binding sites occur in the enteric nervous plexuses of the human colon[43] and this could explain why the motor stimulating responses to TKs are partially inhibited by tetrotodoxin, atropine and hexamethonium[45].

Despite the wealth of information regarding the actions of TKs on gut motility there is relatively little information as to possible alterations of the TK system in GI disease. Evidence, however, is, accumulating to suggest that some of the motor changes associated with intestinal anaphylaxis, infection, inflammation and stress are related to functional alterations of intrinsic enteric or extrinsic primary afferent neurons releasing TKs[48]. The inference that TKs are involved in a number of motor disturbances raises the possibility that TK receptor-selective antagonists could therapeutically be exploited for the correction of disordered gut motility.

The available TK antagonists can be roughly grouped into two main categories: peptidic (obtained from modification of TK amino acid sequence) and non peptidic [for review see[49]]. Selective antagonists to each type of TK receptor have been discovered, but - since $NK_2$-receptor activation in animal and human bowel increases motility and may give rise to muscle spasm - $NK_2$-antagonist are being developed as antispasmodic compounds. And indeed $NK_2$-antagonists are spasmolytic in the rat small intestine in as much as they prevent the increase in small intestinal transit caused by a $NK_2$-agonist[50][50], but lack of any constipating activity[51]. Amongst the selective $NK_2$-antagonists, two compounds are now available for human studies: phase II clinical trials with the non peptide derivative, SR-48,968[52] are ongoing while clinical investigation is being planned with the polycyclic exapeptide derivatives (MEN-10627 and MEN-11420)[53].

*Gut selective calcium-channel blockers*

Several calcium-channel blockers currently in use for the treatment of cardiovascular disorders have recently been tested for their effects on GI motility. The rationale for this approach centres on the concept that

calcium-channel blockers are at least as potent in inhibiting intestinal smooth muscle as in relaxing vascular smooth muscle[54].
Calcium channels can be viewed as macro molecular pores allowing the passage of calcium ions from the extracellular space into cells (Figure 2) and can be divided into two major categories: the voltage-operated channels (VOCs) and the receptor-operated channels (ROCs).

PHYSIOLOGICAL PROCESSES REGULATING CALCIUM FLUXES ACROSS CELLULAR MEMBRANES

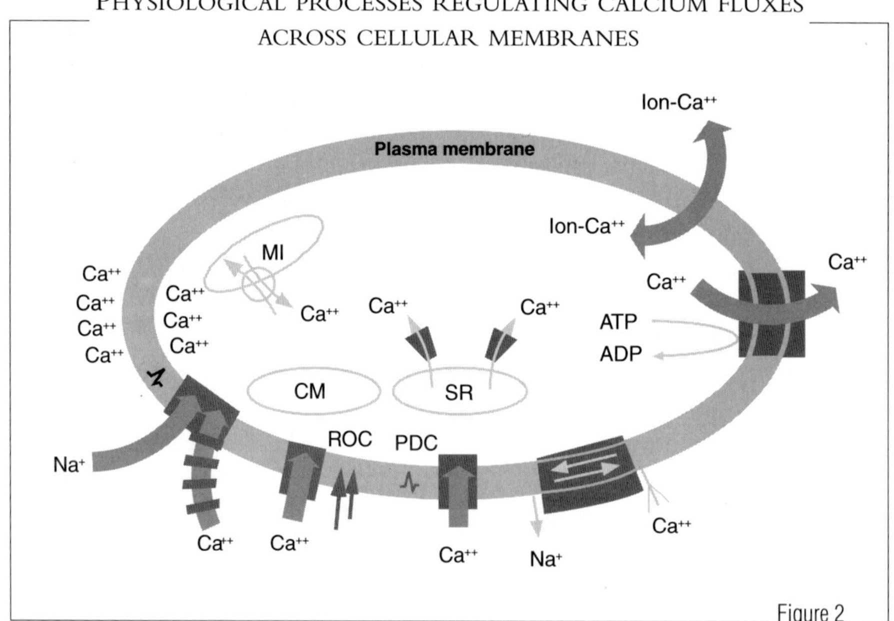


Figure 2

Calcium omeostasis in the smooth muscle. Calcium influx can occur through the potential-dependent (PDCs or VOCs) and receptor-operated (ROCs) calcium channels. Additionally, calcium influx can occur as one component of a plasmalemmal sodium-calcium exchange process that can operate in either direction. Calcium pumping is represented by a plasmalemmal calcium-ATPase, but calcium sequestration (and release) can take place at several intracellular sites, including calmodulin (CM), mitochondria (MI), sarcoplasmic reticulum (SR) and the internal surface of the plasma membrane.

Activation of VOCs is due to changes in membrane potential, while ROCs are voltage insensitive and[55] respond to membrane-mediated alterations other than a change in potential. Studies from smooth muscle cells isolated from guinea-pig taenia coli[56] have shown that -like in cardiac and vascular smooth muscle cells -VOCs could be subdivided in L-type (long lasting) and T-type (transient) on the basis of the characteristics of the $Ca^{2+}$ current within the channel. N-type (neuronal) VOCs with intermediate characteristics have been detected in enteric neurons[57].

Calcium-channel blockers represent a heterogeneous group of agents that differ from a chemical, pharmacological and therapeutic point of view. Since more than 70 different drugs are claimed to act as calcium antagonists, an "ad hoc" Committee tried to establish a classification based on the site of action[58] which anyway fails to include some special agents. A fully satisfactory subdivision is attained by considering the cellular mechanism of action of these compounds. The so-called calcium-entry blockers or slow channel blockers prevent the slow influx of extracellular calcium through specific channels in the membrane. In contrast, calmodulin-antagonists, such as trifluoroperazine and structurally related antipsychotic drugs, decrease the cellular effects of calcium without lowering the intracellular calcium concentration. They block the calcium-dependent processes by interfering with the regulatory protein calmodulin which subserves most of the calcium-dependent functions. The calcium-blocking agents (namely verapamil, nifedipine and diltiazem), which are available and widely used for the treatment of cardiovascular diseases, all inhibit the entry of calcium into cells and may affect smooth muscle tone of many organs throughout the body, including the GI tract.

The mechanisms by which calcium-channel blockers can inhibit GI motility include:

1. a direct action on the smooth muscle, by inhibiting the calcium entrance into the cells through blockade of VOCs[54];
2. modulation of transmitter release from nerve terminals[59], and
3. stimulation of water absorption[60] with consequent decrease of lower GI motility.

There are more detailed studies on the effects of calcium-channel blockers in the esophagus than in other parts of the gastrointestinal tract[61]. This results from the fact that the esophagus lends itself more easily to evaluation. On the contrary, there is only fragmentary information concerning the effects of these drugs on small and large bowel motility in humans [for review see[62]]. On the whole, after administration of calcium-channel blockers postprandial motility was found to be reduced and oro-caecal and colonic transit delayed[62]. Both nifedipine (20 mg sublingually) and nicardipine (10 mg intravenously) reduce the colonic motor response to a standard meal in IBS patients[63,64]. Nifedipine (20 or 40 mg orally) can also inhibit the abnormal motor response to distension in IBS patients[65]. Finally, an increase in rectal sensory threshold was detected after nicardipine (20 mg) in patients but not in healthy subjects[66].

Different attempts could be made in order to minimise the cardiovascular untoward effects of calcium-channel blockers, thus allowing their potential to be exploited in patients with IBS. One could be the development of pharmaceutical preparations delivering the drug to the colon, e.g. a pH-dependent release preparation and another the design of new agents having only a local action on the gut. While no site-specific preparations of calcium-channel blockers are available, some gut selective drugs have been developed and are being used as antispasmodics in IBS. Among these, pinaverium bromide is the most widely known compound. Current evidence indicates that this drug relaxes GI smooth muscle mainly through specific inhibition of $Ca^{2+}$ influx through POCs that exist on the surface membranes of smooth muscle cells[67]. Its in vivo selectivity for the GI tract appears to be due mainly to its pharmacokinetic properties. Because of its low absorption, typical for quaternary ammonium compounds, and its efficient hepato-biliary excretion, most of the orally-administered dose of pinaverium bromide remains within the GI tract[68]. As a matter of fact, not only systemic[69] but also local[70] administration of the drug was found to be effective in reducing meal - or neostigmine-induced colonic motility. Interestingly enough, while two small clinical trials with diltiazem and verapamil in IBS have given disappointing results, pinaverium bromide (50 mg t.i.d.) was found to be better than placebo in improving abdominal pain and constipation [for review see[72]], an effect most likely due to the observed acceleration of colonic transit time[72].

Otilonium bromide is another smooth muscle relaxant found by the Poynard's meta-analysis[73] to be effective in the treatment of IBS symptom complex. Besides being an antimuscarinic, the drug interferes with $Ca^{2+}$ mobilisation, blocking both the cation entry and its release from intracellular stores[74]. Recent experiments[75], performed on isolated rat chromaffin cells, suggest that otilonium bromide binds to VOCs. Because of its poor GI absorption[76], which underlines the lack of untoward effects, otilonium bromide is largely available at intraluminal level. Autoradiographic studies have shown the drug to be accumulated in the colonic and rectal smooth muscle[77].

## Motor-stimulating drugs

Although GI motility has been yet stimulated through the use of dopamine antagonists or of direct or indirect cholinergic drugs, recent evidence strongly suggests that blockade of CCK-receptors and stimulation of motilin receptors are also promising avenues. Since drugs acting on 5-HT receptors, like cisapride, are presently the best available motor stimulating compounds, new derivatives are being developed as gastrokinetic drugs.

*CCK-receptor antagonists*

It is well known that minute amounts of CCK are able to affect gastrointestinal motility under all the possible in vivo and in vitro experimental conditions in both animals and humans[78], thus suggesting this action on the gut to be one of the physiological actions of the peptide. Gastric emptying of both liquids and solids is significantly delayed by CCK and its synthetic derivatives (like for instance CCK-OP and the amphibian peptide caerulein)[79]. The mechanism through which CCK inhibits gastric emptying probably involves a drop in intragastric pressure due to relaxation of the proximal stomach together with a contraction of the antropyloric region, where the peptide decreases the motility index and the basal frequency of the electric rhythm. As far as the small and large intestine is concerned, CCK has a mixture of stimulatory and inhibitory effects on gut motility, although the stimulatory ones are largely predominant. In the first part of the duodenum, the peptide has an inhibitory effect on the motility index and Basic Electric Rhythm (BER) frequency, which resembles its relaxant effect on the sphincter of Oddi. In the small bowel CCK induces motility patterns of the fed state, while in the colon it stimulates electrical spike activity associated with segmenting contractions[80]. In

line with this concept, recent data suggest than endogenous CCK would exert an inhibitory effect on the propulsive motility in the ascending colon[81]. Physiological doses of CCK, however, fail to modify phasic contractility, tone or transit in healthy subjects[82,83] and therefore suggest that endogenous CCK does not play a major physiological role in the regulation of the interdigestive and postprandial colonic motility. It is now well established that CCK exerts its physiological effects through binding with specific receptors located on target cells. At least two different receptors mediate CCK biological actions: $CCK_A$ and $CCK_B$-receptors[84,85]. The $CCK_A$-receptor mediates most of the activities of CCK in the gastrointestinal system. It is present on the pancreatic acinar cells, gallbladder as well as alimentary tract muscle, neurones in the myenteric plexus, vagal afferents from the GI tract and also in certain brain nuclei. The $CCK_B$-receptor is mainly a brain receptor and probably modulates the actions of CCK in the Central Nervous System (CNS). Extensive evidence now indicates that $CCK_A$-receptors are also present in the brain and $CCK_B$-receptors in the periphery[86]; however the original nomenclature still holds. A third receptor was initially believed to represent a third subtype of CCK receptor and named "gastrin" receptor as it was characterised on isolated canine parietal cells; this receptor has subsequently been shown to be identical to the $CCK_B$-receptor [86], and therefore this receptor is also referred to as $CCK_B$/gastrin receptor.
Ten classes of CCK-antagonists including hundreds of compounds have been described[87]. These antagonists have been used successfully in animals to confirm the classical actions of CCK as well as to explore novel activities including its role as a neuropeptide[78]. At present, out of the six $CCK_A$-receptor antagonists so far tested in humans, only three are still under development for potential clinical applications: the two proglumide derivatives loxiglumide and its active enantiomer dexloxiglumide (presently in Phase III) and the indolyl derivative SR 27897B (currently in Phase II), since the substitute benzodiazepine derivatives devazepide and FK-480, and the aspartic acid derivative 2-NAP have been discontinued for gallstone formation and acute renal failure, respectively. Only one abstract dealing with SR-27897B is available in the literature. Indeed almost all the published clinical investigations have been performed with loxiglumide.

Bearing in mind the inhibitory effect of CCK on gastroduodenal motility, one could predict that $CCK_A$-receptor blockade alone would result in an acceleration of emptying rate. This prokinetic activity of $CCK_A$-antagonists is rarely observed however, at least in the experimental animals. In fact, while $CCK_A$-receptor antagonists constantly block CCK-induced inhibition of gastric motility[79], their effect on basal gastric emptying is variable and strictly depends on the experimental conditions. Amongst these, the nature (solid or liquid) and composition of the test meal seem to be the most important ones[88]. Results from human studies[89-95] are in line with those obtained in experimental animals (Table 1).

EFFECT OF $CCK_A$-ANTAGONISTS ON BASAL GASTRIC EMPTYING IN HEALTHY VOLUNTEERS

| Author, year ref | Type of meal | Antagonist | Dose | Effect |
|---|---|---|---|---|
| Meyer et al. 1989[89] | Guar liquid meal | Loxiglumide | 30 mg/Kg p.o. | 0 |
| | 5% glucose solution | Loxiglumide | 30 mg/Kg p.o. | 0 |
| | Mixed liquid meal | Loxiglumide | 30 mg/Kg p.o. | + |
| Liddle et al. 1989[90] | Mixed solid/liquid meal | Devazepide | 10 mg p.o. | 0 |
| Corazziari et al. 1990[91] | Mixed solid meal | Loxiglumide | 800 mg p.o. | 0 |
| Fried et al. 1991[92] | 20% glucose solution | Loxiglumide | 10 mg/Kg i.v. | + |
| | Mixed liquid meal | Loxiglumide | 10 mg/Kg i.v. | + |
| Cantor et al. 1992[93] | Mixed liquid meal | Devazepide | 10 mg p.o. | + |
| Schwizer et al. 1997[94] | Mixed solid/liquid meal | Loxiglumide | 10 mg/Kg•h | + |
| Kreiss et al. 1998[95] | Mixed solid/liquid meal | Lintitript | 15 mg p.o. | + |

+ Acceleration of emptying rate    **0** No effect on emptying rate

Table 1

The effect of loxiglumide on gastric emptying in man was first evaluated by means of radioopaque markers ingested with three different meals[89]. Although loxiglumide significantly accelerated the emptying of the markers after a liquid test meal, no effect was evident when they were ingested with the guar or glucose meals. These apparent contrasting effects can be easily explained taking into account that only the mixed meal releases endogenous CCK and shows that loxiglumide has no intrinsic effect on gastric emptying. However, Fried et al.[92] were able to evidence with this $CCK_A$-antagonist an acceleration of emptying rate (evaluated by gamma scintigraphy) not only of a mixed liquid meal (Ensure®) but also of a glucose meal. Besides the different technique of gastric emptying measurement (radiography versus scintigraphy), the different glucose concentration (5% versus 20%) and caloric content (100 kcal versus 400 kcal) of the two glucose meals as well as the dose (30 mg/kg versus 10 mg/kg/h) and route of administration (oral versus intravenous) of loxiglumide may help to explain discrepancies in findings. It is worth mentioning that Corazziari and his coworkers[91], by using another technique (ultrasonographic measurement of the antral volume) and a solid meal, were unable to confirm the gastrokinetic effect of loxiglumide. On the other hand, in one study[90] devazepide (10 mg orally) proved to be unable to modify gastric emptying of either solids and liquids whereas in another investigation[93] the same dose was found capable of significantly accelerating the early emptying rate of a liquid mixed meal.

In patients with functional dyspepsia and delayed gastric emptying not only was loxiglumide able to accelerate emptying rate but also did improve dyspeptic symptoms[96,97]. In a double-blind, placebo-controlled trial[97], short-term administration of the drug (400 mg t.i.d. for 8 weeks) resulted in symptomatic improvement also in those patients whose gastric emptying was not accelerated by the $CCK_A$-receptor antagonist.

The effects of loxiglumide on small bowel transit time and colonic transit time were studied in healthy volunteers by means of the $H_2$ breath test and radioopaque markers, respectively[89]. In experiments, where intestinal transit was evaluated, the CCK-antagonist was infused intravenously (10 mg/kg/h) starting 60 min before intraduodenal administration of the test meal whereas, in those concerning colonic transit, the compound (800 mg) was given three times daily for 7 days.

Compared with placebo, small bowel transit was not significantly affected by loxiglumide whereas the colonic one was significantly accelerated. In line with this findings, dexloxiglumide was found capable of accelerating colonic transit in an experimental model of constipation in humans[98,99].

On the basis of the above results, a double-blind, randomized, placebo-controlled, crossover study was performed in order to investigate the efficacy of loxiglumide in geriatric patients with chronic constipation[100]. After a baseline phase, a 3-week period of treatment with either loxiglumide (800 mg t.i.d.) or placebo was started, followed by 1-week wash-out period and another 3-week period of treatment with either placebo or loxiglumide. Compared with placebo colonic transit time was significantly accelerated and the number of bowel movements were significantly increased by the drug[100]. Loxiglumide also decreased the need for enema use and did not modify NTB-PABA test, thus showing that improvement of constipation was not due to drug-induced pancreatic insufficiency.

Since CCK is thought to be implicated in the genesis of gastrocolic response[101], the effect of CCK-antagonism on colonic motor response to intragastric fat was studied in healthy humans[102]. Basal motility index (MI) in the sigmoid colon was higher during loxiglumide infusion (10 mg/kg/h) than during placebo. Intragastric administration of soya oil caused a significant increase of MI above baseline during placebo infusion but did not change the already elevated MI during loxiglumide administration. These data confirm that endogenous CCK acts as mediator of gastrocolic response and demonstrate that the peptide has an inhibitory action on basal colonic motility, thus explaining the favourable effects of CCK-antagonism in chronic constipation.

In addition to constipation, another possible therapeutic application of $CCK_A$-antagonists is IBS. Exogenous administration of CCK at doses in the physiological range it was then showed that ileal motility in response to this stimulation was greater in patients with IBS than in healthy controls[103]. The first observation that CCK may be involved in the pathophysiology of IBS comes, however, from earlier studies that showed that CCK administration to IBS patients is able to exacerbate the symptoms of the disease[104]. In addition to symptoms, particularly abdominal pain, CCK can also produce some of the believed motility disorders of the disease[105]. A further confirmation of these earlier findings comes from a very recent study were an exaggerated and prolonged CCK release in response to a fat meal was elicited in IBS patients[106].

A pilot therapeutic study using loxiglumide in IBS seem to indicate a therapeutic potential of $CCK_A$-antagonists in IBS and therefore would confirm an involvement of CCK in the pathophysiology of IBS[107]. The mechanism by which loxiglumide might be clinically beneficial is currently under investigation. Despite evidence indicating that a $CCK_A$-mediated mechanism do not play a major role in the regulation of the interdigestive and postprandial motility of the left colon[82], loxiglumide at clinical doses interferes with the gastrocolic reflex and ileal motility, and is able to selectively slow proximal colonic transit time in IBS patients[108]. In addition, at the same clinical doses loxiglumide significantly decreases the postprandial increase of rectal sensations and pain in IBS patients. Interestingly enough, these changes were not paralleled by relevant motility changes [D'Amato, personal communication].

*Motilin receptor agonists*

Motilin seems to affect mainly, but not exclusively, the proximal part of the gastrointestinal tract[109]. The peptide has no significant influence upon gut contractile activity during the digestive state. Conversely, in the interdigestive state it induces the cyclic recurrent episodes of caudal moving bands of strong contractions that move from the lower esophageal sphincter to the terminal ileum. Exogenous motilin infusion was shown to increase gastric emptying in humans[109], but this peptide is not obviously suitable for use as a gastrokinetic because of its short half-life and the need of intravenous administration.

Little attention has been paid to a possible role for motilin in the regulation of motility in the large intestine. It was reported that the peptide increases colonic myoelectric activity and pressures as well as initiates a premature giant MMC in the caecum of the dog[109]. These effects have however been considered pharmacologic rather than physiological ones. The recent discovery of motilin receptors in colonic smooth muscle[110], with a density higher than that found in the antrum and duodenum, shed new light on the physiological role of motilin and opened new perspectives for the therapeutic applications of drugs acting on motilin receptors.

Motilin binding sites were found on the smooth muscle layers of the gastric antrum, duodenum and colon, but no positive binding reaction was detected in that of the caecum. Specific binding sites were particularly abundant in the circular muscle layers, with low concentrations in the longitudinal muscle layers of the gastric antrum, duodenum and colon[111]. Specific motilin receptors have been identified on the GI muscle (including the colonic one) of several animal species[84,112].

Ten years ago it was shown for the first time that erythromycin mimics the effect of motilin on gastrointestinal motility[113]. Erythromycin and related 14-member macrolide compounds inhibit the binding of motilin to its receptors on gastrointestinal smooth muscle membranes and may therefore act as motilin agonists[114,115]. The contractile activity of these drugs is similar to that induced by motilin and cannot be blocked by atropine or tetrodotoxin (TTX), thus suggesting a direct effect upon smooth muscle cells[115]. In isolated colonic smooth muscle[110], erythromycin displaced $^{125}$I-labeled motilin, thus suggesting the two substances to bind the same receptors. In the rabbit, this macrolide antibiotic is able to simulate mechanical and electrical activity of the colon in a dose-dependent manner with a mechanism dependent on the influx of extracellular calcium[116].

While the gastric motor effect of erythromycin in both healthy subjects and patients with gastroparesis is well established[84,112], conflicting data have been reported for small and large bowel motility. Indeed, Bradette et al.[117] found that while in the interdigestive period erythromycin induces in the sigmoid region a post-prandial motility pattern, it fails to modify post-prandial contractile profiles and Jameson et al.[118] were unable to find out any affect on sigmoid manometric pattern. However, in chronically constipated subjects given intravenous erythromycin (500 mg/h) Bassotti et al.[119] found a significant increase of segmental contractile activity in the sigmoid, but not transverse and descending colon. Similarly, although some investigations[120,121] found an acceleration of intestinal and/or colonic transit time after erythromycin in healthy volunteers, others[118,122,123] were unable to confirm this finding. However, an acceleration of transit time has been observed in patients (with chronic constipation, intestinal pseudo-obstruction or diabetes or surgically-induced ileus) in whom it was delayed[124-126]. Both Asler et al.[127] and Sharma et al.[128] found a significant decrease in transit time of the right colon, thus suggesting a shift in faecal distribution. Taken together, these data suggest that this macrolide antibiotic could be helpful in the treatment of constipation.

### MOTILINOMIMETICS UNDER DEVELOPMENT

| Author, year | Compound | Company | Structural features | $pK_d$ |
|---|---|---|---|---|
| Depoortere et al., 1990 | EM-523 | Takeda, Japan | 14; enol | 8.40 |
| Sakai et al., 1993 | EM-574 | Takeda, Japan | 14; enol | 7.94 |
| Hanyu et al., 1993 | KW-5139 | Kyowa, Japan | [Leu13]-po-motilin | 9.18 |
| Nellans et al., 1994 | A-81229 | Abbott, USA | 14; enol | 8.14 |
| Takanashi et al., 1994 | GM-611 | Chugai, Japan | 14; enol | 8.38 |
| Greenwood et al., 1994 | LY-267108 | Lilly, USA | 12; enol | ND |
| Eeckhout et al., 1994 | KC-11458 | Solvay, Germany | 12; enol | ND |
| Macielag et al., 1995 | OHM-11638 | Ohmeda, USA | Motilin fragment analogue | 8.94 |
| Maes et al., 1996 | ABT-229 | Abbott, USA | 12; enol | ND |

For references see Scarpignato, 1997[88]

**ND** Not Determined

Table 2

While screening a number of erythromycin derivatives, Omura et al.[129] discovered a group of compounds with a loss in antibiotic potency, but an increased potency to induce contractions and to mimic motilin. For this reason Itoh & Omura[130] proposed to give the name motilides to all macrolides with a) a direct contractile effect in vitro on rabbit duodenal segments; b) the capacity to induce in vivo phase III activity in dogs. Peeters[112] proposed to use the name motilinomimetics for any compound able to interact with the motilin receptor, because the discovery of the prokinetic properties has also stimulated a renewed interest into motilin. Motilinomimetics may therefore in the future consist of two classes of compounds: motilides (macrolide derivatives) and motilin analogues. Several derivatives, devoid of antibacterial activity but endowed with affinity for motilin receptors, have been synthesised (Table 2) and are presently under study [for review see[88]]. Further development will depend on the lack of antimicrobial activity and the absence of fading of the prokinetic effect during prolonged administration.

*5-HT$_4$-receptor agonists*

Most of the 5-hydroxytryptamine (serotonin, 5-HT) present in the adult human body is located in the gastrointestinal tract. The vast majority is contained in enteroendocrine cells, the rest exists mainly in myenteric interneurons separated from the mucosa by an intraenteric barrier. Physiological studies suggest that 5-HT plays a vital role in mediating both sensory and reflex responses to gastrointestinal stimuli and, thus, this transmitter is closely implicated in gut reactions[131]. Several studies have shown that 5-HT is implicated in the motor control of the gut [for review see[132]], but how serotonin modulates this function in health and disease is still not well understood. In bowel preparations, 5-HT indirectly causes smooth muscle contraction through acetylcholine release from excitatory (cholinergic) neurones. 5-HT also directly activates smooth muscle although this mechanism seems to be less important[133].

The use of selective agonists and antagonists allowed to establish that the biological actions of 5-hydroxytryptamine (5-HT) are mediated by at least 4 types of receptors: 5-HT$_1$-like, 5-HT$_2$, 5-HT$_3$ and the recently described 5-HT$_4$-receptor[131,133]. It is well known that metoclopramide is an effective, albeit weak, antagonist of 5-HT$_3$-receptors which have been found only associated with peripheral autonomic, afferent and enteric neurons[134]. The effectiveness - as antiemetic and motor stimulating compounds - of some selective 5-HT$_3$-antagonists (like for instance ondansetron, granisetron and tropisetron), devoid of any effect at dopamine receptors, suggested that blockade of these sites plays an important role in the mechanism of action of metoclopramide[135]. However, the lack of correlation between the potency of these compounds as 5-$HT_3$-receptor antagonists and their ability to stimulate gastrointestinal motility is consistent with the idea that mechanisms other than blockade of 5-$HT_3$-receptors should be involved in their motor stimulating activity[133]. Rather, an agonistic activity at level of 5-$HT_4$-receptors, located on nerve terminals of both cholinergic interneurons and motor neurons and whose stimulation increases Ach release, seems to be the key mechanism of established (e.g. cisapride) and new prokinetic compounds [for review see[136]].

Although there are several, relatively selective 5-$HT_4$-agonists in the substituted benzamide group (e.g. renzapride, zacopride, clebropride), most of the available clinical trials have evaluated cisapride, whose stimulatory action on the bowel motility is well known[88]. As far as its mode of action is concerned, it is at least difficult to associate the "enterokinetic action"of cisapride with 5-$HT_4$ activation[137], since in the human isolated ascending and sigmoid colon 5-$HT_4$-receptors have been found to inhibit the contractile activity of the circular muscle[138]. Conversely from the human stomach[139], the drug proved to be incapable of releasing acetylcholine from the human colon[140]. 5-$HT_4$-receptors, however, seem to be involved in the intestinal secretory activity of serotonin[141].

Although cisapride may be useful in some patients with constipation, it could actually represent the prototype of "enterokinetic compounds" for the management of delayed colorectal transit. Two of such compounds, namely prucalopride and tegaserod, display a strong stimulatory action on the bowel and are now under phase II and phase III clinical trials, respectively. Prucalopride (compound marked R-09387) is a dihydrobenzo-furancarboxamide, endowed with a potent, although partial, agonistic activity towards 5-$HT_4$-receptors[142]. In a placebo-controlled study in healthy volunteers, the drug was found capable of significantly increasing colonic transit time as well as the mean number of bowel movements per week[143], an effect confirmed by two recent large trials[144,145] in patients with chronic constipation. Tegaserod (HTF-919) is another partial 5-$HT_4$-agonist, belonging to aminoguanidine-indole derivatives[146]. Preliminary investigations found an acceleration of small bowel and colonic transit[147] as well as an improvement in bowel function after short-term drug administration in constipation-predominant IBS patients [Rüegg & McLeod, personal communication]. The drug, like other 5-$HT_4$-agonists (Table 3), also possesses an antagonistic action toward 5-$HT_3$-receptors. The matter is rather puzzling since - on the contrary - some 5-$HT_3$-antagonists display agonistic properties at level of 5-$HT_4$-receptors, some are devoid of such an effect while tropisetron (ICS 205-930) actually behaves (at high doses) as a 5-$HT_4$-antagonist[133]. Whatever the receptor subtype involved, novel drugs acting on 5-HT receptors are all capable of affecting upper or/and lower gastrointestinal motility and, provided their action be confirmed in patients, new prokinetic compounds belonging to this class of drugs will be soon available for clinical use.

5-$HT_4$-RECEPTOR LIGANDS CURRENTLY UNDER CLINICAL DEVELOPMENT

| Drug | Company | Status | Receptor Activity | |
|---|---|---|---|---|
| | | | 5-$HT_4$ | 5-$HT_3$ |
| Mosapride | Dainippon | Phase I/II | Agonist | - |
| Fabesetron | Pharma | Phase II | Antagonist | Antagonist |
| SB-207266 | Fujisawa | Phase I/II | Antagonist | - |
| Lintopride | SKB | Phase II | Agonist | Antagonist |
| Zacopride | Synthelabo | Phase III | Agonist | Antagonist |
| Tegaserod | Synthelabo | Phase III | Partial agonist | Antagonist |
| Prucalopride | Novartis Pharma | Phase III | Partial agonist | - |

For references see Scarpignato, 1997[88]

Table 3

## Drugs affecting visceral perception

Over the last decade, the role of visceral sensitivity has been largely recognized in the pathophysiology of functional digestive disorders, particularly in the IBS [for review see[148,149]]. These studies have highlighted the role of afferent pathways arising from the gut as a possible target for new treatments intended to relieve pain or modify altered reflexes present in such patients[150]. These pharmacological targets have been identified mainly by studies on animal models of visceral hyperalgesia of various origins including local inflammation. Locally, several mediators are of paramount importance for sensitization of nerve endings: 5-hydroxytryptamine, bradykinin, TKs, calcitonin gene-related peptide, and neurotrophins. Selective antagonists to various subtypes of their receptors are currently available and have been shown to be active in these animal models. Other substances, such as somatostatin, opioid peptides, CCK, oxytocin, and adenosine, modulate the transmission of nociceptive inputs from the gut to the brain and are of clinical interest[150].

Visceral hypersensitivity could theoretically result from either mechanoreceptor dysfunction (peripheral mechanism) or aberrant processing of afferent input at spinal or brain centres (central mechanism). The latter possibility seems to be a very likely one. It was indeed shown that sympathetic autonomic activation enhances perception of gut distention in normal individuals[151] and that focusing attention to the gut amplifies the magnitude of the perceived signals arising from the gut, whereas distraction attenuates them[152]. Thus, it is conceivable that under certain conditions normal visceral afferent signals are magnified via modulatory mechanisms and converted into symptoms. In dyspepsia, for instance, this pathophysiological process would develop when the stomach fails to relax appropriately to accommodate its content or perhaps when there is retardation of its emptying. Such a hypothesis would encompass symptoms arising with normal gastric emptying (patient feels what is in fact normal accommodation) or delayed gastric emptying (patient feels gastric distention to a greater extent than normal individuals) or perhaps even when food is maldistributed within the stomach and stretches a particular region[153].

Visceral hypersensitivity may therefore determine symptoms either by making patients aware of normal motor events or by exaggerating perception of abnormal events. Drugs affecting visceral perception represent therefore a logic therapeutic approach in FGID[154,155].

Amongst them antidepressants, 5-$HT_3$-antagonists, K-opioid agonists and somatostatin analogs have been extensively studied in both healthy volunteers and patients with FGID.There is also some indirect evidence suggesting that $CCK_A$-receptor antagonists (e.g. loxiglumide), besides affecting GI motility, may also reduce visceral perception.

*Antidepressants*
These drugs are often included in management algorithms for FGID, especially IBS, The tricyclic antidepressants (e.g. amitriptyline, imipramine, doxepin) and more recently, the serotonin reuptake inhibitors (e.g. fluoxetine, paroxetine, sertraline) have a role in controlling pain via central analgesia[156], as well as the associated depressive symptoms. These drugs should be therefore considered for unremitting pain and impaired daily function, with or without coexistent symptoms of major or atypical (masked) depression. On the contrary, anxiolytics, such as benzodiazepines, do not relieve pain and may lead to dependence. Even with doses lower than the conventional ones complete remission or improvement of bowel symptoms is observed[157], provided the treatment period be sufficiently long (i.e. at least 3 months). Tricyclic antidepressants may cause or aggravate constipation in patients with IBS because of their anticholinergic side effects, and are thus best avoided in the subgroup with pain and constipation

Because of their complex pharmacological properties (both central and peripheral), antidepressants may exert useful actions at more than one site along the brain-gut axis.Two recent studies showed that imipramine can prolong orocecal and whole gut transit times in diarrhea-predominant and control subjects, while paroxetine reduced orocecal transit times with no effect on whole gut transit times[158,159]. Although, as the Authors acknowledge, demonstration of altered transit by antidepressants does not imply therapeutic usefulness, the above studies have shown that antidepressants can alter motor function independently of mood effects, since the antidepressants were taken only for 4 to 5 days. As regards modulation of afferent information from the gut by antidepressants, two recent preliminary reports[160,161] indeed suggest that this is a possible mechanism of action. The latter study, carried out in healthy humans, reported that imipramine can increase pain and sensation thresholds to esophageal balloon distention. Thus, antidepressants seem to have analgesic and neuromodulatory properties independent of their psychotropic effects, and these effects may occur sooner and at lower doses that is the case when these drugs are used for the treatment of depression[162,163].

*5-HT$_3$-receptor antagonists*

5-HT$_3$-receptors are present throughout the enteric nervous system on both sensory and motor neurones and their activation results in measurable changes in GI motility and transit [for review see[164]]. However, there is no consensus with respect to the effect of 5-HT$_3$-receptor antagonists on visceral perception.

While ondansetron was found capable of reducing esophageal sensitivity in patients with NCCP[165], its effect on gastric perception are controversial. Indeed, whereas it reduced nausea and gastric sensitivity to distention during intraduodenal lipid infusion[166], no effects on both sensitivity and compliance were seen in other experimental conditions[167,168]. Similarly, a lack of effect on rectal sensitivity was reported in healthy subjects[169] and IBS patients[168-170]. Granisetron however does reduce either rectal sensitivity and postprandial motility in patients with IBS[171]. A recent investigation[172] with alosetron showed that also this 5-HT$_3$-receptor antagonist increases the compliance of the colon to distension in these patients. This pharmacological effect could therefore contribute to changes in perception of colonic distension and explain the observed symptom improvement in IBS[173]. Here again, alosetron did not affect perception of gastric distention in healthy volunteers[174].

It is worthwhile to emphasize that discrepancies in findings are not easy to explain only on the basis of the different experimental conditions (e.g. healthy subjects versus patients, different modalities and duration of visceral stimulation, different evaluation of patient's perception, different routes of drug administration, etc.). Indeed, pharmacological differences exist amongst the different compounds[133,175], that could account for the conflicting results observed either in experimental and clinical studies. Although - on the basis of the available data - it not possible to draw any definite conclusion on the effect of 5-$HT_3$-receptor antagonists on the visceral perception in the GI tract, it seems that such an effect, if present, is confined to the lower gut and is more evident in patients with FGID than in healthy subjects.

*k-receptor agonists*

Inhibition of somatic and visceral pain is a general feature of opioid agonists, which unfold their antinociceptive effects by different opioid receptors located peripherally as well as centrally. Recently, k-opioid receptor agonists have been proposed as a new pharmacological approach to the treatment of functional gut disorders[176,177] on the basis that k-opioid receptors are thought to be located on vagal and non-vagal afferent pathways. Activation of these receptors causes a decrease in calcium currents, resulting in increased nociceptive thresholds and attenuation of neuronal excitability[178]. Peripherally acting k-opioid agonists would also have the advantage of avoiding the central side effects of opioids as well the potent inhibitory effect on gut motility exerted by μ- and δ-opioid agonists

Fedotozine has been shown to suppress afferent visceral activity in several animal models[176], such as experimental ileus, acetic-acid induced colonic hypersensitivity, colo-gastric inhibitory reflex. In humans, fedotozine decreases sensitivity to distention in the stomach[179] and colon[180], without modifying gastric and colonic compliance or somatic sensitivity.

More importantly, oral fedotozine (30 mg t.i.d.) was reported to reduce dyspeptic symptoms and epigastric pain in functional dyspepsia[181] and abdominal pain in patients with IBS[182]. In the latter study, fedotozine also improved the quality of life. However, additional studies with fedotozine in IBS have been disappointing and it is presently unknown whether the drug will be further developed.

*Somatostatin analogs*

Somatostatin and its stable analogs such as octreotide have antinociceptive effects in various animal models and have been shown to induce analgesia in humans[183]. This observation raised the question as to whether somatostatin and its analogs also affect intestinal visceral perception.

While several investigations have shown an inhibitory effect of octreotide on rectal sensation[184-187] conflicting results have been reported as far as gastric perception is concerned. In an early study[188], octreotide was found to increase the threshold for fullness during distention, while a subsequent investigation[189] found no effect of octreotide on either perception or discomfort thresholds. In patients with IBS, however, the peptide does increase thresholds of colonic visceral perception without modifying muscle tone or compliance[190] (Figure 3). As regards the clinical use of somatostatin analogs, the inconvenient route of administration (octreotide is administered subcutaneously) and high cost limit at present their use. New, orally active, somatostatin analogs are now under development[191].

### *$CCK_A$-receptor Antagonists*

Many studies have evaluated the role of CCK in stimulating gut afferents (mainly vagal afferents), and it is clearly established that CCK is involved in a great number of intestino-intestinal activating or inhibitory reflexes (for review see[192]). However, only few studies have evaluated its role in the mediation of nociceptive messages from the upper and lower parts of the gut.

Recently, it has been shown that CCK and $CCK_A$-receptors are involved in the induction of meal-like fullness and nausea associated with intraduodenal lipid infusion and gastric distention (Table 4) in both healthy subjects[193] and patients with FD[194]. This effect is blocked by loxiglumide[193].

Similarly, in IBS patients in whom CCK infusion mimicks their usual pain[105], oral loxiglumide was able to reduce the number of subjects experiencing anorectal and sigmoid pain after a fatty meal [D'Amato, personal communication], whose intake is followed by an exagerrated release of endogenous CCK[106]. It must be pointed out that $CCK_A$-receptor antagonists are endowed with many pharmacological effects on GI motility that should be taken into account when examining their action on visceral perception.

Therefore, the antinociceptive properties of CCK antagonists has to be evaluated in experiments measuring visceral perception during gastric or intestinal distention.

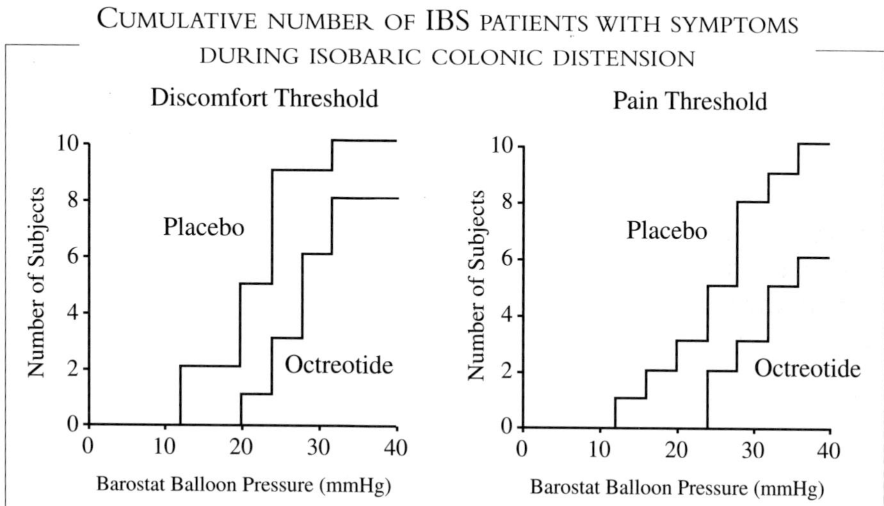


Figure 3

Cumulative numbers of IBS patients who experienced discomfort and pain during isobaric intracolonic distension after injection of either placebo or octreotide. The curves obtained in IBS patients following octretide administration show a significant ($p<0,01$ at the $X_2$ test) shift toward higher pressures compared to those following placebo.
Reproduced from Bradette M, Delvaux M, Straumont G, et al.[190]

SENSATIONS REPORTED DURING GASTRIC DISTENTIONS AFTER DIFFERENT TREATMENT

| | FULLNESS | | DISCOMFORT | |
|---|---|---|---|---|
| | Pressure | Meallike | Pain | Nausea |
| SA-P | 97 | 3 | 92 | 8 |
| SA-LOX | 92 | 8 | 94 | 6 |
| LI-P | 26[a] | 74[a] | 30[a] | 70[a] |
| LI-LOX | 67[b] | 33[b] | 60[c] | 40[c] |

Significantly different
[a] from SA-P (P< 0,001)
[b] from LI-P (but not from SA-LOX) (P< 0,05)
[c] from SA-LOX (P< 0,05) and from LI-P (P= 0,05).

**SA** isotonic saline
**P** placebo
**LOX** loxiglumide
**LI** intralipid

Table 4

Data show percentages of distentions during which a particular sensation was reported by the subjects.
Reproduced from Feinle C, D'Amato M, Read NW[193].

## Conclusions

Drugs affecting motility and perception in the gut are now available and several new ones are being developed. All the above compounds belong to a long line of drugs that have been touted as potential breakthroughs in the treatment of FGID. However, none of the other "magic bullets"has withstood the objective scrutiny of controlled clinical trial testing, and it is difficult to imagine that these new agents will be any different. Further work is needed to determine the predictive value of objective abnormalities for the efficacy of a given drug in the individual patient. This is the crucial point to define a rational strategy in clinical practice, especially to establish if functional investigation is needed before a drug affecting motility or perception be given.

### *REFERENCES*


1. Kellow JE, Delvaux M, Azpiroz F, et al. *Principles of applied neurogastroenterology: physiology/motility-sensation*. Gut 1999;45 (Suppl II):II17-II24.
2. Talley NJ, Stanghellini V, Heading RC, et al. *Functional gastroduodenal disorders*. Gut 1999;45 (Suppl II): II37-II42.
3. Drossmann DA, Creed FH, Fava GA, et al. *Psychosocial aspects of the functional gastrointestinal disorders*. Gastroenterol Int 1995;8:47-90.
4. Parsons ME, Garner AG. *Review article: Drug development in gastroenterology. The changing view of Industry*. Aliment Pharmacol Ther 1995;9:457-463.
5. Malagelada JR. *Functional dyspepsia. Insights on mechanisms and management strategies*. Gastroenterol Clin NA 1996;25:103-12.
6. Drossman DA, Whitehead WE, Camilleri M. *Irritable bowel syndrome: a technical review for practice guideline development*. Gastroenterology 1997;112:2120-37.
7. Müller-Lissner S, Coremans G, Dapoigny M, et al. *Motility in Irritable Bowel Syndrome*. Digestion 1997;58:196-202.
8. Morisset J, Geoffrion L, Larose L et al. *Distribution of muscarinic receptors in the digestive tract organs*. Pharmacology 1986;22:189-95.
9. Eglen RM, Hegde SS, Watson N. *Muscarinic receptor subtypes and smooth muscle function*. Pharmacol Rev 1996;48:531-65.

10. Lepor H, Rigaud G, Shapiro E, et al. *Muscarinic cholinergic and alpha2-adrenergic receptors in the epithelium and muscularis of the human ileum.* Surgery 1990;107:461-7.
11. Kerr PM, Hillier K, Wallis RM, Garland CJ. *Characterization of muscarinic receptors mediating contractions of circular and longitudinal muscle of human isolated colon.* Br J Pharmacol 1995;115:1517-24.
12. Gomez A, Martos F, Bellido I, et al. *Muscarinic receptor subtypes in human and rat colon smooth muscle.* Biochem Pharmacol 1992;43:2413-19.
13. Kopp R, Lambrecht G, Mutschler E, et al. *Human HT-29 colon carcinoma cells contain muscarinic $M_3$ receptors coupled to phosphoinositide metabolism.* Eur J Pharmacol 1989;172:397-405.
14. Thomas EA, Baker SA, Ehlert FJ. *Functional role for the $M_2$ muscarinic receptor in smooth muscle of guinea pig ileum.* Mol Pharmacol 1993;44:102-10.
15. Reddy H, Watson N, Ford APDW, Eglen RM. *Characterization of the interaction between muscarinic $M_2$ receptors and beta-adrenoceptor subtypes in guinea-pig isolated ileum.* Br J Pharmacol 1995;114:49-56.
16. Eglen RM, Reddy H, Watson N, Challis RAJ. *Muscarinic acetylcholine receptor subtypes in smooth muscle.* Trends Pharmacol Sci 1994;15:114-19.
17. Wallis RM. *Pre-clinical and clinical pharmacology of selective muscarinic $M_3$ receptor antagonists.* Life Sci 1995; 56: 861-8.
18. Alabaster VA. *Discovery and development of selective $M_3$ antagonists for clinical use.* Life Sci 1997;60:1053-1060.
19. Wallis RM, Napier CM. *Muscarinic antagonists in development for disorders of smooth muscle function.* Life Sci 1999;64:395-401.
20. Feinberg M. *The problems of anticholinergic adverse effects in older patients.* Drugs Aging 1993;3:335-48.
21. Houghton LA, Rogers J, Whorwell PJ, et al. *Zamifenacin (UK-76,654), a potent gut $M_3$ selective muscarinic antagonist, reduces colonic motor activity in patients with irritable bowel syndrome.* Aliment Pharmacol Ther 1997;11:561-8.
22. Micheletti R, Schiavone A, Giachetti A. *Muscarinic $M_1$ receptors stimulate a nonadrenergic noncholinergic inhibitory pathway in the isolated rat duodenum.* J Pharmacol Exptl Ther 1988,244:680-4.
23. Schiavone A, Sagrada A, Micheletti R, Giachetti A. *Pharmacological characterization of muscarinic receptors involved in McN-A-343-induced effects on intestinal motility and heart rate in conscious dogs.* Br J Pharmacol 1988;94:566-72.
24. Hakonarson H, Herrick DJ, Grunstein MM. *Mechanism of impaired beta-adrenoceptor responsiveness in atopic sensitized airway smooth muscle.* Am J Physiol 1995;269:L645-L652.

25. Bayliss WM, Starling EH. *The movements and innervation of the small intestine.* J Physiol (Lond) 1899;24:99-143.
26. McIntyre AS, Thompson DG. *Review article: Adrenergic control of motor and secretory function in the gastrointestinal tract.* Aliment Pharmacol Ther 1992;6: 125-42.
27. De Ponti F, Garoni C, Cosentino M, et al. *Adrenergic mechanisms in the control of gastrointestinal motility: from basic science to clinical applications.* Pharmacol Ther 1996;69:59-78.
28. Emorine L, Blin N, Strosberg AD. *The human $\beta_3$-adrenoceptor: the search for a physiological function.* Trend Pharmacol Sci 1994; 15: 3-7.
29. Manara L, Croci T, Landi M. *$\beta_3$-adrenoceptors and intestinal motility.* Fund Clin Pharmacol 1955;9:332-42.
30. De Ponti F, Gibelli G, Croci T, et al. *Functional evidence of atypical $\beta_3$-adrenoceptors in the human colon using the beta -3-selective adrenoceptor antagonist, SR 59230A.* Br J Pharmacol 1996b;117:1374-6.
31. Krief S, Lonnqvist F, Raimbault S, et al. *Tissue distribution of $\beta_3$-adrenergic receptor mRNA in man.* J Clin Invest 1993;91:344-9.
32. Berkowitz DE, Nardone NA, Smiley RM, et al. *Distribution of $\beta_3$-adrenoceptor mRNA in human tissues.* Eur J Pharmacol (Mol Pharmacol Section) 1995;289:223-8.
33. Howe R. *$\beta_3$-adrenergic agonists.* Drugs Future 1993;18:529-49.
34. Giudice A, Croci T, Bianchetti A, Manara L. *Inhibition of rat colonic motility and cardiovascular effects of new gut-specific beta-adrenergic phenylethanolaminotetralines.* Life Sci 1989;44:1411-7.
35. De Ponti F, Cosentino M, Costa A, et al. *Inhibitory effects of SR 58611A on canine colonic motility: Evidence for a role of beta -3-adrenoceptors.* Br J Pharmacol 1995;114:1447-53.
36. Delvaux M, Louvel D, Peronnet P, et al. *Effect of SR 58611A, an agonist at the adrenergic beta-3 receptor, on rectal sensory thresholds in healthy volunteers.* Gastroenterology 1995;108:A589.
37. Holzer P, Holzer-Petsche U. *Tachikinins in the Gut. Part I. Expression, release and motor function.* Pharmacol Ther 1977;73:173-217.
38. Guard S, Watson SP. *Takchykinin receptor types: classification and membrane signalling mechanisms.* Neurochem Int 1991;18:149-65.
39. Maggi CA. *The mammalian tackykinin receptors.* Gen Pharmacol 1995;26:911-44.
40. Holzer-Petsche U. *Tachikinin receptors in gastrointestinal motility.* Regul Peptides 1995;57:19-42.
41. Gates-TS, Zimmerman-RP, Mantyh-CR, et al. *Substance P and substance K receptor*

*binding sites in the human gastrointestinal tract: Localization by autoradiography*. Peptides 1988;9:1207-19.

42. Maggi CA, Patacchini R, Santicioli P, et al. *Human isolated small intestine: motor response of the longitudinal muscle to field stimulation and exogenous neuropeptides.* Naunyn Schmiedeberg's Arch Pharmacol 1989; 339: 415-23.
43. Maggi CA, Patacchini R, Santicioli P, et al. *Human isolated ileum: motor responses of the circular muscle to field stimulation and exogenous neuropeptides.* Naunyn Schmiedeberg's Arch Pharmacol 1990;341:256-61.
44. Giuliani S, Barbanti G, Turini D, et al. *$NK_2$ tachykinin receptors and contraction of circular muscle of the human colon: Characterization of the $NK_2$ receptor subtype.* Eur J Pharmacol 1991;203:365-70.
45. Kölbel CB, Mayer EA, Holtmann G, et al. *Effects of neurokinins on human colonic motility*. Neurogastroenterol Motil 1995;6:119-27.
46. Croci T, Aureggi G, Manara L, et al. *Functional neurotensin and tachykinin $NK_2$ receptors in human colon strips*. Gastroenterology 1997;112:A716.
47. Korman LY, Sayadi H, Bass B, et al. *Distribution of vasoactive intestinal polypeptide and substance P receptors in human colon and small intestine.* Dig Dis Sci 1989;34:1100-08.
48. Holzer P, Holzer-Petsche U. *Tachykinins in the gut. Part II. Roles in neural excitation, secretion and inflammation.* Pharmacol Ther 1997b;73:219-63.
49. Maggi CA, Patacchni R, Rovero P, Giachetti A. *Tachykinin receptors and tachykinin receptor antagonists.* J Auton Pharmacol 1993;13:23-93.
50. Tramontana M, Maggi CA, Evangelista S. *Spasmolytic effect of the $NK_2$-receptor-selective antagonist MEN 10,627 in rat small intestine.* Jpn J Pharmacol 1994;65:281-3.
51. Croci T, Emonds Alt X, Manara L. *SR 48968 selectively prevents faecal excretion following activation of tachykinin $NK_2$ receptors in rats.* J Pharmac Pharmacol 1994; 46:383-5.
52. Emonds Alt X, Advenier C, Soubrie P, et al. *SR 48968: non peptide antagonist of the tachykinin $NK_2$-receptor.* Drugs Future 1995;20:701-7.
53. Quartara L, Rovero P, Maggi CA. *Peptide-based tachykinin $NK_2$ receptor antagonists.* Med Res Rev 1995;15:139-55.
54. Godfraind T, Miller R, Wibo M. *Calcium antagonism and calcium entry blockade.* Pharmacol Rev 1986;38:321-416.
55. Pietrobon D, Di Virgilio F, Pozzan T. *Structural and functional aspects of calcium homeostasis in eukaryotic cells.* Eur J Biochem 1990;193:599-622.
56. Yoshino M, Someya T, Nishio A, Yabu H. *Whole-cell and unitary Ca channel currents in mammalian intestinal smooth muscle cells: evidence for the existence*

*of two types of Ca channels*. Pflügers Arch (Eur J Physiol) 1988;411:229-31.

57. Ahmad S, Rausa J, Jang E, Daniel EE. *Calcium channel binding in nerves and muscle of canine small intestine*. Biochem Biophys Res Comm 1989;159:119-25.
58. Spedding M, Paoletti R. *Classification of calcium channels and sites of action of drugs modifying channel function*. Pharmacol Rev 1992;44:363-7.
59. Lecchini S, Marcoli M, De Ponti F, et al. *Selectivity of $Ca^{2+}$ channel blockers in inhibiting muscular and nerve activities in isolated colon*. Br J Pharmacol 1991;102:735-41.
60. Donowitz M, Levin S, Powers G, et al. *$Ca^{2+}$ channel blockers stimulate ileal and colonic water absorption*. Gastroenterology 1985,89:858-66.
61. Traube M, McCallum RW. *Calcium-channel blockers and the gastrointestinal tract*. Am J Gastroenterol 1984;79:892-6.
62. De Ponti F, Giaroni C, Cosentino M, et al. *Calcium-channel blockers and gastrointestinal motility: Basic and clinical aspects*. Pharmacol Ther 1993; 60:121-48.
63. Narducci F, Bassotti G, Gaburri M, et al. *Nifedipine reduces the colonic motor response to eating in patients with the irritable colon syndrome*. Am J Gastroenterol 1985;80:317-9.
64. Prior A, Harris SR, Whorwell PJ. *Reduction of colonic motility by intravenous nicardipine in irritable bowel syndrome*. Gut 1987;28:1609-12.
65. Blume M, Schuster M, Tucker H. *Effect of nifedipine on colonic motility in irritable bowel syndrome*. Gastroenterology 1983;84:1109A.
66. Sun WM, Edwards CA, Prior A, et al. *Effect on oral nicardipine on anorectal function in normal human volunteers and patients with irritable bowel syndrome*. Gut 1990; 35:885-90.
67. Beech DJ, MacKenzie I, Bolton TB, Christen MO. *Effects of pinaverium on voltage-activated calcium channel currents of single smooth muscle cells isolated from the longitudinal muscle of the rabbit jejunum*. Br J Pharmacol 1990;99:374-378.
68. Christen MO. *Pinaverium bromide: A calcium antagonist with selectivity for the gastrointestinal tract*. Today's Ther Trends 1995;13:47-62.
69. Fioramonti J, Frexinos J, Staumont G, Bueno L. *Inhibition of the colonic motor response to eating by pinaverium bromide in irritable bowel syndrome patients*. Fund Clin Pharmacol 1988;2:19-27.
70. Passaretti S, Sorghi M, Colombo E, et al. *Motor effects of locally administered pinaverium bromide in the sigmoid tract of patients with irritable bowel syndrome*. Int J Clin Pharmacol Ther Toxic 1989;27:47-50.
71. Pace F, Coremans G, Dapoigny M, et al. *Therapy of irritable bowel syndrome - An overview*. Digestion. 1995;56:433-42.
72. Froguel E, Chaussade S, Roche H, et al. *Effects of an intestinal smooth muscle calcium*

*channel blocker (pinaverium bromide) on colonic transit time in humans.* J Gastrointest Motil 1990;2:176-9.

73. Poynard T, Naveau S, Mory B, Chaput J. *Meta-analysis of smooth muscle relaxants in the treatment of irritable bowel syndrome.* Aliment Pharmacol Ther 1994;8: 499-510.
74. Maggi CA, Manzini S, Meli A. *Octylonium bromide: a smooth muscle relaxant which interferes with calcium ions mobilization.* Arch Int Pharmacodyn Ther 1983;264:305-23.
75. Gandia L, Lopez MG, Villarroya M, et al. *Blocking effects of octyilonium on $Ca^{2+}$ channels and secretion in rat chromaffin cells.* Eur J Pharmacol 1996;298:199-205.
76. Capurso L, Tarquini M, Casini A, et al. *Plasma pharmacokinetics of 300 mg of octylonium bromide solution after endoscopic application.* Curr Ther Res 1991;50:539-45.
77. Amenta F, Baroldi P, Ferrante F, Napoleone P, et al. *Autoradiographic localization of octylonium bromide binding sites in the rat gastrointestinal tract.* Arch Int Pharmacodyn Ther 1991;311:5-19.
78. Grider JR. *Role of cholecystokinin in the regulation of gastrointestinal motility.* J Nutr. 1994;124 (Suppl):1334S-1339S.
79. Scarpignato C, Varga G, Corradi C. *Effect of CCK and its antagonists on gastric emptying.* J Physiol (Paris) 1993;87:291-300.
80. Snape WJ, Matarazzo SA, Cohen S. *Effect of eating and GI hormones on human colonic myoelectrical and motor activity.* Gastroenterology 1978;75:373-8.
81. Fossati-Marchal S, Coffin B, Flourié B, et al. *Effects of cholecystokinin octapeptide (CCK-OP) on the tonic and phasic motor activity of the human colon.* Gastroenterology 1994;106:A499.
82. Niederau C, Faber S, Karaus M. *Cholecystokinin's role in regulation of colon motility in health and in irritable bowel syndrome.* Gastroenterology 1992;102:1889-98.
83. O'Brien MD, Camilleri M, Thomforde GM, et al. *Effect of cholecystokin octapeptide and atropine on human colonic motility, tone, and transit.* Dig Dis Sci 1997;42:26-33.
84. Scarpignato C. *Cholecystokinin antagonists and motilides: pharmacology and potential in the treatment of gastroesophageal reflux disease and other digestive motor disorders.* Front Gastrointest Res 1992;20:90-128.
85. Boden P, Hall MD, Hughes J. *Cholecystokinin receptors.* Cell Mol Neurobiol 1995; 15:545-559.
86. Wank SA. *Cholecystokinin receptors.* Am J Physiol 1995;269:G628-G646.
87. D'Amato M, Rovati LC. *Cholecystokinin-A receptor antagonists: therapies for gastrointestinal disorders.* Exp Opin Invest Drugs 1997;6:819-36.
88. Scarpignato C. *Pharmacological stimulation of gastrointestinal motility: where we*

*are and where are we going?* Dig Dis 1997;15 (Suppl 1):112-36.

89. Meyer BM, Werth BA, Beglinger C, et al. *Role of cholecystokinin in regulation of gastrointestinal motor functions.* Lancet 1989;2:12-5.
90. Liddle RA, Gertz BJ, Kanayama S, et al. *Effects of a novel cholecystokinin (CCK) receptor antagonist, MK-329, on gallbladder contraction and gastric emptying. Implications for the physiology of CCK.* J Clin Invest 1989;84:1220-5.
91. Corazziari E, Ricci R, Biliotti D, et al. *Oral administration of loxiglumide (CCK antagonist) inhibits postprandial gallbladder contraction without affecting gastric emptying.* Dig Dis Sci 1990;35:50-4.
92. Fried M, Erlacher URS, Schwizer W, et al. *Role of cholecystokinin in the regulation of gastric emptying and pancreatic enzyme secretion in humans.* Gastroenterology 1991;101:503-11.
93. Cantor P, Mortensen PE, Myhre J, et al. *The effect of the cholecystokinin receptor antagonist MK-329 on meal-stimulated pancreaticobiliary output in humans.* Gastroenterology 1992;102:1742-51.
94. Schwizer W, Borovicka J, Kunz P, et al. *Role of cholecystokinin in the regulation of liquid gastric emptying and gastric motility in humans: studies with the CCK antagonist loxiglumide.* Gut 1997;41:500-4.
95. Kreiss C, Schwizer W, Borovicka J, et al. *Effect of lintitript, a new $CCK_A$ receptor antagonist, on gastric emptying of a solid-liquid meal in humans.* Regulatory Peptides 1998;74:143-9.
96. Li Bassi S, Rovati LC, Giacovelli G, et al. *Effects of loxiglumide, a cholecystokinin antagonist in non-ulcer dyspepsia.* Gastroenterology 1990;98:A77.
97. Chua AS, Bekkering M, Rovati LC, Keeling PW. *Clinical efficacy and prokinetic effect of the $CCK_A$ antagonist loxiglumide in nonulcer dyspepsia.* Ann NY Acad Sci 1994;713:451-3.
98. Meier R, D'Amato M, Pullwitt A, et al. *Effect of a $CCK_A$ receptor antagonist in an experimental model of delayed colonic transit time in man.* Gastroenterology 1994;106:A538.
99. Meier R, Beglinger C, Giacovelli G, D'Amato M. *Effect of the $CCK_A$ receptor antagonist dexloxiglumide on postprandial gallbladder emptying and colonic transit time in healthy volunteers.* Gastroenterology 1997;112:A788.
100. Meier R, Beglinger C, Thurmshirn M, et al. *Therapeutic effects of loxiglumide, a cholecystokinin antagonist, on chronic constipation in elderly patients: a prospective, randomised, double-blinded, controlled trial.* J Gastroenter Mot 1993;5:129-35.
101. Renny A, Snape WJ, Sun E, et al. *Role of cholecystokinin in the gastrocolic response to a fat meal.* Gastroenterology 1983;85:17-21.

102. Jehle EC, Blum AL, Fried M. *Role of cholecystokinin in the regulation of basal colonic motility and the gastrocolic response.* Gastroenterology 1990;98:A361.
103. Kellow JE, Millar LJ, Phillips SF. *Dysmotility of the small intestine is provoked by stimuli in the irritable bowel syndrome.* Gut 1988;29:1236-43.
104. Harvey RF, Read AE. *Effect of cholecystokinin on colonic motility and symptoms in patients with the irritable bowel syndrome.* Lancet 1973;1:1-3.
105. Roberts-Thomson IC, Fettman MJ, Jonsson JR, Frewin DB. *Responses to cholecystokinin octapeptide in patients with functional abdominal pain syndromes.* J Gastroenterol Hepatol 1992;7:293-7.
106. Sjolund K, Ekman R, Lindgren S, Rehfeld JF. *Disturbed motilin and cholecystokinin release in the irritable bowel syndrome.* Scand J Gastroenterol 1996;31:1110-14.
107. Cann PA, Rovati LC, Smart H, Spiller RC, et al. *Loxiglumide a $CCK_A$ antagonist.* In: Irritable Bowel Syndrome: a pilot multicentre clinical study. N York Acad Sci 1994.
108. Barrow L, Blackshaw PE, Wilson CG, et al. *Selective slowing of proximal colon transit in irritable bowel syndrome by the cholecystokinin-receptor antagonist, loxiglumide.* Eur J Gastroenterol Hepatol 1994;6:381-7
109. McIntosh CHS, Brown JC. *Motilin: isolation, secretion, actions and pathophysiology.* Front Gastrointest Res 1990;17:307-52.
110. Hasler WL, Heldsinger A, Owyang C. *Erythromycin contracts rabbit colon myocytes via occupation of motilin receptors.* Am J Physiol 1992;262:G50-G55.
111. Sakai T, Satoh M, Sonobe K, et al. *Autoradiographic study of motilin binding sites in the rabbit gastrointestinal tract.* Regul Peptides 1994;53:249-57.
112. Peeters T. *Erythromycin and other macrolides as prokinetic agents.* Gastroenterology 1993;105:1886-99.
113. Tomomasa T, Kuruome T, Arai H. *Erythromycin induces migrating motor complex in human gastrointestinal tract.* Dig Dis Sci 1986;31:157-61.
114. Kondo Y, Torii K, Itoh Z. *Erythromycin and its derivatives with motilin-like biological activities inhibit the specific binding of 125I-motilin to duodenal muscle.* Biochem Biophys Res Comm 1988;150:877-82.
115. Peeters T, Matthijs G, Depoortere I. *Erythromycin is a motilin receptor agonist.* Am J Physiol 1989;257:G470-G474.
116. Costa A, De Ponti F, Gibelli G, et al. *In vivo characterization of the colonic prokinetic effect of erythromycin in the rabbit.* Pharmacology 1977;54:64-7.
117. Bradette M, Poitras P, Boivin M. *Effect of motilin and erythromycin on the motor activity of the human colon.* J Gastrointestin Motil 1993; 5: 247-51.
118. Jameson JS, Roger J, Misiewicz JJ, et al. *Oral or intravenous erythromycin has no effect*

*on human distal colonic motility*. Aliment Pharmacol Ther 1992;6:589-95.

119. Bassotti G, Betti C, Imbimbo BP, et al. *Erythromycin and edrophonium chloride do not stimulate colonic propagated activity in chronically constipated subjects*. Gastroenterology 1991;100:A419.
120. Lehtola J, Jauhonen P, Kesaniemi A, et al. *Effect of erythromycin on the oro-caecal transit time in man*. Eur J Clin Pharmacol 1990;39:555-8.
121. Landry C, Vidon N, Sogni P, et al. *Effects of erythromycin on gastric emptying, duodeno-caecal transit time, gastric and biliopancreatic secretion during continuous gastric infusion of a liquid diet in healthy volunteers*. Eur J Gastroenterol Hepatol 1995; 7:797-802.
122. Minocha A, Gallo SH. *Effect of erythromycin on orocecal transit time in normal healthy male subjects: a double-blind placebo controlled study*. Can J Gastroenterol 1995;9:195-8.
123. Ueberschaer B, Ewe K, Alles U, Schmidtmann I. *Effect of 4 x 250 mg erythromycin on human gastrointestinal transit*. Z Gastroenterol 1995;33:340-34.
124. Minami T, Nishibayashi H, Shinomura Y, Matsuzawa Y. *Effects of erythromycin in chronic idiopathic intestinal pseudo-obstruction*. J Gastroenterol 1996;31:855-9.
125. Minocha A, Katragadda R, Rahal PS, Ries A. *Erythromycin shortens orocaecal transit time in diabetic male subjects: A double-blind placebo-controlled study*. Aliment Pharmacol Ther 1995;9:529-33.
126. Altomare DF, Rubini D, Pilot MA, et al. *Oral erytromycin improves gastrointestinal motility and transit after subtotal but not total gastrectomy for cancer.* Br J Surg;84:1017-21.
127. Hasler A, Heldsinger A, Soudah H, Owyang C. *Erythromycin promotes colonic transit in humans: mediation via motilin receptors*. Gastroenterology 1990;98:A358.
128. Sharma SS, Bhargava N Mathur SC. *Effect of oral erythromycin on colonic transit in patients with idiopathic constipation*. A pilot study. Dig Dis Sci 1995;40:2446-9.
129. Omura S, Tsuzuki K, Sunazuka T, et al. *Macrolides with gastrointestinal motor stimulating activity*. J Med Chem 1987;30:1941-3.
130. Itoh Z, Omura S. *Motilide, a new family of macrolide compounds mimicing motilin*. Dig Dis Sci 1987;32:915.
131. Read NW, Gwee KA. *The importance of 5-hydroxytryptamine receptors in the gut*. Pharmacol Ther 1994;62:159-73.
132. Talley NJ. *Review article: 5-hydroxytryptamine agonists and antagonists in the modulation of gastrointestinal motility and sensation: clinical implications*. Aliment Pharmacol Ther 1992;6:273-89.
133. Costall B, Naylor RJ. *5-hydroxytryptamine: new receptors and novel drugs for gastrointestinal motor disorders*. Scand J Gastroenterol 1990;25:769-87.
134. Fernandez AG, Massingham R. *Peripheral receptor populations involved in the*

*regulation of gastrointestinal motility and the pharmacological actions of metoclopramide-like drugs*. Life Sci 1985;36:1-14.

135. Fozard JR. *5-$HT_3$ receptors and cytotoxic drug-induced vomiting*. Trends Pharmacol Sci 1987;8:44-5.
136. Eglen RM, Hegde SS. *5-hydroxytryptamine (5-$HT)_4$ receptors: physiology, pharmacology and therapeutic potential*. Exp Opin Invest Drugs 1996;5:373-88.
137. Tonini M. *Recent advances in the pharmacology of gastrointestinal prokinetics*. Pharmacol Res 1996;33:217-26.
138. Tam FS-F, Hillier K, Bunce KT. *Characterization of the 5-hydroxytryptamine receptor type involved in inhibition of spontaneous activity of human isolated colonic circular muscle*. Br J Pharmacol 1994;113:143-50.
139. Schuurkes JAJ, Meulemans AL, Obertop H, Akkermans LMA. *5$HT_4$ receptors on the human stomach*. J Gastrointest Motil 1991;3:119.
140. Burleigh DE, Trout SJ. *Evidence against an acetylcholine releasing action of cisapride in the human colon*. Br J Clin Pharmacol 1995;20:475-8.
141. Borman RA, Burleigh DE. *Evidence for the involvement of a 5-HT-4 receptor in the secretory response of human small intestine*. Br J Pharmacol 1993; 110:927-8.
142. Briejer MR, Ghoos EJ, Schuurkes JAJ. *Serotonin 5HT-4 receptors mediate the R-093877-induced changes in contractile patterns in the canine colon*. Gastroenterology 1997;112:A705.
143. Poen AC, Felt-Bersma RJF, Meuwissen SGM. *A placebo controlled study to evaluate the effects of repeated oral doses of R-093877 on gastrointestinal transit and anorerectal manometry in healthy volunteers*. Gastroenterology 1997;112:A807.
144. Otten MH, Schneider H, WurzerH, et al. *A Double-Blind, Placebo-Controlled Evaluation of Safety and Efficacy of 12-Week, Twice-Daily Treatment with Prucalopride in Patients with Chronic Constipation*. Gastroenterology 1999;116: A1055.
145. Felt-Bersma RJF, Bouchoucha M, Wurzer H, et al. *Effects of a New Enterokinetic Drug, Prucalopride, on Symptoms of Patients with Chronic Constipation: A Double-Blind, Placebo-Controlled, Multicenter Study in Europe*. Gastroenterology 1999; 116:A992.
146. Buchheit KH, Gamse R, Giger R, et al. *The serotonin 5-HT-4 receptor. 2. Structure-Activity studies of the indole carbazimidamide class of agonist*. J Med Chem 1995; 38:2331-8.
147. Prather CM, Camilleri M, McKinzie S, et al. *HTF919, a Partial 5$HT_4$ Agonist, Accelerates Small Bowel Transit in Patients with Constipation-Predominant Irritable Bowel Syndrome*. Gastroenterology 1999;116:A1066-A1067.
148. Mayer EA, Raybould HE. *Role of visceral afferent mechanisms in functional bowel disorders*. Gastroenterology 1990;99:1688–1704.

149. Mayer EA, Gebhart GF. *Basic and clinical aspects of visceral hyperalgesia.* Gastroenterology 1994;107:271–93.
150. Bueno L, Fioramonti J, Delvaux M, Frexinos J. *Mediators and pharmacology of visceral sensitivity: from basic to clinical investigations.* Gastroenterology 1997;112:1714-43.
151. Iovino P, Azpiroz F, Domingo E, Malagelada JR. *The sympathetic nervous system modulates perception and reflex responses to gut distension in humans.* Gastroenterology 1995;108:680-6.
152. Accarino AM, Azpiroz F, Malagelada JR. *Attention and distraction: effects on gut perception.* Gastroenterology 1997;113:415-22.
153. Troncon LEA, Bennett RJM, Ahluwalia NK, Thompson DG. *Abnormal intragastric distribution of food during gastric emptying in functional dyspepsia patients.* Gut 1994;35:327-32.
154. Mönnikes H. *Pharmacotherapy of altered brain-gut interactions.* In: Corazziari E, editor. NeUroGastroenterology. Berlin: de Gruyter 1996;85-108.
155. De Ponti F, Malagelada JR. *Functional gut disorders: from motility to sensitivity disorders. A review of current and investigational drugs for their management.* Pharmacol Ther 1998;80:49-88.
156. Onghena P, Houdenhove BV. *Antidepressant-induced analgesia in chronic non-malignant pain: a meta-analysis of 39 placebo-controlled studies.* Pain 1992;49:205-19.
157. Clouse RE, Lustman PJ, Geisman RA, Alpers DH. *Antidepressant therapy in 138 patients with irritable bowel syndrome: A five-year clinical experience.* Aliment Pharmacol Ther 1994;8:409-16.
158. Gorard DA, Libby GW, Farthing MJG. *Influence of antidepressants on whole gut and orocaecal transit times in health and irritable bowel syndrome.* Alim Pharmacol Ther 1994;8:159-66.
159. Gorard DA, Dewsnap PA, Medbak SH,et al. *Central 5-hydroxytryptaminergic function in irritable bowel syndrome.* Scand J Gastroenterol 1995;30:994-9.
160. Su X, Chapleau MW Gebhart GF. *Effect of antidepressants on mechanosensitive pelvic nerve afferent fibers innervating the colon of the rat.* Gastroenterology 1997;112:A833.
161. Peghini P, Katz P, Castell D. *Imipramine decrease oesophageal pain perception in human male volunteers.* Gut 1998;42:807-13.
162. AGA Patient Care Committee. *American Gastroenterological Association medical position statement: irritable bowel syndrome.* Gastroenterology 1997;112:2118-9.
163. AGA Patient Care Committee. *Irritable bowel syndrome: a technical review for practice guideline development.* Gastroenterology 1997;112:2120-37.
164. Camilleri M, von der Ohe MR. *Drugs affecting serotonin receptors.* Balliére's Clin Gastroenterol 1994;8:301-19.

165. Stark, MJr, Maher K, Gupta P, et al. *Visceral afferent blockade with ondansetron (Zofran®) increases nociceptive thresholds in patients with chest pain of undetermined etiology (CPUE).* Am J Gastroenterol 1991;86:1305.

166. Feinle C, Read NW. *Ondansetron reduces nausea induced by gastroduodenal stimulation without changing gastric motility.* Am J Physiol 1996;271:G591-G597.

167. Wilmer A, Tack J, Coremans G, Janssens J et al. *Effect of ondansetron, a 5-HT$_3$-receptor antagonist, on perception of gastric distensionand gastric compliance in healthy man.* Gastroenterology 1993;104:A603.

168. Zighelboim J, Talley NJ, Philllips SF, et al. *Visceral perception in irritable bowel syndrome. Rectal and gastric responses to distension and serotonin type 3 antagonism.* Dig Dis Sci 1995;40:819-27.

169. Goldberg PA, Kamm MA, Setti-Carraro P, et al. *Modification of visceral sensitivity and pain in irritable bowel syndrome by 5-HT$_3$ antagonism (ondansetron).* Digestion 1996;57:478-83.

170. Hammer J, Phillips SF, Talley NJ, Camilleri M. *Effect of a 5-HT$_3$ antagonist (ondansetron) on rectal contractility and compliance in health and the irritable bowel syndrome.* Aliment Pharmacol Ther 1993;7:543-51.

171. Prior A, Read NW. *Reduction of rectal sensitivity and postprandial motility by granisetron, a 5-HT$_3$ receptor antagonist, in patients with irritable bowel syndrome.* Aliment Pharmacol Ther 1993;7:175-80.

172. Delvaux M, Louvel D, Mamet J-P, et al. *Effect of alosetron on responses to colonic distension in patients with irritable bowel syndrome.* Aliment Pharmacol Ther 1998;12:849-55.

173. Bardhan K, Bodemar G, Geldof H, et al. *A double-blind placebo-controlled study to evaluate the efficacy of alosetron in the treatment of irritable bowel syndrome.* Gastroenterology 1996;110:A630.

174. Zerbib F, Bruley Des Varannes S, Oriola RC, et al. *Alosetron does not affect the visceral perception of gastric distension in healthy subjects.* Aliment Pharmacol Ther 1994;8:403-7.

175. Banner SE, Sanger GJ. *Differences between 5-HT$_3$ receptor antagonists in modulation of visceral hypersensitivity.* Br J Pharmacol 1995;114:558-62.

176. Junien JL, Riviere P. *Review article. The hypersensitive gut-peripheral kappa agonists as a new pharmacological approach.* Aliment Pharmacol Ther 1995;9:117-26.

177. Corazziari E. *Role of opioid ligands in the irritable bowel syndrome.* Can J Gastroenterol 1999;13 (Suppl A):71A-75A.

178. Junien JL, Wettstein JG. *Role of opioids in peripheral analgesia.* Life Sci 1992;51: 2009-18.

179. Coffin B, Bouhassira D, Chollet R, et al. *Effect of the kappa agonist fedotozine on perception of gastric distension in healthy humans.* Aliment Pharmacol Ther 1996; 10:919-25.
180. Delvaux M, Louvel D, Lagier E, et al. *The kappa agonist fedotozine relieves hypersensitivity to colonic distension in patients with irritable bowel syndrome.* Gastroenterol 1999;116:38-45.
181. Fraitag B, Homerin M, Hecketsweiler P. *Double-blind dose-response multicenter comparison of fedotozine and placebo in treatment of nonulcer dyspepsia.* Dig Dis Sci 1994;39:1072-77.
182. Dapoigny M, Abitbol JL, Fraitag B. *Efficacy of peripheral kappa agonist fedotozine versus placebo in treatment of irritable bowel syndrome. A multicenter dose-response study.* Dig Dis Sci 1995;40:2244-8.
183. Paice JA, Kroin JS, Penn RD. *Analgesic effect of octreotide: therapeutic potential.* In: Scarpignato C, editor. Octreotide: from Basic Science to Clinical Medicine. Basel: Karger 1996;270-80.
184. Plourde V, Lembo T, Shui Z, et al. *Effects of the somatostatin analogue octreotide on rectal afferent nerves in humans.* Am J Physiol 1993;265:G742-G751.
185. Hasler WL, Soudah HC, Owyang C. *A somatostatin analogue inhibits afferent pathways mediating perception of rectal distention.* Gastroenterology 1993;104:1390-7.
186. Hasler WL, Soudah HC, Owyang C. *Somatostatin analog inhibits afferent response to rectal distention in diarrhea-predominant irritable bowel patients.* J Pharmacol Exp Ther 1994;268:1206-11.
187. Chey WD, Beydoun A, Roberts DJ, et al. *Octreotide reduces perception of rectal electrical stimulation by spinal afferent pathway inhibition.* Am J Physiol 1995;269:G821-G826.
188. Mertz H, Walsh JH, Sytnik B, Mayer EA. *The effect of octreotide on human gastric compliance and sensory perception.* Neurogastroenterol Motil 1995;7:175-85.
189. Bourgeois S, Coulie B, Tack J, Janssens J. *The somatostatin-analogue octreotide does not affect visceral perception of the fundus in man.* Gastroenterology 1997;112:A1134.
190. Bradette M, Delvaux M, Staumont G, et al. *Octreotide increases thresholds of colonic visceral perception in IBS patients without modifying muscle tone.* Dig Dis Sci 1994;39:1171-8.
191. Nelson-Pearcy C, Hammond PJ, Gwilliam ME, et al. *Effect of a new oral somatostatin analog (SDZ CO 611) on gastric emptying, mouth to cecum transit time, and pancreatic and gut hormone release in normal male subjects.* J Clin Endocrinol Metab 1994;78:329-36.
192. Wettstein JG, Bueno L, Junien JL. *CCK antagonists: pharmacology and therapeutic*

*interest*. Pharmacol Ther 1994;62:267–82.

193. Feinle C, D'Amato M, Read NW. *CCKA-receptors modulate gastric sensory and motor responses to gastric distension and duodenal lipid*. Gastroenterology 1996;110:1379-85.
194. Feinle C, Meyer O, D'Amato M, Fried M. *CCKA-receptor blockade alleviates dyspeptic symptoms during gastric distension and duodenal lipid in patients with functional dyspepsia*. Gastroenterology 1999;116:A992.

*Address for correspondence*

**SCARPIGNATO C, MD, DSC, PharmD, FCP, FACG**
Laboratorio di Farmacologia Clinica
Dipartimento di Medicina Interna
Università di Parma
Ospedale Maggiore
Via Volturno 39 43100 Parma Italia
Fax: +39 0521 292499
E-mail: scarpi@tin.it

# PROBIOTICS IN HUMAN HEALTH
## COLONIZATION OF THE GASTROINTESTINAL TRACT, NUTRITIVE AND THERAPEUTIC ASPECTS

*G Panichi*

### Colonization of the gastrointestinal tract with bacterial flora

Colonization of the Gastrointestinal (GI) tract occurs within a few days of birth. The type of delivery, the composition of the diet, and the maternal bacterial flora all contribute to the initial colonization. Time needed for bacteria to colonize the large bowel is about two weeks and does not differ between breast- and bottle-fed newborns.

Of the various aerobes, the Gram negative (G-) E. Coli and the Gram positive (G+) Streptococcus are usually the first bacteria to colonize the GI tract and might reach a concentration of $10^8$ - $10^{10}$ per g faeces. At the same time, several species of anaerobes, such as Bifidobacterium, Clostridium, and Bacteroides colonize the GI tract.

After these first two weeks in the breastfed infants, as far as concerns the aerobes, there is a reduction of E. Coli and Streptococcus and, as far as concerns the anaerobes, of Clostridium and Bacteroides accompanied by a marked increase in Bifidobacterium that tend to predominate. In bottle-fed infants, no such redistribution characterized by a fall of G- and G+ aerobes and of G- anaerobes and Clostridium and a rise of G+ Bifidobacterium anaerobes is observed. In these infants, the composition of bacterial flora is more complex and the relative concentration of G+ and G- aerobes and anaerobes is variable. The relatively simple flora of the breast-fed newborns remains stable until normal feeding is started after weaning. A few days after weaning E. Coli, Streptococcus, Clostridium and Bacteroides appear and the difference between breast-fed and formula-fed infants vanishes.

This initial period lasts about one year, until the child's diet stabilizes with the standard everyday life feeding and the microflora, which has become modified to that of an adult, will remain unchanged unless specific impaired conditions occur[1].

The presence of more than 400 bacteria species in the human intestine is clear evidence that the microflora colonizing the GI tract constitute a complex eco-system made up of aerobes and anaerobes (Table 1).

PREDOMINANT MICROORGANISMS OF THE INTESTINAL MICROFLORA

| **Aerobes** | | **Anaerobes** | |
|---|---|---|---|
| Gram + | Gram – | Gram + | Gram – |
| • Streptococci | • Enterobacteriaceae | • Peptostreptococci | • Bacteroides |
| • Staphylococci | | • Clostridia | • Veillonellae |

Table 1

Considering that the microflora is about 40-55% of the total weight of the endoluminal content, on average 200-500 g, and has a concentration of $10^{10}$ - $10^{12}$ UFC per g it can be seen that, in the human GI tract, the bacteria outnumber the cells of the entire organism. Studies performed in animals and humans have led to the conclusion that: "the composition of intestinal microflora is the result of a complex series of relationships between the organisms and the endogenous bacteria as well as among the bacteria themselves". It has also been demonstrated that any bacterium can colonize a germ-free animal, but it is not as easy for such an event to take place in a normocompetent animal with a normal endogenous microflora. Human intestinal microflora is relatively stable, but it is easy for the strains of the endogenous species to be substituted by others of the same, but genetically different, species.

A large proportion of the endogenous intestinal microflora is multilayered and adheres to the intestinal walls. The first layer of bacteria is strictly adherent to the epithelial cells; the subsequent layers are superimposed one upon the other and all layers are embedded in a substance called mucus, composition and origin of which, whether from the epithelium or the bacteria, has not been yet clarified[1].

Relevant factors that regulate and affect the intestinal microflora are:

- physico-chemical conditions
- interactions between the host and the endoluminal bacteria
- interactions between the bacteria
- antibiotics, probiotics, and prebiotics
- diet, to a certain extent
- anatomical conditions of the intestinal lumen.

## Probiotics

Until recently, probiotics were considered those microorganisms used mainly in the cheese industry to enhance the milk fermentation process. Today, we consider a probiotic "a live microbial feed supplement (vital and capable of reproducing) that, ingested per os, beneficially affects the host by improving endoluminal microflora balance". A brief list of probiotic organisms that are ingested by humans in fermented foods and pharmaceutical preparations is shown in Table 2.

MICROORGANISMS USED AS PROBIOTICS IN FOOD, LIVESTOCK, AGRICOLTURE

| | |
|---|---|
| Saccharomyces boulardii | Streptococcus salivarius spp. thermophilus |
| Lactobacillus acidophilus | |
| Lactobacillus plantarum | Bifidobacterium bifidum |
| Lactobacillus GG | Bifidobacterium infants |
| Lactobacillus casei spp. rhamnosus | Enterococcus faecium |
| Lactobacillus brevis | Lactococcus lactis spp. lactis |
| Lactobacillus delbrueckii spp. bulgaricus | Lactococcus spp. cremoris |

Table 2

One nutritional benefit of probiotics has been studied mainly by assessing the role of fermentation by Lactobacillus on alimentary products. General parameters investigated concern the effect of fermentation on quantity, digestion and absorption of nutrients. It has been shown that the proteolytic effect of yoghurt is followed by more free aminoacids that are more easily absorbed than after milk. Several studies in animals have shown that different products such as acidified milk, fermented milk, and yoghurt enhance the growth of microflora much more than standard milk. In addition probiotics synthetize vitamins. There is general agreement that products derived from milk fermented by means of live and reproducing probiotics are more abundant in vitamins, minerals, proteins, carbohydrates and, furthermore, improve intestinal absorption[2].
Probiotics are also indicated in the treatment of some intestinal disorders (Table 3).

INTESTINAL PATHOLOGICAL CONDITIONS FOR WHICH PROBIOTICS MAY BE INDICATED

- ✓ Intestinal Infections and dismicrobisms
- ✓ Inflammatory Bowel Disease
- ✓ Hepatic encephalopathy
- ✓ Carcinogenesis

Table 3

The probiotics used in the treatment of pathological conditions should ideally have some specific properties. They should be of human origin since some beneficial effects are species-specific; they should also be resistant to gastric acid and bile digestion and they should survive using, for their metabolism, the substances present in the lumen. It is not clear whether the property to adhere to the intestinal epithelium is a prerequisite to prolong their presence within the intestinal lumen; the property of adherences seems, however, necessary to prolong their survival.

## Intestinal infections and dysmicrobism

The use of several types of probiotics has long since been claimed in the treatment of a variety of intestinal infections and dysmicrobisms. Gotz et al.[3] reported that when a preparation of Lactobacillus is administered before treatment with ampicillin a reduction of 14% to 0% is observed in diarrhoea in patients treated for various infections. Zychowicz et al.[4] have used probiotics in the treatment of 31 children affected by Salmonella and Shigella-induced diarrhoea; 43% of the Salmonella and 67% of the Shigella infected patients became asymptomatic much earlier than non treated patients; with prolonged administration of acidified milk all patients healed without harbouring the infectious microrganisms.

Lactobacillus, Bifidobacterium, Enterococcus, and Streptococcus have been used in the prophylaxis of traveller's diarrhoea secondary to enterotoxigenic E. Coli. However, neither Lactobacillus (L.) acidophilus nor Enterococcus faecium displayed a favourable probiotic effect in a group of Austrian tourists[5]. Nonetheless, the occurrence of diarrhoea was reduced from 71% to 43% of tourists visiting Egypt and treated prophylactically with capsules containing S. Thermophilus, L. Bulgaricus, L. Acidophilus and B. Bifidum.

Isolauri et al.[7] assessed the efficacy of L. Casei spp. GG in the treatment of acute diarrhoea in 71 children aged of 4-45 months. Results of this randomized placebo controlled trial showed that L. GG, as a fermented milk or lyophilized powder, is of benefit to reduce the duration of diarrhoea.

Raza et al.[8] in Pakistan reported, in a prospective, double blind, placebo controlled trial performed in hospital children affected by diarrhoea, that treatment with L. GG significantly reduced the symptomatology of the group treated with the active compound. Lactobacillus spp. have been used with non univocal results also in the treatment of pseudomembranous colitis. L. acidophilus NCDO 1748 as lyophilized powder has not been of benefit in the treatment of pseudomembranous colitis, whereas L. GG eradicated Clostridium difficile in 5 patients and prevented subsequent relapses[9]. However, not all Lactobacillus act on intestinal pathogens. In 23 healthy volunteers infected with an enterotoxigenic E. Coli strain the administration of a marketed compound containing L. acidophilus and L. bulgaricus did not affect the incubation period, number of bowel movements or duration of the infection[10]. Saccaromices boulardi has been used in the attempt to prevent Cl. difficile - induced diarrhoea. In a double blind trial performed in 180 patients, diarrhoea was present in 9.5% of the patients treated with probiotics and 22% of those treated with placebo.The study indicates that the prophylactic use of the probiotic reduces the occurrence of diarrhoea associated with C. difficile infection, but S. boulardi cannot avoid the colonization and development of the pathogen[11].

### Inflammatory bowel diseases

Up to now, few and contrasting data have become available on the therapeutic role of probiotics in Inflammatory Bowel Diseases (IBD). Fabia et al.[12] reported a significant reduction in the concentration of Lactobacillus in the mucosa of patients with active ulcerative colitis. Favier et al.[13] reported a decrease in faecal concentration of Bifidobacterius in patients with Crohn's disease; Malin et al.[14] have shown that the oral administration of a probiotic, L. GG, in Crohn's disease patients, was followed by an intestinal IgA immune response. Of interest is the recent study by Campieri and Gionchetti[15] who assessed the therapeutic role of a new compound made up of 4 Lactobacillus strains, 3 Bifidobacterius strains, and 1 Streptococcus strain containing 300 billion live lyphilized bacteria per gramme. This compound has been tested with promising results in maintenance treatment of patients with ulcerative colitis and in a group of patients with active chronic pouchitis. These encouraging results indicate that probiotics should be further investigated for their possible therapeutic role in the treatment of IBD.

### Hepatic encephalopathy

Hepatic encephalopathy is a neurological disorder associated with hepatic failure and accompanied by elevated serum levels of ammonia. Ammonia is produced in the intestine from urea by bacterial urease and, once absorbed, is metabolized and detoxified by the liver. In patients with reduced liver function the altered ammonia metabolism leads to hyperammonia ; the administration of L. acidophilus reduces the activity of intestinal bacteria urease and lowers the serum levels of ammonia[2].

## Carcinogenesis

Probiotics added to the diet have been shown to inhibit the production of chemical substances that stimulate colon tumours and to inhibit the translocation of tumoural cells in rodents[16]. An antitumoural action of L. acidophilus has been shown in experimental studies. Diet with oral supplementation of bile resistant human L. acidophilus caused a marked reduction of three different bacterial enzymes: ß-glucoronidase, oxidoreductase, and nitroreductase in the faeces of animals and humans. The above - mentioned enzymes catalyse the conversion of procarcinogens into carcinogens within the intestinal lumen. Additional studies on a chemical carcinogen, 1,2 dymethilhydralazine, active in the development of colon cancer, have shown that this carcinogen produced by intestinal bacteria with ß-glucoronidase is drastically reduced after the administration of human L. acidophilus; the supplementation of this probiotic in the diet can prolong the latency induction period and delay the growth of the tumour.
Overall, the evidence of an antitumoural effect by probiotics via inhibition of carcinogenesis is not overwhelming, but opens new perspectives on the hypothesis that, at least in some specific conditions, their presence in the diet or their use as fermentative compounds of milk derivatives, may have a protective anticarcinogenetic role.

## Conclusions

The shift from antibiotics to probiotics represents an extraordinary change in therapeutic strategy of several disease entities. The term probiotic was first used by Lilly and Stilwell in 1965[17] to describe any compound or microrganism able to improve the intestinal microflora equilibrium in breeding animals. Subsequently Fuller[18] called probiotics those microrganisms that added alive, in human alimentation were of benefit to men's well being. Today, we consider probiotics all those live microrganisms that, added in due quantity in the diet, have beneficial effects on our health status. It is evident that probiotics should be devoid of any pathogenic effect and undesirable side - effects. A recent study[19] performed in Finland compared 12 strains of Lactobacillus isolated from 5192 haemocultures between 1989 and 1994 with strains used in probiotic peparations and had shown that none of those isolated from haemocultures were identical with the marketed probiotics.

Widespread resistance to antibiotics and the aim to succeed in the control of infectious diseases with a more ecological strategy should prompt us to further investigate probiotics. It would also be of interest to investigate their efficacy in those diseases secondary to an alteration in normal intestinal microflora by exogenous pathogens, or following the interaction between the host and endogenous microflora and even between the endogenous microrganisms themselves.

## *REFERENCES*


1. Panichi G. *Fattori che influenzano la flora intestinale normale.* Ann Ist Sup Sanità 1986;22:771-82.
2. Gorbach SL. *Lactic acid bacteria and human health.* Ann Med 1990;22:37-41.
3. Gotz V, Romankiewicz JA, Moss J, Murray HW. *Prophylaxis against ampicillin-associated diarrhea with a Lactobacillus preparation.* Amer J Hosp Pharm 1979;36:754-61.
4. Zychowicz C, Surazynmska A, Sietwierska B, Ciephin Ska T. *Effect of Lactobacillus acidophilus cultures on the carrier state of Shigella and Salmnella organisms in children.* Ped Polska 1974;49:997-1003.
5. Kollaritsch H, Wiedermann G. *Traveller's diarrhoea among Austrian tourists: epidemiology, clinical features and attempts at nonantibiotic drug prophylaxis.* In: Pasini W, editor. Proceedings of the second international conference on tourist health Rimini. Who 1990;74-82.
6. Black AT, Andersen PC, Orskou F, et al. *Prophylactic efficacy of Lactobacilli on traveller's diarrhea.* In: Steffe R, editor. Travel medicine Conference on international travel medicine Zurich. Berlin: Springer 1989;333-5.
7. Isolauri E, Juntunen M, Rautanen T, et al. *A human Lactobacillus strain (L casei sp GG) promotes recovery from acute diarrhea in children.* Pediatrics 1991;88:90-6.
8. Raza S, Graham SM, Allen SJ, et al. *Lactobacillus GG promotes recovery from acute*

*nonbloody diarrhea in Pakistan.* Ped Infect Dis J 1995;14:107-11.
9. Gorbach SL, Chang T, Goldin B. *Successful treatment of relapsing Clostridium difficile colitis with Lactobacillus GG.* Lancet 1987;ii:1519.
10. Clements ML, Levine MM, Black RE, et al. *Lactobacillus prophylaxis for diarrhea due to enterotoxigenic E. coli.* Antimicrob Agents Chemother 1981;20:104-8.
11. Surawicz CM, Elmer G, Speelman P, et al. *Prevention of antibiotic-associated diarrhea by Saccharomyces boulardii: a prospective study.* Gastroenterology 1989;9:981-8.
12. Fabia R, Arrajaba, Jumansson ML, et al. *Impairment of bacterial flora in human ulcerative colitis and experimental colitis in the rat.* Digestion 1993; 54:248-55.
13. Favier L, Neut C, Mizon L, et al. *Fecal B-D-galacto sidase production and Bifidobacteria are decreased in Crohn's disease.* Dig Dis Sci 1997;42:817-22.
14. Malin M, Suomalainen H, Saxelin M, Isolauri E. *Promotion of IgA immune response in patients with Crohn's disease by oral bacteriotherapy with Lactobacillus GG.* Ann Nutr Metab 1996;40:137-45.
15. Campieri M, Gionchetti P. *Probiotics in inflammatory bowel disease: new insight to pathogenesis or a possible therapeutic alternative?* Gastroenterology 1999;116:1246-9.
16. MacFarlane GT, Cummings JH. *Probiotics and prebiotics: can regulating the activities of intestinal bacteria benefit health?* Br Med J 1999;318:999-1003.
17. Lilly DM, Stillwel RM. *Probiotics: growth promoting factors produced by microorganisms.* Science 1965;47:747-8.
18. Fuller R. *Probiotics in human medicine.* Gut 1991;32:439-42.
19. Saxelin M, Rautelin H, Salminen S, Makela PM. *Safety of commercial products with viable lactobacillus strains.* Inf Dis Clin Prac 1996;5:331-3.

*ADDRESS FOR CORRESPONDENCE*

**PANICHI G, MD**
Dipartimento Malattie Infettive e Tropicali
Università di Roma "La Sapienza"
Viale del Policlinico
00161 Roma Italia
Fax: +39 06 4957855
E-mail: profpan@tin.it

# PROBIOTICS IN INFLAMMATORY BOWEL DISEASE

*EC Zucconi, P Gionchetti, A Venturi, F Rizzello, R Johansson, U Helwig, M Campieri*

## Intestinal microflora

The Gastrointestinal (GI) tract can be described as a reservoir with an internal surface area similar to that of a tennis court, approximately 200-250 $m^2$ separating $10^{13}$ eucaryotic cells from $10^{14}$ bacterial cells.
The intestinal epithelium, microflora and mucosal immune system constitute a complex ecosystem in a delicate balance, responsible for GI integrity[1]. There are considerable variations in the bacterial pattern and concentration between the different levels of the GI tract. The stomach normally contains a small number of bacteria ($10^3$ cfu/g) and the local microflora is predominantly Gram positive and aerobic.
The small bowel represents a zone of transition between the sparse population of the stomach and the very dense population of the colon. The concentration and pattern of the microflora in the proximal small bowel are similar to those of the stomach, whilst in the distal ileum, Gram-negative begin to outnumber the Gram-positive and the bacterial concentration increases significantly. However, the most dramatic change occurs across the ileo-caecal valve: the total number of micro-organisms increases up to one million fold ($10^{11}$-$10^{12}$), and anaerobes outnumber aerobes in the ratio of 1000:1[2]. The gut represents an enormously complex ecosystem containing over 400 bacterial species, in which a delicate balance exists between the indigenous microflora and the host. The exact mechanisms by which the intestinal microflora interact with the intestinal immune system are not well understood. On the one hand, the presence of microflora is crucial for the maturation of the immune system and the development of normal intestinal morphology, and maintains a chronic and immunologically balanced inflammatory response, the so-called "physiologic inflammation"[3,4]. On the other, in order to maintain this delicate balance, the host has acquired various protective mechanisms against bacterial attachment

and translocation, which include:

- the barrier provided by the epithelial layer
- mechanical factors, such as desquamation and peristalsis
- factors which interfere with bacterial attachment such as mucus layer and secretory IgA, which represent the primary immune barrier against the pathogen.

More recently, the presence at the mucosal level of antimicrobial peptides has been suggested.
The microflora displays important functions including a nutritive, metabolic, immunologic and protective role, and it has been suggested to regard flora as part of the human body.
Fermentation of non-digestible dietary substrates is a major metabolic function of colonic microflora, and Short-Chain Fatty Acids (SCFA), the metabolic endpoint of carbohydrate fermentation, serve as energy substrates for colonocytes. Colonic microflora also play a key role in metabolizing primary bile acid. As already mentioned, the intestinal flora play a crucial role in the intestinal immune system homeostasis.
Finally, experimental evidence suggests that intestinal flora also have some protective functions such as uptake and detoxification of toxic chemicals, a barrier effect against translocation of potentially pathogenic bacteria and inhibition of the proliferation of clostridia, E.coli and shigella, strains that become pathogenic when overgrown.

## Probiotics

At the beginning of this Century, Nobel prize winner Eelie Metchnikoff first hypothesized that large numbers of lactobacilli could inhibit the growth of some unhealthy bacterial species[5]. The use of the term probiotic, however, dates from 1974 when Parker used it to describe organisms and substances which contribute to intestinal microbial balance. This definition was revised by Fuller who defined probiotic as a live feed supplement which beneficially affects the host animal by improving its microbial balance[6]. This definition stresses the importance of viability and avoids the broad term of substances which can even include antibiotics.

More recently, Schaafsma defined probiotic as living organisms, which upon ingestion, in certain numbers, exert health benefits beyond inherent basic nutrition[7]. This revision emphasises the need for sufficient populations of live microrganisms, and further indicates that benefits can include both improvement of microbial balance and other health effects, such as immunomodulation.

The probiotic preparations currently on the market are mainly based on lactic acid bacteria (lab) which include lactobacilli, streptococci and bifidobacteria. These three genera have been shown to be important components of the GI microflora and are all relatively harmless. They metabolise carbohydrates by fermentation, producing lactic acid as the major end-products (homofermentative strains) or as a significant component in a mixture of end-products (heterofermentative strains).

There are some basic requirements for strain selection. It is important that probiotic strains be of human origin, because some health-promoting effects may be species-specific. Other requisites include acid and bile resistance and the ability to be metabolically active within the intestinal lumen, where they should survive but not persist in the long-term. There is no general consensus among research work as to whether or not a probiotic must adhere to the intestinal mucosal surface in order to exert its effects. Moreover strains must be antagonistic against pathogenic bacteria and the strains should be safe and tested for human use.

Finally, an ideal probiotic organism should be viable after storage and maintain its beneficial properties after processing and culture.

Therefore, the probiotic concept remains controversial, primarily because the mechanisms by which probiotic microrganisms antagonise unwanted GI microrganisms or exert other beneficial effects to the host in vivo have not yet been identified.

The hypothesized mechanisms of action include the so-called "colonisation resistance", a complex of actions including production of antibiotic-like substances and hydrogen peroxide, competition for adhesion receptors (many pathogens must adhere to the gut wall to colonise and produce disease), and competition for nutrients.

Another mechanism of action is considered the stimulation of the immune system and, particularly, of phagocytic activity, natural killer activity, proliferation of lymphocytes, production of cytokines such as

gamma interferon (IFN) and production of sIgA.
Despite the increasing interest in the use of probiotics by the general public and industry who see them as natural cures, acceptance of these products by the medical world has been slow: this is due to the few convincing data to support the many health-promoting claims. Probiotics have been proposed for the treatment of acute diarrhoea in infants and adults, for antibiotic associated diarrhoea, for functional diarrhoea and Inflammatory Bowel Disease (IBD). Unfortunately most studies have been small, uncontrolled, poorly documented and have lacked precise definitions of end-points. Most available probiotic organisms are classified as foods.
There is a plethora of data on probiotics from in vitro and animal studies, however, these claims need to be tested in humans with carefully controlled studies on clearly defined selected strains.

## Role of microflora in IBD

Although the causes of IBD remain unclear, substantial progress has been made in the identification of pathophysiologic mechanisms of chronic intestinal inflammation.
There are currently three theories on the aetiology of IBD:

- the presence of a persistent infection with a specific pathogen;
- the presence of an impaired mucosal barrier;
- the presence of an abnormal host immune response to ubiquitous agents.

Therefore, the fundamental question regarding the aetiology of IBD is: does chronic, recurring inflammation reflect an appropriate response to a persistent abnormal stimulus or an abnormally aggressive and prolonged response to a normal stimulus?
In either situation, the microbial components of the lumen provide the persistent antigenic drive to induce and perpetuate chronic enterocolitis. A body of clinical and experimental evidence suggests a role for intestinal microflora, at least in the perpetuation on the inflammatory process in IBD.
As far as concerns the clinical observations, first of all, the distal ileum

and the colon are the areas with the highest bacterial concentrations and represent the sites of inflammation in IBD. Also, pouchitis occurs in the presence of bacterial overgrowth and dysbiosis.
Enteric bacteria and their phlogistic products, have been detected deep in the inflamed mucosa in Crohn's disease.
Recently, convincing evidence of tolerance breakdown to the normal commensal flora in active IBD has emerged, supporting the theory that hyperreactivity to ubiquitous antigen from the intestinal microflora is implicated, at least in the perpetuation of IBD[8,9].
Decreasing the bacterial concentration with antibiotics or faecal stream diversion decreases activity in Crohn's disease and to a lesser extent in ulcerative colitis; pouchitis also improves with antibiotic treatment.
Finally, Rutgeerts et al.[10] recently showed that intestinal contents trigger post-operative recurrence of Crohn's disease in the terminal ileum. Experimental studies have shown that purified bacterial products can initiate and perpetuate experimental colitis and that antibiotics decrease inflammation in several animal models.
The importance of luminal bacteria is further emphasised by the absence of spontaneous colitis in some transgenic and knock-out animal models of colitis in the presence of germ-free conditions[11].

## Use of highly concentrated probiotics in IBD

We recently had the possibility to use a new probiotic preparation, VSL-3, containing 500 billions/g of viable lyophilized bacteria, of 4 strains of lactobacilli (casei, plantarum, acidophilus and delbruekii subsp. bulgaricus), 3 strains of bifidobacteria (longum, breve and infantis), and 1 strain of streptococcus thermophilus.
This product possesses two main innovative characteristics: the very high bacterial concentration, and the presence of a consortium of bacterial species.
The rationale of this preparation is based mainly on theoretical speculations and on evidence coming from in vitro studies:

- the choice of strains for VSL-3 was again based on the results of in vitro studies performed by the microbiologist who developed this product;

- most of the strains used for VSL-3 demonstrated a high survival ability in culture at very low pH and, therefore, can pass through the entire gut at very high concentrations.

*Probiotics and ulcerative colitis*

Firstly, we carried out a pilot study using VSL-3 in patients allergic or intolerant to salazopyrin (SASP) or amino salicylic acid (5-ASA), considering as a primary endpoint the colonic probiotic colonization, and as a secondary endpoint the clinical evaluation[12].

Patients recruited for the study had a recent relapse, within 3 months, and a past history of at least two relapses per year. Twenty patients received 6 g/day of VSL-3 for 12 months.

As far as concerns the primary endpoint, stool culture and determination of faecal pH were performed at baseline, after 10, 20, 40, 60, 75, 90 days and then after 6 and 12 months. Faecal samples were evaluated for the determination of concentration of total anaerobes and aerobes, enterococci, streptococci, clostridia, coliforms, bacterioides, lactobacilli and bifidobacteria. Microbiological determination showed a significant increase in concentration of lactobacilli, bifidobacteria and Streptococcus Thermophilus, which was evident already after 10 days and remained constant throughout the entire treatment period. No significant modifications were seen in the concentrations of the other bacterial species. Faecal pH was significantly reduced by the treatment with VSL-3. As far as concerns the second endpoint, clinical assessment was performed at baseline and every 2 months; the endoscopic assessment was conducted at baseline and 6 and 12 months, or in the case of relapse. Of the 20 patients treated, 4 had a relapse, 1 was lost to follow-up and 15 remained in remission.

During the clinical study no side effects were reported and all the patients showed good compliance. The microbiological data show that the strains contained in VSL-3 are able to colonize the gut only during the period ofVSL-3 administration.

These preliminary data suggest the efficacy of probiotics in maintaining remission in ulcerative colitis patients allergic or intolerant to SASP and 5-ASA. However, further double-blind studies on larger populations must be carried out.

*Probiotics and pouchitis*

Pouchitis, a non-specific inflammation of the ileal reservoir, is the most common long-term complication following pouch surgery for ulcerative colitis. Its cumulative frequency largely depends on the duration of the follow-up and is about 50% at ten years.

The aetiology is still unknown and is likely to be multifactorial, but bacteria are thought to play an important role, as suggested by the efficacy of antibiotic treatment. In most cases, patients have a chronic relapsing disease and, so far, no maintenance study has been carried out. Recently, a reduced faecal concentration of lactobacilli and bifidobacteria has been shown in patients with active pouchitis, suggesting that this syndrome could be due to instability of the microflora. We carried out a study aimed at evaluating the efficacy of this new oral probiotic preparation versus placebo as maintenance treatment for chronic relapsing pouchitis[13].

As far as concerns the inclusion criteria, patients had to have a chronic relapsing pouchitis, defined as a disease with at least 3 relapses per year. The presence of a score 0, after 1-month antibiotic treatment, in the clinical and endoscopic portion of the pouchitis disease activity index by Sandborn et al.[14], which includes clinical, endoscopic and acute histological criteria. No other forms of treatment were allowed. The study was a randomized double-blind trial.

Forty patients who went into remission (with a pouchitis disease activity index of 0) after 1 month of antibiotic treatment with ciprofloxacin 1 g plus rifaximin 2 g per day, were randomized to receive VSL-3 6 g daily or a placebo identical in appearance for 9 months.

Clinical assessment was carried out upon entry and thereafter every month; endoscopic and histological assessments were performed upon entry and thereafter every two months; stool culture was done before and after antibiotic treatment and subsequently every month.

Relapse was defined as an increase of at least 2 points in the clinical portion of the pouchitis activity index.

As far as concerns the clinical result, of the 20 patients who received the placebo, all relapsed, 8 within two months, 7 within 3 months and the remaining 5 within 4 months. In contrast, 17 of the 20 patients treated with VSL-3 were still in remission after 9 months. These 17 patients,

after suspension of the treatment, relapsed within 4 months.
As far as concerns the microbiological results, patients treated with VSL-3 showed a significantly increased faecal concentration of lactobacilli, bifidobacteria and streptococcus salivarius compared both with concentrations present before and after antibiotic treatment. The significant increase was already present after 1 month and remained stable throughout the study. No significant changes were observed for bacteroides, coliforms, clostridia, enterococci and total aerobes and anaerobes compared to baseline levels. One month after withdrawal of treatment, faecal concentrations of the strains administered with VSL-3 were reduced to the values present before the beginning of the antibiotic treatment.

In conclusion, apart from rotavirus diarrhoea, there is no convincing evidence from well designed, double-blind trials on the effectiveness of probiotics in the prevention or treatment of infective colitis. With regard to IBD, there is clinical and experimental evidence that microflora play a role in the pathogenesis. Results obtained with high concentration of probiotics further suggest a potential role for probiotics in the treatment of IBD.

## *REFERENCES*

1. Tancrede C. *Role of human interflora in health and disease.* Eur Clin Microbiol Infect Dis 1992;11:1012-5.
2. Simon GL, Gorbach SL. *Intestinal flora in health and disease.* Gastroenterology 1984;86:174-93.
3. Kenworthy R. *Observations on the reaction of the intestinal mucosa to bacterial challenge.* J Clin Pathol 1971;24:138-42.
4. Mahida YR, Rose F, Chan WC. *Antimicrobial peptides in the gastrointestinal tract.* Gut 1997;40:161-3.
5. Merchnikoff E. *The prolungation of life. Optimistic Studies.* London: Heineman; 1907.
6. Fuller R. *Probiotics in human medicine.* Gut 1991;32:439-42.
7. Schaafsma G. *Significance of probiotics in human diets.* In: SOMED 21st International

Congress on Microbial Ecology and Disease, Paris; October 28-30 1996. Paris: Institute Pasteur; 1996; 117 (abstract).

8. Klasen IS, Melief MJ, van Halteren AG et al. *The presence of peptidoglycan-polysaccharide complexes in the bowel wall and the cellular responses to these complexes in Crohn's disease.* Clin Immunol Immunopathol 1994;71:303-8.
9. Duchmann R, Kaiser I, Hermann E et al. *Tolerance exists towards resident intestinal flora but is broken in active inflammatory bowel disease (IBD).* Clin Exp Immunol 1995;102:448-55.
10. Rutgerts P Hiele M, Geboes K et al. *Controlled trial of metronidazole treatment for prevention of Crohn's recurrence after ileal resection.* Gastroenterology 1995;108:1617-21.
11. Madsen KL, Tavernini MM, Doyle JSG et al. *Lactobacillus spp prevents development of enterocolitis in interleukin-10-gene deficient mice.* Gastroenterology 1997;112:A1030.
12. Venturi A, Gionchetti P, Rizzello F, et al. *Impact on the faecal flora composition of a new probiotic preparation. Preliminary data on maintenance treatment of patients with ulcerative colitis (UC) intolerant or allergic to 5-aminosalicylic acid (5-ASA).* Aliment Pharmacol Ther 1999. In press.
13. Gionchetti P, Rizzello F, Venturi A et al. *Maintenance treatment of chronic pouchitis: a randomised placebo-controlled, double-blind trial with a new probiotic preparation.* Gastroenterology 1998;114:A985.
14. Sandborn WJ, Tremaine WJ, Batts KP et al. *Pouchitis after ileal pouch-anal anastomosis: a Pouchitis Disease Activity Index.* Mayo Clin Proc 1994;69:409-15.

*ADDRESS FOR CORRESPONDENCE*

**CAMPIERI M, MD**
Dipartimento di Medicina Interna e Gastroenterologia
Università di Bologna
O. P. S. Orsola
Via Massarenti 9 40138 Bologna Italia
Fax: +39 051 392538
E-mail: campieri@med.unibo.it

# Antibiotics in diverticular disease of the colon

*L Capurso, C Papi*

Diverticular disease of the colon is very common in Western societies and its frequency is strikingly correlated with advancing age[1]. Estimates based on necroscopy or radiologic findings indicate that it occurs in about 10% of the population in the United States, the United Kingdom and Australia[2]; by contrast, the disease is rarely observed in less industrialized countries and in Japan[3].

Uncommon before the age of 40 years, diverticular disease of the colon is currently found in one third to one half of all autopsies of subjects over 60 years of age[2,3].

The hypothesis drawn from these observations is that the high frequency of diverticular disease in Western societies results from a low fibre consumption by an aging population.

The dietary fibre hypothesis is largely supported by epidemiological observations and case-control studies[3]. Most rural populations in underdeveloped countries eat 50-70 g fibre per day; by contrast, the mean non-starch polysaccharide intake in Western populations is 15-25 g/day[2,3]. Diverticular disease has been classified according to the clinical severity into asymptomatic diverticular disease and symptomatic diverticular disease (uncomplicated and complicated disease) (Table 1)[4].

The majority of patients harbouring diverticula remain asymptomatic; only 20% will develop symptoms and signs of illness, but only a minority of patients, probably 4 to 5%, will develop major complications, 1-2% require hospitalization and 0.5% require surgery.

Probably less than 0.01% of patients die from complications related to diverticular disease (Tables 2, 3)[5].

Symptoms attributed to diverticula (abdominal pain or discomfort, bloating, disturbances of bowel habits) are also features of Irritable Bowel Syndrome (IBS), and it has been suggested that IBS is a prediverticular stage or that diverticular disease of the colon and IBS may coexist in many people and when bowel symptoms occur with diverticulosis coli they may be due to a coexistent IBS rather that to diverticula itself [6,7].

This hypothesis is supported by the fact that many patients with symptomatic diverticular disease show colonic motility patterns similar to those with IBS[8], and patients with asymptomatic disease have colonic myoelectric activity similar to that of normals[9].

### CLINICAL CLASSIFICATION OF DIVERTICULAR DISEASE[4]

**Asymptomatic diverticular disease**

**Symptomatic diverticular disease**

*Uncomplicated*
- Mild forms

*Complicated*
- Microperforation with serosal inflammation (severe diverticular disease)
- Pericolic abscess
- Diffuse (purulent or faecal) peritonitis
- Fistula
- Obstruction
- Bleeding

Table 1

### NATURAL HISTORY OF DIVERTICULAR DISEASE OF THE COLON

| | |
|---|---|
| 100 | patients with colonic diverticula |
| 20% | ➠ symptoms and signs of disease |
| 4-5% | ➠ major complications |
| 1-2% | ➠ hospitalization |
| 0.5% | ➠ surgery |
| 0.01% | ➠ death |

Table 2

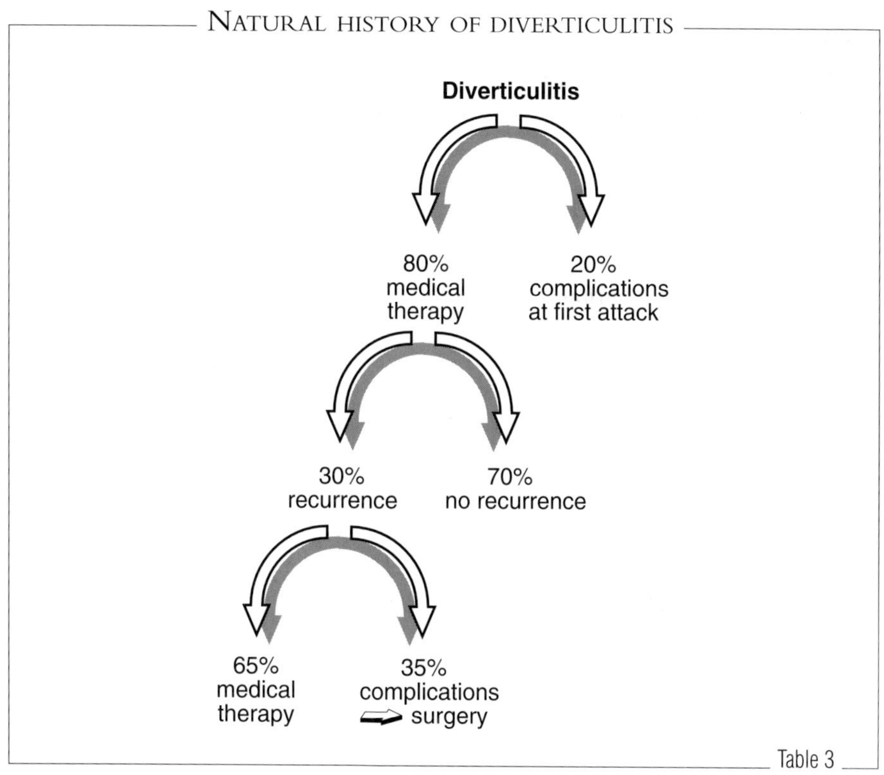


Table 3

## Treatment of diverticular disease of the colon

Treatment of diverticular disease is aimed at the relief of symptoms and to prevent major complications[4]. Current views on the epidemiology and pathogenesis of diverticular disease and IBS provide the rationale for the treatment of these disorders with high fibre diets and fibre supplementation.

Bran and bulking agents are commonly used in the treatment of symptomatic diverticular disease but their real efficacy is still controversial. Although some controlled clinical trials have shown a benefit of high-fibre diets in obtaining symptomatic relief[10-13], other studies failed to show positive results[14-16]. A recent meta-analysis failed to show a therapeutic advantage of fibre supplementation, as compared to placebo, in IBS patients[17]. Moreover, there is no evidence that high fibre diets or fibre supplementation prevent major complications of diverticular disease[2].

Anticholinergic drugs and spasmolytic agents such as mebeverine are widely used in the treatment of symptomatic diverticular disease. The observed hypermotility of the sigmoid colon in many symptomatic patients provides the rationale for using these drugs. However, the efficacy of antispasmodics has never been clearly documented[2]. A recent meta-analysis, however, suggests a therapeutic advantage of antispasmodics as compared to placebo in patients with IBS[17].

Broad spectrum antibiotics are commonly used in the treatment of diverticulitis. The bacterial spectrum involved includes aerobic (Escherichia coli, Proteus, Klebsiella, Enterococcus) and anaerobic (Bacteroides, Clostridium, Bifidobacterium, Peptostreptococcus) bacteria. A combination of an aminoglycoside plus clyndamycin given parenterally is usually effective. Alternatively, a third generation cephalosporin can be used. Most patients with diverticulitis respond to conservative management such as "bowel rest", nasogastric suction, analgesics, intravenous fluid therapy and antibiotics (Table 3).

In uncomplicated disease, when an inflammatory component is excluded by definition, there is no apparent rationale for using antibiotics. However, in a subset of patients with more severe symptoms, when an inflammatory component is clinically suspected, a course of antibiotics, such as metronidazole, is advisable[4]. Poorly absorbable antibiotics are considered of little value because the critical site of antibiotic effect is the pericolic tissue rather than the luminal surface[2].

However, some observations suggest a possible role of gut microflora in determining symptoms related to diverticular disease such as abdominal pain/discomfort and bloating. Bacterial metabolism is the sole source of $H_2$ and $CH_4$[18,19]; these gases can play a role in determining symptoms such as bloating and pain due to "air trapping". Antimicrobial therapy could reduce bacterial mass and bacterial gas production. Interactions between dietary fibre, bacterial metabolism and colonic functions are complex and not yet fully elucidated. It is well known that fibre increases stool bulk and affects colonic transit time in several ways: by water holding, by proliferation of bacteria and by the products of bacterial fermentation (such as Short Chain Fatty Acids (SCFA))[20] . It has long since been assumed that fibre exerts its effect on bowel habits by retaining water in the gut and stimulating peristalsis through increased bulk. However, water holding is an "in vitro" property of fibre which is inversely related to faecal bulking and colonic transit time in vivo. This is not surprising because virtually all fibre is broken down in the gut by intestinal bacteria. Moreover water holding can be equated to solubility of fibre and soluble fibre (such as glucomannan) are more rapidly degraded by gut microflora[20]. This view is supported by a recent study in which it has been shown that antimicrobial therapy determines a rise in mean faecal weight in subjects on a constant fibre intake, probably reducing bacterial degradation of fibre[21]. Thus poorly absorbable antibiotics may act on gut microflora reducing fibre degradation and enhancing the effects of undegraded fibre on colonic functions. These observations provide a rationale for using antibiotics in uncomplicated symptomatic disease.

In a multicentre double blind placebo controlled trial[22], 168 outpatients with symptomatic uncomplicated diverticular disease of the colon, were randomly assigned to two different treatment schedules: 84 patients received fibre supplementation (glucomannan (Dicoman 5®) 2 g/day) plus rifaximin (Normix®) 400 mg b.i.d. for 7 days every month, and 84 patients received glucomannan 2 g/day plus placebo two tablets b.i.d for 7 days every month.

Clinical evaluation has been performed upon admission and at 3-month intervals for 12 months considering 6 clinical variables:

1. upper abdominal pain/discomfort
2. bloating
3. lower abdominal pain/discomfort
4. tenesmus
5. diarrhoea
6. abdominal tenderness.

Each symptom was graded using a simple score system (0=no symptoms, 1=mild, 2=moderate, 3=severe); a global symptomatic score, calculated from the sum of each symptom score, was assigned to each patient at every clinical evaluation.

Results have been analysed considering the global symptomatic score in the two groups of treatment and the evolution of the severity of each symptom at each clinical evaluation.
Both treatments are effective in reducing the score after the first three months of treatment; however, patients treated with rifaximin show a significant reduction in the score as compared to patients treated with placebo at 6, 9 and 12 months ($p<0.05$; $p<0.001$; $p<0.001$, respectively) (Figure 1).

Figure 1

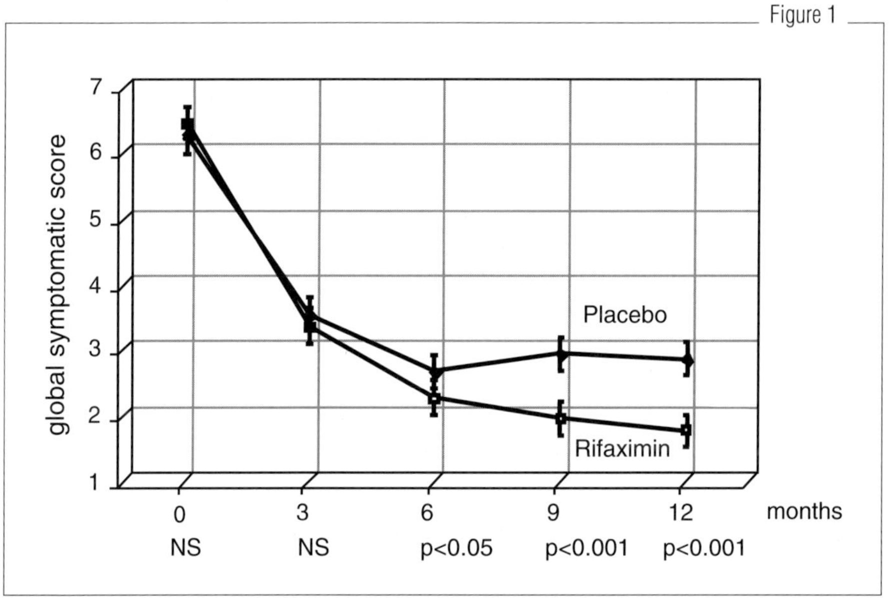


Global symptomatic score in the two treatment groups.

After 12 months of treatment 68.9% of patients in the rifaximin group are symptom-free or mildly symptomatic (global score = 0-1) as compared to 39.5% in the placebo group ($p=0.001$) (Figure 2).
This means a 30% improvement with rifaximin, as compared to fibre supplementation only, in the long-term treatment. Some symptoms such as bloating, abdominal pain and abdominal tenderness appeared to be significantly affected by antibiotic treatment as compared to placebo. The results of this study suggest that cyclic administration of rifaximin can be

of some advantage in the relief of symptoms in patients with symptomatic uncomplicated diverticular disease.

Figure 2

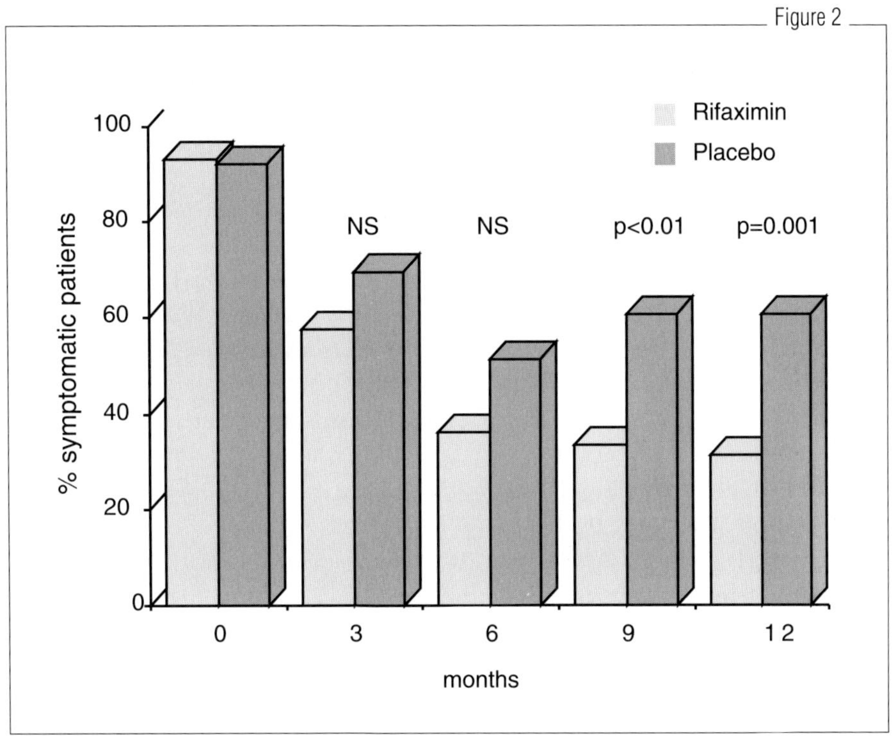


Percentage of symptomatic patients in the two treatment groups at each interval.

An intringuing question is the possible role of poorly absorbable antibiotics in preventing inflammatory complications of diverticular disease. At the present time, there is no clinical evidence that antibiotics can prevent diverticulitis. In our study[22], 4 patients developed diverticulitis in one year, 2 in the rifaximin group and 2 in the placebo group. Considering the relatively low occurrence rate of inflammatory complications of diverticular disease, studies in order to identify a 50% reduction of the one-year complications rate, considering a predicted rate of 3-5% in patients treated with fibre supplementation only, should include 380 to 758 patients per group of treatment.

## *REFERENCES*


1. Parks TG. *Natural history of diverticular disease of the colon.* Clin Gastroenterol 1975;4:53-69.
2. Almy TP, Howell DA. *Diverticular disease of the colon.* N Engl J Med 1980;302:324-31.
3. Painter NS, Burkitt DP. *Diverticular disease of the colon, a 20th Century problem.* Clin Gastroenterol 1975;4:3-21.
4. Torsoli A, Inoue M, Manousos O, Smith A,Van Steensel CJ. *Diverticular disease of the colon: Data relevant to treatment.* Gastroenterol Int 1991;4:3-20.
5. Naitove A, Almy TP. *Diverticular disease of the colon.* In: Sleisenger, Fordtran, editors. Gastrointestinal disease.Philadelphia; WB Saunders Company; 1989;1419-34.
6. Thompson WG, Patel DG, Tao N, Nair RC. *Does uncomplicated diverticular disease produce symptoms?* Dig Dis Sci 1982;27:605-8.
7. Thompson WG, Patel DG. *Clinical picture of diverticular disease of the colon.* Clin Gastroenterol 1986;4:903-16.
8. Ritchie L. *Similarity of bowel distension characteristics in the irritable bowel syndrome and diverticulosis.* Gut 1977; 18: 990-5.
9. Gold MH, Carlson GM, Mathias JR. *Colonic myoelectric activity in diverticulosis.* Gastroenterology 1979;76:1139-44.
10. Brogribb AJM. *Treatment of symptomatic diverticular disease with a high fiber diet.* Lancet 1977;i:664-6.
11. Ornstein MH, Littlewood ER, Baird IM, et al. *Are fiber supplements really necessary in diverticular disease of the colon? A controlled trial.* Br Med J 1981;282:1353-6.
12. Weinreich J. *The treatment of diverticular disease.* Scand J Gastroenterol 1982;79(Suppl):128-9.
13. Ewerth S, Ahlberg J, Holmstrom B, et al. *Influence on symptoms and transit time of Vi Siblin R in diverticular disease.* Acta Chir Scand 1980;500(Suppl):40-59.
14. Solotof JI, Gudmand Hoyer E, Kreg B, et al. *A double blind trial of wheat bran on symptoms of irritable bowel syndrome.* Lancet 1976;i:270-2.
15. Hodgson WJB. *The placebo effect: is it impotrtant in diverticular disease?* Am J Gastroenterol 1977;67:157-62.
16. Longstreth GF, Fox DD, Youkeles L, et al. *Psyllium therapy in the irritable bowel syndrome.* Ann Int Med 1981;95:53-6.
17. Ferrario F, Ciaco A, Papi C, et al. *L'approccio razionale alla terapia della sindrome del colon irritabile.* Gastroenterol Int (Ed Italiana) 1994;5:93-8.

18. Levitt MD, French P, Donaldson RM. *Use of hydrogen and methane excretion in the study of intestinal flora* [abstract]. J Lab Clin Med 1968;72:988-94.
19. Engel RR, Levitt MD. *Intestinal tract gas formation in newborns* [abstract]. In: Program for meeting of American Pediatric Society and Society for Pediatric Research; 1970;266.
20. Macfarlane GT, Cummings JH. *The colonic flora, fermentation and large bowel digestive function.* In: Phillips SF, Pemberton JH, Shorter RG, editors. The large intestine: physiology, pathophysiology and disease. New York: Raven Press; 1991.
21. Kurpad AV, Shetty PS. *Effects of antimicrobial therapy on fecal bulking.* Gut 1986;27:55-8.
22. Papi C, Ciaco A, Koch M, et al. *Efficacy of Rifaximin in the treatment of symptomatic diverticular disease of the colon. A multicentre double-blind placebo controlled trial.* Aliment Pharmacol Ther 1995;9:33-9.

*ADDRESS FOR CORRESPONDENCE*

**CAPURSO L, MD**
Via Paolo Frisi, 44
00197 Roma Italia
Fax: +39 06 33062641

# ANTIBIOTICS IN CROHN'S DISEASE

*ML Scribano, C Prantera*

Crohn's Disease (CD) is a chronic intestinal inflammatory disease of unknown origin, mainly treated with steroids and/or other immunosuppressive drugs. Many experienced clinicians employ different types of antibiotics in their clinical practice, and consider their use helpful for improving symptoms and inducing remission of active phases.

## Rationale for the use of antibiotics in Crohn's disease

Other chronic intestinal diseases characterized by diarrhoea such as Whipple's disease and tropical sprue are successfully treated with antibiotics. CD lesions are usually located in upstream valves, and it is well known that bacteria overgrow in areas where the flow of bowel content slows down[1]. The diversion of faecal stream heals CD lesions[2]. Rutgeerts et al. have shown that patients in whom a terminal ileostomy was constructed proximally to ileo-colo anastomosis did not experience recurrent disease until the ileostomy was closed[3].

Antibiotics are successfully employed in the treatment of perianal fistulae and seem to be helpful in the management of entero-enteric and enterocutaneous fistulae[4,5].

Moreover, some mycobacterial diseases such as intestinal tuberculosis and Johne's disease, a chronic enteritis of ruminants caused by Mycobacterium paratuberculosis, show pathological characteristics similar to those of CD[6].

## Data in favour of an infective cause of Crohn's disease

Epidemiological data from studies on family clustering in France, and on small outbreaks among village residents and cohabitants in England, seem to point towards an infective factor[7,8]. Mycobacterium paratuberculosis has been the mainly accused factor, because it is the cause of Johne's disease and essentially because of certain convincing evidence collected over the last fifteen years[9,10]. An equal weight of evidence, however, argues against the hypothesis that CD is caused by Mycobacterium paratuberculosis or other mycobacterial species[11].

In conclusion, the probability that some type of Mycobacterium is responsible for CD has not, so far, been adequately substantiated.

## Antimycobacterial therapy

Many antibiotics active against mycobacteria in a single or multiple regimen have been attempted in CD; anecdotal reports have generally reported success in treating CD patients with different antimycobacterial agents. Open and controlled trials have given contrasting results. The results vary between the completely negative trials of Shaffer et al.[12] and Swift et al.[13], in which a classic antitubercular therapy was employed, and the trial employing clarithromycin with positive results[14]. In the middle are two trials from Ireland and Italy that demonstrated a certain efficacy of clofazimine alone and of a combination of rifampicin, ethambutol, clofazimine and dapsone[15,16].

The complexity of CD, as well as differences in the drugs employed, in the length of treatment, and the evaluation of results, makes any conclusive comment impossible.

## Role of intestinal flora

Some authors have hypothesised that while the primary mechanisms of intestinal injury remain unknown, commensal bacteria with their products enhance and perpetuate the inflammatory activity in CD[17]. As in the case of an infected wound, so the intestinal flora might perpetuate the inflammatory process colonising the initial lesion induced from the primary agent of CD which has broken through the epithelial barrier. An increase in intestinal permeability in CD patients, demonstrated in recent studies[18], may lead to the absorption of toxic bacterial products and of bacteria themselves from the lumen; in fact, an increase in intestinal permeability predicted relapse of symptoms in 76% of 72 CD patients followed for 1 year[18]. Not only the increased intestinal permeability but also bacterial overgrowth over the lesions account for bacteria penetration of the gut wall. There may be several reasons for bacterial overgrowth in the CD bowel:

- faecal stasis
- wall lesion that impairs motility and/or
- intestinal narrowing and stricture.

Elevated antibody levels directed against the normal intestinal bacteria, such as E. coli, Bacteroides and other species, have been shown in the serum of CD patients. This fact implies that intraluminal bacteria can translocate across the intestinal wall[19]. Moreover, a variety of products from the gut flora have inflammatory properties and might have an impact on the local immune system. In conclusion, there is substantial evidence that the intestinal microflora and its products may enhance and perpetuate the inflammatory response of CD, and that they are responsible for the frequent septic state of these patients.

## Antibiotic treatment in Crohn's disease

Despite the absence of a definite role of antibiotics as first line treatment of CD, they are employed in the management of such complications as abscesses and toxic state in order to reduce the overgrowth of bacteria in the gut lumen, to improve symptoms such as diarrhoea, pain and meteorism. Nevertheless, the results are sometimes conflicting.

*Metronidazole*

Of the various antibiotics, metronidazole is the most employed. This imidazole compound, active against some parasites and most anaerobic bacteria, is now widely used in treating perianal CD.

In a randomised crossover trial - the Cooperative CD Study in Sweden- metronidazole was compared with sulfasalazine; both drugs were equally effective, but only when the colon was involved; it is interesting to note that metronidazole was effective in patients who failed on sulfasalazine, but the reverse was not observed[20]. In a trial from Birmingham, metronidazole alone or combined with cotrimoxazole had little therapeutic value in active CD[21]. Remission rates at 16 weeks in a Canadian study were 36% with 10 mg/kg/day of metronidazole and 27% with the double dosage; metronidazole was more effective when the colon was involved[22].

These studies indicate that metronidazole is active in Crohn's colitis and ileocolitis, but not when located in the small bowel. The small group of patients with colitis who were included in the arm on metronidazole in the trial from Birmingham could account for the negative results[21]. Recently, a trial was performed on metronidazole in the prevention of recurrence in Crohn's ileitis following surgery[23]. The antibiotic, started on the seventh day after surgery for a 3-month period, decreased the severity of early endoscopic recurrence in the neo-terminal ileum, in comparison to placebo, and also seemed to delay the symptomatic recurrence at 1 year .

***Side effects*** Metronidazole is generally well tolerated, even at the dosage of 20 mg/kg. Side effects vary between 10 and 20% according to the dosage and duration of treatment. The more frequent adverse events are gastrointestinal intolerance, neurotoxicity and metallic taste. Peripheral neuropathy, as a side effect, has been reported in 50 to 85% of patients on long-term metronidazole treatment[4].

*Ciprofloxacin*

Ciprofloxacin is a quinolone derivative that exhibits a selective suppressive effect on the intestinal microflora. E. coli and aerobic Enterobacteriaceae are especially sensitive to this antibiotic, which, in contrast, has little effect on Bacteroides and Clostridium spp.

Ciprofloxacin was anecdotally reported to be effective in the long-term treatment of 10 cases of active perianal CD[5] and 4 cases of CD with ileal localisation[24]. Two larger open studies employed ciprofloxacin and metronidazole in the treatment of active CD. In the first, from Italy, 52% of patients achieved a complete remission (Crohn's Disease Activity Index - CDAI<150), 19% were considered failures and 13% withdrew because of side effects[25]. The second study was a Canadian retrospective analysis of 72 patients; twenty-nine patients were concurrently receiving steroids[26]. Of the non-steroid treated group, 67% of patients had a clinical response. Three controlled trials have been published on ciprofloxacin in active CD. The first enrolled 89 patients, concomitantly treated with steroid and metronidazole, who were randomised to receive placebo or ciprofloxacin[27]. Endoscopic and clinical failures occurred in 11 patients on ciprofloxacin and in 12 in the control group. The high rate of success which is normally achieved with steroid treatment does not allow a reliable evaluation of drug efficacy. The second study was a randomized controlled trial on the efficacy and safety of 12 weeks' treatment with metronidazole plus ciprofloxacin versus systemic steroid in 41 patients with active CD[28]. Ten of the 22 patients on antibiotics (45%) and 12 of the 19 on steroid (63%) had a CDAI of less than 150 at the end of the study. Six patients on antibiotics (27%) and two on steroid (11%) were withdrawn because of side effects. The authors concluded that, despite the high incidence of side effects, this antibiotic combination can be an alternative to steroid in the treatment of acute CD. The best results in terms of efficacy and side effects were observed at 6 weeks. The third trial, published as an abstract, showed that ciprofloxacin is as effective as mesalazine in treating mild to moderate flare-up of CD[29].

*Side effects* The percentage of side effects is different in the few published studies. One trial reported a 59% incidence of adverse events related to the 2 antibiotics[28]. In another controlled study, a 16% incidence of side effects was observed, but patients also received other concomitant drugs[27]. The percentage of side effects depends on the dosage and duration of treatment. Side effects are of gastrointestinal origin, but skin reactions, a not infrequent increase in transaminase levels, a case of high serum amylase, and a possibly related case of transient ischaemic attack have also been described[25].

## Conclusions

At the present time, until the exact cause and mechanism of CD have been identified, drugs that interfere with the immune response as well as antibiotics will be essential in the armamentarium of CD therapies. A combination of metronidazole with ciprofloxacin seems to be useful in treating active CD phases, as an alternative to or in combination with steroid. CD localized in the colon and in the ileum seems to be more sensitive to these antibiotics. Today, a treatment with 1 g/day of each of these 2 antibiotics for a period of 6 weeks appears to be advisable. Side effects and bacterial resistance are of concern in their long-term use.

### *References*


1. Rutgeerts P, Ghoos Y, Van Trappen G, et al. *Ileal dysfunction and bacterial overgrowth in patients with Crohn's disease.* Eur J Clin Invest 1981;11:199-206.
2. Burman JH, Thompson H, Cooke WT, et al. *The effects of diversion of intestinal contents on the progress of Crohn's disease of the large bowel.* Gut 1971;12:11-5.

3. Rutgeerts P, Goboes K, Peeters M, et al. *Effect of faecal stream diversion on recurrence of Crohn's disease in the neoterminal ileum.* Lancet 1991;338:771-4.
4. Brandt LJ, Bernstein LH, Boley SS, et al. *Metronidazole therapy for perianal Crohn's disease: a follow-up study.* Gastroenterology 1982;83:383-7.
5. Turunen U, Farkkila M, Valtonen V, et al. *Long-term outcome of ciprofloxacin treatment in severe perianal or fistulous Crohn's disease.* Gastroenterology 1993;104:A793.
6. Chiodini RJ, Van Kruiningen HJ, Merkal RS, et al. *Ruminant paratuberculosis (Johne's disease): the current status and future prospects.* Cornell Vet 1984;74:218-62.
7. Van Kruiningen HJ, Colombel JF, Cartun RW, et al. *An in-depth study of Crohn's disease in two French families.* Gastroenterology 1993;104:351-60.
8. Allan RN, Pease P, Ibbotson JP. *Clustering of Crohn's disease in a Cotswold village.* Q J Med 1986;59:473-8.
9. Chiodini RJ, Van Kruiningen HJ, Merkal RS, et al. *Characteristics of an unclassified Mycobacterium species isolated from patients with Crohn's disease.* J Clin Microbiol 1984;20:966-71.
10. Thayer WR, Coutu JA, Chiodini RJ, et al. *Possible role of mycobacteria in inflammatory bowel disease. II. Mycobacterial antibodies in Crohn's disease.* Dig Dis Sci 1984;29:1080-5.
11. Graham DY, Markesich DC, Yoshimura HH. *Mycobacteria and inflammatory bowel disease. Results of culture.* Gastroenterology 1987;92:436-42.
12. Shaffer JL, Hughes S, Linaker BD, et al. *Controlled trial of rifampicin and ethambutol in Crohn's disease.* Gut 1984;25:203-5.
13. Swift GL, Srivastava ED, Stone R, et al. *Controlled trial of anti-tuberculous chemotherapy for two years in Crohn's disease.* Gut 1994;35:363-8.
14. Graham DY, Al-Assi MT, Robinson M. *Prolonged remission in Crohn's disease following therapy for Mycobacterium paratuberculosis.* Gastroenterology 1995;108:A826.
15. Afdhal NH, Long A, Lennon J, et al. *Controlled trial of antimycobacterial therapy in Crohn's disease. Clofazimine versus placebo.* Dig Dis Sci 1991;36:449-53.
16. Prantera C, Kohn A, Mangiarotti R, et al. *Antimycobacterial therapy in Crohn's disease: results of a controlled, double-blind trial with a multiple antibiotic regimen.* Am J Gastroenterol 1994;89:513-8.
17. Beeken WL, Kanich RE. *Microbial flora of the upper small bowel in Crohn's disease.* Gastroenterology 1973;65:390-7.
18. Wyatt J, Vogelsang H, Hubl W, et al. *Intestinal permeability and the prediction of relapse in Crohn's disease.* Lancet 1993;341:1437-9.
19. Macpherson A, Khoo UY, Forgacs I, et al. *Mucosal antibodies in inflammatory bowel disease are directed against intestinal bacteria.* Gut 1996;38:365-75.
20. Ursing B, Alm T, Barany F, et al. *A comparative study of metronidazole and sulfasalazine*

*for active Crohn's disease: the Cooperative Crohn's Disease Study in Sweden. II. Result.* Gastroenterology 1982;83:550-62.

21. Ambrose NS, Allan RN, Keighley MRB, et al. *Antibiotic therapy for treatment in relapse of intestinal Crohn's disease: a prospective randomized study.* Dis Colon Rectum 1985;28:81-5.
22. Sutherland L, Singleton J, Sessions J, et al. *Double blind, placebo controlled trial of metronidazole in Crohn's disease.* Gut 1991;32:1071-5.
23. Rutgeerts P, Hiele M, Geboes K, et al. *Controlled trial of metronidazole treatment for prevention of Crohn's recurrence after ileal resection.* Gastroenterology 1995;108:1617-21.
24. Peppercorn MA. *Is there a role for antibiotics as primary therapy in Crohn's ileitis?* J Clin Gastroenterol 1993;17:235-7.
25. Prantera C, Kohn A, Zannoni F, et al. *Metronidazole plus ciprofloxacin in the treatment of active, refractory Crohn's disease: results of an open study.* J Clin Gastroenterol 1994;19:79-88.
26. Greenbloom SL, Steinhart AH, Greenberg GR, et al. *Ciprofloxacin and metronidazole: combination antibiotic therapy for ileocolonic Crohn's disease.* Clin Invest Med 1995;18:48.
27. Turunen U, Farkkila M, Hakala K, et al. *Ciprofloxacin treatment combined with conventional therapy in Crohn's disease. A prospective, double blind, placebo controlled study.* Gut 1995;37:193.
28. Prantera C, Zannoni F, Scribano ML, et al. *An antibiotic regimen for the treatment of active Crohn's disease: a randomized, controlled clinical trial of metronidazole plus ciprofloxacin.* Am J Gastroenterol 1996;91:328-32.
29. Colombel JF, Lemann M, Cassagnou M, et al. *Ciprofloxacin vs mesalazine in the treatment of active Crohn's disease.* Gut 1996;39 (Suppl 3):A188.

*ADDRESS FOR CORRESPONDENCE*

**PRANTERA C, MD**
Divisione di Gastroenterologia
Azienda Ospedaliera S. Camillo-Forlanini
Via Portuense 332 00149 Roma Italia
Fax: +39 06 5562249
E-mail: prantera@tin.it

# Psychological therapy of chronic gastrointestinal disease

*GA Fava*

Since the early fifties, there has been a steady growth in psychotherapy research. Use of control groups, standardized assessments, follow-up evaluations, blind raters have built the research evidence necessary to verify the effectiveness of psychotherapeutic approaches in a number of psychiatric and medical disorders[1].

In many controlled studies, no significant differences between psychotherapeutic modalities emerged. This suggested the presence of some common and non-specific therapeutic ingredients that even very different psychotherapeutic techniques may share. Such ingredients include attention to the patient, disclosure of psychological distress and feelings, high arousal, interpretation (and thus rationalization) of symptoms, and the rituals associated with the psychotherapeutic setting[2]. Psychotherapy research has shown that the benefits of psychotherapy are maximal when a specific technique is used in the setting of a well-specified psychiatric disorder. For instance, behavioural therapies were found to be most effective in phobic and anxiety disorders, whereas cognitive therapies had a higher impact on depressive disorders[3]. At times, different psychotherapeutic approaches are combined [e.g., Cognitive Behavioural Treatment (CBT)]. The heading cognitive-behavioural has characterized the most effective approaches in psychiatric disorders[3]. The cognitive hypothesis proposes that emotions of any kind arise from a person's idiosyncratic interpretation of the meaning of situations and events[4]. Such emotions may result in physical sensations and symptoms and/or in misinterpretation of health-related information. Cognitive therapy is aimed at changing beliefs about the consequences of the problem and at suggesting alternative interpretations. Behavioural therapies are aimed at modifying maladaptive behaviour (e.g., avoidance in phobias) and include techniques such as exposure in vivo, relaxation and biofeedback.

Several psychotherapeutic approaches have been proposed to alleviate psychological distress and improve physical symptoms in Gastrointestinal (GI) disorders, particularly of the functional type. Such approaches have included CBT, relaxation training, hypnosis, and brief dynamic psychotherapy (the forming of an intense relationship with the patient, linking symptoms to feelings, and then understanding the relationship of symptoms to problems or emotional difficulties in the patient's life). At times, a combination of these treatment modalities has been attempted. The majority of the controlled investigations showed the superiority of psychological treatments associated with conventional medical treatment compared to medical therapy alone. No significant differences between treatment modalities emerged, suggesting a strong impact of non-specific ingredients of psychotherapy[5,6]. These investigations, however, considered GI disorders as homogeneous entities, even though they often dealt with patients who were refractory to conventional gastroenterologic approaches.

These studies, however, have limited impact on clinical practice, unless they are filtered by a sequential approach. Psychotherapy is a time-consuming process that requires considerable motivation, that can be attained only by selected patients. Furthermore, the majority of patients with functional GI disorders respond to conventional medical treatment in conjunction with explanation and reassurance[3]. In one of the most important psychotherapy trials on Irritable Bowel Syndrome (IBS), Guthrie et al.[7] included only patients with continuous symptoms for at least one year, who attended a GI clinic for at least 6 months and who were unresponsive to conventional medical treatment.

These criteria provide a reasonable gastroenterologic background for further exploring the psychological dimension in patients with chronic GI disorders. Obviously, such criteria should be supplemented by customary clinical judgement (e.g., marked depressive features, impaired quality of life).

## Psychological assessment of patients

In the controlled studies available, patients with chronic GI disorders were treated as if psychological mechanisms were homogeneous in the patients. Research evidence just shows the contrary: patients are very heterogeneous as to psychopathology and psychometric dimensions[8]. Often referral to a psychiatrist becomes a source of frustration for the gastroenterologist.

This is also because current diagnostic criteria used in clinical psychiatry such as DSM-IV[9], fail to provide a satisfactory description of psychosomatic syndromes and problems[10]. In particular, the failure of the DSM classification of somatoform disorders to provide proper identification, prognostic indications, and therapeutic implications for the somatizing patient in medical practice, has been emphasized[8]. This failure has led to the development of an alternative diagnostic and conceptual framework by our international group of psychosomatic investigators[11].

A set of 12 diagnostic criteria (DCPR) for use in psychosomatic research has been developed (Tables 1-12). These criteria are currently undergoing cross-national validation. However, some preliminary data on 70 consecutive patients with functional GI disorders in an Italian tertiary care facility (M/F=24/46; age=39.8 ± 15.4 years) may be worth reporting here.

Both DSM-IV and DCPR diagnoses were used. DSM somatoform disorders (undifferentiated, somatization disorder, hypochondriasis) were present in 20 cases (29%), whereas DCPR persistent somatization was observed in 28 (40%). An overlap between the two types of diagnosis occurred in only 8 patients (17%). Furthermore, the DCPR allowed us to characterize other clinical phenomena related to somatization, such as alexithymia (41 cases; 59%) and functional somatic symptoms secondary to a psychiatric disorder (24 cases; 35%). The latter diagnosis (Table 1) enables us to identify a psychiatric disorder that preceded the onset of functional somatic symptoms and included the specific symptoms involved within its manifestations (e.g., panic disorder and cardiac symptoms). Such hierarchical rule was found to be of clinical and predictive value[12].

In these cases, treatment of the primary psychiatric disorder (whether pharmacological or psychological or both) according to well-defined guidelines is likely to entail disappearance or considerable decrease of bowel symptoms. Other cases (Table 2) would present clinical characteristics that are likely to respond to psychotherapy instead of drug treatment[8]. Another example may involve the persistent somatizers (Table 3). Kellner[13] suggested that it may be advantageous to conceptualize a somatizing patient as someone in whom psychophysiological symptoms have clustered.

These patients are more likely to respond to explanation, reassurance, and support by the treating physician than by complex and time-consuming psychotherapeutic techniques[3]. Similar considerations apply to health anxiety (Table 4), conversion symptoms (Table 5), alexithymia (Table 6), type A behaviour (Table 7), disease phobia (Table 8), thanatophobia (Table 9), illness denial (Table 10), anniversary reaction (Table 11), irritable mood (Table 12).

| DIAGNOSTIC CRITERIA FOR FUNCTIONAL SOMATIC SYMPTOMS SECONDARY TO A PSYCHIATRIC DISORDER (A THROUGH D ARE REQUIRED) |
|---|
| **A.** Symptoms of autonomic arousal (e.g., palpitations, sweating, tremor, flushing) or functional medical disorder (e.g., irritable bowel syndrome, fibromyalgia, neurocirculatory asthenia), causing distress, or repeated medical care, or resulting in impaired quality of life. |
| **B.** Appropriate medical evaluation does not disclose any organic pathology to account for the physical complaints. |
| **C.** A psychiatric disorder (which includes the involved somatic symptoms within its manifestations) preceding the onset of functional somatic symptoms (e.g., panic disorder and cardiac symptoms). |
| **D.** Even though health anxiety may occur, the patient does not meet the criteria for hypochondriasis or disease phobia. |

Table 1

Revised from Fava GA, Freyberger HJ, Bech P et al.[11]

## Diagnostic criteria for demoralization (A through C are required)

**A.** A feeling state characterized by the patient's consciousness of having failed to meet his or her own expectations (or those of others) or being unable to cope with some pressing problems. The patient experiences feelings of helplessness, or hopelessness, or giving up.

**B.** The feeling state should be prolonged and generalized (at least one month duration).

**C.** The feeling closely antedated the manifestations of a medical disorder or exacerbated its symptoms.

Table 2

Revised from Fava GA, Freyberger HJ, Bech P et al.[11]

## Diagnostic criteria for persistent somatization (A and B are required)

**A.** Functional medical disorder (e.g., fibromyalgia, fatigue, oesophageal motility disorders, non ulcer dyspepsia, irritable bowel syndrome, neurocirculatory asthenia, urethral syndrome), duration of which exceeds 6 months, causing distress, or repeated medical care, or resulting in impaired quality of life.

**B.** Additional symptoms of autonomic arousal (involving also other organ systems) and exaggerated side effects from medical therapy are present, indicating low sensation or pain thresholds and high suggestibility.

Table 3

Revised from Fava GA, Freyberger HJ, Bech P et al.[11]

## DIAGNOSTIC CRITERIA FOR HEALTH ANXIETY (A AND B ARE REQUIRED)

**A.** Generic worry about illness, concern about pain and bodily preoccupations (tendency to amplify somatic sensations) of less than 6 months' duration.

**B.** Worries and fears readily respond to appropriate medical reassurance, even though new worries may ensue after some time.

Table 4

Revised from Fava GA, Freyberger HJ, Bech P et al.[11]

## DIAGNOSTIC CRITERIA FOR CONVERSION SYMPTOMS (A THROUGH C ARE REQUIRED)

**A.** One or more symptoms or deficits affecting voluntary motor or sensory function, characterized by lack of anatomical or physiological plausibility, and/or absence of expected physical signs or laboratory findings, and/or inconsistent clinical characteristics. If symptoms of autonomic arousal or functional medical disorder are present, conversion symptoms should be prominent, causing distress, or repeated medical care, or resulting in impaired quality of life.

**B.** At least 2 of the following features are present:

1. ambivalence in symptom reporting (e.g., the patient appears relaxed or unconcerned as he/she describes distressing symptoms),
2. hystrionic personality features (colourful and dramatic expression, language and appearance; demanding dependency; high suggestibility; rapid mood changes),
3. precipitation of symptoms by psychological stress, the association of which the patient is unaware,
4. history of similar physical symptoms experienced by the patient, or observed in someone else, or wished on someone else.

**C.** Appropriate medical evaluation does not disclose any organic pathology to account for the physical complaints.

Table 5

Revised from Fava GA, Freyberger HJ, Bech P et al.[11]

## Diagnostic criteria for alexithymia

At least 3 of the following 6 characteristics should be present:

1. inability to use appropriate words to describe emotions
2. tendency to describe details instead of feelings (e.g. circumstances surrounding an event rather than the feelings)
3. lack of a rich fantasy life
4. thought content associated more with external events rather than fantasy or emotions.
5. unawareness of the common somatic reactions that accompany the experience of a variety of feelings
6. occasional but violent and often inappropriate outbursts of affective behavior

Table 6

Revised from Fava GA, Freyberger HJ, Bech P et al.[11]

## Diagnostic criteria for Type A behavior (A and B are required)

**A.** At least 5 of the following 9 characteristics should be present:

1. excessive degree of involvement in work and other activities subject to deadlines
2. steady and pervasive sense of time urgency
3. display of motor-expressive features (rapid and explosive speech, abrupt body movements, tensing of facial muscles, hand gestures) indicating sense of being under the pressure of time
4. hostility and cynicism
5. irritable mood
6. tendency to speed up physical activities
7. tendency to speed up mental activities
8. high intensity of desire for achievement and recognition
9. high competitiveness

**B.** The behavior elicits stress-related physiologic responses that precipitate or exacerbate symptoms of a medical condition.

Table 7

Revised from Fava GA, Freyberger HJ, Bech P et al.[11]

## DIAGNOSTIC CRITERIA FOR DISEASE PHOBIA (A THROUGH C ARE REQUIRED)

**A.** Persistent, unfounded fear of suffering from a specific disease (e.g., AIDS, cancer), with doubts remaining despite adequate examination and reassurance.

**B.** Fears tend to manifest themselves in attacks rather than in costant, chronic worries as in hypochondriasis. Panic attacks may be an associated feature.

**C.** The object of fears does not change with time and duration of symptoms exceeds 6 months.

Table 8

Revised from Fava GA, Freyberger HJ, Bech P et al.[11]

## DIAGNOSTIC CRITERIA FOR THANATOPHOBIA (A THROUGH C ARE REQUIRED)

**A.** Attacks with the sense of impending death and/or conviction of dying soon, even though there is no objective medical reason for such fear.

**B.** Marked and persistent fear and avoidance of news which reminds of death (e.g., funerals, obituary notices). Exposure to these stimuli almost invariably provokes an immediate anxiety response.

**C.** The avoidance, anxious anticipation and distress interfere significantly with the person's level of functioning.

Table 9

Revised from Fava GA, Freyberger HJ, Bech P et al.[11]

### Diagnostic criteria for illness denial (A and B are required)

**A.** Persistent denial of having a physical disorder and of the need of treatment (e.g., lack of compliance, delayed seeking medical attention for serious and persistent symptoms, counterphobic behavior), as a reaction to the symptoms, signs, diagnosis or medical treatment of a physical illness.

**B.** The patient has been provided a lucid and accurate appraisal of the medical situation and management to be followed.

Table 10

Revised from Fava GA, Freyberger HJ, Bech P et al.[11]

### Diagnostic criteria for anniversary reaction (A through C are required)

**A.** Symptoms of autonomic arousal (e.g., palpitations, sweating, tremor, flushing) or functional medical disorder (e,g,, irritable bowel syndrome, fibromyalgia, neurocirculatory asthenia) or conversion symptoms causing distress, or repeated medical care, or resulting in impaired quality of life.

**B.** Appropriate medical evaluation unconvers no organic pathology to account for the physical complaints.

**C.** Symptoms began when the patient reached the age or in the occasion of the anniversary when a parent or very close family member developed a life-threatening illness and/or died. The patient is unaware of such association.

Table 11

Revised from Fava GA, Freyberger HJ, Bech P et al.[11]

DIAGNOSTIC CRITERIA FOR IRRITABLE MOOD
(A THROUGH C ARE REQUIRED)

**A.** A feeling state characterized by irritable mood which may be experienced as brief episodes, in particular circumstances, or it may be prolonged and generalized. It requires an increased effort of control over temper by the individual or results in irascible verbal or behavioral outbursts.

**B.** The experience of irritability is always unpleasant for the individual and overt manifestation lacks the cathartic effect of justified outbursts of anger.

**C.** The feeling elicits stress-related physiologic responses that precipitate or exacerbate symptoms of a medical disorder.

Table 12

Revised from Fava GA, Freyberger HJ, Bech P et al.[11]

## Referral for psychotherapy

It is conceivable, even though yet to be tested in controlled studies, that patients with chronic GI diseases who are properly screened and selected may offer a better response to brief psychotherapy than unselected patients. Diagnostic developments in psychosomatic diagnosis may thus pave the way for more targeted psychotherapeutic efforts in altered brain-gut mechanisms. Controlled studies may then determine whether a specific technique (e.g., CBT) is more likely to yield successful results than others. Until more research evidence is at hand, gastroenterologists should not dismiss the considerable therapeutic potential of psychotherapy in the setting of chronic GI diseases.

### *REFERENCES*

1. Bergin AE, Garfield SL, editors. *Handbook of psychotherapy and behavior change.* New York: Wiley; 1994.

2. Frank JD, Frank JB. *Persuasion and healing.* Baltimore: The Johns Hopkins University Press; 1991.
3. Fava GA. *Psychotherapy research: clinical trials versus clinical reality.* Psychother Psychosom 1986;46:6-12.
4. Salkovskis P. *The cognitive-behavioral approach.* In: Creed F, Mayou R, Hopkins A, editors. Medical symptoms not explained by organic disease. London: Royal College of Psychiatrists and Royal College of Physicians; 1992;70-84.
5. Drossman DA, Creed FH, Fava GA, et al. *Psychosocial aspects of the functional gastrointestinal disorders.* Gastroenterol Int 1995;8:47-90.
6. Friedli K, King MB, Lloyd M, Horder J. *Randomised controlled assessment of nondirective psychotherapy verus routine general-practitioner care.* Lancet 1997;350:1662-5.
7. Guthrie E, Creed F, Dawson T, Tomenson B. *A controlled trial for psychological treatment for the irritable bowel syndrome.* Gastroenterology 1991;100:450-7.
8. Fava GA, Freyberger H, editors. *Handbook of psychosomatic medicine.* Madison, CT: International Universities Press; 1998.
9. *Diagnostic and statistical manual of mental disorders* (DSM-IV). Washington, DC: American Psychiatric Association (APA);1994.
10. Fava GA. *The concept of psychosomatic disorder.* Psychother Psychosom 1992;58:1-12.
11. Fava GA, Freyberger HJ, Bech P, et al. *Diagnostic criteria for use in psychosomatic research.* Psychother Psychosom 1995;63:1-8.
12. Fava GA, Porcelli P. *Multisomatoform disorder.* (Letter to the Editor). Arch Gen Psychiatry 1998;55:756.
13. Kellner R. *Psychosomatic syndromes and somatic symptoms.* Washington: American Psychiatric Press; 1991.
14. Taylor GJ, Bagby RM, Parker JDA. *Disorders of affect regulation.* Cambridge: Cambridge University Press; 1997.

*Address for correspondence*

**FAVA GA, MD**
Dipartimento di Psicologia
Università di Bologna
Viale Berti Pichat 5
40127 Bologna Italia
Fax: +39 051 243086

# Cognitive behavioural treatment for functional gastrointestinal disorders

*BB Toner*

This paper has two general aims:

1. to provide a rationale for the use of Cognitive Behavioural Therapy (CBT), for functional Gastrointestinal (GI) disorders
2. to provide practical information concerning the application of cognitive behavioural therapy for functional gastrointestinal disorders.

Over the past 17 years, there have been 12 controlled studies involving cognitive and/or behavioural techniques in the treatment of functional gastrointestinal disorders. All of these studies have focused on Irritable Bowel Syndrome (IBS). In general, results support the efficacy of CBT strategies for the treatment of IBS. However, most of the published treatments for IBS have been taken from theoretical approaches developed for work with individuals who presented to mental health professionals with largely depressive- or anxiety-related problems. There has been little theoretical or empirical work that has identified and integrated the specific psychosocial issues of individuals with IBS into a treatment model. Our team in Toronto was the first to apply cognitive-behavioural principles to IBS patients using a specific cognitive-behavioural model for IBS. Although initial data from our group appear promising, further refinement of CBT tailored specifically to IBS patients is needed. We find that an introduction of the gate theory of pain is very helpful in highlighting the association between thoughts, feelings, behaviour and painful GI symptoms. The presence of many unhelpful cognitions have been identified in individuals with IBS. These cognitions can serve to open up the gate, that is make the pain more central or more intense. Factors that can close the gate include coping strategies such as controlling thoughts of pain through attention diversion. We have recently developed a scale for assessing cognitions of individuals with IBS. The following themes are presented to serve as suggested content areas for CBT in individual or group format. These are based on themes that have been identified in the literature as well as from our own clinical work as especially relevant for IBS patients. Contingent on the formulation of presenting or emerging issues and goals, the order of inclusion of these themes can be changed to fit the particular needs of a given individual or group. These include:

1. establishing an association between thoughts, feelings, behaviour and bowel symptoms
2. pain management
3. bowel-performance anxiety
4. anger and assertion
5. shame
6. social approval
7. control.

## Review of studies on cognitive behavioural treatment for functional gastrointestinal disorders

In reviewing literature CBT for IBS, it is important to highlight that the term CBT, as used in this work, does not represent one specific approach or set of techniques, but rather refers to many different compositions drawn from a large pool of cognitive and behavioural strategies. While most of the previous studies do not give a rationale for the use of CBT strategies, we expect that CBT strategies would focus on an exploration of how certain cognitions and behaviours may impact on GI symptoms and associated psychosocial distress[1].

Within the past 17 years, there have been 12 controlled studies involving cognitive and/or behavioural techniques in the treatment of IBS[1-12]. Most studies have used a multicomponent behavioural or CBT package. Treatment packages have included various combinations of cognitive therapy, stress management training, contingency management, relaxation techniques, educational components, biofeedback, assertiveness training, pain management and bowel habit training.

In general, results support the efficacy of CBT strategies for the treatment of IBS. Specifically, three studies found that CBT packages improved GI symptoms and psychological distress relative to symptom monitoring control conditions[2,3,7]. Three studies reported superior improvement[4,5] or similar improvement[2] in various GI symptoms relative to antispasmodics and/or bulking agents. One study found improvement in abdominal symptoms, coping strategies and avoidance behaviour relative to a waiting list control group[11]. Toner et al.[1] randomized 101 IBS patients to cognitive-behavioural group therapy (including progressive relaxation), an attentional placebo control (psycho-educational group therapy) and a standard medical care condition. Results indicated that the CBT group therapy significantly improved depressive symptoms, need for social desirability and GI symptom diary scores including abdominal pain, tenderness, diarrhoea, constipation, and bloating. These psychological and GI symptoms did not improve in the control groups. Three studies using cognitive therapy alone found: significant improvement in IBS symptoms, depression and anxiety relative to symptom monitoring[9]; significant improvement in IBS symptoms and depression relative to an attention-placebo control[10]; and a third study showed improvement on GI symptoms in both individual and group cognitive therapy compared with a symptom monitoring group[12].

## Developing a cognitive behavioural model for IBS

Most of the published treatments for IBS have been taken from theoretical approaches developed for work with individuals who presented to mental health professionals with largely depressive- or anxiety-related problems. There has been little theoretical or empirical work that has identified and integrated the specific psychosocial issues of individuals with IBS into a model for treatment. Consequently, to date, there are few psychological approaches that are tailored to the needs of this population. Our group was the first to adapt cognitive-behavioural principles to IBS patients using a specific cognitive-behavioural model for IBS[13] with both group and individual formats. Although preliminary data appear promising, further refinement of CBT tailored specifically to IBS patients are needed.

Specifically, one area that needs to be further developed and incorporated into the treatment model is an appreciation of the cognitive and emotional distress associated with having a debilitating chronic illness in a society where there is insufficient knowledge and empathy as well as substantial stigma and trivialization associated with a so-called functional somatic disorder. Accordingly, it is important to highlight that, when a person with IBS is referred to a health professional, he/she may come into the office with the belief that the care giver does not think their symptoms are "real" or serious, but "all in their head". The therapeutic alliance is enhanced by validating the reality of the symptoms and also challenging society's view of the artificial dualism of functional/organic components of illness. Another area that needs to be considered is the influence of gender on IBS. For example, despite the repeated documentation of gender differences in patients with IBS (ratio of 3 women to every man), there has been little attention devoted to gender issues in the conceptualization and treatment of IBS[13].

The cognitive-behavioural model presented here has been adapted by our group in Toronto[13] from a model developed by Sharpe et al.[14] for functional somatic syndromes. Central to the cognitive-behavioural model is the way the person thinks about his/her bowel symptoms. If the bowel symptoms are attributed to disease or organic cause, then the person may seek out medical consultation for a medical explanation of his/her difficulties. A large percentage of people who consult a physician are reassured by the negative findings. A small percentage of patients (or their physicians) are not reassured and may be referred to a specialist for more extensive investigations. Some patients may still feel that something has been missed or overlooked by the specialist and seek out other GI specialists or consult various non-medical therapists in the persistent search for more extensive investigation.

According to our cognitive-behavioural model, IBS symptoms and distress are perpetuated by an interaction between psychological, social and physiological factors. Cognitions such as "there must be a medical explanation for this pain", lead to certain behaviours (further medical consultations), increased attention and hypervigilance of bodily sensations, increased anxiety and arousal which may lead to a heightened sensitivity to pain. During this process, sensations become intense which may then lead to further thoughts that something must have been overlooked, leading to further physiological arousal and self scrutiny which amplifies bodily sensations. Independent of the predisposed factors associated with the symptoms, cognitions about the illness and the associated anxiety serve to maintain and amplify the symptoms. Accordingly, this model highlights that how the individual approaches his/her IBS psychologically (i.e., by hypervigilance to bodily symptoms and attribution of illness) serve to amplify symptoms and interferes with coping and quality of life.

Consistent with an information processing model, people selectively attend to those cognitions and perceptions that confirm their explanatory hypotheses while selectively ignoring information or sensory input that is inconsistent with their beliefs[15]. Accordingly, other possible contributing factors such as life stressors, psychological distress, overwork, interpersonal conflict or loss may be minimized or selected out of their conceptualization of their IBS symptoms. There is some empirical support for this model from the work of Drossman et al.[16] who found that individuals with IBS who sought out specialized consultation for their symptoms (i.e., IBS patients) were significantly more likely to minimize psychological and stress-related factors in their lives relative to a comparison group of individuals with IBS who did not consult specialists for their symptoms (i.e., IBS non-patients). More recently, in a prospective study, Levy et al.[17] found that IBS patients were less likely to report an association between IBS symptoms and stressors relative to IBS non-patients.

## Introducing the role of psychological treatment to patients

Physicians often encounter difficulties in encouraging patients to pursue psychological treatments for functional GI disorders[18]. Many patients interpret referrals to psychologists or psychiatrists as insulting and as indicating the physician does not believe there is something really wrong[19]. The physician and therapist must first acknowledge to the patient the possibility of these concerns. They can then counter the implication that the patient's symptoms are imaginary or are caused by "mental" problems with a careful explanation of our knowledge of the connection between the mind and body. Once this concept has been explained, patients are better able to comprehend the rationale underlying the use of psychotherapies such as CBT for functional GI disorders. These concerns must be addressed if a positive therapeutic alliance is to be established between the patient and health professional[19].

The term "brain-gut connection" has been used to help patients better understand the specific mind-body association between psychological factors and bowel function. It is now widely recognized by clinicians and researchers that the mind and body are linked. This means, quite simply, that they do not operate independently of each other, but there is an interactive effect between them (Seeing the mind and body as separate is often referred to as "mind-body dualism"). We have physical sensations and we react cognitively and behaviourally to these sensations. These reactions, in turn, have further effects on our phyiology, which affect our cognitions, etc.[20-25]. This is the basis for the psychological treatment of functional GI disorders. Because the mind and body are linked, psychological treatments can improve symptoms. To say that all functional GI symptoms are "in the patient's head" is really falling back into this faulty mind/body split. Functional GI disorders are real problems. Although no structural or biochemical abnormalities have been found, to date, to explain patients' symptoms, they are no less real. Ultimately, even if a physical basis is discovered, it will still be important to recognize the interaction between the mind and body to help alleviate symptoms and/or suffering for many patients[26-30].

It should be explained to patients that:

1. emotions and stress can influence the symptoms of functional GI disorders
2. psychological treatments can improve these symptoms.

The mechanisms for these connections might be conceptualized as follows: the brain receives input from many sources. Some information comes from the outside world, while other information comes from the gut, which has a nervous system that sends signals to the brain. Circuits in the brain that process emotions and thinking are connected to other circuits that control pain or discomfort. The brain processes this information and sends signals to the gut, or intestines. The nervous system in the gut responds to the brain's input. For instance, under conditions of stress or anxiety, the brain may send messages to the gut that affect its function or make it more sensitive to pain. Psychosocial factors may also influence the way in which symptoms are experienced. Consistent with this line of thinking, studies have found a high prevalence of anxiety and depression in patients with IBS[1,31]. One way psychological treatments help affect symptoms is by improving methods of coping with stress, likely resulting in fewer signals being sent to the intestines and symptom improvement[18].

## Assessing cognitions

A review of the literature indicates that there are no standardized measures available that have been designed to assess cognitions of Functional Bowel Disorder (FBD) patients. Accordingly, it is difficult to assess the efficacy of CBT when there is no adequate measure of change in the primary measures of conceptual and clinical importance (i.e., cognition). Our group in Toronto recently addressed this need by developing a reliable and valid instrument to assess the cognitions of patients diagnosed with FBD[32,33]. In developing this instrument, we began with a set of 204 items based on cognitions recorded in thought diaries of patients diagnosed with FBD. These items were then examined for redundancy, ambiguity, clarity and relevance, resulting in a list of 99 candidate items. We further refined the list by generating some possible items based on our own clinical and research experience, and by submitting the list for review to a multidisciplinary team of international experts who are involved in the research and treatment of FBD. This resulted in a final list of 95 candidate items, which were administered, along with a set of validating questionnaires, to a new sample of 75 FBD patients in Canada and the United States.

The findings indicate that the final 25-item scale has high reliability (Cronbach's alpha = .93; inter-item correlation = .36); high concurrent criterion validity evidenced by the correlation of the scale with a global rating of life interference due to bowel symptoms ($r=.71$; $p<.001$); acceptable convergent validity evidenced by the correlation of the scale with the Dysfunctional Attitudes Scale ($r=.38$; $p<.01$); high content validity and face validity; and no social desirability contamination ($r=.15$; ns). Therefore, the Cognitive Scale for Functional Bowel Disorders is a valid and reliable scale which can be used as an outcome measure in evaluating the efficacy of different forms of psychotherapeutic intervention for FBD, and can also serve as a helpful assessment tool for health professionals working with patients diagnosed with FBD.

## Application of CBT for IBS: suggested themes

The following themes are presented to serve as suggested content areas for individual or group sessions. These are based on themes that have been identified in the literature as well as in our own clinical work as relevant for most IBS clients. Contingent on the formulation of presenting or emerging issues and goals, the order and inclusion of themes can be changed to fit the particular needs of a given individual or group. These include: establishing an association between thoughts, feelings, behaviours and bowel symptoms; bowel-performance anxiety; pain management; anger and assertion; shame; social approval and control[32,33]. While space does not permit one to cover all of the themes here, I will highlight the first two themes to illustrate how they may be used in sessions.

## Association among thoughts, feelings, behaviour and IBS

The major focus of CBT is the systematic evaluation of the perceptions, thoughts, belief systems and assumptions which underly behaviour and which are connected closely to feelings, behaviours and physiological reactions. The first step in this process is to identify the specific patterns of thinking, behaving and feeling that are associated with IBS. For example, an individual with IBS may develop some bothersome bowel symptoms during a period of illness or environmental stress. If these symptoms are potentially embarassing, such as excessive gas or bowel urgency, the person may develop certain beliefs that interfere with spontaneous behaviours. For example, the person may come to believe that certain social events or situations are not "safe" because there is not a washroom easily available. The individual may then become reluctant to engage in social events away from home, and avoid or escape from such situations. This pattern of behaviour can make an individual feel depressed, anxious or angry. These feelings in themselves contribute to physiological arousal, and increase the likelihood and severity of bowel symptoms. We find that an introduction of gate theory of pain is very helpful in highlighting the association between thoughts, feelings and behaviours and painful GI symptoms.

The gate theory[34] helps us understand how thoughts, feelings and behaviour affect pain. The gate theory of pain states that pain messages originate at the site of bodily damage, injury or disease and are then passed through a mechanism that works like a "gate to the brain". The brain then interprets the pain message, and it is at this point that pain is experienced. The pain "gate" can be partly or fully opened or closed, determining the amount of pain experienced.

Factors that can open the gate (make pain more central or more intense) include, for example, thoughts that focus attention on the pain, and boredom because of minimal involvement in life activities. Feelings that can open the gate include depression, anxiety, anger. Behaviours can also open the gate, such as an inappropriate activity level or lack of pleasant activities. Factors that can close the gate (make pain less central or less intense) include coping strategies such as controlling pain thoughts through attention diversion. Examples of attention diversion are distraction, imagery, and relaxation. Cognitive restructuring strategies, such as altering the self-talk to messages such as "I can handle this, I've handled it before" versus "I can't stand another second of this pain" are also useful. Pain can also be reduced by changing activity patterns, such as engaging in pleasurable activities.

## Bowel performance anxiety

An especially important theme is that of bowel performance anxiety. This theme manifests itself in the worry that the bowels will not function, or perform, properly, and much attention is paid to managing food and environment to mimimize the likelihood of bowel distress. Many IBS patients experience considerable concern about how they might function and appear in social situations. Many of their concerns are similar to those who present for treatment of social anxiety. In addition to fears about negative evaluation, patients frequently have concerns that bowel symptoms will negatively affect their capacity to function and enjoy a broad variety of situations. Many patients forego taking on challenges or engaging in new activities because of their predictions that they will be negatively affected by their IBS symptoms. The case of Ms. ZA. speaks to this concern[1]. Ms. ZA. experienced a very distressing occurrence a couple of years previously while eating at an unfamiliar hotel restaurant. She had almost lost control of her bowels and had been unable to find a bathroom. Ms. ZA., a fastidious person, had been horrified by the experience and had since been very reluctant to go to unfamiliar places. She listed the following situations as progressively more anxiety-producing, because of her concern about having to suddenly find a bathroom:

1. eating alone at her desk at work
2. eating alone at the local food court where bathrooms were close and available
3. eating at the local food court with a friend sympathetic to her bowel problems
4. eating at a strange restaurant with a sympathetic friend
5. eating at a strange restaurant with coworkers who were unaware of her bowel problems.

In treatment, Ms. ZA. was encouraged to systematically encounter these situations, from the least to the most anxiety-producing, in order to gain some evidence about whether her experiences were consistent with her (catastrophic) expectations. The objective was twofold: to gain some firsthand experience that challenged her negative expectations were, in fact, unhelpful, and to demonstrate that she could manage to endure some anxiety and concurrent sensations of bowel urgency without having an "accident".

During each situation, Ms. ZA. was encouraged to write thought records before and after the event, so she could see whether or not her negative expectations were realized. As she listed anxious expectations prior to the situation, she also worked to counter each anxiety by adaptive response. For example, for the worry that her friend would think it was "weird" to have to get up and go to the bathroom two or three times during the meal, she developed the response that her friend had given many indications that she respected and liked her, and that those feelings would not totally disappear because of her need to go to the bathroom frequently. She also practiced some breathing exercises as a way to calm herself and delay her need to use the bathroom. She would often find that if she gave herself enough time to get used to a situation, her sense of bowel urgency would dissipate. As she practiced encountering situations that she had previously avoided, she became more confident and more willing to go beyond familiar and "safe" settings. She began to take pride in her accomplishments, and after some weeks of practising, reported that she was able to accept an invitation from her coworkers to go out after work to a bar that she had never gone to before.

## Conclusions

This paper has provided the rationale for the use of CBT for IBS based on both theoretical and research perspectives. It provided a review of CBT studies for IBS and suggested a model for CBT for IBS. Practical information concerning the application of CBT was discussed. In particular, themes were suggested as possible content areas for therapy sessions. Future work will need to further refine the CBT model and specific CBT techniques and strategies to increase the efficacy of CBT for functional GI disorders.

### *References*


1. Toner BB, Segal ZV, Emmott S, et al. *Cognitive-behavioural group therapy for patients with irritable bowel syndrome.* Internat J Group Psychother 1998;48:215-43.
2. Bennett P, Wilkinson S. *A comparison of psychological and medical treatment of the irritable bowel syndrome.* Br J Clin Psychol 1985;24:215-6.
3. Lynch PM, Zamble E. *A controlled behavioral treatment study of irritable bowel syndrome.* Behav Ther 1989;20:509-23.
4. Corney RH, Stanton R, Newell R, et al. *Behavioral psychotherapy in the treatment of irritable bowel syndrome.* J Psychosom Res 1991;35:461-9.
5. Shaw G, Srtgastava ED, Sadlier M, et al. *Stress management for irritable bowel syndrome: a controlled trial.* Digestion 1991;50:36-42.
6. Rumsey N. *Group stress management programmes vs. pharmacological treatment in the treatment of the irritable bowel syndrome.* In: Keaton KW, Creed F, Goeting NLM, editors. Current approaches towards confident management of irritable bowel syndrome. Lyme Regis, UK: Lyme Regis; 1991;33-9.
7. Neff DF, Blanchard EB. *A multi-component treatment for irritable bowel syndrome.* Behav Ther 1987;18:70-83.

8. Blanchard EB, Schwarz SP, Neff DF, Gerardi MA. *Prediction of outcome from the self-regulatory treatment of irritable bowel syndrome*. Behav Res Ther 1981;26:187-90.
9. Green B, Blanchard EB. *Cognitive therapy for irritable bowel syndrome.* J Consult Clin Psychol 1994;62:576-82.
10. Payne A, Blanchard EB. *A controlled comparison of cognitive therapy and self-help support groups in the treatment of irritable bowel syndrome.* J Consult Clin Psychol 1995;63:779-86.
11. Van Dulmen MA, Fennis JFM, Bleijenberg G. *Cognitive-behavioral group therapy for irritable bowel syndrome: effects and long-term follow-up.* Psychosom Med 1996;58:508-14.
12. Vollmer A, Blanchard EG. *Controlled comparison of individual versus group cognitive therapy for irritable bowel syndrome.* Behav Ther 1998;29:19-33.
13. Toner BB. *Cognitive-behavioral treatment of functional somatic syndromes: integrating gender issues.* Cogn Behav Pract 1994;I:157-78.
14. Sharpe M, Peveler R, Mayou R. *The psychological treatment of patients with functional somatic symptoms: a practical guide.* J Psychosom Res 1992;36:515-29.
15. Barsky AJ, Geringer E, Woods CA. *A cognitive-educational treatment for hypochondriasis.* Gen Hosp Psych 1988;10:322-7.
16. Drossman DA, McKee DC, Sandler RS. *Psychosocial factors in the irritable bowel syndrome: a multivariate study of patients and non-patients with irritable bowel syndrome.* Gastroenterology 1988;95:701-8.
17. Levy RL, Cain KC, Jarrett M, Heitkemper MM. *The relationship between daily life stress and gastrointestinal symptoms in women with irritable bowel syndrome.* J Behav Med 1997;20:177-93.
18. Toner BB, Levy RL. *How to legitimize psychological treatment for functional gastrointestinal disorders* (Unpublished manuscript).
19. Toner BB, Rutter C. *Psychologic treatments of IBS.* In: Blackhouse S, Dancey CP, editors. Treating IBS. London, U.K.: Robinson; 1995;77-100.
20. Drossman DA. Presidential Address: *Gastrointestinal illness and the biopsychosocial model.* Psychosom Med 1998;60:258-67.
21. Mayer EA, Berghart GF. *Basic and clinical aspects of visceral hyperalgesia.* Gastroenterology 1994;107:271-93.
22. Drossman DA. *Psychosocial factors in the care of patients with gastrointestinal disorders.* In: Yamada T, editor. Textbook of gastroenterology. Philadelphia, JB Lippincott; 1995;620-7.
23. Camilleri M, Ford MJ. *Functional gastrointestinal disease and the autonomic nervous system: a way ahead?* Gastroenterology 1994;106:1114-8.

24. Mayer EA, Raybould HE. *Role of visceral afferent mechanisms in functional bowel disorders*. Gastroenterology 1990;99:1688-704.
25. Mayer EA. *Functional bowel disorders and the visceral hyperalgesia hypothesis*. In: Mayer EA, Raybould HE, editors. Basic and clinical aspects of chronic abdominal pain. New York: Elsevier; 1993;3-38.
26. Toner BB, Garfinkel PE, Jeejeebhoy KN. *Psychological factors in irritable bowel syndrome*. Can J Psychiatry 1990;35:158-161.
27. Toner BB, Garfinkel PE, Jeejeebhoy KN, et al. *Self-schema in irritable bowel syndrome*. Psychosom Med 1990;52:149-55.
28. Toner BB, Koyama E, Garfinkel PE, et al. *Social desirability and irritable bowel syndrome*. Int J Psychiatry Med 1992;22:99-103.
29. Drossman DA. *The functional gastrointestinal disorders and their diagnosis: a coming of age*. In: Drossman DA, Richter JE, Talley NJ, et al., editors. Functional gastrointestinal disorders: diagnosis, pathophysiology and treatment. Boston: Little, Brown Co; 1994;1-23.
30. Drossman DA, Creed FH, Fava GA, et al. *Psychosocial aspects of the functional gastrointestinal disorders*. Gastroenterol Int 1995;8:47-90.
31. Walker EA, Roy-Byrne PO, Katon WJ. *Irritable bowel syndrome and psychiatric illness*. Am J Psychiatry 1990;147:565-72.
32. Toner BB, Segal ZV, Emmott S, Myran D. *Cognitive-behavioral treatment for irritable bowel syndrome: the brain-gut connection*. New York: Guilford Press; 1999.
33. Toner BB, Stuckless N, Downie FP, et al. *Development of a cognitive scale for functional bowel disorders*. Psychosom Med 1998;60:492-7.
34. Melzack R, Wall PD. *Pain mechanisms: a new theory*. Science 1965:150:971-80.

*ADDRESS FOR CORRESPONDENCE*

**TONER BB, PhD**
Centre for Addiction and Mental Health
250 College Street
Toronto, Ontario M5T 1R8 Canada
Fax: +1 416 979 6811
E-mail: tonerb@cs.clarke-inst.on.ca

# Hypnosis for irritable bowel syndrome

*PJ Whorwell*

It is well known that the conventional treatment for Irritable Bowel Syndrome (IBS) is far from satisfactory although a number of different drugs are in development which may, hopefully, change this situation.

For many patients, IBS is not particularly severe and once they understand the nature of the condition and realise that it is not life threatening, they can often cope with the problem reasonably well. Unfortunately, in some patients the disorder becomes much more intrusive and they suffer greatly from their symptoms which can affect all aspects of their lives. Their quality of life deteriorates, they lose time off work or even have to give up work completely, they become chronic attenders in primary and secondary care clinics and their life becomes dominated by their condition. Why some patients become so severely affected by their disease is unknown but is probably related to other factors such as coping capacities and psychological status. How much it is just related to severity of symptoms remains to be determined as it is well known that different people seem to cope with illness differently, a good example being the "common cold". Whatever the cause, these patients with severe IBS become a major drain on health service and economic resources and are especially hard to manage.

In the early 1980's, we decided to establish whether hypnotherapy may have a possible beneficial effect in severe intractable IBS. A controlled trial was set up in which 30 patients were randomised to receive either hypnotherapy or a control visit where they were given equal attention but no active hypnosis[1]. They were treated at weekly intervals for 12 weeks and at the end of the trial compared in terms of scores for pain, distension, bowel dysfunction and general well being. All these parameters improved significantly (Figure 1) and in a further study the improvement was shown to be long lasting[2]. It is also well known that patients with IBS suffer from a number of extra-colonic symptoms[3] such as backache, lethargy, bladder and gynaecological symptoms which some individuals can find as intrusive as the bowel symptoms of IBS[4].

Figure 1

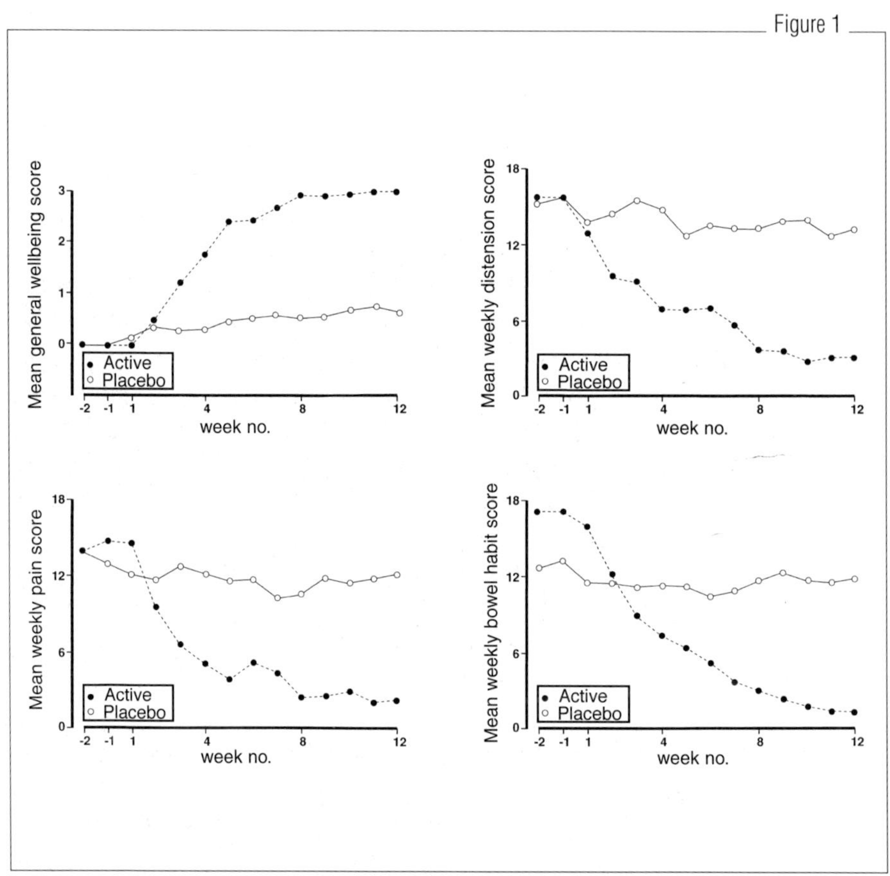


Symptom scores in patients and controls undergoing hypnotherapy for IBS.

Furthermore, the quality of life of these individuals can be considerably reduced[5]. In a more recent study, we have examined the effect of hypnotherapy on these parameters with further encouraging results[6]. There was a significant reduction of many of the extra-colonic symptoms (Figure 2) and quality of life (Figure 3) also significantly improved. Some of the patients were permanently out of work because of their problem and those receiving hypnosis returned to work more than controls. It was also noted that patients consulted their General Practitioner's less frequently, not only for their IBS but also for other reasons, following their hypnotherapy.

Figure 2

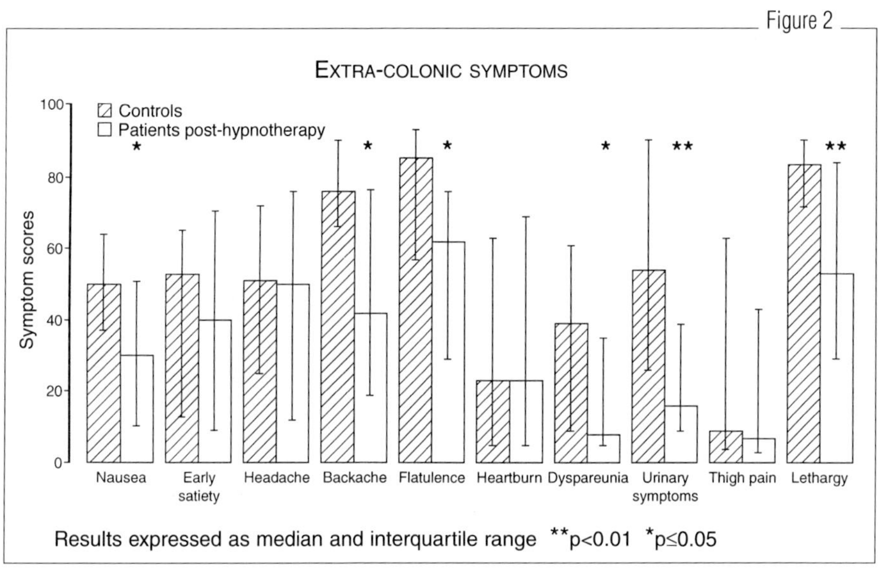


Change in extra-colonic symptoms following hypnotherapy.

Figure 3

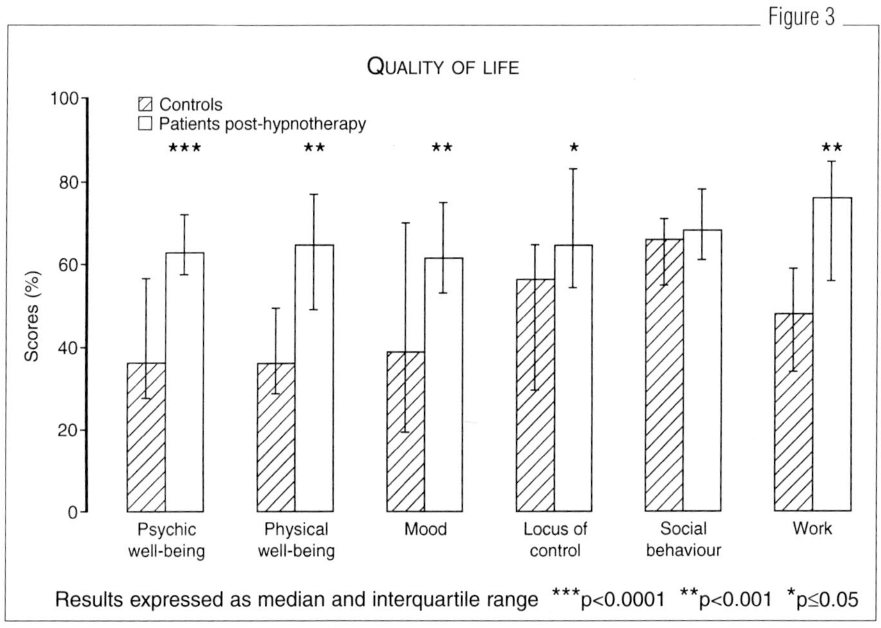


Change in quality of life following hypnotherapy.

The mechanism by which hypnotherapy helps these patients must remain speculative at this time but, undoubtedly, there must be a powerful psychotherapeutic component to a treatment of this type. However, we do have some evidence that hypnosis can influence both motility and visceral sensitivity both of which have been incriminated in the pathogenesis of IBS although the latter is more fashionable at the current time.
Figure 4 shows the effect of hypnotic induction on fasting colonic motility and, as can be seen, this can have quite a striking effect.

Figure 4

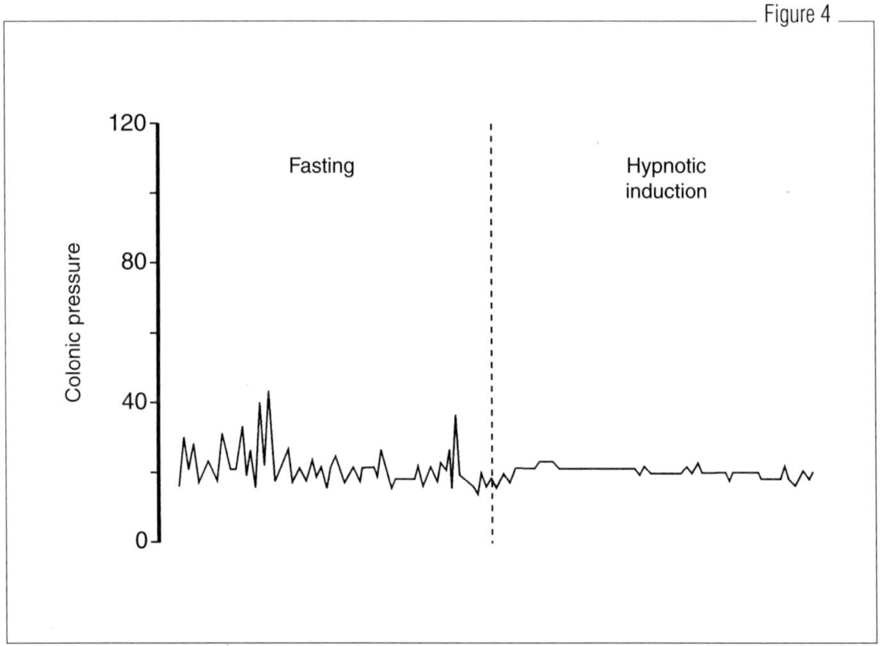


Change in fasting colonic motility during hypnosis

In a study on visceral sensitivity[7], a group of patients had this assessed before and after a three-month course of hypnotherapy and those demonstrating hypersensitivity at the beginning showed a significant reduction in this measurement at the end of treatment. What is possibly more interesting is that this observation was also observed outside the hypnotised state suggesting that a more fundamental "resetting" of visceral sensation had taken place (Figure 5).

Figure 5

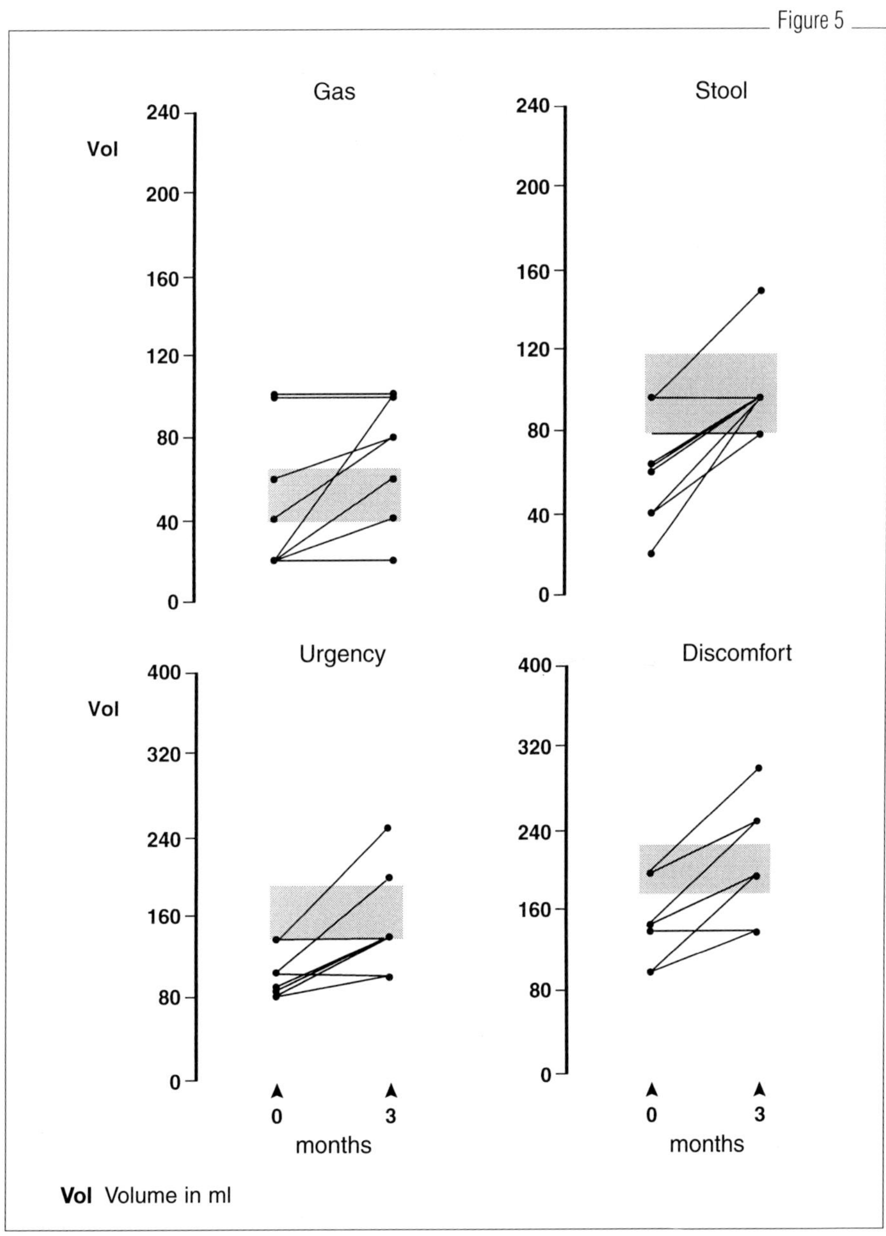


Change in visceral sensitivity following a 3-month course of hypnotherapy. Note change towards more normal values during endoluminal distension (shaded areas).

All these data suggest that hypnosis is a very good treatment for severe IBS and it is tempting to speculate that milder patients might do even better. The major problem with hypnosis is that it is very time consuming and labour intensive and, therefore, very costly to provide. Another problem is that although it is a surprisingly easy technique for the practitioner to learn, it is much more difficult to put into practice. Many doctors find it hard to cope with an approach to the patient which employs the repetitive use of a few words, instructions to "get better" and the inability of hide behind the prescription pad - if a drug does not work you can blame the drug, if hypnosis does not work, you blame yourself. The technique of hypnosis is well described and will not be dealt with here[8]. However, it is our firm belief that to obtain satisfactory results in IBS, it must be focused on the gut[9]. It is not good enough just to hypnotise the patient, tell them they are going to feel less anxious and cope better and expect their IBS to settle down. The patient has to be provided with a reasonably good model of their IBS and various strategies on how they can modify their IBS in a positive way. Thus, they should be given a fairly in depth tutorial (depending on educational and intellectual status) on the possible mechanisms involved in the pathogenesis of IBS and how they might be able to modify them. This then allows them to use the various hypnotic skills, mostly visual and tactile, that they are about to learn to approach their IBS in what we call a "gut focused" approach. After the tutorial visit the patient is then seen at weekly intervals for formal hypnotherapy sessions. New concepts and strategies are introduced reasonably slowly and an audiotape, equivalent to a hypnotherapy session, is given to them with instructions to use it once a day, if possible. The patient is given 12 treatments and, near the end, these can be spread out a little over time to avoid the course ending too abruptly. After the treatment is finished, patients are at liberty to telephone for an occasional "top up" session if they feel the need for a little more help.

In recent years, we have built up a hypnotherapy unit which provides treatment for IBS patients within the structure of the National Health Service. It is currently staffed by 6 non-medically qualified, full-time hypnotherapists under the supervision of a manager and ultimately supervised by the author. This has several advantages: non-medically qualified therapists are less expensive to employ, are often more

dedicated and committed to the therapy and, lastly, are just as successful, in terms of outcome, as their medically qualified counterparts[10].
All patients going through the unit are followed-up after 1 year and our most recent figure for the percentage of people still well after this time is 69%. It is also of interest to note that even the IBS treatment failures say that they are glad to have had the hypnotherapy as they feel it often helps them to cope with their problem even though it may not have relieved their symptoms.

## Conclusions

Hypnotherapy appears to be an effective treatment for severe intractable IBS. Unfortunately, it is very time consuming and costly to provide but when looking at cost benefit ratios it is important to bear in mind that the relief of symptoms is long lasting. Despite this, it is probably unrealistic to ever expect hypnotherapy to become a practical solution for the vast majority of patients with less severe symptoms.

### *References*


1. Whorwell PJ, Prior A, Faragher EB. *Controlled trial of hypnotherapy in the treatment of severe refractory irritable bowel syndrome.* Lancet 1984;II:1232-4.
2. Whorwell PJ, Prior A, Colgan SM. *Hypnotherapy in severe irritable bowel syndrome: further experience.* Gut 1987;28:423-5.
3. Whorwell PJ, McCallum M, Creed FH, Roberts CT. *Non colonic features of irritable bowel syndrome.* Gut 1986;27:37-40.
4. Maxton DG, Morris JA, Whorwell PJ. *Ranking of symptoms by patients with irritable bowel syndrome.* Br Med J 1989;299:1138-9.
5. Wells NEJ, Hahn BA, Whorwell PJ. *Clinical economics review-irritable bowel syndrome.* Aliment Pharmacol Ther 1997;11:1019-30.
6. Houghton LA, Heyman D, Whorwell PJ. *Symptomatology, quality of life and economic features of irritable bowel syndrome and the effect of hypnotherapy.* Aliment Pharmacol Ther 1996;10:91-5.

7. Prior A, Colgan SM, Whorwell PJ. *Changes in rectal sensitivity following hypnotherapy for irritable bowel syndrome.* Gut 1990;31:896-8.
8. Waxman D. *Hartland's medical and dental hypnosis.* 3rd edn. London: Ballière Tindall; 1989.
9. Whorwell PJ. *Hypnosis and the gastrointestinal system.* [Editorial]. Br J Hosp Med 1991;45:27-9.
10. Taylor EE, Whorwell PJ. *Cost effective provision of hypnotherapy in a hospital setting: a practical solution.* Br J Med Econom 1993;6:75-9.

*ADDRESS FOR CORRESPONDENCE*

**WHORWELL PJ, MD**
Department of Medicine
University Hospital of South Manchester
Nell Lane, West Didsbury
Manchester M20 2LR, United Kingdom
Fax: +44 161 434 5194

# Assessment of treatment outcome in the functional gastrointestinal disorders

*KB Klein*

The Functional Gastrointestinal Disorders (FGIDs) are common, associated with considerable suffering and disability, and costly to society. As such they deserve truly effective treatment. However, because their pathogenesis is not well-understood, because there are no objective markers of efficacy, and because placebo response rates may be high, devising appropriate treatments and determining whether they are effective is not a simple matter[1]. Randomized Controlled Trials (RCTs) are the only reliable way of establishing efficacy.

This paper will focus on a centrally important aspect of RCTs in the functional GI disorders-the trial's outcome measures.

## Requirements for meaningful primary outcome measures

The RCT is a scientific experiment. As in any experiment, its validity depends on proper design and appropriate data analysis. Unless the outcome measures can satisfy the following basic criteria, the results of the clinical trial, no matter how "positive" they appear, will not provide compelling evidence that the treatment is of use.

### *The clinical trial must use a single primary outcome measure*

A key requirement for a meaningful clinical trial is that it be designed around a single predetermined parameter, the "primary outcome measure", on which the success of the trial rises or falls. The study's sample size is based on the expected behavior of this measure in the placebo group and the minimal increment above the placebo response in the experimental treatment group that is felt to be clinically meaningful. The "primary efficacy analysis"- the analysis that determines whether the experimental intervention is considered successful or not - is around this measure.

Additional parameters, the "secondary efficacy measures", may provide evidence in support of the success shown in the primary measure, may reflect various facets of the possible benefits of the intervention, may provide insights into the mechanism of action of the therapy, and may allow the generation of hypotheses to be tested in subsequent studies. But secondary efficacy measures must have a subsidiary role. In general, inferential statistical testing is done only on the primary efficacy measure. If such testing is done on secondary measures, an adjustment must be made for the effects of doing multiple comparisons. It is never appropriate to do a "statistical fishing expedition" by testing all measures collected in the RCT to try to find some result that is "significant".

*The measure must be relevant to the desired result of therapy*

The primary outcome measure must be relevant to the fundamental treatment goal.

Thus, one must have this goal clearly in mind in designing the trial and choosing the outcome measure. Such goals may be rather different depending on the patient population being studied (e.g., newly diagnosed vs refractory), the presumed effect of the test therapy (e.g., "peripheral analgesic" vs motility-modifying), and the "customer" for whom the trial is undertaken (patient, physician, third party payer, or employer).

*The measure must truly reflect what it is meant to*

Calling a scale a "Functional Dyspepsia Severity Index" does not automatically mean that it is measuring the severity of dyspepsia. Numerous scales have been constructed to measure abdominal pain. Clearly they do not all measure the same thing or behave in the same way. One must have confidence that the measures being employed in the RCT accurately quantitate the outcome of interest. Ensuring that the measure is "valid" is a complex and time-consuming undertaking, but important to making the results of the RCT meaningful.

*The measure must have appropriate properties for use in a treatment trial, and be correctly analyzed*

Of particular importance, it must be shown to be sensitive to change in the patient's condition over the relatively brief duration of the RCT. Furthermore, it must be analyzed correctly - for example, transforming an ordinal scale into numerical equivalents and calculating and comparing mean scores is not appropriate[2].

## Unsatisfactory primary outcome measures

A number of measures that have been commonly used in treatment trials of the functional GI disorders are poorly suited as primary outcome measures.

*Physiological measures*
The symptoms of the functional GI disorders are intrinsically subjective, and notoriously poorly correlated with GI physiology. Thus, despite the attraction of "objectively" measurable parameters such as transit time, motility, visceral sensitivity, and sphincter pressure these are inappropriate as primary outcome measures. A treatment that "normalizes" motility or that decreases visceral hypersensitivity on barostat testing but does not improve actual symptoms is of little use to the patient. In some circumstances, physiological parameters may be useful as secondary measures. They may support the presumed basis for the effect of a treatment, but they can not be considered surrogates for efficacy.

*"Objective" clinical measures*
A number of scales have been designed to describe and quantitate such things as stool form and frequency. While these may be of value in some types of research, they are not useful as primary outcome measures in treatment trials. They deal with only a specific component of the functional GI disorder symptom complex, which is of variable importance to an individual patient. Furthermore, they do not necessarily have direct clinical implications, and may not predict an overall response to treatment. As secondary measures, they may have a role in some circumstances. For example, like physiological measures, they may provide some insight into the possible mechanism of action of an intervention.

*Psychological measures*
The fields of psychology and psychiatry have the most experience and sophistication in developing scales that quantify non objectively

measurable states. Well-known examples of such scales are those for depression (e.g., the HAM-D and MADRAS) and anxiety (e.g., the HAM-A and STAI). A number of such scales have been extensively validated and shown to be responsive to change in the context of an RCT. These instruments are well suited for clinical trials in patients with clearly-defined psychopathology. However, they are not appropriate as primary outcome measures in treatment trials of the functional GI disorders unless the target population is characterized by a clear psychopathological diagnosis in addition to the functional GI disorder. In that case, the study becomes one of the treatment of the psychopathology in patients who also have a functional GI disorder.

*Composite scores*

One approach to the variability and multiplicity of symptoms in the functional GI disorders has been to try to capture each element of the symptom complex in separate rating scales, and combine these into a single score. This approach acknowledges the importance of having a single primary endpoint. However, such composite scales are generally arbitrarily constructed, without justification for the importance each component receives. For example, mucous in the stool may be given the same weight as abdominal pain, whereas for most patients with Irritable Bowel Syndrome (IBS) belly pain is a much more central feature of their condition.

Since composite scores are made up of fixed contributions from each sub-scale, they cannot accommodate the varying therapeutic needs of different patients. Furthermore, such scales are usually "validated" (if at all) by showing that scores are correlated with the overall clinical impression. It remains to be shown that they have any advantages over the simpler and widely used clinical global rating scales.

*Quality of life measures*

There has been much interest in recent years in "disease-specific" quality of life instruments. Indeed, for IBS, at least three IBS-specific quality of life scales have recently been developed[3-5]. Disease-specific QoL scales are said to be more sensitive in a particular condition than are "generic" measures such as the SF-36. However, to date, no quality of life instruments for the FGIDs have been widely used and none has been shown to be sensitive to changes in the patient's medical condition.

Particularly because some of the subscales of such instruments reflect areas that might be expected to change slowly even when the condition markedly improves (e.g. body image, interpersonal relationships, sexual functioning) it would be predicted that health-related QoL measures may not show the responsiveness one would like to see in a typical treatment trial. Quality of life scales are perhaps best used as outcome measures in very long-duration trials or trials with long-term follow-up, particularly in studies where a treatment has previously been found to be effective, and the question is whether it leads to any improvement in quality of life. As primary outcome measures in short term efficacy studies, it is not clear that these scales will be sensitive to change, or even if they will have any advantages over Clinical Global Impression (CGI)-type scales, which have a long track record of successful use in RCTs.

## An approach to the selection of primary outcome measures

*Is there an ideal outcome measure for all treatment trials in the functional GI disorders?*

Particularly for conditions such as the functional GI disorders, which have no objective markers, it is not easy to define what constitutes effective therapy.

Furthermore, not everyone would agree on what a desirable therapeutic outcome should be. Different patients with the same diagnosis may have quite different treatment goals. And patient-centered goals might be different from those of other relevant parties such as the physician, the payer for medical care, the employer, and the patient's family. All of these perspectives may provide legitimate - though very different - endpoints - for an intervention. However, a given treatment may not be capable of achieving them all, and it is very unlikely that a single clinical trial could be designed to assess such a multitude of endpoints simultaneously. How then should one select the primary outcome measure for a treatment trial in any of the functional GI disorders?

## Clinical outcome measures

Most RCTs in the functional GI disorders focus on some aspect of clinical improvement. Depending on the patient population being studied, the nature of the therapeutic intervention, and the specific goal of successful therapy, several types of instruments are suitable for the primary outcome measure.

*Clinical global impression scales*

The symptoms that result in a diagnosis of one of the functional GI disorders are varied, and interact in complex ways. Thus, there is a strong argument for a primary outcome measure that allows the patient (and/or an observer) to integrate the contribution of a disparate group of symptoms in a single global clinical rating. Indeed, this parallels usual clinical practice where one of the first - and most important - questions the physician asks the patient is, "how are you feeling?," or "how have you been doing since I saw you last?" The response to these questions involves, at least implicitly, the patient's weighing all aspects of how he/she is feeling and functioning and integrating them into a single overall answer. This sort of summary measure has been formalized in the "CGI" (Clinical Global Impressions) scales[6]. They were originally developed by the US National Institute of Mental Health about thirty years ago for use in schizophrenia studies, but since then have been widely and successfully used in many therapeutic areas. Though never formally validated or studied for inter-rater reliability, these scales have high face validity and have the virtue of being simple, brief, and easy to understand across languages and cultures. They are Likert-type scales, with seven descriptors. The investigator-rated "severity of illness" scale goes from "normal" to "among the most extremely ill." The patient- or investigator-rated "global improvement" scale ranges from "very much improved" through "no change" to "very much worse" (Table 1).

The severity of illness scale is administered at baseline and periodically during the course of the trial.

The global improvement scale, which has the benefit of "normalizing" the baseline severity of symptoms for each patient, is administered periodically during the study, or, in short trials, at the end of the treatment period. There tends to be a high correlation between the severity of illness and global improvement scales, and between patient and observer ratings.

If CGI-type scales are used for the primary outcome measure, they should be supported by appropriately chosen secondary measures to help understand the basis of any improvement seen.

LIKERT-TYPE GLOBAL OUTCOME SCALES[6]

| Severity of illness scale | | Clinical global improvement scale | |
|---|---|---|---|
| 1 | Normal, not at all ill | 1 | Very much improved |
| 2 | Borderline ill | 2 | Much improved |
| 3 | Mildly ill | 3 | Minimally improved |
| 4 | Moderately ill | 4 | No change |
| 5 | Markedly ill | 5 | Minimally worse |
| 6 | Severely ill | 6 | Much worse |
| 7 | Among the most extremely ill | 7 | Very much worse |

Table 1

### *Pain scales*

Pain is a key feature of most of the functional GI disorders, and for many patients is the most troublesome symptom. Thus it is not surprising that the assessment of pain has been a common outcome measure in clinical trials in the functional GI disorders, particularly in IBS and functional dyspepsia. Pain measures that have been used include: absolute scales, change relative to baseline, "worst pain" experienced over a fixed time interval (ranging from one day to two weeks), "average pain" experienced during various intervals, "integrated" measures of "intensity x time", and number of pain-free days[1]. Unfortunately, many of these measures were developed without an appreciation of the complexity of the human experience of pain[7] or an adequate understanding of the various issues around clinical pain measurement[8,9].

Clinical trials usually focus on some aspect of pain "intensity," ignoring the fact that pain is multi-dimensional. In addition to intensity, pain can be rated as to its quality, unpleasantness, and the effect it has on the patient's physical and psychological functioning[9,10]. Pain scales rating each of these dimensions may be ordinal (e.g., mild, moderate, strong, very strong), or cardinal (e.g., visual analog scales). Despite theoretical arguments, visual analog scales probably have no real advantages over descriptive scales, either cardinal or ordinal, and they tend to be a bit more confusing to patients and more subject to errors. In any case, in general, ordinal and visual analog scales perform similarly, as an example in nonulcer dyspepsia (NUD) demonstrates[11]. In several other therapeutic areas, a great deal of thought has gone into constructing pain scales that have the appropriate clinical and psychometric properties for use in clinical trials. Such scales are available that have good internal consistency, reliability, objectivity, and validity[12], and have been able to distinguish active drugs from placebo in clinical trials[13]. Just as there are advantages to letting the observer or the patient integrate all aspects of his/her condition in a clinical global impressions scale, similar scales with a focus on pain relief have been successfully used in pain research studies[13].

*Others*

Though not as well studied as global impression or pain scales, other measures have been successfully used as sensible primary outcome measures in RCTs for conditions with no objectively measurable endpoints. Such scales include those that characterize daily functioning, well-being, or patient-determined "adequate relief" of symptoms[14].

## Non-clinical outcome measures

As mentioned previously, treatment trials may reasonably have a focus that is other than strictly clinical, and, by some perspectives, such "alternative" treatment goals are even more important than traditional clinical ones. Examples include lessening medical care resource utilization, decreasing health care expenditures, reducing time lost from and increasing efficiency at work, and improving family satisfaction. A focus on each of these outcomes requires rather different clinical trial designs and very different outcome measures. In general, it would be unrealistic to expect that a study designed with a primary clinical endpoint can also convincingly demonstrate any of these non-clinical advantages.

## Clinical vs statistical significance in the efficacy measure

There is a well-recognized difference between a "statistically significant difference" and a "clinically significant" difference in an outcome measure. For example, in a very large clinical trial of an antihypertensive medication it could be that the experimental intervention lowered the systolic blood pressure by a mean of 2 mmHg more than did placebo. By the appropriate inferential statistical test, this difference could be statistically significant - that is, unlikely to have occurred by chance. However, a difference of only 2 mmHg would be considered clinically unimportant.

Clinical significance is a matter of judgement, not something that can be derived scientifically. A "clinically significant difference" can operationally be taken to mean a difference that would lead to the use of the test treatment in practice.

A clinically significant difference may vary with the condition being treated and the nature and cost of the therapy. For example, an inexpensive once-a-day tablet which modestly improves the primary efficacy measure relative to placebo may be appropriate to employ in treating patients. However, intensive one-to-one psychodynamic psychotherapy which results in only the same modest improvement may be too costly to be of practical use.

Whatever the increment of what is considered clinically significant, it must be clearly decided, preferably with some cogent justification, prior to the start of the trial. A small statistically significant difference that, after the data are analyzed, is declared "clinically significant" is always suspect. The smaller the difference that is felt to be clinically meaningful, the larger the number of patients that must be enrolled in the study to avoid a Type II error. Finally, it is not enough to simply show that an experimental therapy shows a clinically and statistically significant advantage over placebo. At least two other factors must be considered before one could recommend the treatment. First is the safety profile. No matter how effective a treatment proves to be, unless it can be shown to be safe, and to have a clinically favorable "efficacy/safety ratio", it should not be used in practice. Thus carefully assessing safety in the RCT is as important as employing sound outcome measures. Second, both the efficacy and safety must be put in perspective by an appreciation of the cost of treatment.

## Conclusions

Choosing a clearly-defined primary outcome measure with appropriate validation and psychometric properties is essential in the process of planning a randomized clinical trial for any of the functional GI disorders (Table 2).

| KEY STEPS IN THE SELECTION AND APPLICATION OF OUTCOME MEASURES FOR CLINICAL TRIALS IN THE FUNCTIONAL GI DISORDERS | |
|---|---|
| 1 | Choose a primary efficacy measure based on the patient population being studied, the expected effects of the therapeutic intervention, and the outcome of particular interest. |
| 2 | Choose secondary efficacy measures that will both compliment and support the results in the primary measure. |
| 3 | Design the clinical trial with the primary efficacy measure in mind. |
| 4 | Base a sample size calculation on the known characteristics of the primary efficacy measure (e.g., expected variability if a continuous measure) and the minimum difference between the active treatment and placebo groups that would be considered clinically relevant. |

Table 2

The measure should be tailored to the basic question one is trying to answer. The nature of the question and how it is to be framed, in turn, will be influenced by the presumed mechanism of action of the experimental intervention, the patient population chosen for study, as well as other considerations. Once the measure is chosen, the overall design of the RCT can be developed and a sample-size calculation done. For many RCTs with a primary clinical focus, acceptable primary outcome measures include CGI scales or other scales with a global and patient-centered perspective, or appropriately constructed and applied measures of pain. Such measures must be valid, responsive to change within the fairly short duration of a clinical trial, and be analyzed appropriately.

The success or failure of the RCT rests on inferential statistical testing of the primary outcome measure in the experimental and control (usually placebo) groups. However, it is advisable to have secondary efficacy measures in the study as well. In general, these are chosen to help explain the efficacy demonstrated with the primary measure, or to generate hypotheses for further study. The results of such secondary measures should be analyzed with descriptive, not inferential, statistics.

RCTs with non-clinical endpoints may answer specific questions. Such questions include whether the test treatment can lessen health resource utilization, save money, reduce days lost from work and improve productivity at work. In general, the design and primary outcome measures of such studies are rather different from those of clinically-oriented trials. The statistical analyses and standards of proof may be different as well.

## REFERENCES


1. Klein KB. *Controlled treatment trials in the irritable bowel syndrome: a critique.* Gastroenterology 1988;95:232-41.
2. MacKenzie CR, Charlson ME. *Standards for the use of ordinal scales in clinical trials.* Br Med J 1986;292:40-3.
3. Hahn BA, Kirchdoerfer LJ, Fullerton S, Mayer E. *Evaluation of a new quality of life questionnaire for patients with irritable bowel syndrome.* Aliment Pharmacol Ther 1997;11:547-52.
4. Houghton LA, Heyman DJ, Whorwell PJ. *Symptomatology, quality of life and economic features of irritable bowel syndrome - the effect of hypnotherapy.* Aliment Pharmacol Ther 1996;10:91-5.
5. Patrick DL, Drossman DA, Frederick IO et al. *Quality of life in persons with irritable bowel syndrome: development and validation of a new measure.* Dig Dis Sci 1998;43:400-11.
6. National Institute of Mental Health. CGI. *Clinical Global Impressions.* In: Guy W, editor. ECDEU Assessment for Psychopharmacology. Rockville, MD: Rev. ed.; 1976;217-22.

7. Melzack R. Wall PD. *The challenge of pain*. 2nd ed. London: Penguin Books; 1988.
8. Turk DC, Kerns RD. *Conceptual issues in the assessment of clinical pain*. Int J Psych Med 1983;13:57-68.
9. Chapman CR, Casey KL, Dubner R et al. *Pain measurement: an overview.* Pain 1985;22:1-31.
10. Gracely RH. *Evaluation of multi-dimensional pain scales.* Pain 1992;48:297-300.
11. Nyren O, Adami HO, Bates S et al. *Self-rating of pain in nonulcer dyspepsia: a methodological study comparing a new fixed-point scale and the visual analogue scale.* J Clin Gastroenterol 1987;9:408-14.
12. Gracely RH, McGrath P, Dubner R. *Ratio scales of sensory and affective verbal pain descriptors.* Pain 1978;5:5-18.
13. Max MB, Lynch SA, Muir J et al. *Effects of desipramine, amitriptyline, and fluoxetine on pain in diabetic neuropathy*. N Engl J Med 1992;326:1250-6.
14. Mangol AW, Hahn BA, Heath AT et al. *Adequate relief as an endpoint in clinical trials in irritable bowel syndrome.* J Int Med Res 1998;26:76-81.

*ADDRESS FOR CORRESPONDENCE*

**KLEIN KB, MD**
International Drug Development Consulting
7470 NE Manual Road
Bainbridge Island, Washington 98110 USA
Fax: +1 206 780 2907
E-mail: iddlkbk@cs.com

# PHARMACOECONOMICS GASTRO-OESOPHAGEAL REFLUX DISEASE AND IRRITABLE BOWEL SYNDROME

*GP Zara, M Eandi*

## Pharmacoeconomic aspects

Safety and efficacy are not the only parameters of interest in the choice of medical technology; costs are playing an important role. There is a growing interest in "value for money", which can be assessed economically by comparing the costs and the consequences of alternative courses of action[1].

Pharmacoeconomics is the description and analysis of the costs and consequences of drug therapy to health care systems and society. The value of pharmacoeconomics has been advocated by governments and academics all over the world, as a way of reconciling unlimited demands for medicines with a limited ability to fund their supply.

All the aspects of the use of medicines may be allocated costs; by convention, the costs of any given disease are categorized under three principal headings:

- *Direct costs* comprise the expenditures incurred by the health-care system in managing the disease. Consultation with health care professionals, preventive measures, diagnostic tests, medications and in- and out-patient care are all examples of direct costs. In some studies, the latter also include personal spending by patients on the management of their disease;
- *Indirect costs* are the production losses that arise through absence from work due to ill health. At the extremes such losses can stem from short-term absences of just a few days or permanent exit from the labour force because of severe disability or premature death;
- *Costs covering the pain*, namely, immobility and other physical and psychological deficits experienced by patients as a consequence of ill health.

These intangible costs are difficult to translate into monetary terms and are rarely featured as financial values in cost of illness studies. However, their significance to patients is increasingly being recognized, particularly in conditions such as Irritable Bowel Syndrome (IBS), and are captured through quality of life measurements. The consequences of drug therapy include benefits for both individual patients and society at large, which may be quantified in terms of health outcome and quality of life, in addition to purely economic impact[2].

Using these cost categories as a basis, the global cost of a particular therapeutic regimen may usually be considered to be the sum of the individual costs, each multiplied by its frequency during the course of therapy. Thus, the drug acquisition cost, i.e., the headline cost most often associated with the administration of a drug, may actually assume various degrees of significance in the global cost analysis, depending on the relative cost of the drug, the cost of administration equipment, labour charges, and so on. Furthermore, it must be appreciated that even quite minor differences in the value of each of the cost variables between countries, or even between districts within national boundaries, may result in significant differentials in the global cost of a particular treatment regimen in different geographical areas.

A number of different economic evaluation methods may be used: cost-minimization (only costs examined when there are no differences in the consequences); cost-effectiveness (in which cost/success unit is assessed; for example, cost/year-life-gained); cost-utility [cost/utility unit, for example cost/QALY (quality-adjusted life years)]; cost-benefit (where both costs and outcomes are considered in monetary units). The health economic construction placed on any given set of symptoms or diseases is, to a large extent, a function of the health care system concerned. Therefore, any pharmacoeconomic analysis must consider the perspective of a given decision-maker (society, third party payer, hospital or patients[3]).

There are several therapeutic strategies that are effective and well tolerated in the treatment of the diseases. Thus, consideration of cost and cost-effectiveness are important for deciding between therapies. A useful first step in developing disease management strategies is the determination of the frequency and costs of these conditions, and of the component of health care that contribute most to overall costs.

Gastrointestinal disorders account for almost 10% of all contacts between patients and general practitioners, although this level of clinical workload represents the tip of a large iceberg of morbidity in the community. Epidemiological surveys have shown that 1-year community prevalence of dyspepsia and reflux symptoms is of the order of 40%, that around 20% of the general population meet the criteria for IBS, and the rectal bleeding is experienced by approximately 20% of the general population each year. However, only a minority of individuals with these symptoms seek medical advice, with the proportion ranging from around 25% for dyspepsia to 40% per annum for rectal bleeding. The health economic consequences of "hidden" gastrointestinal disease are difficult to quantitate[4].

A recent study of the costs of Acid-Related Disorders (ARD) to health maintenance organizations in USA has shown that the ARDs prevalence (5.8%) increases with advancing age. Gastro-Oesophageal Related Disorders (GORD) are the most common ARD. Annual per person attributable costs were US$ 1183, US$ 471, US$ 431, respectively, for peptic ulcer disease, GORD, and gastritis/dyspepsia (Figure 1).

Figure 1

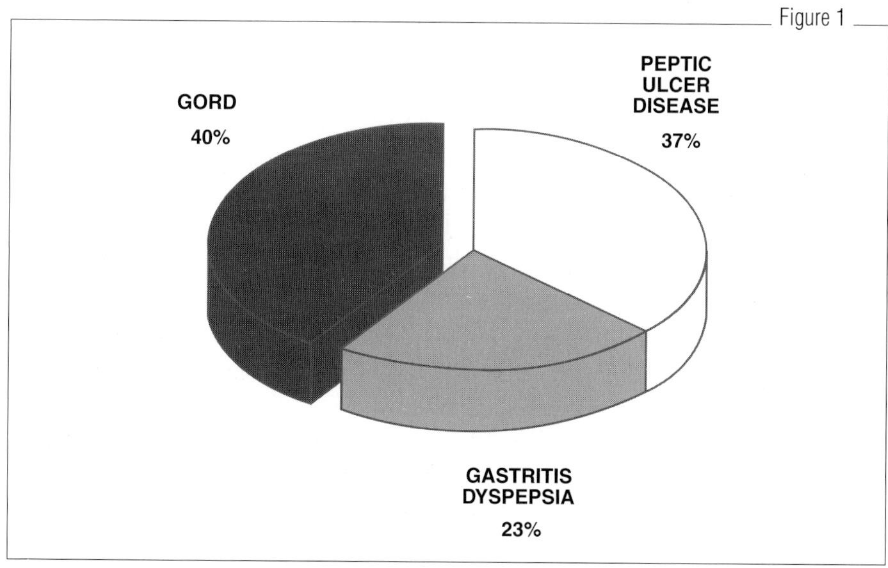


Annual health plan costs for each acid-related disorder.
Modified from Levin TR, Schmittdiel JA, Kuntz K et al.[5]

Excess inpatient costs for peptic ulcer disease explain its high costs. Outpatient costs were somewhat higher for GORD than for the other two diseases. Pharmacy costs were relatively low for each condition[5].

## Gastro-oesophageal reflux disease

In several studies the efficacy of different drug treatment strategies in reflux oesophagitis is analysed with the help of modelling techniques. In an English study, based on two large multicentric clinical trials, Bate[6] analysed drug costs and effectiveness of omeprazole, ranitidine and cimetidine in the treatment of reflux oesophagitis. Three effectiveness measures were used:

- Endoscopically confirmed healing
- Asymptomatic patient
- Complete success defined as endoscopically confirmed healing and asymptomatic patient.

The author concluded that the cost per treatment success, regardless of effectiveness measure, was lower for treatment with omeprazole 20 mg/day than for ranitidine 300 mg/day and for cimetidine 400 mg 4 times daily. The main limitations of the Bate study are: first, it considers only drug costs and health-care costs more widely; and second, the very short period of one acute episode does not allow for the inclusion of the costs and adverse effects associated with recurrence of oesophagitis beyond the first event. In an extension of the earlier study Bate and Richardson[7] compared the initial treatment of oesophagitis with omeprazole vs ranitidine beyond the first acute event to a period of 1 year. The daily dose was incremented over time for patients that were not healed. The authors concluded that over a 1-year period the treatment of 100 patients would cost £41515 for ranitidine vs £31417 for omeprazole. The main concern of this study is that the analysis was conducted exclusively in terms of a comparison of two drugs, but it is known from clinical experience that higher grades of disease can relapse. Therefore, the logic of this approach is that we should be less interested in economic comparison of the drugs per se and more interested in the cost-effectiveness of the overall management strategies and the ways in which these drugs could be used optimally in those strategies[8].

The Swedish study of Lindberg[9] compared initial treatment with either ranitidine or omeprazole over a 12-week period, where direct health care costs and indirect costs were compared to outcomes in terms of weeks without oesophagitis. The model used in the analysis assumed that patients would be managed in the same way as they would have been in a clinical trial (Table 1).

COST-EFFECTIVNESS ANALYSIS OF DIFFERENT STRATEGIES IN REFLUX OESOPHAGITIS. TOTAL TIME FOR ANALYSIS WAS 12 WEEKS

| **Cost items** | **Treatment strategy** | |
|---|---|---|
| | *Omeprazole* | *Ranitidine* |
| **Drug cost only** | | |
| Mean cost per patient | 1386 | 1609 |
| Mean number of weeks healed oesophagitis | 6.75 | 3.71 |
| Cost per week (SEK) with healed oesophagitis | 205 | 434 |
| **Drug cost + cost of gastroscopy (direct and indirect costs)** | | |
| Mean cost per patient | 4201 | 4230 |
| Mean n. weeks healed oesophagitis | 6.75 | 3.71 |
| Cost per week (SEK) with healed oesophagitis | 622 | 1140 |

Table 1

Modified from Lindberg G[9].

The analysis showed that omeprazole 20 mg once daily is clearly more cost-effective than ranitidine 150 mg twice daily in the treatment of reflux oesophagitis. Omeprazole is more effective with regard to healing of oesophagitis, and it leads to a lower average cost of treatment. Sensitivity analyses showed that this conclusion was valid for all reasonable changes in the cost factors. The main limitation of this study is the duration of the study that is short at only 12 weeks. In fact, it is common knowledge that once diagnosed with erosive reflux oesophagitis, patients require lifelong therapy. Ideally, this therapy should heal oesophagitis, relieve reflux symptoms, prevent complications.

However, the optimal treatment strategy remains controversial. After initial healing maintenance therapy with proton pump inhibitors (PPI) prevents relapse in a vast majority of patients[10,11]. Surgical therapy for complicated GORD (stricture and severe oesophagitis) remains an alternative to long-term PPI because of concern over long-term safety and cost of PPI therapy. Additionally, laparoscopic fundoplication can now be performed with less morbidity and cost than with the open technique and is being increasingly performed as definitive treatment of reflux oesophagitis[12]. In a recent paper, Viljakka et al.[13] compared the lifelong costs of surgical vs medical treatment of severe GORD in Finland and their calculations showed Nissen fundoplication to be less costly than continuous, lifelong medication with PPI or 300 mg ranitidine daily, irrespective of the patient's gender or age. Only treatment with ranitidine, 150 mg/day, was cheaper than surgery in females over 60-65 years and males over 55-59 years. However, this dose is insufficient to maintain normal oesophageal mucosa in most patients with GORD. The surgical costs included pre- and post-operative endoscopy, preoperative 24-h oesophageal pH monitoring and manometry, the stay in hospital, management of complications (wound infection, post-operative pneumonia etc.), sick leave, and calculated financial loss due to fatal outcome. The main message from this study is that when medical management of erosive oesophagitis requires a regimen of continuous PPI, Nissen fundoplication is a less costly alternative in the long run.

A cost effectiveness analysis of medical vs surgical treatment in patients with severe or refractory oesophagitis was carried out by Van Den Boom et al. in The Netherlands[14]. Effectiveness of both medical and surgical treatment was established by means of meta-analysis of published papers until 1996. In particular, in the comparison of medical maintenance treatment with omeprazole vs the (laparascopic) Nissen fundoplication, effectiveness was defined as the ability of the respective treatments, to retain patients in full remission of oesophagitis during a certain period of time, expressed in patient-years. Costs were estimated using a modelling technique. Only direct medical costs due to treatment were regarded. All the other types of costs were ignored. From this analysis, it appears that surgery (Nissen fundoplication) is a cost-effective treatment option as compared with omeprazole treatment if this medical treatment is to last longer than approximately 4 years. If effectiveness is solely expressed in terms of keeping patients in full remission of their oesophagitis, changing to surgery will lead to substantial savings from this point in time. A laparoscopic Nissen procedure might be even more cost effective, due to a substantial reduction in hospital stay. For the authors, the laparoscopic Nissen fundoplication is more cost effective than medical treatment if this treatment is to last longer than approximately 17 months.

An American study by Heudebert et al.[15] substantially confirmed the results of the Dutch study.

The authors used a decision analytic modeling technique (Markov-cycle tree simulation model) to compare two strategies, medical vs surgical treatment, for the management of patients with erosive oesophagitis. Utilities varied by the quality of life associated with each health state and as such are considered to be quality-adjusted. For example, a patient who remained symptom-free for the 5-year period accumulated 5 QALY utility units, whereas another patient who had oesophagitis symptoms after 2 years of perfect health accumulated 4.7 QALYs. All cost estimates represent the reimbursement for all medications, outpatient-based procedures and hospital costs, assuming a private insurance coverage.

This cost-utility simulation model shows that for middle-aged individuals with moderate to severe symptomatic oesophagitis, long-term treatment with omeprazole and laparoscopic Nissen fundoplication are equally effective for up to 5 years. The difference in cost favours use of PPI until at least 10 years have elapsed. For older patients (age 55 or older), the use of a PPI seems the traditional choice because in this case the surgical strategy seems to be sensitive to small changes in motility and long-term morbility, outcomes that are more likely to occur with increasing age. Conversely, for younger and otherwise healthy patients, the choice of laparoscopic Nissen fundoplication may be appropriate for two important reasons:

1. from a patient's point of view, the prospect of requiring daily medication for the next 30-40 years might be considered both burdersome and impractical,
2. from the point of view of a third-party payer, the longer the patient has to live, the more likely laparoscopic Nissen fundoplication will become equivalent or cheaper than the PPI-first strategy.

## Irritable bowel syndrome

IBS represents one of the most common conditions encountered by the gastroenterologist and general internist alike. It has been estimated that there are between 2.4 and 3.5 million visits to physicians yearly in the United States by patients with IBS[16]. In England and Wales, some information has been obtained from the fourth national study of morbidity in general practice during the course of a year. For 1995, the study indicates a current total 846,349 consultations per annum; this is equivalent to an average of 1.6 contacts each year per patient seeking help from general practice for IBS. This also represents about 10% of the total primary care workload resulting from diseases of the digestive system and at an average cost per consultation of £15.49 in 1994/95 results in an expenditure of £13.1 million per year[17]. However, this estimate should be treated with caution because there is no way of gauging how accurately IBS is being diagnosed and classified in the primary care setting and whether there is a tendency to over- or under-diagnose the condition.

In a recent paper, Talley et al. estimated the direct medical costs of a well-defined cohort of individuals with IBS compared with controls from the same community. Given that the population of people older than 20 years of age in Olmsted County Minnesota, USA in 1992 was roughly 75,000 and the prevalence of IBS was 18%, the authors estimated the total excess charges for IBS alone were approximately $4 million for

1992 in Olmsted County. Extrapolating to the population of U.S., white persons would result in excess charges of $8 billion for IBS yearly. The overall median charges incurred by subjects with IBS was $742 compared with $429 for controls and $614 for subjects with some gastrointestinal symptoms.
The charges were 1.6 times higher in subjects with IBS relative to those without symptoms. This study, however, did have a limitation: the results represent only a proportion of the total socioeconomic impact of IBS in the community. However, the general conclusion of the study was that people with functional bowel complaints accrued more medical charges than others without symptoms[18].
The difficulties encountered in quantifying the amount and cost of the general practitioner's time consumed by IBS equally confound attempts to measure the expenditure on medicines prescribed by family doctors to treat the disorder. In the United Kingdom, in an attempt to overcome these problems, a market research study was undertaken using the DIN-LINK database[17]. This database is constructed from the computerized record-keeping of approximately 360 general practitioners working in 100 practices in the UK. The results, which are projected up from the sample to yield national (UK) data indicate that nearly 1.7 million prescriptions were written for IBS in that year. If this figure is multiplied by the average net ingredient cost per prescription for gastrointestinal disorders, which is estimated at £5.10, and a spending cost of almost £1 per prescription is added, this yields a total expenditure on GP-prescribed medication for IBS of £10.1 million. If this figure is ajusted for the estimated patient population, the final figure is £12.5 million.
In a recent survey conducted by consultant general gastroenterologists in the North of England, it was estimated that the in-patient and out-patient costs for the hospital sector of the National Health System was approximately £20 million per year. Furthermore, the annual expenditure on IBS by the UK National Health System is estimated to be £45.6 million. This figure is equivalent to just 0.1% of total NHS annual spending and represents approximately £90 per consultation/sufferer[17]. However, we must keep in mind that the various cost estimates are constructed from imperfect databases and are, if anything, probably conservative.

## Conclusions

Against this background, further research into the economics of IBS and all gastrointestinal diseases would be worthwhile. Such data would provide an indication of the magnitude of the burden in relation to other diseases and, thereby, supply useful information which could, for example, help determine research priorities. A better understanding of the distribution of the costs within health-care spending would also allow a clearer identification of areas warranting closer attention in the attempt to achieve greater efficiency in health-care spending[18]. It should, however, be emphasized that cost of illness data alone are inappropriate for determining whether further resources should be allocated to providing treatments for gastrointestinal diseases. Decisions, in this respect, depend on the availability of treatment options, their cost and their effectiveness, not on the size of the economic burden generated by the disorders.

### *References*

1. Jonsson B, Karlsson G. *Economic evaluation in gastrointestinal disease.* Scand J Gastroenterol 1996;220:44-51.
2. Cooke J, Doreau C, Eandi M. *Pharmacoeconomic aspects of antibacterial treatment with cefotaxime.* J Chemother 1997;9(Suppl 2):34-44.
3. Drummond MF, Stoddard GL, Torrance GW. *Methods for the economic evaluation of health care programmes.* Oxford: Oxford University Press; 1987.
4. Jones RH. *Clinical economics review: gastrointestinal disease in primary care.* Aliment Pharmacol Ther 1996;10:233-9.
5. Levin TR, Schmittdiel JA, Kuntz K, et al. *Costs of acid-related disorders to a Health Maintenance Organization.* Am J Med 1997;103:520-8.
6. Bate CM. *Cost-effectiveness of omeprazole in the treatment of reflux esophagitis.* Br J Med Econ 1991;1:53-61.
7. Bate CM, Richardson PDL. *A one-year model for the cost-effectiveness of treating reflux oesophagitis.* Br J Med Econ 1992;2:5-11.
8. Sridhar S, Huang J, O'Brien BJ, Hunt RH. *Clinical economics review: cost-effectiveness*

*of treatment alternatives for gastro-oesophageal reflux disease.* Aliment Pharmacol Ther 1996;10:865-73.

9. Lindberg G. *Omeprazole vs ranitidine in reflux esophagitis in Sweden.* PharmacoEcon 1994;5(Suppl 3):27-34.
10. Klinkenberg-Knol EC, Festen HPM, Jansen JBMF, et al. *Long term treatment with omeprazole for refractory reflux esophagitis: efficacy and safety.* Ann Intern Med 1994;121:161-7.
11. Dent J, Yeomans ND, Mackinnon M, et al. *Omeprazole versus ranitidine for prevention of relapse in reflux esophagitis: a controlled double-blind trial of their efficacy and safety.* Gut 1994;35:590-8.
12. Rattner DW, Brooks DC. *Patient satisfaction following laparoscopic and open antireflux surgery.* Arch Surg 1995;130:289-93.
13. Viljakka M, Nevalainen J, Isolauri J. *Lifelong costs of surgical versus medical treatment of severe gastroesophageal reflux disease in Finland.* Scand J Gastroenterol 1997;32:766-72.
14. Van Den Boom G, Go PMMYH, Hameeteman W, Dallemagne B. *Cost effectiveness of medical versus surgical treatment in patients with severe or refractory gastroesophageal reflux disease in The Netherlands.* Scand J Gastroenterol 1996;31:1-9.
15. Heuderbert GR, Marks R, Mel Wilcox C, Centor RM. *Choice of long-term strategy for the management of patients with severe esophagitis: a cost-utility analysis.* Gastroenterology 1997;122:1078-86.
16. Sandler RS. *Epidemiology of irritable bowel syndrome in the United States.* Gastroenterology 1990;99:409-15.
17. Wells NEJ, Hahn BA, Whorwell PJ. *Clinical economic review: irritable bowel syndrome.* Aliment Pharmacol Ther 1997;11:1019-30.
18. Talley NJ, Gabriel SE, Harmsen WS, et al. *Medical costs in community subjects with irritable bowel syndrome.* Gastroenterology 1995;109:1736-41.

*Address for correspondence*

**EANDI M, MD**

Dipartimento di Anatomia Farmacologia e Medicina Legale

Università di Torino

Via P. Giuria 13 10125 Torino Italia

Fax: +39 011 6707788

E-mail: mario.eandi@unito.it

# AUTHOR INDEX

# SUBJECT INDEX

Page numbers in *italics* indicate *tables* or *figures*

## A



## B

## D

## H

## Q



## S